Frontiers in Anti-Infective Agents

(Volume 3)

21ˢᵗ Century Challenges in Antimicrobial Therapy and Stewardship

Edited by

Islam M. Ghazi

&

Michael J. Cawley

Phialdelphia College of Pharmacy
Univeristy of the Sciences Philadelphia
Philadelphia
USA

Frontiers in Anti-Infective Agents

Volume # 3

21st Century Challenges in Antimicrobial Therapy and Stewardship

Editors: Islam M. Ghazi & Michael J. Cawley

ISSN (Online): 2705-1080

ISSN (Print): 2705-1072

ISBN (Online): 978-981-14-6183-5

ISBN (Print): 978-981-14-3383-2

ISBN (Paperback): 978-981-14-6182-8

Published by Bentham Science Publishers Pte. Ltd. Singapore. All Rights Reserved.

need for a court order if at any point you breach any terms of this License Agreement. In no event will any delay or failure by Bentham Science Publishers in enforcing your compliance with this License Agreement constitute a waiver of any of its rights.

3. You acknowledge that you have read this License Agreement, and agree to be bound by its terms and conditions. To the extent that any other terms and conditions presented on any website of Bentham Science Publishers conflict with, or are inconsistent with, the terms and conditions set out in this License Agreement, you acknowledge that the terms and conditions set out in this License Agreement shall prevail.

Bentham Science Publishers Pte. Ltd.
80 Robinson Road #02-00
Singapore 068898
Singapore
Email: subscriptions@benthamscience.net

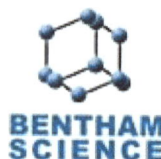

BENTHAM SCIENCE

CONTENTS

PREFACE

The field of infectious diseases is rapidly evolving in response to challenges posed by the continuing increase in bacterial resistance. Practitioners should be up to date with recent data, novel approaches and top-notch practices. This book is not intended to be a review of the management of specific disease states, the purpose of the book is to raise awareness about selected topics that are recent and represent novel strides in the field. It is intended to be of appropriate length and depth to appeal to a wide basis readership.

The book is designed to address selected topics that are of importance in the practice of infectious diseases including updates and subject comprehensive compilation of data not covered in details elsewhere. The book will start by illustrating the global picture of resistance influencing antimicrobial use and therapeutic decisions, discussing possible reasons for the spread of resistance, possibly the use animal farming and agriculture, injudicious prescription patterns and other factors. The pharmacology and antibiotic classes will be discussed, emphasizing the new agents demonstrating advances, gaps to be covered and future targets. Given the paucity of antimicrobial pipelines, the role of pharmaceutical formulation with be discussed to demonstrate how innovative drug delivery methods can improve efficacy, safety and achieve targeted drug delivery. Alternative routes of administration (other than oral and intravenous) will be detailed as means of enhancing the penetration of antimicrobials to the site of action and improving clinical outcomes.

Understanding how pathogens develop resistance has a strong impact on the selection of therapeutic agents and addressing difficult to treat infections, three chapters will address the molecular basis of resistance in Gram-positive, -negative and fungi, respectively. Timely diagnosis and prescription of appropriate spectrum antibiotics are crucial to achieve positive clinical outcomes. The use of advanced technology to aid in rapid diagnosis will be the subject of chapter to explain the available tools and how to integrate them in clinical practice. A chapter will address the remaining therapeutic options for difficult to treat infections (case studies, animal research, *in vitro* models and expert opinion). The future of antimicrobial agents' development, agents on the horizon and unmet medical needs will be elucidated. The next chapter will discuss the initiatives by organization, societies and authorities to combat antimicrobial resistance and rationale for the use of antibiotics. In light of limited data on the subject, understanding dosing principals in patients maintained on renal replacement therapy and ECMO (extracorporeal circuit) is an interesting and required topic. A chapter will address practice issues related to antimicrobial stewardship to raise awareness and foster collaboration and strengthen aspects of interprofessional education.

The target audience will include advanced medical, pharmacy and nursing students interested in infectious diseases, infectious diseases trainees (residents and fellows), infectious diseases practitioners and interested general practitioners. On behalf of all the chapter authors, we hope to spread the word to the clinicians and promote the best practices in the discipline of infectious diseases.

Islam M. Ghazi & Michael J. Cawley
Phialdelphia College of Pharmacy
Univeristy of the Sciences
Philadelphia
USA

List of Contributors

Abrar K. Thabit Pharmacy Practice Department, Faculty of Pharmacy, King Abdulaziz University, Jeddah, Saudi Arabia

Adebowale O. Adeluola Department of Pharmaceutical Microbiology and Biotechnology, Faculty of Pharmacy, College of Medicine campus, University of Lagos, Lagos, Nigeria

Addison Pang Providence Health & Services, Portland, OR, USA

Ahmed F. El-Yazbi Department of Pharmacology and Toxicology, Faculty of Pharmacy, Alexandria University, Egypt
Department of Pharmacology and Toxicology, Faculty of Medicine and Medical Center, the American University of Beirut, Beirut, Lebanon

Alaa Abouelfetouh Department of Microbiology and Immunology, Faculty of Pharmacy, Alexandria University, Alexandria, Egypt

Alyssa Christensen Providence Health & Services, Portland, OR, USA

Benjamin Georgiades Shionogi Inc, Florham Park, NJ, USA

Diaa Alrahmany Inpatient Pharmacy, Sohar Hospital, Sultanate of Oman

Elisa Morgan Doylestown Hospital, 595 W State St, Doylestown, PA, 18901, USA

Elsayed Aboulmagd Department of Microbiology and Immunology, Faculty of Pharmacy, Alexandria University, Alexandria, Egypt

Enas A. Almohammadi Pharmacy Practice Department, Faculty of Pharmacy, King Abdulaziz University, Jeddah, Saudi Arabia

Hadeel N. Alshaikh Pharmacy Practice Department, Faculty of Pharmacy, King Abdulaziz University, Jeddah, Saudi Arabia

Islam M. Ghazi Phialdelphia College of Pharmacy, Univeristy of the Sciences Philadelphia, Philadelphia, USA

Janise Philllips Department of Pharmacy Services, Houston Methodist Willowbrook, Houston, Texas, USA

Jonathan C. Cho Mountain View Hospital, Las Vegas, NV, USA

Kamilia Abdelraouf Center of Anti-infective Research and Development, Hartford Hospital, Hartford, Connecticut, USA

Kolawole S. Oyedeji Department of Medical Laboratory Science, University of Lagos, Lagos, Nigeria

Lamia S. Alzahrani Pharmacy Practice Department, Faculty of Pharmacy, King Abdulaziz University, Jeddah, Saudi Arabia

Lucia Rose Cooper University Hospital, Camden, NJ, 08103, USA

Madeline King University of the Sciences - Philadelphia College of Pharmacy, Philadelphia, PA, 19104, USA

Mervat A. Kassem Department of Microbiology and Immunology, Faculty of Pharmacy, Alexandria University, Alexandria, Egypt

Michael J. Cawley Philadelphia College of Pharmacy/University of the Sciences, Philadelphia, PA, USA

Morgan Anderson Advocate Aurora Health, Downers Grove, IL, USA

Nesrine Rizk Division of Infectious Diseases, Department of Internal Medicine and Medical Center, the American University of Beirut, Beirut, Lebanon

Nisrine Haddad Department of Pharmacy, the American University of Beirut Medical Center, Beirut, Lebanon

Nizar Attallah Department of Nephrology, Cleveland Clinic Abu Dhabi, Abu Dhabi, UAE

Pardeep Gupta Department of Pharmaceutics, University of the Sciences, Philadelphia, USA

Rebecca L. Dunn Fisch College of Pharmacy, The University of Texas at Tyler, Tyler, TX, USA

Rim W. Rafeh Department of Pharmacology and Toxicology, Faculty of Medicine and Medical Center, the American University of Beirut, Beirut, Lebanon

Sean Nguyen Shionogi Inc, Florham Park, NJ, USA

Takova D. Wallace-Gay Fisch College of Pharmacy, The University of Texas at Tyler, Tyler, TX, USA

Vaishnavi Parikh Department of Pharmaceutics, University of the Sciences, Philadelphia, USA

Viktorija O. Barr Rosalind Franklin University, North Chicago, IL, USA
T2Biosystems, Lexington, MA, USA

Wasim S. El Nekidy Department of Pharmacy, Cleveland Clinic Abu Dhabi, Abu Dhabi, UAE

CHAPTER 1

Global Landscape of Microbial Resistance

Elsayed Aboulmagd*, Mervat A. Kassem and **Alaa Abouelfetouh**

Department of Microbiology and Immunology, Faculty of Pharmacy, Alexandria University, Alexandria, Egypt

Abstract: Antimicrobial agents are considered one of the most useful and successful forms of chemotherapeutics in the history of medicine. Unfortunately, resistance to such antimicrobial agents is widespread globally which represents a major challenge faced by the health authorities. Some species of microorganisms are intrinsically resistant to the effects of certain antimicrobial agents whereas the selective pressure of antimicrobials can cause others to acquire the resistance due to mutation of the target sites or horizontal gene transfer. The increased dissemination of microbes resistant to antibiotics may be caused by misuse/overuse of antibiotics, non-human use of antimicrobials or pharmaceutical manufacturing effluents. The emergence and spread of antimicrobial resistance influence many sectors in the healthcare system which will be negatively reflected on the whole community and can lead to many consequences which include high morbidity and mortality rates, loss of protection for patients and increased healthcare costs. The continuously increasing rate of antibiotic resistance to almost all traditional antimicrobial agents boosted the urgent need for the development of new non-traditional therapeutics. In addition, innovative strategies should be applied to reduce the emergence of new resistant pathogens. There are many alternative approaches and treatment options at different stages of investigation and development to combat multidrug-resistant pathogens including: development of new antibiotics, phage therapy, monoclonal antibodies, probiotics and anti-virulence factors. Because antibiotic resistance is a cross-border problem and microbes travel freely, international cooperation and coordination are required to solve such a problem. The use of antimicrobial agents should be optimized and misuse and overuse of such vital drugs should be avoided, and stewardship antibiotic programs should be implemented for the proper utilization of antibiotics. In addition, the non-human use of antimicrobial agents in agriculture and animal husbandry should be as limited as possible to reduce the unnecessary use that accelerates the development of antimicrobial resistance. In addition, global public awareness programs are urgently needed to educate everyone about the hazards and consequences of antimicrobial resistance and how such problems could be countered.

* **Corresponding author Elsayed Aboulmagd:** Department of Microbiology and Immunology, Faculty of Pharmacy, Alexandria University, Alexandria, Egypt; Tel: +2-03-5424642; Fax: +2-03-4873273; E-mail: elsayed20@hotmail.com

Islam M. Ghazi & Michael J. Cawley (Eds.)

Keywords: Antimicrobial resistance, antibiotic misuse, selective pressure, gene transfer, intrinsic resistance, acquired resistance, economic cost, antimicrobial stewardship, alternative therapy, phage therapy, probiotics.

The discovery of antibiotics in the first half of the 20th century made treating and preventing infections a real possibility, saving the lives of millions worldwide [1]. Following the discovery of penicillin, more antimicrobials joined the market and started being used in clinical practice. However, clinically relevant microorganisms soon started developing resistance to most antimicrobials, threatening once again the lives of those undergoing surgeries, organ transplantation or receiving chemotherapeutic agents [2]. In 1945, Alexander Fleming warned about the development of antimicrobial resistance (AMR) where he said "It is not difficult to make microbes resistant to penicillin in the laboratory by exposing them to concentrations not sufficient to kill them, and the same thing has occasionally happened in the body. The time may come when penicillin can be bought by anyone in the shops." Because microorganisms know no boundaries, AMR is currently a global problem causing a staggering loss in lives and resources.

AMR develops when the microorganisms causing infections are no longer inhibited or killed by the agents that were effective in treating these infections. This leads to the emergence of "superbugs" capable of wide-spreading in the absence of competition from susceptible microorganisms already killed by exposure to the antimicrobials. These superbugs can also cause serious infections that are difficult to treat or are even untreatable [3]. Contrary to what was believed, that increased resistance can be energetically costly which limits the capacity of the resistant strain to survive in the absence of the antibiotic pressure [4], some of the super-resistant bugs are more virulent and show increased transmissibility [5]. The consequences are terrifying, with a reported annual death rate of 700000 lives in 2014. This figure is expected to increase to 10 million deaths, or one person dying every three seconds by 2050. The global economic waste is projected to amount to $100 trillion or a loss of $10,000 per person of 2016's population by 2050 if the present spreading mechanisms remain unchecked, especially in low and middle-income countries [3].

Microbes can become resistant to antimicrobials naturally over the course of time due to genetic mutations as well as the horizontal transfer of resistance genes among different microbes [6]. As a matter of fact, the first penicillinase conferring penicillin resistance was discovered before penicillin became publicly available for use [7]. However, the extensive use of the antimicrobials in the last century and their subsequent disposal in the environment selected for antimicrobial-resistant microbes in a manner that far outweighed the effect of natural selection for survival purposes [6, 7]. A review of the available annotated bacterial genome sequences suggests the presence of over 20000 potential resistance genes [5]. Only a fraction of these genes is currently associated with resistance phenotypes [6].

GLOBAL NATURE OF AMR PROBLEM

It would be naive to presume that the problem of AMR is restricted to those regions of the world where resistance levels are high or that the problem can be contained. That is for the simple reason that travelers to regions with high AMR prevalence can return home colonized with a superbug. Moreover, resistant strains can be carried on the body of an aircraft or transported goods, crossing the borders between high risk and lower risk regions [8].

AMR has recently been reported in 500,000 patients from 22 countries [9], with children up to 12 months of age and the elderly being more vulnerable to resistant infections, and men being more susceptible than women [10]. The rates and trends of resistance are different between countries. Among the Organization for Economic Co-operation and Development (OECD) countries, resistance grew from 14% in 2005 to 17% in 2015 for eight high-priority antibiotic-bacterium combinations, with Turkey, Greece and Korea showing seven times higher average resistance rates (35%) than Iceland, Netherlands and Norway (5%) (Fig. **1**). Resistance to second and third-line antibiotics is expected to increase in 2030 by 70% relative to 2005 in OECD countries. In low and middle- income countries such as Brazil, Indonesia and Russia, resistance rates are between 40% and 60%, which is far greater than the average rate of 17% encountered among OECD countries. These high levels are projected to grow from four to seven times higher than OECD countries by 2050 [10].

Gram-negative bacteria pose the highest threat, following the development of resistance to carbapenems [1]. In developing countries, neonatal infections due to *E. coli* and *Klebsiella* spp. were found to be highly resistant to the WHO recommended regimens of gentamicin and ampicillin, with percentages as high as 71% resistance to gentamicin among *Klebsiella* spp. and 50% among *E. coli* [11]. Ampicillin resistance levels were higher, at 60-70% among *E. coli* and 100% among *Klebsiella* spp [12]. The spread of extended-spectrum β-lactamase producing Enterobacteriaceae strains made the use of cephalosporins to treat such infections impractical, shifting the medical attention towards carbapenem prescription as first-line drugs for cases of sepsis [13, 14]. However, carbapenem resistance among Enterobacteriaceae (CRE) due to the presence of β-lactamases [*e.g.* New Delhi metallo-β-lactamase (NDM) or extended spectrum β-lactamase

(ESBL) and/or carbapenemases (*e.g. Klebsiella pneumoniae* carbapenemase (KPC)] has been increasingly reported worldwide [6, 15].

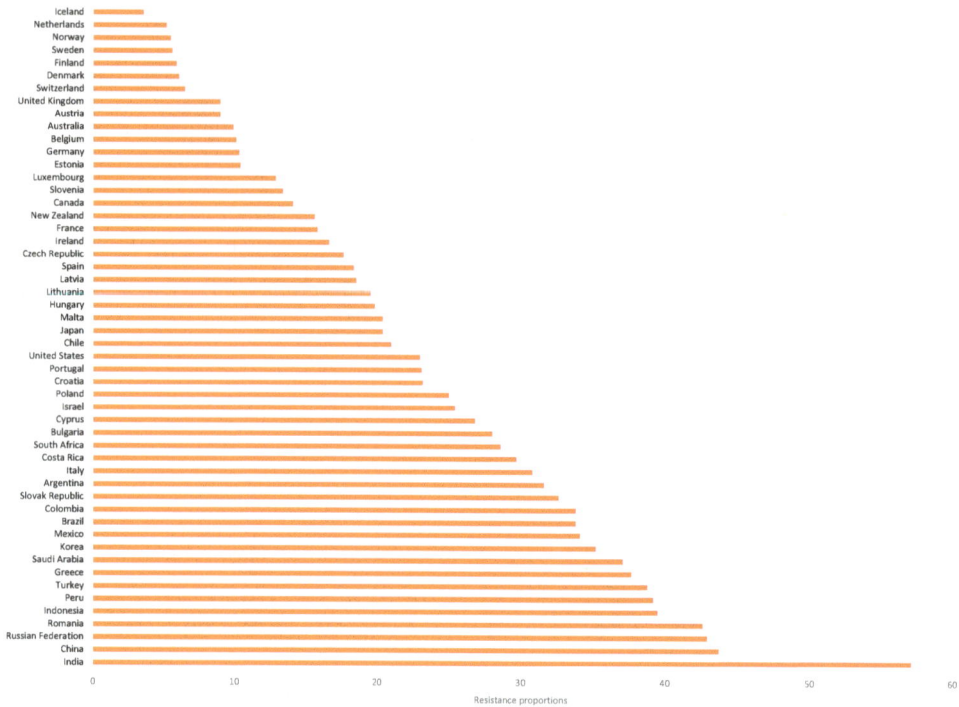

Fig. (1). Average resistance proportions for eight priority antibiotic-bacterium combinations in 2015 [10].

In the USA, the prevalence of CRE, mostly *Klebsiella* spp., increased from 0% to 1.4% between 2001 and 2010 [16]. In Europe, the European Antimicrobial Resistance Surveillance Network reported rare carbapenem resistance among *E. coli* isolates, yet it was above 10% among *Klebsiella pneumoniae* and even higher among *Acinetobacter baumannii* and *Pseudomonas aeruginosa* [17]. The development of pan resistance among *A. baumannii* isolates decreased their susceptibility towards carbapenems making the management of such infections notably worrisome [14]. Carbapenem resistance among *A. baumannii*, *P. aeruginosa* and Enterobacteriaceae marks them as pathogens of critical priority on the WHO list of targets for the discovery of new antibiotics [18].

In the developed world, newer antibiotics and stricter infection control regimens are used to fight infections due to gram-positive bacteria. The prevalence of bacteremia due to methicillin-resistant *Staphylococcus aureus* (MRSA), figuring as a high priority pathogen on the WHO list [18], is decreasing between 2014 and

2017 in close to one-third of European countries, yet it remained higher than 25% in 30% of the countries mainly in central and southern Europe in 2017 [17]. The rates of decline were higher in the USA between 2005 and 2011, where a study in nine metropolitan areas reported a decrease in the adjusted national incidence rates of invasive MRSA infections by 54.2% among hospital-onset infections, 27.7% among healthcare-associated community-onset infections and by 5% among community-associated infections [19]. Nevertheless, community-associated MRSA infections seem to pose less of a threat in Europe than they do in the USA [20]; however, high nasal carriage and infection rates have been reported among humans who have contact with livestock, particularly pigs in many European countries, suggesting a role for pigs as a reservoir for MRSA transmission to humans [21 - 23].

On the other hand, in Africa and Asia, the prevalence rates were generally higher and the figures were derived from individual studies rather than national surveillance systems. A study conducted in eight Asian countries showed that the highest rates of hospital-associated *S. aureus* infections due to MRSA were reported in Sri Lanka at 86.5% and the lowest rate was 22.6% in India, with an average of 67.4%. The rates were lower in community-associated infections with an average of 25.5% and the highest rate of 38.8% again in Sri Lanka and the lowest rate of 2.5% in Thailand (Fig. **2**) [24]. In most African countries, MRSA prevalence was below 50% but seemed to be increasing between 2000 and 2011 [25], except in South Africa that showed a decreasing trend from 36% in 2006 [26] to 24% between 2007 and 2011 [27]. The prevalence was lowest in Madagascar 6% between 2001 and 2005 [28], and highest in Ethiopia (55%) in 2006 [29] and Egypt (52%) then Algeria (45%) between 2003 and 2005 [30]. In Botswana, the prevalence varied between 23% and 44% between 2000 and 2007 [31, 32], and in Tunisia it increased from 16 to 41% between 2002 and 2007 [25] (Fig. **3**).

The full extent of the global problem is not completely understood. In 2015, the WHO launched the Global Antimicrobial Resistance Surveillance System (GLASS) to standardize AMR surveillance worldwide. The system liaises with national and regional surveillance systems to gather data about enrolled countries, regarding their surveillance programs and AMR data on *Acinetobacter* spp., *E. coli*, *K. pneumoniae*, *Neisseria gonorrhoeae*, *Salmonella* spp., *Shigella* spp., *S. aureus* and *Streptococcus pneumoniae*, all of which figure on the WHO list of high-risk pathogens [18, 33]. These pathogens cause infections that are increasingly becoming antibiotic-resistant, necessitating the use of last resort agents which are sometimes less effective, more dangerous and not always available, especially in low resource settings, putting additional strain on healthcare budgets [33]. The system also incorporates data from other surveillance systems that can impact AMR in humans such as those monitoring antimicrobial consumption and resistance in the food chain in a One Health approach [34]. GLASS is expected to help estimate the real disease burden of bacterial infections, and to use evidence-based data to advise policymakers on the treatment and control measures and to evaluate the effectiveness of these measures to avoid the spread of resistance [33]. The system doesn't monitor TB, HIV or malaria for which WHO already has well-established monitoring systems that have been generating data for years [9].

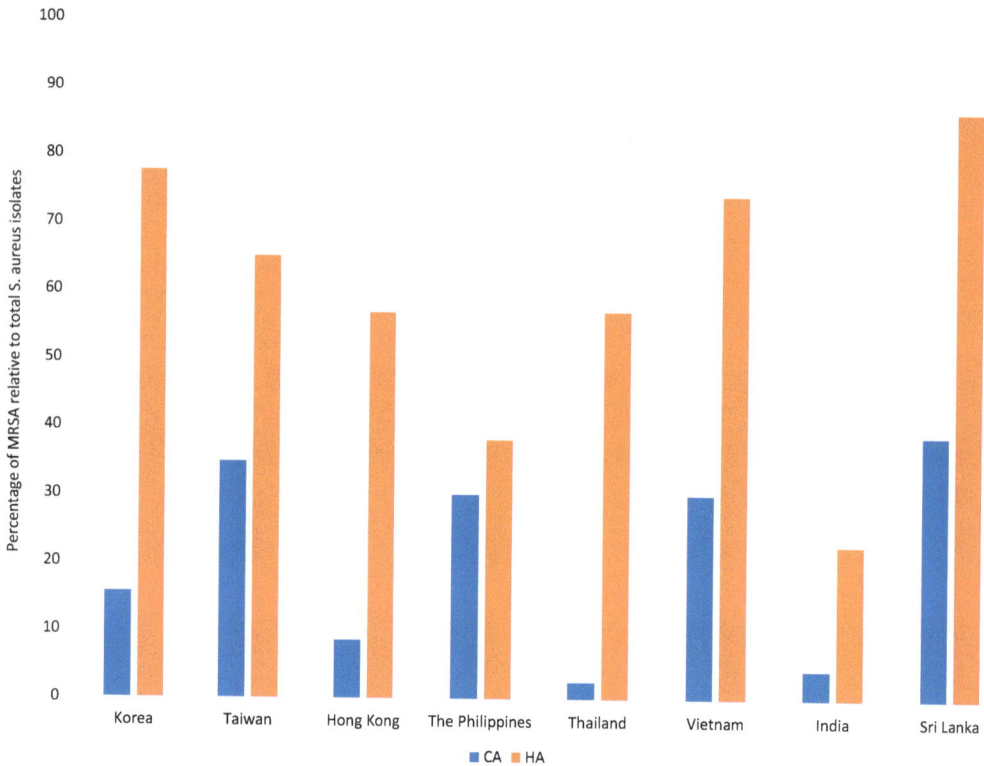

Fig. (2). Prevalence of MRSA among *S. aureus* isolates from community-associated (CA) and hospital-associated (HA) infections in Asia [24].

A total of 25 (48%) high-income, 20 (38%) middle-income and 7 (14%) low-income countries are enrolled in the GLASS system as of 2018 [9]. The first GLASS report, released in January 2018, included national surveillance data from 40 countries, whereas 22 countries reported their levels of antibiotic resistance in 2016 [9, 33]. The quality of data and state of completeness of data reporting differ between countries, as many countries are still challenged regarding their infrastructure capacity and fund availability. However, the pathogens reported the most as being antibiotic-resistant are *E. coli*, *K. pneumoniae*, *S. aureus*, *S. pneumoniae* then *Salmonella* spp. Between zero and 82% of the isolates suspected of causing bloodstream infections were resistant to at least one of the antibiotics recommended to treat such infections. Resistance to ciprofloxacin ranged between 8% and 65% among *E. coli* causing urinary tract infection in reporting countries [9].

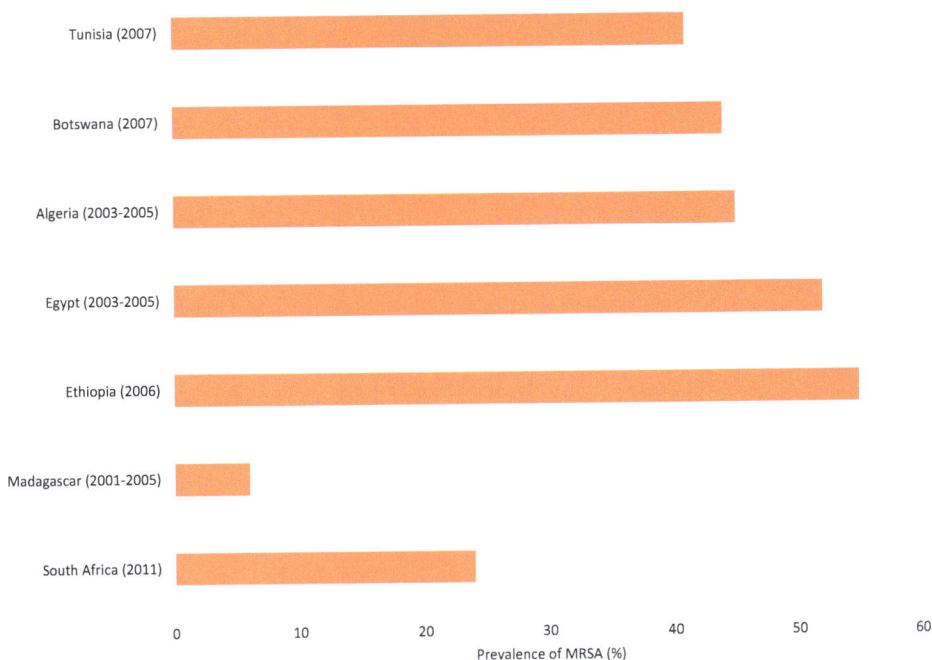

Fig. (3). Prevalence of MRSA in Africa [25].

CAUSES OF AMR

Antibiotic Misuse as a Driver of Resistance

A number of factors have been associated with the increase in worldwide resistance. These include the increase in surgical operations, the world geriatric population, the substandard levels of sanitation and infection control in hospitals in developing countries and the low cost of older antibiotics which made antibiotics an open-access resource that is often abused [1, 6, 35]. Irrational prescription and the lack of regulations governing over-the-counter sales of antibiotics in many low and middle-income countries are further aggravating the problem, with patients having access to antibiotics even without a prescription, leading to misuse, including overuse and sometimes underuse [2, 6].

Inappropriate antibiotic use takes different forms, including antibiotics taken for the wrong indication, such as when antibiotics are prescribed, whether under patient pressure or otherwise, or in many cases self-administered to treat viral infections or self-limited diseases [36, 37]. It is estimated that up to 50% of the antibiotics are prescribed inappropriately, including the wrong antibiotic choice, incorrect dosing or wrong duration of treatment [38], which could be linked to limited diagnosing capabilities, especially in developing countries [39]. Moreover, self-medication, especially in developing countries, is very concerning as it may lead to unsuccessful therapy due to similar reasons [40]. Another form of antibiotic misuse is represented by the failure of the patients to comply with the antibiotic regimen, manifesting as dose missing or stopping the antibiotic prematurely when the patient starts to feel better or can't tolerate the side effects [39, 41]. In most of these cases, the use of the wrong antimicrobial agent or the wrong dose exposes the bugs to concentrations of antimicrobials insufficient to kill them, which promotes resistance development [36].

Misuse can also take the form of or lead to the overuse of antimicrobials. A direct relationship and strong correlation exist between antibiotic consumption and the prevalence of antibiotic resistance [42]. In the case of *P. aeruginosa*, an important nosocomial pathogen that endangers the lives of cystic fibrosis patients, the lengthy antibiotic use has been linked to the development of antibiotic resistance [6, 43].

The world human consumption of antibiotics increased by 36% between 2000 and 2010, three- quarters of this increase occurred in Brazil, Russia, India, China and South Africa (BRICS) [44]. India's retail sales volume represented 23% of BRICS' volume, probably owing to the under-regulation of the over-the-counter sale of antibiotics in India [45]. Moreover, China was responsible for 57% of the increase in antibiotic sales in the hospitals among BRICS countries, which could be explained by the dependence of some hospitals on pharmaceutical sales to increase their revenue [45, 46]. Another factor expanding antibiotic consumption in some developing countries is poor to no antibiotic sales/use regulations, allowing antibiotic purchase without medical prescription and sometimes even through unregulated supply chains [47]. This phenomenon is compounded by the economic growth and prosperity in the above-mentioned countries [45] and in high-income countries, patients sometimes put pressure on physicians to prescribe an antibiotic conforming to what patients consider the norm [48]. Moreover, the use of poor quality and/or counterfeit antimicrobials, especially in low and middle-income countries, has dire consequences for communities and healthcare settings. The presence of low concentrations of the active pharmaceutical ingredients in the falsified medicines will expose the pathogens to sub-lethal antimicrobial concentrations that may lead to the evolution of an MDR mutant

[49]. The consumption of two last-resort antibiotics: carbapenems and polymyxin was notably high at 45% and 13%, respectively, together with broad-spectrum cephalosporins, broad-spectrum penicillins and fluoroquinolones [45]. However high the rates of antibiotic consumption are, access to antibiotics isn't equitable, with many patients in rural and resource-poor areas lacking proper access to the antibiotics they need, which results in more deaths than those caused by antibiotic resistant infections [1, 3, 50].

The rising consumption of antibiotics in humans and animals together with the high levels of antibiotic waste polluting the environment drive resistance development [51 - 53]. This occurs through the killing of the susceptible clones, selecting for resistant mutants that thrive and dominate the population, a good example of the Darwinian notion of selection and survival [6, 51]. The use of broad-spectrum antibiotics may exacerbate the problem by selecting for multidrug-resistant strains [51]. This is hardly surprising regarding that half of the antimicrobials used in human healthcare and even higher levels among livestock in countries that are members of OECD are inappropriate [54]. This occurs mostly when patients receive antibiotics to treat viral infections or for self-limited conditions [36, 37]. Moreover, the prolonged use of antibiotics, in particular broad-spectrum ones, can lead to the death of susceptible normal intestinal microbiota allowing the super-growth of hard to treat *Clostridium difficile* [55]. The incidence of such infections was 453000 cases in 2011 in the USA alone, with a mortality rate of about 6.4% [56].

Use of Sub-therapeutic Concentrations of Antibiotics in Animals as Growth Promoters

Animal husbandry is another area where antibiotics are massively used as growth promoters in sub-therapeutic concentrations as well as for disease prevention, especially when the animals are kept in poor conditions. Livestock consumes about 70% of the antibiotics that are medically important for humans in the USA and about 50% in other countries around the world [57]. In the USA, about three-quarters of these antibiotics are also used to treat human pathogens and about half of the remaining agents are structurally similar to human antibiotics [58, 59]. The consumption of antibiotics in animals by 2030 is expected to increase by 67% globally and to nearly double in BRICS countries [60]. In India, it is expected to increase by 312% to meet the growing demands for meat and animal products for human consumption as a result of rising incomes in China and Southeast Asia [60]. The use of antibiotics in sub-therapeutic concentrations in agriculture has been linked to the increase in the prevalence of antibiotic resistance genes [61]. The benefit of using antibiotics as growth promoters is questionable in modern farming and tends to vary with the age, species and lineage of the animal as well as the sanitary and management conditions [62]. Consequently, the European Union has already forbidden the use of antibiotics as growth promoters, and in the USA, the FDA is taking action to limit the use of sub-therapeutic doses of medically important antibiotics in livestock [57].

Antibiotics as Environmental Waste

Another contributor to the problem is the way the factories manufacturing the Active Pharmaceutical Ingredients (API) of antibiotics dispose of their waste [57]. There are few to no standards governing the disposal of API effluent around the world [63]. China and India are examples where a significant amount of APIs are being manufactured. This may be due to lower production cost which is generally a reflection of more relaxed standards [57, 64]. It is estimated that more than 50% of the antibiotics produced in China are released in the rivers [65]. The situation is disconcerting, especially that ciprofloxacin concentration in an Indian river where 90 manufacturers of APIs disposed of their effluent was 1000 fold higher than the concentration toxic to bacteria and was greater than the expected serum concentration in patients taking ciprofloxacin [66, 67]. Even when the effluent was treated, in some cases the level of antibiotic was still considerably high following treatment [68]. Such environments laden with antibiotics or their APIs can act as reservoirs for resistance genes [52, 53]. Moreover, insufficient treatment of water released from other sources, such as livestock, agriculture and healthcare settings, *etc.* compounds the problem, posing a considerable environmental risk and impacting different ecosystems [69]. Regarding the current lack of binding regulations of waste disposal in many countries, efforts are being made to determine the levels of antibiotics in waste that would drive resistance development [70].

Selective Pressure, Gene Transfer and Mutation

In addition to selective pressure induced and encouraged by frequent or irrational administration of antibiotics, both horizontal transfer of the genes encoding antibiotic resistance by transferring plasmids and vertical transfer by mutation of the target sites of the different antimicrobial agents play an essential role in the evolution and spread of microbial resistance [71]. Moreover, the administration of an antibiotic may not only select for resistance to such a drug but also to other antimicrobials of the same class which are structurally related.

TYPES AND MECHANISMS OF AMR

Some microorganisms are intrinsically resistant to the action of certain antimicrobials, whereas others become tolerant to previously inhibitory concentrations of antimicrobials, the former is referred to as intrinsic resistance and the latter as acquired resistance [72].

Intrinsic Resistance

Intrinsic resistance occurs as a result of inherent, and mostly chromosomally mediated, particular traits in the microorganism that make them unresponsive to the action of the antimicrobial. These characteristics include: (1) reduced affinity or lack of target site as exemplified in the insensitivity of Mycoplasma devoid of cell wall to the action of the β-lactams, (2) production of inactivating enzymes such as the β-lactamases produced by some gram-negative bacteria to hydrolyze β-lactams or the enzymes that alter the structure of the antibiotic to prevent its binding to the target such as aminoglycoside acetyltransferases, (3) decreased permeability seen in vancomycin resistance among members of the Enterobacteriaceae as a result of the outer membrane acting as a permeability barrier, and finally (4) efflux systems among gram-positive and gram-negative bacteria which together with decreased permeability result in reduced drug uptake [72 - 76]. Overexpression of some efflux pumps can render previously susceptible bacteria resistant to clinically useful antibiotics [77, 78]. Some efflux pumps have narrow substrate specificity (for example, the tetracycline pumps), but many transport a wide range of structurally dissimilar substrates and are known as multidrug resistance (MDR) efflux pumps [79]. Some of these mechanisms can also be disseminated to susceptible microorganisms through horizontal gene transfer rendering them MDR as well. Table **1** shows some selected intrinsic resistance mechanisms. Another form of phenotypic resistance is provided by the persister cells. These are cells that represent 10^{-6} to 10^{-4} of the population and that survive antimicrobial chemotherapy [80]. They are especially important in a biofilm setting, where, following antimicrobial chemotherapy, surviving planktonic persisters are killed by the immune system, whereas biofilm persister cells encased in the extracellular matrix of the biofilm escape. Once the antimicrobial is discontinued, these cells re-establish the biofilm that sheds more planktonic cells causing a relapse of the infection [81]. The cyclical use of one, and preferably two different antimicrobials, has been suggested to treat such infections. The first application of the antimicrobial is meant to kill the majority of the population, leaving the persisters to grow and potentially lose the persister phenotype allowing for eradication when the second antimicrobial is applied [82].

Table 1. Selected examples of intrinsic resistance mechanisms [74].

Antimicrobial	Intrinsically Resistant Microorganism	Mechanism
Aminoglycosides	*Anaerobic bacteria* *Enterococci*	Lack/insufficient oxidative metabolism to drive drug uptake
β-lactams: Ampicillin Imipenem Aztreonam Cephalosporins	*Klebsiella* spp. *Stenotrophomonas maltophila* Gram-positive bacteria *Enterococci*	Production of β-lactamases Production of β-lactamases Lack of target (penicillin binding proteins, PBPs) Lack of target (penicillin binding proteins, PBPs)
Vancomycin	Gram-negative bacteria Lactobacilli and Leuconostoc	Lack of permeability through outer membrane Lack of target (cell wall precursor)
Metronidazole	*Aerobic bacteria*	Inability to activate the drug by anaerobic reduction
Sulphonamides, trimethoprim, tetracycline, or chloramphenicol	*P. aeruginosa*	Reduced intracellular concentration resulting from reduced uptake

Acquired Resistance

For most known classes of antimicrobials, their use in clinical practice predisposed for the development of resistance. The length of time it takes for resistance to develop is a factor of the complexity of the acquired resistance mechanism [72, 83]. For penicillin, it took a couple of years for resistance to develop as a result of the product of one gene, whereas for vancomycin it took the enterococci 29 years to acquire the five genes required for high-level vancomycin resistance [72, 84, 85].

Acquired resistance can be either the result of mutations in chromosomal genes or the acquisition of foreign DNA coding for antibiotic resistance genes, often obtained from intrinsically resistant organisms present in the environment through horizontal gene transfer (HGT) [86, 87]. Such changes in the bacterial genome may alter the nature of proteins expressed by the organism and consequently the structural and functional features of the bacteria leading to resistance against a particular antibiotic [88]. Table **2** shows some selected acquired resistance mechanisms.

Bacterial cells can mutate their genes, at a mutation rate of 1 in 10^7. Some strains are hypermutable (mutators) with a mutation rate that is up to 1000 fold higher than in normal cells, mainly due to defects in DNA repair and proofreading mechanisms [89, 90]. A notable example is *P. aeruginosa* isolated from cystic fibrosis patients where mutators can represent 20% of the population [91]. When such mutations confer resistance to a particular antibiotic and in the presence of selective pressure due to the exposure to such antibiotics, all susceptible cells are killed allowing the resistant ones to thrive and dominate the population. Resistance development following exposure to sub-therapeutic concentrations of an antibiotic is an illustrative example of the role of selective pressure in resistance development [72]. Selective pressure was also demonstrated in the transition from methicillin susceptibility to resistance among *S. aureus* isolated from hospitalized patients postoperatively, due to mutation in the PBPs [92, 93]. Quinolone resistance in *E. coli* can be caused by point mutations in the *gyrA* gene or the *parC* gene leading to changes in at least seven and three amino acids, respectively. On the other hand, a single point mutation in the *rpoB* gene is associated with complete resistance to rifampin [94]. Mutations within the coding sequences of the porin channels in the outer membrane of gram-negative bacteria possibly reduce the permeation rates of bulky drug molecules without affecting those of smaller nutrient molecules. Clinically important bacterial pathogens like *Serratia marcescens, Salmonella enterica, K. pneumonia* and *P. aeruginosa*, have utilized this reduced drug uptake system to resist important antimicrobial agents, such as the β-lactams, fluoroquinolones, aminoglycosides, as well as chloramphenicol [95]. In prokaryotic genomes, mutations also frequently occur due to base changes caused by exogenous agents, DNA polymerase errors, deletions, insertions and duplications. Moreover, a mutation increases the prevalence of genetic recombination, providing diversity to antibiotic resistance mechanisms [96, 97].

Table 2. Selected examples of acquired resistance mechanisms [72].

Antibiotic Class	Mechanism
β-lactams	Production of β-lactamases, mutation of PBPs
Vancomycin	Horizontal acquisition of *vanHAX* genes reprogramming D-Ala-D-Ala to D-Ala-D-Lac or D-Ala-D-Ser
Macrolides of the erythromycin class	Overexpression of efflux pumps and enzymatic modification of the drug
Tetracyclines	Overexpression of efflux pumps
Aminoglycosides	Enzymatic modification of the drug
Fluoroquinolones	Mutation of gyrase and topoisomerase genes

Acquisition of foreign DNA material through HGT is one of the most important drivers of bacterial evolution and it is frequently responsible for the development of AMR. Methicillin resistance among *S. aureus* can occur when the pathogen acquires *mecA* encoding PBP2' or PBP2a that has a lower affinity towards the β-lactams [92, 93, 98]. Bacteria acquire external genetic material through three main strategies: transformation, transduction and conjugation.

Transformation is the uptake of short fragments of naked DNA by naturally transformable bacteria. This DNA is normally present in the external environment due to the death and lysis of another bacterium. Transformation is perhaps the simplest type of HGT. Bacteria capable of taking up DNA from the environment are termed "competent." Some microorganisms, such as many streptococci and *A. baumannii*, are competent at a specific stage in their growth [99, 100].

Transduction involves the transfer of DNA from one bacterium into another *via* bacteriophages. In this case, the phage particles are packaged with bacterial DNA instead of phage. Although it is uncommon, there have been examples of antibiotic resistance genes, and even entire mobile genetic elements, being mobilized by transduction [101].

Conjugation is considered the main mechanism of HGT, it involves the transfer of DNA *via* sexual pilus and requires cell-to-cell contact. DNA fragments that contain resistance genes from resistant donors can then make previously susceptible bacteria express resistance as coded by the newly acquired resistance genes. This mechanism of transfer permits genetic exchange between many different bacterial genera [102]. The emergence of resistance in the hospital environment often involves conjugation and is likely to occur at high rates in the gastrointestinal tract of humans under antibiotic treatment. As a rule, conjugation uses mobile genetic elements as vehicles to share valuable genetic information, although direct transfer from chromosome to chromosome has also been well characterized [103]. The most important mobile genetic elements are plasmids that mediate the lion's share of resistance, transposons and integrons [104, 105].

Multidrug Resistance Caused by Altered Physiological States

The antibiotic susceptibility of bacterial cells is also affected by their physiological states. Even high concentrations of antibiotics do not kill all of the bacterial population, leaving behind a persister population that is genetically identical to the susceptible cells. The presence of persisters is one of the mechanisms explaining the increased resistance of biofilms to antibiotics [106]. The presence of persisters is now thought to be an example of the strategy whereby bacteria naturally generate mixtures of phenotypically different populations so that one of them can be advantageous to a changing environmental demand [107].

CONSEQUENCES OF AMR

Treatment Failure and Loss of Activity

A direct consequence of AMR development is that antimicrobial agents lose their activity towards microbes. A case in point is gonorrhea that was treatable by penicillin till the 1980s when *Neisseria gonorrhea* developed resistance to both penicillin and tetracycline, then to quinolones in the mid-2000s, necessitating the use of third-generation cephalosporins to which the bacterium is currently developing resistance [108, 109].

High Morbidity and Mortality and Ensuing Economic Cost

AMR can seriously compromise the health and life of many patients [1], mainly because of the initial use of antimicrobials to which the infectious agent is resistant and the resulting delay in starting the right therapy [110, 111]. This burden is often borne by low and middle-income countries where patients can't afford to use more expensive second and third-line drugs when treatment fails as a result of the infectious agent becoming resistant to the action of first-line antimicrobials [45]. AMR can also lead to the inability to carry out surgical procedures in the elderly and other vulnerable populations because of the high risk of untreatable infections, once more raising morbidity and mortality rates [1]. It is expected that AMR will become one of the leading causes of death by the year 2050 [3, 112].

A measure of increasing morbidity is the lengthier hospital stay and need for intensive care for patients suffering from infections due to resistant bugs [113, 114]. This amounts to 1.29 fold increase in the length of hospital stay in case of MRSA bacteremia [115], 2.6 fold in case of extended spectrum beta-lactamase producing strains of *K. pneumoniae* and 1.7 fold in case of carbapenem-resistant *P. aeruginosa* [116], and an added cost of $10,000 to $40,000 to treat such infections [117, 118], attributable to patient isolation with extra measures for infection control, prolonged treatment and laboratory testing and more expensive antibiotics [119]. In addition, AMR increased the risk of death by 1.2 in the case of pneumonia and bloodstream infections [120]. In neonates, the increased risk of death is even higher and can reach as high as twice the risk in infections with susceptible strains [121]. In Europe alone, it is estimated that complications associated with antibiotic resistance cost €9 billion annually [122]. In the USA, AMR costs about $20 billion and $35 billion for excess direct healthcare costs and loss of productivity due to infection, respectively [123]. On a global scale, the lost productivity associated with AMR infections is projected to be 2% to 3.5% and to amount to a cumulative $100 trillion by 2050 [3, 112].

HOW TO MITIGATE THE AMR PROBLEM?

Due to the dryness of new antimicrobials' pipelines, containment and prevention of antibiotic resistance should be a major priority. Since human health is directly connected to the environment and animal health, and due to the strong relationship between the development of antibiotic resistance and using of antibiotics in agriculture, any containment program should adopt a One Health approach [38, 124].

Surveillance and Antimicrobial Stewardship

The size, severity and widespread nature of AMR make it imperative to find solutions to curb its spread. Seeing as antibiotic misuse/overuse is at the root of the problem, antibiotic use needs to be regulated, especially in those countries where people can purchase an antibiotic even without a prescription. As a first step, there is an immediate need for robust surveillance and tracking systems to monitor the extent of antibiotic use on local and global levels. WHO launched the GLASS system in 2015 to achieve this goal and published its first report in 2018 with updates to follow regularly (Fig. 4) [33]. This requires the commitment of policymakers to put in place and enforce antimicrobial stewardship to prevent the unnecessary and often excessive use of antibiotics in humans [125]. Another measure to extend the life span of antimicrobials is to restrict or control the use of certain agents, especially last resort ones and/or to rotate the use of antimicrobials [126]. In this respect, the use of information and communication technology in the form of e-health can help prescribers make the proper antibiotic choice and decide on the right dose and duration [127]. In line with antimicrobial stewardship measures, there is a need to restrict the use of antibiotics in agriculture and animal husbandry as growth promoters or to prevent infections rather than to treat actual ones and to shift to agents not medically important for humans [3].

These measures need the national commitment of local health authorities to devise national action plans, and because microbes know no borders international cooperation is also needed to bring about the successful implementation of such plans. WHO is already coordinating such efforts on regional and global levels [3, 128]. All action plans require a multi-sectoral One Health approach involving humans, animals, and environmental health [124]. The aim of the plan is to ensure ongoing successful treatment *via* the preservation of the usefulness of the existing antimicrobial agents and the effective prevention of infections caused by multi-resistant pathogens. As of May 2017, one-third of the WHO member states had already developed their action plans to tackle AMR with another third working on theirs [129]. To achieve these goals, it is important to improve awareness of AMR and to reduce the incidence of infection [128]. Raising awareness can occur *via* campaigns to educate the general public on the risks of antibiotic misuse and ensuing resistance. These campaigns can also reduce patients' pressure on prescribers to prescribe antibiotics even when they are not called for as in the treatment of viral infections like the common cold [37].

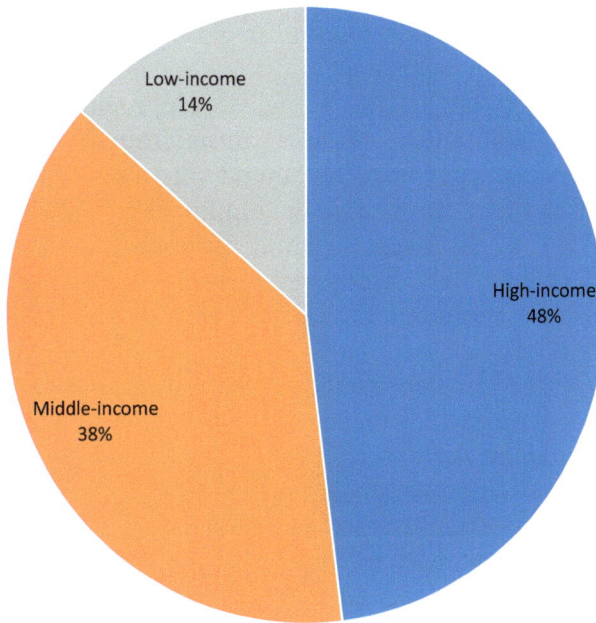

Fig. (4). Distribution of countries enrolled in the GLASS system (2018) [33].

Reducing the incidence of infection by improving hygiene and sanitation, the application of stricter infection control measures in healthcare settings and efficient vaccination programs will undoubtedly decrease the need for antimicrobial agents [3]. To help reduce antibiotic overuse, an improvement in diagnostics is called for to expedite antibiotic sensitivity testing and to properly and rapidly identify resistant bacteria. This has the potential to help physicians stop prescribing antibiotics "just in case" one is needed when the diagnostics are not available or are too expensive to afford in some resource-limited settings [3].

Chemical Modifications and Discovery of New Antibiotics

The discovery of penicillin in 1928 started a golden age of antibiotic discovery that lasted till the 1960s, with enough new agents still being discovered till the

1980s to overcome the ever occurring problem of antibiotic resistance [130, 131]. However, since the 1980s and with the exception of some new drug discoveries between 2011 and 2016 [37, 132], the interest of the pharmaceutical companies to discover new entities has waned [130], and very few agents have been approved for the treatment of infectious diseases [133]. A potential hypothesis is that pharmaceutical companies acquire large financial incentives from the increased demand on their agents when they become last resort options due to pathogens acquiring resistance to most other agents. By this time the last resort antibiotic might be already out of patent protection or close to being so which limits the incentive to invest in newer agents. In addition, because antibiotics are used for relatively short periods due to the rapid development of MDR pathogens, investment in the development of new antimicrobial agents is no longer profitable. There is an urgent need to amend this situation. Governments are encouraged to invest in research and development of new antimicrobials, to reward such innovative discoveries while limiting the unnecessary use of antibiotics to preserve the newly discovered ones. This requires cumulative global efforts with the United Nations and the G20 (Group of Twenty) taking active roles to ensure the success of such initiatives. A "market entry reward" of about one billion USD is suggested to celebrate the successful introduction in the market of new drugs, this is to ensure that these antimicrobials can be made available to anyone who needs them regardless of whether they come from a high or limited resource country. It is also to ensure that the new drugs won't be over-marketed or overpriced to cover the expenses that went into drug discovery and still make them profitable. This is especially true considering that the total profit from sales of patented antibiotics is 4.7 billion USD annually which is equivalent to one top-selling anticancer drug, reducing the attractiveness to pharmaceutical companies to invest in antimicrobials. However, to make the "market entry reward" initiative successful, governments must review and adjust their purchasing and distribution systems [3].

The majority of the new agents target gram-positive bacteria, leaving the resistant gram-negative pathogens that figure as a critical priority on the WHO list of priority pathogens with few effective treatment options. The complex nature of the cell wall of gram-negative bacteria makes it especially difficult to find new agents that can permeate the cell wall and stay inside [131]. Most of the new agents in the clinical pipelines are modifications of older agents with a narrow therapeutic spectrum against one or a few specific pathogens and aim to overcome resistance problems [131]. As of May 2017, only 51 antibiotics, including combinations, and 11 biologicals, mainly monoclonal antibodies and endolysins to be used as adjuncts to antibiotic therapy, are in the different phases of the clinical pipeline, with 16 targeting critical priority pathogens, including carbapenem-resistant *A. baumannii*, carbapenem-resistant *P. aeruginosa* and carbapenem-resistant Enterobacteriaceae. Of the 16, three are considered innovative and only one is developed for oral formulation. Oral preparations are especially needed in low resource countries for the treatment of infections in outpatients. Also of the 16 agents, five agents are in phase 3, one in phase 2 and ten in phase 1. With the potential of 14% of the agents in phase 1 to be approved for use in clinical practice, only one to two agents out of these ten are expected to reach the market. The narrow spectrum of action of these agents makes it hard to use them for the empirical treatment of severe infections during that window of time before the antimicrobial susceptibility results become available and where the choice of the right antibiotic could prove life-saving [131]. Because of the challenges that face the discovery of new antimicrobial agents and the huge investment and long period needed to sponsor such discoveries, it is paramount to maintain the efficacy of the already present antimicrobial agents through the development of new combination therapies [134 - 136]. A cocktail of antibiotics is nowadays recommended for the treatment of TB to decrease resistance development. However, for a variety of reasons, strains of *Mycobacterium tuberculosis* resistant to four or more agents have occurred to the extent that there are now strains that are totally drug resistant [137 - 139].

Alternative Approaches to Treat Resistant Infections

Nowadays, there are many alternative approaches and treatment options at different stages of investigation and development to combat different bacterial infections caused by MDR pathogens [140, 141].

Virulence factors are a group of molecules and structures that enable microorganisms to initiate and establish microbial infections and diseases. Drugs with anti-virulence potential are considered attractive candidate drugs to control MDR pathogens. These anti-virulence drugs can interfere with vital processes essential for microbial pathogenesis such as adherence, invasion, colonization, biofilm formation, intracellular replication, damage of host tissues and evasion of host immune system [142].

Quorum sensing inhibition is another potential approach for combating bacterial pathogens by disrupting the communication between bacterial cells [39, 143]. Inhibition of quorum sensing doesn't kill the bacterial cells, resulting in no selective pressure and hence the rate of emergence of microbial resistance will be low [143].

Vaccines are used primarily as a prophylactic tool to prevent infectious diseases, reduce the severity of the disease and raise the threshold load of pathogenic microorganisms required for induction of infection. The development of new vaccines to different pathogens could play an important role in limiting the spread of microbial resistance by reducing and preventing the need for antimicrobial agents [144, 145].

Bacteriophages and phage lytic proteins are emerging as potentially attractive non-conventional therapeutic agents to eradicate resistant bacteria and combat the development of newly arising multidrug-resistant pathogens [146, 147]. They are safe, highly specific thus minimizing the chance of secondary infections, able to effectively eradicate bacterial biofilm and environmentally friendly [147]. In addition, phage-antibiotic combinations showed promising and significant synergistic activity against different resistant pathogens [40, 147 - 149].

Probiotics are living "good" microorganisms that have many benefits for human health. They minimize, either alone or in combination with antibiotics, the risk of different bacterial infections and the need for antibiotics. Therefore, probiotics reduce the emergence and spread of antibiotic resistance [150]. Moreover, there are currently many other alternative approaches at different research levels such as monoclonal antibodies [142], antimicrobial peptides [143], immune stimulants [144], antibiofilms [145] and new antibiotic combinations [146]. The possible side effects and limitations of such alternative therapies are depicted in Table **3**.

Table 3. Side effects and/or limitations of alternative therapies against multidrug-resistant pathogens.

Alternative Therapies	Side Effects and/or Limitations
- Monoclonal antibodies [151]	Headache, myalgia and dizziness [152]
- Quorum sensing inhibitors [151]	Low selectivity, increase microbial survival ability, more difficult to eradicate microbes [153]
- Antimicrobial peptides [151]	Cytotoxicity, hemolytic activity, immunogenicity [154]
- Bacteriophages and phage lytic proteins [151]	Fever due to release of endotoxin [146]
- Antibiofilms [151]	Cytotoxicity [155]
- Probiotics [151]	Gastrointestinal symptoms [156], itchy rash, allergy [157]
- Vaccines [151]	Rapid development of resistance in some bacterial species [158]
- Antibiotic combinations [151]	High cost, increased risk of side effects, superinfection, antagonism [159]

CONCLUSION

Antimicrobial resistance is a global problem that jeopardizes the achievements of modern medicine and is a harbinger to the return to a time when simple infections were fatal. Injudicious antibiotic use in human healthcare as well as animal husbandry, together with the slowdown in the discovery of new antimicrobials are at the root of the problem. Regulating antimicrobial use and encouraging the discovery of novel agents and alternative therapies seem the way forward to win the human fight against pathogenic microbes.

CONSENT FOR PUBLICATION

Not applicable.

CONFLICT OF INTEREST

The authors confirm that the contents of this chapter have no conflict of interest.

ACKNOWLEDGEMENTS

Declared none.

REFERENCES

[1]   Laxminarayan R, Matsoso P, Pant S, *et al*. Access to effective antimicrobials: a worldwide challenge. Lancet 2016; 387(10014): 168-75.
        [http://dx.doi.org/10.1016/S0140-6736(15)00474-2] [PMID: 26603918]

[2]   Laxminarayan R, Duse A, Wattal C, *et al*. Antibiotic resistance-the need for global solutions. Lancet Infect Dis 2013; 13(12): 1057-98.
        [http://dx.doi.org/10.1016/S1473-3099(13)70318-9] [PMID: 24252483]

[3]   Review on antimicrobial resistance. Tackling drug-resistant infections globally: final report and recommendations 2016.

[4]   Andersson DI, Hughes D. Antibiotic resistance and its cost: is it possible to reverse resistance? Nat Rev Microbiol 2010; 8(4): 260-71.
        [http://dx.doi.org/10.1038/nrmicro2319] [PMID: 20208551]

[5]   Liu B, Pop M. ARDB--antibiotic resistance genes database. Nucleic Acids Res 2009; 37(Database issue): D443-7.
        [http://dx.doi.org/10.1093/nar/gkn656] [PMID: 18832362]

[6]   Davies J, Davies D. Origins and evolution of antibiotic resistance. Microbiol Mol Biol Rev 2010; 74(3): 417-33.
        [http://dx.doi.org/10.1128/MMBR.00016-10] [PMID: 20805405]

[7]   Abraham EP, Chain E. An enzyme from bacteria able to destroy penicillin. Nature 1940; 146: 837.
        [http://dx.doi.org/10.1038/146837a0]

[8]   European Centre for Disease Prevention and Control. Factsheet for experts - Antimicrobial resistance. https://ecdc.europa.eu/en/antimicrobial-resistance/facts/factsheets/experts

[9]   High levels of antibiotic resistance found worldwide, new data shows. https://www.who.int/mediacentre/news/releases/2018/antibiotic-resistance-found/en/

[10]   Organization for Economic Co-operation and Development (OECD). Stopping antimicrobial resistance would cost just USD 2 per person a year 2018. http://www.oecd.org/ health/stopping-antimicrobial-resistance-would-cost-just-usd-2-per-person-a-year.htm

[11]   Zaidi AK, Huskins WC, Thaver D, Bhutta ZA, Abbas Z, Goldmann DA. Hospital-acquired neonatal infections in developing countries. Lancet 2005; 365(9465): 1175-88.

[http://dx.doi.org/10.1016/S0140-6736(05)71881-X] [PMID: 15794973]

[12]   Waters D, Jawad I, Ahmad A, *et al.* Aetiology of community-acquired neonatal sepsis in low and middle income countries. J Glob Health 2011; 1(2): 154-70.
[PMID: 23198116]

[13]   Viswanathan R, Singh AK, Ghosh C, Dasgupta S, Mukherjee S, Basu S. Profile of neonatal septicaemia at a district-level sick newborn care unit. J Health Popul Nutr 2012; 30(1): 41-8.
[http://dx.doi.org/10.3329/jhpn.v30i1.11274] [PMID: 22524118]

[14]   Saleem AF, Ahmed I, Mir F, Ali SR, Zaidi AK. Pan-resistant Acinetobacter infection in neonates in Karachi, Pakistan. J Infect Dev Ctries 2009; 4(1): 30-7.
[http://dx.doi.org/10.3855/jidc.533] [PMID: 20130376]

[15]   Nordmann P, Naas T, Poirel L. Global spread of Carbapenemase-producing Enterobacteriaceae. Emerg Infect Dis 2011; 17(10): 1791-8.
[http://dx.doi.org/10.3201/eid1710.110655] [PMID: 22000347]

[16]   Vital signs: carbapenem-resistant Enterobacteriaceae. MMWR Morb Mortal Wkly Rep 2013; 62(9): 165-70.
[PMID: 23466435]

[17]   European Centre for Disease Prevention and Control (2018). Surveillance of antimicrobial resistance in Europe 2017.

[18]   WHO. Global priority list of antibiotic-resistant bacteria to guide research, discovery, and development of new antibiotics 2017. http://www.who.int/medicines/publications/ global-priority-li-t-antibiotic-resistant-bacteria/en/

[19]   Dantes R, Mu Y, Belflower R, *et al.* National burden of invasive methicillin-resistant *Staphylococcus aureus* infections, United States, 2011. JAMA Intern Med 2013; 173(21): 1970-8.
[PMID: 24043270]

[20]   Johnson AP. Methicillin-resistant *Staphylococcus aureus*: the European landscape. J Antimicrob Chemother 2011; 66 (Suppl. 4): iv43-8.
[http://dx.doi.org/10.1093/jac/dkr076] [PMID: 21521706]

[21]   Van Cleef BA, Broens EM, Voss A, *et al.* High prevalence of nasal MRSA carriage in slaughterhouse workers in contact with live pigs in The Netherlands. Epidemiol Infect 2010; 138(5): 756-63.
[http://dx.doi.org/10.1017/S0950268810000245] [PMID: 20141647]

[22]   Krziwanek K, Metz-Gercek S, Mittermayer H. Methicillin-Resistant *Staphylococcus aureus* ST398 from human patients, upper Austria. Emerg Infect Dis 2009; 15(5): 766-9.
[http://dx.doi.org/10.3201/eid1505.080326] [PMID: 19402964]

[23]   Huber H, Koller S, Giezendanner N, Stephan R, Zweifel C. Prevalence and characteristics of meticillin-resistant *Staphylococcus aureus* in humans in contact with farm animals, in livestock, and in food of animal origin, Switzerland, 2009. Euro Surveill 2010; 15(16): 19542.
[PMID: 20430001]

[24]   Song JH, Hsueh PR, Chung DR, *et al.* Spread of methicillin-resistant *Staphylococcus aureus* between the community and the hospitals in Asian countries: an ANSORP study. J Antimicrob Chemother 2011; 66(5): 1061-9.
[http://dx.doi.org/10.1093/jac/dkr024] [PMID: 21393157]

[25]   Falagas ME, Karageorgopoulos DE, Leptidis J, Korbila IP. MRSA in Africa: filling the global map of antimicrobial resistance. PLoS One 2013; 8(7): e68024.
[http://dx.doi.org/10.1371/journal.pone.0068024] [PMID: 23922652]

[26]   Brink A, Moolman J, da Silva MC, Botha M. Antimicrobial susceptibility profile of selected bacteraemic pathogens from private institutions in South Africa. S Afr Med J 2007; 97(4): 273-9.
[PMID: 17446952]

[27]   Jansen van Rensburg MJ, Whitelaw AC, Elisha BG. Genetic basis of rifampicin resistance in methicillin-resistant *Staphylococcus aureus* suggests clonal expansion in hospitals in Cape Town, South Africa. BMC Microbiol 2012; 12: 46.
[http://dx.doi.org/10.1186/1471-2180-12-46] [PMID: 22448673]

[28]   Randrianirina F, Soares JL, Ratsima E, *et al. In vitro* activities of 18 antimicrobial agents against *Staphylococcus aureus* isolates from the Institut Pasteur of Madagascar. Ann Clin Microbiol Antimicrob 2007; 6: 5.
[http://dx.doi.org/10.1186/1476-0711-6-5] [PMID: 17521424]

[29]   Abera B, Alem A, Bezabih B. Methicillin-resistant strains of *Staphylococcus aureus* and coagulase-negative staphylococus from clinical isolates at Felege Hiwot Refferal Hospital, North West Ethiopia. Ethiop Med J 2008; 46(2): 149-54.
[PMID: 21309204]

[30]   Borg MA, de Kraker M, Scicluna E, *et al.* Prevalence of methicillin-resistant *Staphylococcus aureus* (MRSA) in invasive isolates from southern and eastern Mediterranean countries. J Antimicrob Chemother 2007; 60(6): 1310-5.
[http://dx.doi.org/10.1093/jac/dkm365] [PMID: 17913724]

[31]   Truong H, Shah SS, Ludmir J, *et al. Staphylococcus aureus* skin and soft tissue infections at a tertiary hospital in Botswana. S Afr Med J 2011; 101(6): 413-6.
[PMID: 21920078]

[32]   Wood SM, Shah SS, Bafana M, *et al.* Epidemiology of methicillin-resistant *Staphylococcus aureus* bacteremia in Gaborone, Botswana. Infect Control Hosp Epidemiol 2009; 30(8): 782-5.
[http://dx.doi.org/10.1086/599003] [PMID: 19591580]

[33]   Global antimicrobial resistance surveillance system (GLASS) report. Early implementation 2016-2017. http://www.who.int/glass/resources/publications/early-implementation-report/en/

[34]   Robinson TP, Bu DP, Carrique-Mas J, *et al.* Antibiotic resistance is the quintessential One Health issue. Trans R Soc Trop Med Hyg 2016; 110(7): 377-80.
[http://dx.doi.org/10.1093/trstmh/trw048] [PMID: 27475987]

[35]   Laxminarayan R. Antibiotic effectiveness: balancing conservation against innovation. Science 2014; 345(6202): 1299-301.
[http://dx.doi.org/10.1126/science.1254163] [PMID: 25214620]

[36]   Usluer G, Ozgunes I, Leblebicioglu H. A multicenter point-prevalence study: antimicrobial prescription frequencies in hospitalized patients in Turkey. Ann Clin Microbiol Antimicrob 2005; 4: 16.
[http://dx.doi.org/10.1186/1476-0711-4-16] [PMID: 16202139]

[37]   Laxminarayan R, Malani A, Howard D, Smith DL. Extending the cure: policy responses to the growing threat of antibiotic resistance 2007.

[38]   Centers for Disease Control and Prevention. About Antimicrobial Resistance 2018. https://www.cdc.gov/drugresistance/about.html

[39]   Ayukekbong JA, Ntemgwa M, Atabe AN. The threat of antimicrobial resistance in developing countries: causes and control strategies. Antimicrob Resist Infect Control 2017; 6: 47.
[http://dx.doi.org/10.1186/s13756-017-0208-x] [PMID: 28515903]

[40]   Aminov RI. A brief history of the antibiotic era: lessons learned and challenges for the future. Front Microbiol 2010; 1: 134.
[http://dx.doi.org/10.3389/fmicb.2010.00134] [PMID: 21687759]

[41]   Woodhead M, Finch R. Public education - a progress report. J Antimicrob Chemother 2007; 60 (Suppl. 1): i53-5.
[http://dx.doi.org/10.1093/jac/dkm158] [PMID: 17656383]

[42]   Goossens H, Ferech M, Vander Stichele R, Elseviers M. Outpatient antibiotic use in Europe and association with resistance: a cross-national database study. Lancet 2005; 365(9459): 579-87.
[http://dx.doi.org/10.1016/S0140-6736(05)70799-6] [PMID: 15708101]

[43]   Horrevorts AM, Borst J, Puyk RJ, *et al.* Ecology of *Pseudomonas aeruginosa* in patients with cystic fibrosis. J Med Microbiol 1990; 31(2): 119-24.
[http://dx.doi.org/10.1099/00222615-31-2-119] [PMID: 2106033]

[44]   Van Boeckel TP, Gandra S, Ashok A, *et al.* Global antibiotic consumption 2000 to 2010: an analysis of national pharmaceutical sales data. Lancet Infect Dis 2014; 14(8): 742-50.
[http://dx.doi.org/10.1016/S1473-3099(14)70780-7] [PMID: 25022435]

[45]   Laxminarayan R, Heymann DL. Challenges of drug resistance in the developing world. BMJ 2012; 344: e1567.
[http://dx.doi.org/10.1136/bmj.e1567] [PMID: 22491075]

[46]   Sweidan M, Zhang Y, Harvey K, Yang Y, Shen X, Yao K. Proceedings of the 2nd National Workshop on Rational Use of Antibiotics in China.

[47]   Gartin M, Brewis AA, Schwartz NA. Nonprescription antibiotic therapy: cultural models on both sides of the counter and both sides of the border. Med Anthropol Q 2010; 24(1): 85-107.
[http://dx.doi.org/10.1111/j.1548-1387.2010.01086.x] [PMID: 20420303]

[48]   Antibiotic overuse: the influence of social norms. J Am Coll Surg 2008; 207(2): 265-75.
[http://dx.doi.org/10.1016/j.jamcollsurg.2008.02.035] [PMID: 18656057]

[49]   Hamilton WL, Doyle C, Halliwell-Ewen M, Lambert G. Public health interventions to protect against falsified medicines: a systematic review of international, national and local policies. Health Policy Plan 2016; 31(10): 1448-66.
[http://dx.doi.org/10.1093/heapol/czw062] [PMID: 27311827]

[50]   Daulaire N, Bang A, Tomson G, Kalyango JN, Cars O. Universal access to effective antibiotics is essential for tackling antibiotic resistance. J Law Med Ethics 2015; 43 (Suppl. 3): 17-21.
[http://dx.doi.org/10.1111/jlme.12269] [PMID: 26243238]

[51]   Holmes AH, Moore LS, Sundsfjord A, *et al.* Understanding the mechanisms and drivers of antimicrobial resistance. Lancet 2016; 387(10014): 176-87.
[http://dx.doi.org/10.1016/S0140-6736(15)00473-0] [PMID: 26603922]

[52]   Bengtsson-Palme J, Boulund F, Fick J, Kristiansson E, Larsson DG. Shotgun metagenomics reveals a wide array of antibiotic resistance genes and mobile elements in a polluted lake in India. Front Microbiol 2014; 5: 648.
[http://dx.doi.org/10.3389/fmicb.2014.00648] [PMID: 25520706]

[53]   Flach CF, Johnning A, Nilsson I, Smalla K, Kristiansson E, Larsson DG. Isolation of novel IncA/C and IncN fluoroquinolone resistance plasmids from an antibiotic-polluted lake. J Antimicrob Chemother 2015; 70(10): 2709-17.
[http://dx.doi.org/10.1093/jac/dkv167] [PMID: 26124213]

[54]   Antimicrobial resistance - Policy insights 2016.

[55]   Sun X, Hirota SA. The roles of host and pathogen factors and the innate immune response in the pathogenesis of *Clostridium difficile* infection. Mol Immunol 2015; 63(2): 193-202.
[http://dx.doi.org/10.1016/j.molimm.2014.09.005] [PMID: 25242213]

[56]   Lessa FC, Mu Y, Bamberg WM, *et al.* Burden of *Clostridium difficile* infection in the United States. N Engl J Med 2015; 372(9): 825-34.
[http://dx.doi.org/10.1056/NEJMoa1408913] [PMID: 25714160]

[57]   O'Neill J. Review on antimicrobial resistance. Antimicrobials in agriculture and environment: reducing unnecessary use and waste 2015.

[58]   FDA. Summary report on antimicrobials sold or distributed for use in food-producing animals 2016.

https://www.fda.gov/downloads/forindustry/userfees/animaldruguserfeeactadufa/ucm588085.pdf

[59]   Marshall BM, Levy SB. Food animals and antimicrobials: impacts on human health. Clin Microbiol Rev 2011; 24(4): 718-33.
[http://dx.doi.org/10.1128/CMR.00002-11] [PMID: 21976606]

[60]   Van Boeckel TP, Brower C, Gilbert M, *et al.* Global trends in antimicrobial use in food animals. Proc Natl Acad Sci USA 2015; 112(18): 5649-54.
[http://dx.doi.org/10.1073/pnas.1503141112] [PMID: 25792457]

[61]   Zhu YG, Johnson TA, Su JQ, *et al.* Diverse and abundant antibiotic resistance genes in Chinese swine farms. Proc Natl Acad Sci USA 2013; 110(9): 3435-40.
[http://dx.doi.org/10.1073/pnas.1222743110] [PMID: 23401528]

[62]   Laxminarayan R, Van Boeckel T, Teillant A. The economic costs of withdrawing antimicrobial growth promoters from the livestock sector. OECD Food Agric Fish Work Pap 2015; 78.

[63]   Ågerstrand M, Berg C, Björlenius B, *et al.* Improving environmental risk assessment of human pharmaceuticals. Environ Sci Technol 2015; 49(9): 5336-45.
[http://dx.doi.org/10.1021/acs.est.5b00302] [PMID: 25844810]

[64]   Sum of Us. Bad Medicine: How the pharmaceutical industry is contributing to the global rise of antibiotic-resistant superbugs 2015.

[65]   Zhang QQ, Ying GG, Pan CG, Liu YS, Zhao JL. Comprehensive evaluation of antibiotics emission and fate in the river basins of China: source analysis, multimedia modeling, and linkage to bacterial resistance. Environ Sci Technol 2015; 49(11): 6772-82.
[http://dx.doi.org/10.1021/acs.est.5b00729] [PMID: 25961663]

[66]   Larsson DG, de Pedro C, Paxeus N. Effluent from drug manufactures contains extremely high levels of pharmaceuticals. J Hazard Mater 2007; 148(3): 751-5.
[http://dx.doi.org/10.1016/j.jhazmat.2007.07.008] [PMID: 17706342]

[67]   Larsson DG. Pollution from drug manufacturing: review and perspectives. Philos Trans R Soc Lond B Biol Sci 2014; 369(1656): 20130571.
[http://dx.doi.org/10.1098/rstb.2013.0571] [PMID: 25405961]

[68]   Li D, Yang M, Hu J, Ren L, Zhang Y, Li K. Determination and fate of oxytetracycline and related compounds in oxytetracycline production wastewater and the receiving river. Environ Toxicol Chem 2008; 27(1): 80-6.
[http://dx.doi.org/10.1897/07-080.1] [PMID: 18092864]

[69]   Ng C, Gin KYH. Monitoring antimicrobial resistance dissemination in aquatic systems. Water 2019; 11(71).
[http://dx.doi.org/10.3390/w11010071]

[70]   Bengtsson-Palme J, Larsson DG. Concentrations of antibiotics predicted to select for resistant bacteria: Proposed limits for environmental regulation. Environ Int 2016; 86: 140-9.
[http://dx.doi.org/10.1016/j.envint.2015.10.015] [PMID: 26590482]

[71]   Lerminiaux NA, Cameron ADS. Horizontal transfer of antibiotic resistance genes in clinical environments. Can J Microbiol 219; 65(1): 34-44.
[PMID: 30248271]

[72]   Walsh C. Molecular mechanisms that confer antibacterial drug resistance. Nature 2000; 406(6797): 775-81.
[http://dx.doi.org/10.1038/35021219] [PMID: 10963607]

[73]   Koronakis V, Eswaran J, Hughes C. Structure and function of TolC: the bacterial exit duct for proteins and drugs. Annu Rev Biochem 2004; 73: 467-89.
[http://dx.doi.org/10.1146/annurev.biochem.73.011303.074104] [PMID: 15189150]

[74]   Giguère S. Antimicrobial Drug Action and Interaction: An Introduction. Antimicrobial therapy in

Veterinary Medicine. 4th ed.., Ames 2006.

[75]   Fernández L, Hancock RE. Adaptive and mutational resistance: role of porins and efflux pumps in drug resistance. Clin Microbiol Rev 2012; 25(4): 661-81.
[http://dx.doi.org/10.1128/CMR.00043-12] [PMID: 23034325]

[76]   Nikaido H. Multidrug resistance in bacteria. Annu Rev Biochem 2009; 78: 119-46.
[http://dx.doi.org/10.1146/annurev.biochem.78.082907.145923] [PMID: 19231985]

[77]   Levy SB. Active efflux mechanisms for antimicrobial resistance. Antimicrob Agents Chemother 1992; 36(4): 695-703.
[http://dx.doi.org/10.1128/AAC.36.4.695] [PMID: 1503431]

[78]   Paulsen IT, Brown MH, Skurray RA. Proton-dependent multidrug efflux systems. Microbiol Rev 1996; 60(4): 575-608.
[http://dx.doi.org/10.1128/MMBR.60.4.575-608.1996] [PMID: 8987357]

[79]   Alekshun MN, Levy SB. Molecular mechanisms of antibacterial multidrug resistance. Cell 2007; 128(6): 1037-50.
[http://dx.doi.org/10.1016/j.cell.2007.03.004] [PMID: 17382878]

[80]   Keren I, Kaldalu N, Spoering A, Wang Y, Lewis K. Persister cells and tolerance to antimicrobials. FEMS Microbiol Lett 2004; 230(1): 13-8.
[http://dx.doi.org/10.1016/S0378-1097(03)00856-5] [PMID: 14734160]

[81]   Lewis K. Programmed death in bacteria. Microbiol Mol Biol Rev 2000; 64(3): 503-14.
[http://dx.doi.org/10.1128/MMBR.64.3.503-514.2000] [PMID: 10974124]

[82]   Lewis K. Riddle of biofilm resistance. Antimicrob Agents Chemother 2001; 45(4): 999-1007.
[http://dx.doi.org/10.1128/AAC.45.4.999-1007.2001] [PMID: 11257008]

[83]   Davies J. Bacteria on the rampage. Nature 1996; 383(6597): 219-20.
[http://dx.doi.org/10.1038/383219a0] [PMID: 8805692]

[84]   Arthur M, Courvalin P. Genetics and mechanisms of glycopeptide resistance in enterococci. Antimicrob Agents Chemother 1993; 37(8): 1563-71.
[http://dx.doi.org/10.1128/AAC.37.8.1563] [PMID: 8215264]

[85]   Walsh CT, Fisher SL, Park IS, Prahalad M, Wu Z. Bacterial resistance to vancomycin: five genes and one missing hydrogen bond tell the story. Chem Biol 1996; 3(1): 21-8.
[http://dx.doi.org/10.1016/S1074-5521(96)90079-4] [PMID: 8807824]

[86]   Martinez JL, Baquero F. Mutation frequencies and antibiotic resistance. Antimicrob Agents Chemother 2000; 44(7): 1771-7.
[http://dx.doi.org/10.1128/AAC.44.7.1771-1777.2000] [PMID: 10858329]

[87]   Davies JE. Origins, acquisition and dissemination of antibiotic resistance determinants. Ciba Found Symp 1997; 207: 15-27; discussion -35.

[88]   Forbes BA, Sahm DF, Weissfeld AS. Bailey and Scott's Diagnostic Microbiology. 10th ed., St. Louis: Mosby Inc. 1998.

[89]   Miller JH. Spontaneous mutators in bacteria: insights into pathways of mutagenesis and repair. Annu Rev Microbiol 1996; 50: 625-43.
[http://dx.doi.org/10.1146/annurev.micro.50.1.625] [PMID: 8905093]

[90]   Horst JP, Wu TH, Marinus MG. *Escherichia coli* mutator genes. Trends Microbiol 1999; 7(1): 29-36.
[http://dx.doi.org/10.1016/S0966-842X(98)01424-3] [PMID: 10068995]

[91]   Oliver A, Cantón R, Campo P, Baquero F, Blázquez J. High frequency of hypermutable *Pseudomonas aeruginosa* in cystic fibrosis lung infection. Science 2000; 288(5469): 1251-4.
[http://dx.doi.org/10.1126/science.288.5469.1251] [PMID: 10818002]

[92]   Spratt BG. Resistance to antibiotics mediated by target alterations. Science 1994; 264(5157): 388-93.

[http://dx.doi.org/10.1126/science.8153626] [PMID: 8153626]

[93] Schentag JJ, Hyatt JM, Carr JR, *et al.* Genesis of methicillin-resistant *Staphylococcus aureus* (MRSA), how treatment of MRSA infections has selected for vancomycin-resistant *Enterococcus faecium*, and the importance of antibiotic management and infection control. Clin Infect Dis 1998; 26(5): 1204-14.
[http://dx.doi.org/10.1086/520287] [PMID: 9597254]

[94] Giedraitienė A, Vitkauskienė A, Naginienė R, Pavilonis A. Antibiotic resistance mechanisms of clinically important bacteria. Medicina (Kaunas) 2011; 47(3): 137-46.
[PMID: 21822035]

[95] Achouak W, Heulin T, Pagès JM. Multiple facets of bacterial porins. FEMS Microbiol Lett 2001; 199(1): 1-7.
[http://dx.doi.org/10.1111/j.1574-6968.2001.tb10642.x] [PMID: 11356559]

[96] Gillespie SH. Antibiotic resistance in the absence of selective pressure. Int J Antimicrob Agents 2001; 17(3): 171-6.
[http://dx.doi.org/10.1016/S0924-8579(00)00340-X] [PMID: 11282261]

[97] Rodríguez-Rojas A, Rodríguez-Beltrán J, Couce A, Blázquez J. Antibiotics and antibiotic resistance: a bitter fight against evolution. Int J Med Microbiol 2013; 303(6-7): 293-7.
[http://dx.doi.org/10.1016/j.ijmm.2013.02.004] [PMID: 23517688]

[98] Chu DT, Plattner JJ, Katz L. New directions in antibacterial research. J Med Chem 1996; 39(20): 3853-74.
[http://dx.doi.org/10.1021/jm960294s] [PMID: 8831751]

[99] Smith HO, Gwinn ML, Salzberg SL. DNA uptake signal sequences in naturally transformable bacteria. Res Microbiol 1999; 150(9-10): 603-16.
[http://dx.doi.org/10.1016/S0923-2508(99)00130-8] [PMID: 10673000]

[100] Biswas I. Genetic tools for manipulating *Acinetobacter baumannii* genome: an overview. J Med Microbiol 2015; 64(7): 657-69.
[http://dx.doi.org/10.1099/jmm.0.000081] [PMID: 25948809]

[101] Del Grosso M, Camilli R, Barbabella G, Blackman Northwood J, Farrell DJ, Pantosti A. Genetic resistance elements carrying mef subclasses other than mef(A) in *Streptococcus pyogenes*. Antimicrob Agents Chemother 2011; 55(7): 3226-30.
[http://dx.doi.org/10.1128/AAC.01713-10] [PMID: 21502613]

[102] Davies J. Inactivation of antibiotics and the dissemination of resistance genes. Science 1994; 264(5157): 375-82.
[http://dx.doi.org/10.1126/science.8153624] [PMID: 8153624]

[103] Manson JM, Hancock LE, Gilmore MS. Mechanism of chromosomal transfer of *Enterococcus faecalis* pathogenicity island, capsule, antimicrobial resistance, and other traits. Proc Natl Acad Sci USA 2010; 107(27): 12269-74.
[http://dx.doi.org/10.1073/pnas.1000139107] [PMID: 20566881]

[104] McDermott PF, Walker RD, White DG. Antimicrobials: modes of action and mechanisms of resistance. Int J Toxicol 2003; 22(2): 135-43.
[http://dx.doi.org/10.1080/10915810305089] [PMID: 12745995]

[105] Hall RM, Collis CM, Kim MJ, Partridge SR, Recchia GD, Stokes HW. Mobile gene cassettes and integrons in evolution. Ann N Y Acad Sci 1999; 870: 68-80.
[http://dx.doi.org/10.1111/j.1749-6632.1999.tb08866.x] [PMID: 10415474]

[106] Lewis K. Persister cells and the riddle of biofilm survival. Biochemistry (Mosc) 2005; 70(2): 267-74.
[http://dx.doi.org/10.1007/s10541-005-0111-6] [PMID: 15807669]

[107] Dhar N, McKinney JD. Microbial phenotypic heterogeneity and antibiotic tolerance. Curr Opin Microbiol 2007; 10(1): 30-8.
[http://dx.doi.org/10.1016/j.mib.2006.12.007] [PMID: 17215163]

[108]   Sethi S, Golparian D, Bala M, *et al.* Antimicrobial susceptibility and genetic characteristics of *Neisseria gonorrhoeae* isolates from India, Pakistan and Bhutan in 2007-2011. BMC Infect Dis 2013; 13: 35.
[http://dx.doi.org/10.1186/1471-2334-13-35] [PMID: 23347339]

[109]   CDC Grand Rounds: the growing threat of multidrug-resistant gonorrhea. MMWR Morb Mortal Wkly Rep 2013; 62(6): 103-6.
[PMID: 23407126]

[110]   Lodise TP, McKinnon PS, Tam VH, Rybak MJ. Clinical outcomes for patients with bacteremia caused by vancomycin-resistant enterococcus in a level 1 trauma center. Clin Infect Dis 2002; 34(7): 922-9.
[http://dx.doi.org/10.1086/339211] [PMID: 11880957]

[111]   Tumbarello M, Sanguinetti M, Montuori E, *et al.* Predictors of mortality in patients with bloodstream infections caused by extended-spectrum-beta-lactamase-producing Enterobacteriaceae: importance of inadequate initial antimicrobial treatment. Antimicrob Agents Chemother 2007; 51(6): 1987-94.
[http://dx.doi.org/10.1128/AAC.01509-06] [PMID: 17387156]

[112]   Review on antimicrobial resistance. Tackling a crisis for the health and wealth of nations 2014.

[113]   Fighting Antimicrobial Resistance. http://www.who.int/news-room/fact-sheets/ detail/antimicrobial-resistance

[114]   Holmberg SD, Solomon SL, Blake PA. Health and economic impacts of antimicrobial resistance. Rev Infect Dis 1987; 9(6): 1065-78.
[http://dx.doi.org/10.1093/clinids/9.6.1065] [PMID: 3321356]

[115]   Cosgrove SE, Qi Y, Kaye KS, Harbarth S, Karchmer AW, Carmeli Y. The impact of methicillin resistance in *Staphylococcus aureus* bacteremia on patient outcomes: mortality, length of stay, and hospital charges. Infect Control Hosp Epidemiol 2005; 26(2): 166-74.
[http://dx.doi.org/10.1086/502522] [PMID: 15756888]

[116]   The cost of antibiotic resistance: effect of resistance among *Staphylococcus aureus, Klebsiella pneumoniae, Acinetobacter baumannii,* and *Pseudmonas aeruginosa* on length of hospital stay. Infect Control Hosp Epidemiol 2002; 23(2): 106-8.
[http://dx.doi.org/10.1086/502018] [PMID: 11893146]

[117]   Smith R, Coast J. The true cost of antimicrobial resistance. BMJ 2013; 346: f1493.
[http://dx.doi.org/10.1136/bmj.f1493] [PMID: 23479660]

[118]   http://www.oecd.org/about/secretary-general/g20-health-ministers-meeting-fighting-antimicrobial-resistance.htm

[119]   Mulvey MR, Simor AE. Antimicrobial resistance in hospitals: how concerned should we be? CMAJ 2009; 180(4): 408-15.
[http://dx.doi.org/10.1503/cmaj.080239] [PMID: 19221354]

[120]   Lambert ML, Suetens C, Savey A, *et al.* Clinical outcomes of health-care-associated infections and antimicrobial resistance in patients admitted to European intensive-care units: a cohort study. Lancet Infect Dis 2011; 11(1): 30-8.
[http://dx.doi.org/10.1016/S1473-3099(10)70258-9] [PMID: 21126917]

[121]   Kayange N, Kamugisha E, Mwizamholya DL, Jeremiah S, Mshana SE. Predictors of positive blood culture and deaths among neonates with suspected neonatal sepsis in a tertiary hospital, Mwanza-Tanzania. BMC Pediatr 2010; 10: 39.
[http://dx.doi.org/10.1186/1471-2431-10-39] [PMID: 20525358]

[122]   Oxford J, Kozlov R. Antibiotic resistance--a call to arms for primary healthcare providers. Int J Clin Pract Suppl 2013; (180): 1-3.
[http://dx.doi.org/10.1111/ijcp.12334] [PMID: 24238423]

[123]   Centers for Disease Control and Prevention. Antibiotic Resistance Threats in the United States 2013.

https://www.cdc.gov/drugresistance/pdf/ar-threats-2013-508.pdf

[124] Walsh TR. A one-health approach to antimicrobial resistance. Nat Microbiol 2018; 3(8): 854-5.
[http://dx.doi.org/10.1038/s41564-018-0208-5] [PMID: 30046173]

[125] Doron S, Davidson LE. Antimicrobial stewardship. Mayo Clin Proc 2011; 86(11): 1113-23.
[http://dx.doi.org/10.4065/mcp.2011.0358] [PMID: 22033257]

[126] Shlaes DM, Gerding DN, John JF Jr, *et al.* Society for Healthcare Epidemiology of America and Infectious Diseases Society of America Joint Committee on the Prevention of Antimicrobial Resistance: guidelines for the prevention of antimicrobial resistance in hospitals. Clin Infect Dis 1997; 25(3): 584-99.
[http://dx.doi.org/10.1086/513766] [PMID: 9314444]

[127] Palos C, Bispo A, Rodrigues P, França L, Capoulas M. Optimizing antimicrobial prescription through e-health: setting, dosing, timing and stewardship. Antimicrob Resist Infect Control 2015; 4 (Suppl. 1): O3.
[http://dx.doi.org/10.1186/2047-2994-4-S1-O3]

[128] WHO. Global action on antimicrobial resistance 2015. http://www.wpro.who.int/entity/drug_resistance/resources/global_action_plan_eng.pdf

[129] Berlin Declaration of the G20 Health Ministers. Together Today for a Healthy Tomorrow 2017.

[130] Rolain JM, Abat C, Jimeno MT, Fournier PE, Raoult D. Do we need new antibiotics? Clin Microbiol Infect 2016; 22(5): 408-15.
[http://dx.doi.org/10.1016/j.cmi.2016.03.012] [PMID: 27021418]

[131] WHO. Antibacterial agents in clinical development: an analysis of the antibacterial clinical development pipeline, including tuberculosis. Including Tuberculosis 2017.

[132] Butler MS, Blaskovich MA, Cooper MA. Antibiotics in the clinical pipeline at the end of 2015. J Antibiot (Tokyo) 2017; 70(1): 3-24.
[http://dx.doi.org/10.1038/ja.2016.72] [PMID: 27353164]

[133] Ventola CL. The antibiotic resistance crisis: part 1: causes and threats. P&T 2015; 40(4): 277-83.
[PMID: 25859123]

[134] Aboulmagd E, Alsultan AA, Al Mohammad HI, Al-Badry S, Hussein EM. *In vitro* synergistic activity of amikacin combined with subinhibitory concentration of tigecycline against extended spectrum β-lactamase-producing *Klebsiella pneumoniae.* J Microbiol Antimicrob 2013; 5(5): 44-9.
[http://dx.doi.org/10.5897/JMA13.0262]

[135] Aboulmagd E, Alsultan AA. Synergic bactericidal activity of novel antibiotic combinations against extreme drug resistant *Pseudomonas aeruginosa* and *Acinetobacter baumannii.* Afr J Microbiol Res 2014; 8(9): 856-61.
[http://dx.doi.org/10.5897/AJMR2013.6477]

[136] DRIVE-AB Report. Revitalizing the antibiotic pipeline. Stimulating innovation while driving sustainable use and global access. http://drive-ab.eu/wp-content/ uploads/2018/01/DRIVE-AB-Fin-l-Report-Jan2018.pdf

[137] Shah NS, Wright A, Bai GH, *et al.* Worldwide emergence of extensively drug-resistant tuberculosis. Emerg Infect Dis 2007; 13(3): 380-7.
[http://dx.doi.org/10.3201/eid1303.061400] [PMID: 17552090]

[138] Sotgiu G, Ferrara G, Matteelli A, *et al.* Epidemiology and clinical management of XDR-TB: a systematic review by TBNET. Eur Respir J 2009; 33(4): 871-81.
[http://dx.doi.org/10.1183/09031936.00168008] [PMID: 19251779]

[139] Velayati AA, Masjedi MR, Farnia P, *et al.* Emergence of new forms of totally drug-resistant tuberculosis bacilli: super extensively drug-resistant tuberculosis or totally drug-resistant strains in iran. Chest 2009; 136(2): 420-5.

[http://dx.doi.org/10.1378/chest.08-2427] [PMID: 19349380]

[140] Brunel AS, Guery B. Multidrug resistant (or antimicrobial-resistant) pathogens - alternatives to new antibiotics? Swiss Med Wkly 2017; 147:: w14553.
[PMID: 29185252]

[141] Czaplewski L, Bax R, Clokie M, *et al.* Alternatives to antibiotics-a pipeline portfolio review. Lancet Infect Dis 2016; 16(2): 239-51.
[http://dx.doi.org/10.1016/S1473-3099(15)00466-1] [PMID: 26795692]

[142] Mühlen S, Dersch P. Anti-virulence strategies to target bacterial infections. Curr Top Microbiol Immunol 2016; 398: 147-83.
[http://dx.doi.org/10.1007/82_2015_490] [PMID: 26942418]

[143] Waters CM, Bassler BL. Quorum sensing: cell-to-cell communication in bacteria. Annu Rev Cell Dev Biol 2005; 21: 319-46.
[http://dx.doi.org/10.1146/annurev.cellbio.21.012704.131001] [PMID: 16212498]

[144] Atkins KE, Flasche S. Vaccination to reduce antimicrobial resistance. Lancet Glob Health 2018; 6(3): e252.
[http://dx.doi.org/10.1016/S2214-109X(18)30043-3] [PMID: 29433663]

[145] Lipsitch M, Siber GR. How can vaccines contribute to solving the antimicrobial resistance problem? MBio 2016; 7(3): e00428-16.
[http://dx.doi.org/10.1128/mBio.00428-16] [PMID: 27273824]

[146] Sulakvelidze A, Alavidze Z, Morris JG Jr. Bacteriophage therapy. Antimicrob Agents Chemother 2001; 45(3): 649-59.
[http://dx.doi.org/10.1128/AAC.45.3.649-659.2001] [PMID: 11181338]

[147] Lin DM, Koskella B, Lin HC. Phage therapy: An alternative to antibiotics in the age of multi-drug resistance. World J Gastrointest Pharmacol Ther 2017; 8(3): 162-73.
[http://dx.doi.org/10.4292/wjgpt.v8.i3.162] [PMID: 28828194]

[148] Valério N, Oliveira C, Jesus V, *et al.* Effects of single and combined use of bacteriophages and antibiotics to inactivate *Escherichia coli.* Virus Res 2017; 240: 8-17.
[http://dx.doi.org/10.1016/j.virusres.2017.07.015] [PMID: 28746884]

[149] Chaudhry WN, Concepción-Acevedo J, Park T, Andleeb S, Bull JJ, Levin BR. Synergy and order effects of antibiotics and phages in killing *Pseudomonas aeruginosa* biofilms. PLoS One 2017; 12(1): e0168615.
[http://dx.doi.org/10.1371/journal.pone.0168615] [PMID: 28076361]

[150] Ouwehand AC, Forssten S, Hibberd AA, Lyra A, Stahl B. Probiotic approach to prevent antibiotic resistance. Ann Med 2016; 48(4): 246-55.
[http://dx.doi.org/10.3109/07853890.2016.1161232] [PMID: 27092975]

[151] Worthington RJ, Melander C. Combination approaches to combat multidrug-resistant bacteria. Trends Biotechnol 2013; 31(3): 177-84.
[http://dx.doi.org/10.1016/j.tibtech.2012.12.006] [PMID: 23333434]

[152] Meisel K, Rizvi S. Complications of monoclonal antibody therapy. Med Health R I 2011; 94(11): 317-9.
[PMID: 22204093]

[153] Krzyżek P. Challenges and limitations of anti-quorum sensing therapies. Front Microbiol 2019; 10: 2473.
[http://dx.doi.org/10.3389/fmicb.2019.02473] [PMID: 31736912]

[154] Lei J, Sun L, Huang S, *et al.* The antimicrobial peptides and their potential clinical applications. Am J Transl Res 2019; 11(7): 3919-31.
[PMID: 31396309]

[155]   Andrea A, Molchanova N, Jenssen H. Antibiofilm peptides and peptidomimetics with focus on surface immobilization. Biomolecules 2018; 8(2): E27.
[http://dx.doi.org/10.3390/biom8020027] [PMID: 29772735]

[156]   Rondanelli M, Faliva MA, Perna S, Giacosa A, Peroni G, Castellazzi AM. Using probiotics in clinical practice: Where are we now? A review of existing meta-analyses. Gut Microbes 2017; 8(6): 521-43.
[http://dx.doi.org/10.1080/19490976.2017.1345414] [PMID: 28640662]

[157]   Hungin APS, Mitchell CR, Whorwell P, *et al.* Systematic review: probiotics in the management of lower gastrointestinal symptoms - an updated evidence-based international consensus. Aliment Pharmacol Ther 2018; 47(8): 1054-70.
[http://dx.doi.org/10.1111/apt.14539] [PMID: 29460487]

[158]   Buchy P, Ascioglu S, Buisson Y, *et al.* Impact of vaccines on antimicrobial resistance. Int J Infect Dis 2020; 90: 188-96.
[http://dx.doi.org/10.1016/j.ijid.2019.10.005] [PMID: 31622674]

[159]   Petrosillo N, Capone A, Di Bella S, Taglietti F. Management of antibiotic resistance in the intensive care unit setting. Expert Rev Anti Infect Ther 2010; 8(3): 289-302.
[http://dx.doi.org/10.1586/eri.10.7] [PMID: 20192683]

CHAPTER 2

Innovative Drug Delivery Systems for Antimicrobial Agents

Vaishnavi Parikh and **Pardeep Gupta**[*]

Department of Pharmaceutics, University of the Sciences, Philadelphia, USA

Abstract: In the era of superbugs and antimicrobial resistance to conventional antibiotics, there is an urgent need for alternative drug delivery systems to optimize antimicrobial administration. Traditionally, routes of antimicrobial administration include oral, intravenous, intramuscular, intracerebroventricular, aerosol, rectal, and topical methods. However, more innovative drug delivery systems are required for the treatment of antimicrobial resistance at the cellular level. With recent advances, hefty research has been underway, including the use of nanotechnology and antimicrobial peptides in the fight against multi drug-resistant microorganisms (MDROs). Metal and polymer nanoparticles with or without surface functionalization and antimicrobial peptides act through different mechanisms of actions than conventional antibiotics. Some of these mechanisms of actions are included but are not limited to oxidative and non-oxidative stress, binding to the bacterial membrane, altering cell permeability and integrity, and activation of adaptive immune pathways. This chapter encompasses the cause and effect of multidrug resistance in addition to the nanoparticles, antimicrobial peptides, and gene editing techniques as an alternative or combinatorial antimicrobial combat mechanism for the 21st century.

Keywords: AMPs, Antibacterial, Antimicrobial Peptides, Microbial Resistance, Nanoparticles, Non-Oxidative Stress, Oxidative, Stress.

INTRODUCTION

A key challenge in the treatment of microbial infections is antibiotic resistance. Antibiotics are preferred and cost-effective treatment option against the majority of microbial infections. However, increased resistance of microorganisms against one or more antibiotics decreases the chances to cure less dangerous infections that can turn into life-threatening conditions due to the lack of treatment options. With 80% of antibiotics sold in the USA, of which 70% of these are prescribed incorrectly, and up to half of all antibiotics used in humans used incorrectly, it

---

[*] **Corresponding author Pardeep Gupta:** Department of Pharmaceutics, University of the Sciences, Philadelphia, USA; E-mail: p.gupta@usciences.edu

Islam M. Ghazi & Michael J. Cawley (Eds.)

seems obvious why drug resistance is becoming such a prevalent threat [1]. Among infections in the United States including nursing homes and skilled nursing facilities, about 50% of the *Staphylococcus aureus* were methicillin-resistant; 30% of enterococci vancomycin-resistant, 18% of Enterobacteriaceae drug-resistant strains; 4% of Enterobacteriaceae carbapenem-resistant; 16% of *Pseudomonas aeruginosa* and 50% of *Acinetobacter* species were multi-drug resistant [4 - 10]. This small sample of published data and recent data published by the World Health Organization (WHO) [11] classifying pathogens according to species and type of resistance (critical, high and medium) clearly demonstrates the need for the treatment of these multidrug resistant microorganisms. Carbapenem-resistant, *Acinetobacter baumannii*, *Pseudomonas aeruginosa* and ESBL-producing Enterobacteriaceae are in the critical category. Vancomycin resistant enterococcus faecium, (VREF) and methicillin resistant *Staypylococcus aureus* (MRSA), Clarithromycin resistant *Helicobacter pylori*, Fluoroquinolone resistant *Campylobacter spp,* and *Salmonellae* and cephalosporin and fluoroquinolone resistant *Neisseria gonorrhoeae* are in the high category. Penicillin resistant *Streptococcus pneumoniae*, ampicillin resistant *Haemophilus influenza* and fluoroquinolone resistant *Shigella spp.* are in the medium category [11]. An extensive list of microorganisms posing public health concerns around the world requires immediate attention from the biotech and pharmaceutical industry [12].

Mechanism of Microbial Resistance

Intrinsic resistance and acquired resistance are the two types of resistance at the gene level in microorganisms. Spontaneous mutation of existing genes is the cause of intrinsic resistance, whereas the acquisition of resistant genes from other microorganisms through plasmids, transposons, and integrons is the cause of acquired resistance. Acquired resistance is the predominant factor for the emergence of multidrug resistance among the two [13 - 18]. The acquisition of foreign DNA material involves horizontal gene transfer with three main strategies, namely transformation, transduction, and conjugation. Transformation is the direct incorporation of DNA, which is not a major mechanism in clinically relevant bacteria. However, conjugation involving the transfer of mobile genetic elements through cellular contact in the human gastrointestinal tract is the major reason for the emergence of resistance in healthcare facilities [1]. The changes in protein with biochemistry lead to alteration of targets, generation of passivated enzymes, activation of efflux systems, resistance to antibiotic permeation, generation of biofilms, elimination of specific proteins and production of competitive inhibitor for an antibiotic; one or more of which are responsible mechanisms for resistance to antibiotics. For example, Fluoroquinolone resistance can occur through three different biochemical routes, 1) mutations in genes encoding the target site of fluoroquinolone, DNA gyrase, and topoisomerase, 2) protection of the fluoroquinolone target site by a protein designated as Qnr and 3) over-expression of efflux pumps extruding the drug from cells. One or all of these mechanisms may co-exist. In certain bacterial species, one mechanism is predominantly preferred over the other. For example, the production of β-lactamase is the predominant mechanism seen in gram-negative microorganisms whereas modification of penicillin-binding protein site is a predominant mechanism followed by gram-positive bacteria [1].

Antibiotic resistance mechanisms based on the biochemical route involved in resistance can be categorized as follows:

1. Antimicrobial molecule modification.
2. A barrier to the antibiotic target.
3. Change of target sites.
4. Resistance due to global cell adaptive processes.

Antimicrobial Molecule Modification

The most common bacterial strategy against antibiotics is the production of enzymes that can deactivate the antibiotics by chemical alteration or destruction of the molecule.

Acetylation, phosphorylation, and adenylation are the most frequent biochemical reactions catalyzed by these enzymes rendering the antibiotics unable to interact at the target site. Aminoglycosides, chloramphenicol and streptogramins are among the antibiotics affected by acetylation, aminoglycosides and chloramphenicol are affected by phosphorylation and aminoglycosides and lincosamidesa are affected by adenylation. Multiple aminoglycoside modifying enzymes that covalently modify hydroxyl or amino groups such as acetyltransferase, adenyltransferase or phosphotransferase are classified based on the site of modification. Chloramphenicol acetyltransferase is another example of antibiotic alteration. Chloramphenicol is an antibiotic that inhibits protein synthesis by interaction with the peptidyl-transfer center of the 50S ribosomal subunit. Enzyme induced changes to Chloramphenicol leads to two types, high level (Type A) and low level (Type B) resistance [1].

β-lactamase is a class of enzymes responsible for the destruction of the β-lactam class of antibiotics. Penicillin resistant *S. aureus* infection became widely clinically relevant after plasmid-encoded penicillinase was found to be readily disseminated in this *S. aureus* trait. This led to the discovery of less penicillinase-resistant antibiotic, ampicillin and soon after that a new β- lactamase resistant against ampicillin was found among gram-negative bacteria. The development of the newer generation of β-lactam antibiotics has been followed by the rapid appearance of the deactivating enzyme from then on. To date more than 1000 different β-lactamases have been described [1].

A Barrier to the Antibiotic Target

Many antibiotics with intracellular targets or in thecase of gram-negative bacteria, cytoplasmic membrane, the antibacterial compound must penetrate through the outer cell membrane for its effectiveness. Bacteria have developed different mechanisms to decrease permeability and uptake of antibiotics. These include the change in type, level or function of porins; water-filled channels that allow diffusion of hydrophilic antibiotic molecules and increased expression of efflux pump. β-lactams, tetracyclines and fluoroquinolones are affected by the change in porins. An example of a cell wall barrier is the inactivity of Vancomycin against gram-negativee bacteria due to a lack of permeation through the outer membrane. Mutations in the OprD gene in *P.aeruginosa* is a prime example of porin mediated resistance of carbapenem class of antibiotics. Shift in porin expression from OmpK35 to OmpK36 in *K. pneumoniae* after the therapy with β-lactam antimicrobials correlated with h4-8 fold decrease in their susceptibility to these antimicrobial agents [1].

Substrate specific or broad spectrum specific efflux pumps have been characterized in both gram-positivee and gram-negative bacteria. Five major families of efflux pumps include the major facilitator superfamily (MFS), small multidrug resistance family (SMR), resistance nodulation cell division family (RND), ATP- binding cassette family (ABC), and multidrug and toxic compound extrusion family (MATE). This mechanism of resistance affects a wide range of antimicrobial classes, including protein synthesis inhibitors, tetracyclines, fluoroquinones, carbapenems, polymixins and β-lactams [1]. Tet efflux pumps currently described by more than 20 genes found predominantly in grams positive bacteria from the MFS family have been identified, which extrude tetracyclines and doxycyclines using proton exchange. SMR proteins are small proteins found in both gram-positive and gram-negative bacteria efflux drugs by dimerization using proton motive force for cationic portions of substrates [2]. RND pumps are able to confer resistance to multiple drugs, including tetracyclines, chloramphenicol, fluoroquinolones, novobiocin, some β-lactam antimicrobials by functioning as proton antiporter [1]. ABC family pumps are the largest group of cell membrane proteins involved in the efflux of numerous drugs, including macrolides, by utilizing energy produced from the hydrolysis of ATP [3]. MATE family efflux pumps contribute to multidrug resistance through drug/sodium or proton antiporting [1].

Change of Target Sites

Change of target site or modification of the target site is another common strategy evolved by microorganisms against the antibiotics. Displacement and release of tetracycline from the target protein binding site in *Streptococcus Spp.* and *Campylobacter jejuni* is a classic example where the activity of tetracycline is reduced and protein synthesis resumes. Quinolone resistant protein, Qnr, first found in *K. pneumoniae* is another example of the change of target site where gyrase-cleaved DNA-quinolone complex formation which induces cell death by quinolone molecule is decreased. Resistance to rifampicin, oxazolidones and fluoroquinolones be attributed to another mechanism that is the mutation of the target site. Complete replacement of the antibiotic target site to execute biochemical function is also found to be a strategy for antimicrobial resistance. The activity of most β-lactams, including penicillins, cephalosporins and carbapenem in disruption of cell wall synthesis through the enzyme, PBP is found futile in methicillin-resistant *S. Aureus* [1].

Resistance due to Global Cell Adaptive Processes

Bacteria have devised complex sophisticated mechanisms to survive the hostile environment, including various environmental factors and the human body through the years of evolution. Development of resistance to daptomycin (DAP) and vancomycin (low-level in *S. aureus*) is the most clinically relevant examples of resistance phenotypes that are the result of a global cell adaptive response to the antibacterial attack [1].

The insurmountable issue of microbial resistance to antibiotics can be overcome by the combination of new technologies and natural sources. The continuous evolution of microbial resistance pushes pharmaceutical scientists toward continued research to find new treatment options to combat these pathogens where an understanding of microbial resistance and advances in the drug delivery technologies are very important for the development of more effective antimicrobial materials.

Advances in Drug Delivery Systems

Drug delivery is the science of converting active drug molecules into drug products that are therapeutically efficacious and safe for human use. Some of the challenges in drug delivery include improving the solubility of poorly soluble drugs, stabilizing the drug during its shelf life and different physiological conditions of the body, achieving hydrophilic-lipophilic balance such that drug can be solubilized and absorbed through GI tract, avoiding first-pass metabolism and clearance through the reticuloendothelial system (RES), and reaching the site of action through targeted delivery. Several different advances and novel drug delivery techniques have been achieved over the years through pharmaceutical innovations. Some of the examples of evolution in drug delivery systems include the following.

- Preparation of high energy dosage forms, like solid dispersions, self-emulsifying drug delivery systems, size reduction in nano and micro ranges have been extensively used to improve drug solubility,
- Design of different dosage forms other than that for oral route of action to avoid first-pass metabolism,
- Coating with a polymer like polyethylene glycols to reduce clearance through RES,
- Polymer coatings like polymethacrylates to prevent degradation of drugs sensitive to different pH in the gastrointestinal tract and
- Nanoparticle mediated targeted delivery systems to improve efficacy and reduce side effects.

Similarly, the era of 1944-1970 is considered the golden era in the history of antibiotics, primarily due to the discovery of a variety of classes of antibiotics. As the resistance to antibiotics increased, the use of combinatorial techniques in the 1980s introduced some novel synthetic antibiotics, however, from the same classes. With the biotechnological advance in 1990, the research focused heavily in the area of genome sequencing and gene encoding with a poor yield of new antimicrobial agents. Combined approaches involving natural sources and advanced biotechnology in the era of the 2000s added two new classes of antibiotics by 2010 [19]. Recently, several highly effective means of treating microbial resistance have been developed, including nanoparticles, antimicrobial peptides, and new gene-editing technologies.

Nanotechnology and Nanoengineering

With recent advances, the nanomaterial is a strategy that can prove to be successful against MDROs due to unique properties of nanoparticles (NPs) such as at least one dimension of the material in the nano range, high surface area, high drug loading capacity, surface functionalization and targeted delivery of the drug. Several types of NPs are currently used for drug delivery: liposomal [20], solid lipid (SL) [21, 22], polymer-based, polymer micelles, inorganic nanodrug carriers (including magnetic, mesoporous silica, carbon nanomaterials, and quantum dots), terpenoid-based [23] and dendrimer [24]. Both polymer-based nanoparticles and metallic nanoparticles have been researched extensively and have shown to be efficient against microbial resistance. Different forms of nanoengineered drug delivery systems such as nanofibers, nanosheets, nanohybrids, nano-complexes and nanotubes have been extensively evaluated by researchers.

Nanomaterials can be synthesized by several different pathways including physical, chemical and biological. Physical methods include mechanical milling, ultra-sonication, laser ablation, irradiation, evaporation, and condensation. Chemical methods can be divided into chemical etching, sputtering, laser ablation, and thermal decomposition. The biological methods include synthesis using plant, fungi, bacteria, algae, yeast and actinomycetes for nanoparticle preparation.

Mechanism of Antibacterial activity of Nanomaterials

Since nanoparticles do not present the same mechanisms of action of standard antibiotics, they can be of extreme use against multi drug-resistant (MDR) bacteria [23 - 34]. Nanomaterials have been extensively investigated and reviewed by scientists due to their potential to combat multi drug resistance [35 - 37]. Nanoparticles can exert their antibacterial activity *via* a multitude of mechanisms listed below. The mechanism of action of nanomaterials is also shown in Fig. (**1**).

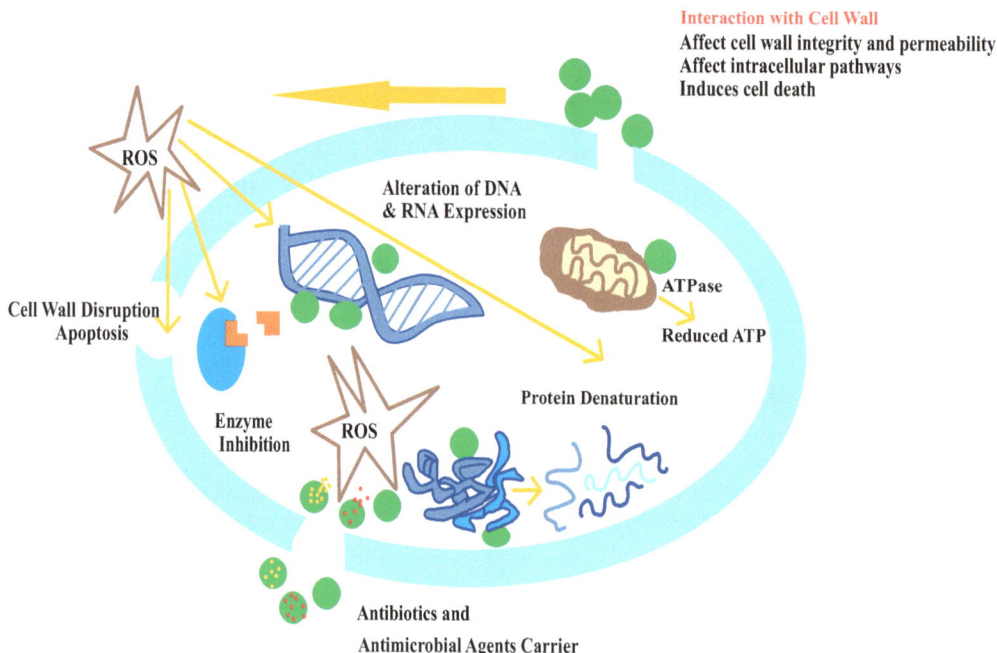

Fig. (1). Mechanism of action of Nanomaterials

exhibits different antimicrobial mechanisms of nanoparticles through Fig. (**1**) direct cell wall disruption through change in permeability and/or 2 induction of intracellular pathways like alteration of DNA and RNA expression, enzyme inhibition and interference with protein functions due to generation of ROS, and transport of antimicrobial agents to enhance their effects

Direct Interaction with the Bacterial Cell Wall

The function of the cell wall is to provide the protection and the shape to the bacterium. Nanoparticles have demonstrated disruption of respiration, one of the major functions of the cell wall [25 - 27]. Nanoparticles can interact with the cell wall through different mechanisms such as electrostatic forces, van der waal's forces, hydrophobic forces and receptor-ligand forces [28 - 31]. Moreover, nanoparticles increase the bacterial cell volume, because honeycomb changes in the cell membrane, and causes cytoplasmic leakage [13]. The nanoparticles thus affect the cell permeability and integrity and also induce the intracellular pathways leading to cell death. The interaction of nanoparticles with microbes depends on the surface of each of them. It is reported that nanoparticles are more effective against gram-positive bacteria in comparison to gram-negative bacteria. This can be attributed to peptide glycan cell wall structure for gram-positive bacteria which is easily permeable in comparison to the lipoprotein structure of the gram-negative bacteria cell wall [13, 32]. Catechin-Cu nanoparticles showing an inhibitory effect on the growth of *E.Coli* and *S.Aureus* is one of the examples of nanoparticles in this category. Catechin- Cu nanoparticles being positively charged, allows direct interaction between the particles and the negatively charged bacteria membranes. In addition, *S. aureus*, a strain representing Gram-positive bacteria, exhibited a lower survival rate in comparison to the *E. coli* strain and was hence lower resistant to the antibacterial effect of the Catechin- Cu nanoparticles [28].

Inhibition of Biofilm Formation

Biofilms are aggregates of one or more species of microbes that rely on the solid surface and extracellular products [33]. Mature biofilms due to rapid multiplication of bacteria form a barrier against antibiotics causing chronic infections. Small size and higher mass to volume ratio of nanoparticles yield a greater interaction with the cell wall rendering destruction of biofilms. Phosphatidylcholine-decorated Au nanoparticles loaded with gentamicin proved to be effective against established biofilms and inhibited biofilm formation of pathogens, including Gram-positive and Gram-negative bacteria [34]. Phosphatidylcholine-decorated Au nanoparticles loaded with gentamicin (GPA NPs) in size range of 180 nm have shown an ability to damage established biofilms and inhibit biofilm formation several bacterial strains. This study presented that GPA NPs inhibited biofilm formation of planktonic *P. aeruginosa, S. aureus, E.Coli,* and *L. monocytogenes* [33]. The coating of silver nanoparticles has also been used on the surface of medical devices to prevent bacterial adhesion and subsequent biofilm formation. Polymeric nanocontainers based on hyperbranched polylysine (HPL), hydrophobically modified by using either glycidylhexadecyl ether or a mixture of stearoyl/palmitoyl chloride, highly stabilized silver nanoparticles in the range of 2-5 nm, Poly (glycolic acid)-based surgical sutures dip-coated with the two different polymeric silver nanocomposites have been used and found to increase efficiency in reduction of bacterial adhesion and biofilm formation [29]. Coatings with combinations of antibiotics and antiseptics like minocycline and rifampin or chlorhexidine and silver-sulfadiazine have been applied to the internal and external surface of catheters. In several studies, these antimicrobial-coated catheters were compared to noncoated catheters, and a reduction of catheter colonization and catheter-related bloodstream infections was found [29].

Trigger Innate as Well as Adaptive Host Immune Responses

Nanoparticles can interact with the innate immune systems through the complement system and mononuclear phagocyte system against microorganisms. Nanoparticles can also be used to deliver antigens as vaccines as part of the adaptive immune system to boost the immunogenicity. It has been reported that conjugation of antigens to nanoparticle surfaces facilitated B-cell activation, due to a higher quantity of antigens that were delivered to antigen-presenting cells (APCs) [30].

Generate Reactive Oxygen Species (ROS)

Reactive oxygen species (O_2), (OH), (H_2O_2), and O_2 from metal ion nanoparticles induce oxidative stress on the bacterial cell wall resulting in changes to cell permeability and lead to bacterial cell membranes damage [13]. Increased gene expression of the oxidative proteins responsible for cell apoptosis and depression of activity of certain periplasmic enzymes essential for maintaining the normal morphology and physiological processes in the bacterial cell are also other mechanisms activated by ROS [34, 38].

Induction of Intracellular Effects

Nanoparticle interactions with cell walls of microorganisms lead to significant alteration of the expression of key proteins and DNA. One study showed that, after entering cells, CuO NPs caused the regulation of proteins involved in nitrogen metabolism, electron transfer, and substance transport. Yamanaka *et al.*

[39] studied the bactericidal action of Ag NPs against *E. coli*, serving as a model microorganism, *via* energy-filtering TEM (EFTEM), two-dimensional electrophoresis (2-DE), and matrix-assisted laser desorption ionization time-of- flight MS (MALDI-TOF MS). The results indicated that the expression of a ribosomal subunit protein, as well as that of certain other enzymes and proteins, is affected by silver ions [40] Similarly; Cui *et al.* [41] examined the antibacterial mechanism of action of Au NPs *via* transcriptomic and proteomic methods. The authors found that Au NPs exert antibacterial activity predominantly in two manners: prevention of joining of a ribosomal subunit with tRNA and collapse of the membrane potential (restraining ATPase activities to reduce the ATP level). TiO_2 NPs allow bacterial DNA compression, degeneration, and fragmentation, thereby reducing the physiological activity of genes [13, 42]. The affinity and binding mode of nano-titanium dioxide and DNA were predicted by molecular docking, which indicated that TiO_2 NPs targeted DNA rich in G–C [13, 43]. In addition, whole-genome analysis can be used to characterize the molecular mechanisms of bacterial apoptosis. Researchers used this technique to analyze the mechanism of NP action against *E. coli* In this study, researchers found the differences in the mechanism of cytotoxicity by zinc oxide (ZnO) nanoparticles and zinc chloride ($ZnCl_2$). The results further indicated that ZnO likely causes the toxicity to *E. coli* through several specific functional gene products synthesis processing, such as translation, gene expression, RNA modification, and structural constituent o ribosome [44].

As a Carrier for Antimicrobial Agents

Achieving the delivery of antimicrobial agents directly intracellularly due to enhanced permeation and retention is greatly helpful in combating pathogens while reducing side effects or toxicity of these antimicrobial agents on other organs. For example, vancomycin-modified mesoporous silica NPs were designed, which made it possible to detect and kill pathogenic gram-positive bacteria selectively over macrophage-like cells, thereby reducing toxicity to ear and kidneys [13, 45]. Nanoparticles can be used as a carrier for antimicrobial agents through several different properties. For example, the small size of nanoparticles can allow intracellular uptake of antimicrobial agents where the average size of these drug molecules are impermeable to intracellular infections. Nanoparticles allow encapsulation of antibiotics, thereby prevent degradation, increase serum concentration, controlled release, and targeted delivery of antimicrobial agents. Both active and passive targeted deliveries have been utilized to provide the protection against systemic side effects or toxicity associated with the higher dose of these antibiotics [46]. Nanoparticle carriers can tackle bacterial threats "passively," through prolonged drug retention at the specific infection site, or "actively," through surface conjugation with active molecules that bind a certain target [46, 47]. A combination of antibiotics in a single type of nanoparticles or a combination of different nanoparticles with the different antimicrobial agents can be used to obtain synergistic effects of these drugs [46]. Data has shown that the combination of gentamicin and chloramphenicol with AgNPs has a better antibacterial effect in multi drug resistant *E. faecalis* than both antibiotics alone [48]. In addition, investigations suggested that nanomaterials used as a drug delivery device in biomedical implants have proven highly effective. TiO_2 nanotubes (TNTs) loaded with antibacterial drugs have shown promising results when used in biomedical implants to control infections due to its properties such as surface roughness, wettability, cellular interaction, drug loading capacity and chemical-physical structure [37].

The multiple simultaneous mechanisms of action against microbes would require multiple simultaneous gene mutations in the same bacterial cell for antibacterial resistance to develop; therefore, it is difficult for bacterial cells to become resistant to nanoparticles [4].

Applications of Nanomaterials

Although nanoparticle-based therapy is an expensive option, it can prove to be beneficial in serious infections where conventional medication fails to improve patient outcomes.

AgNPs are considered the most effective nanomaterial against bacteria but other metallic NPs, such as CuONPs, TiONPs, AuNPs, Fe_3O_2NPs, metal oxides like ZnO, CuO and bimetallic NPs have also demonstrated bactericidal effects [26, 30, 38]. Researches have synthesized AuNPs with bacterial exopolysaccharide (EPS) and functionalized them with antibiotics (levofloxacin, cefotaxime, ceftriaxone, and ciprofloxacin) and demonstrated bactericidal activity against MDR gram-positive and -negative bacteria compared to free drugs with *E. coli* being most susceptible MDR bacteria followed by *K. pneumoniae* and *S. aureus* [45]. Green metallic nanoparticles from various plant sources have also been developed with antibacterial activities. Ag nanoparticles from a variety of sources including extracts from *Phyllanthus amarus*, *isora* fruit, *Artemisia cappilaris*, *aloe vera*, *Acalypha indica* leaves; Au nanoparticles from *Citrullus lanatus* rind; Ag-Au bimetallic nanoparticles from *Plumbago zeylanica*; Ni Nanoparticles from *Ocimum sanctum* leaves, Al_2O_3 nanoparticles from *lemongrass* leaves, Pd nanoparticles from agroforest waste *Moringa oleifera*, Selenium metal nanoparticles from *Bacillus licheniformis*, green synthesized α-Fe_2O_3 nanoparticles from the *Sida cordifolia* plant extract are some of the examples of the green nanoparticles [49, 50].

Apart from metallic nanoparticles, antimicrobial agents are also engineered in the form of nanohybrids, nanoplexes, *etc.* These are hybrids or composites of antibiotics and or other antimicrobial agents complexed with nanoparticles. Different technologies such as hydrophilic-lipophilic liposomes preparation, emulsification and self-emulsifying complexes are used to prepare such materials in the nano-range. For example, ampicillin loaded onto silica covered silver nanoparticles produced a nanohybrid that was potent against ampicillin-resistant *E.Coli* and remained nontoxic towards human cells [51]. Bilayer nano-complexes of oligonucleotide such as transcription factor decoys (TFDs) is demonstrated as another novel mechanism against microbial resistance. TFDs are oligonucleotide copies of the DNA-binding site for transcription factors which competitively inhibit transcription of essential genes when transfected into bacterial cytoplasm. The potential of TFDs against several diseases is evident from the act that single TFD blocks the synthesis of thousands of copies of mRNA [52]. It was also noted that Graphene nanosheets led to bacterial inactivation by the extraction of phospholipid molecules from the cell membrane [13].

PLGA, chitosan, gelatin, polyester adsorbed PEG and several polyalkyl cyano and methyl acrylates are the types of polymers that have been used to prepare nanoparticles. Advantage includes enhanced delivery and significantly higher expression level, improved drug retention, longer systemic drug effect due to reduced RES uptake and improved absorption and permeation. Polymeric nanoparticles are designed to deliver hydrophilic and hydrophobic drug molecules as well as macromolecules such as proteins, peptides, and nucleic acids.

Antimicrobial Peptides (AMP)

Antimicrobial peptides have direct and indirect antimicrobial activity against gram-positive and gram-negative bacteria, fungi, and viruses and are promising next-generation antibiotics that hold great potential for combating MDROs. Antimicrobial peptides are small amphipathic peptides (29 to 42 amino acids) that are cationic (positively charged) in nature [53 - 55]. Insects and plants primarily deploy AMPs as an antibiotic to protect against potential pathogenic microbes, but microbes also produce AMPs to defend their environmental niche. These AMPs produced by microbes should also be considered as antimicrobial agents. Cationic peptides polymyxin B (produced by *Bacillus polymyxa*) and the noncationic glycopeptide vancomycin (produced by *Amycolatopsis orientalis*) include the prominent examples of microbial AMPs that are approved by FDA as antibiotics against, respectively; major multidrug-resistant organisms including *Pseudomonas aeruginosa*, *Acinetobacter baumannii* and *Klebsiella pneumoniae*, MRSA infections. In higher eukaryotic organisms, AMPs can also be referred to as 'host defense peptides', emphasizing their additional immunomodulatory activities. These activities are diverse, specific to the type of AMP, and include a variety of cytokine and growth factor-like effects that are relevant to normal immune homeostasis. In some instances, the inappropriate expression of AMPs can also induce autoimmune diseases, thus further highlighting the importance of understanding these molecules and their complex activities [56].

AMPs typically consist of 10-50 amino acid residues, bear overall positive charge and contain a three-dimensional alignment of amino acid and hydrophobic residues such that structures are uniquely water-soluble [56]. AMPs are found in alpha-helix, beta-sheet and extended structural configurations; *e.g.*, human cathelicidin peptide LL37, bactenecins, defensins, histatin and indolicidin, respectively. AMPs have since been extensively characterized and discovered in virtually all multicellular organisms that have been studied for this activity. Presently, more than 2,500 AMPs have been deposited in the Antimicrobial Peptide Database. It is likely that this list represents only a small fraction of gene-encoded antibiotic proteins produced in nature [57].

Mechanism of Antibacterial activity of Antimicrobial Peptides

Interaction of AMPs with the surface of microorganisms leads to antimicrobial action through a variety of mechanisms as described below [56] and shown in Fig. (2) exhibits mechanism of action of antimicrobial peptides such as electrostatic interactions to change cell wall permeability through pore formation, peptide insertion through membrane, enzymatic disruption of cell membrane; and modulation of immune system.

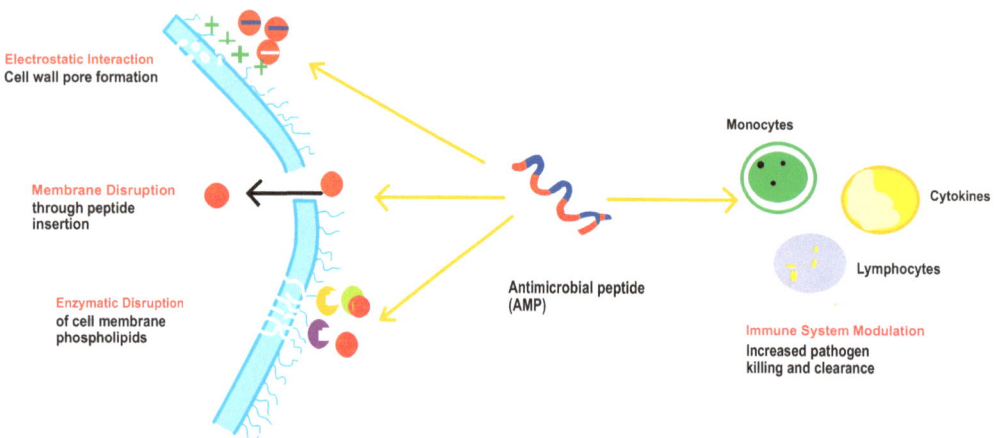

Fig. (2). Mechanism of action of Antimicrobial Peptides.

Bacterial Membrane Disruption through Pore Formation

Cationic surface charge and high ratio of hydrophobic amino acids allow AMPs to bind to negatively charged bacterial membranes through electrostatic interactions. These interactions can lead to non-enzymatic effects like the formation of pores in the bacterial membrane that destroy membrane integrity, promoting lysis of the targeted microbes. This mechanism can be seen with defensins.

Membrane Disruption through the Insertion of Peptide

Some AMPs bind with the bacterial membrane through electrostatic interactions and lead to peptide insertion followed by disruption of the membrane. The human cathelicidin peptide is shown to be effective with this mechanism.

Membrane Disruption through Enzymatic Digestion

Enzymatic digestion mediated membrane disruptions is also one of the cases of the mechanism for the effectiveness of AMPs against microorganisms. Lysozyme induced hydrolysis of the beta-glycosidic linkage between N-acetylmuramic acid and N-acetyl glucosamine in the peptidoglycan of bacterial cell walls, and phospholipase A2 (PLA2) secreted from human platelets induced hydrolysis of bacterial membrane phospholipids causing cell death are the examples of enzymatic disruptions.

Inhibition of Intracellular Functions

Some peptides have also been able to cross the lipid bilayer without causing any damage, but kill bacteria by inhibiting intracellular functions, such as blocking enzyme activity or inhibiting protein and nucleic acid synthesis including AMPs' ability to disrupt the biofilm or inhibit the biofilm formation.

In addition to the antimicrobial activity, AMPs also act as immunomodulators. This involves the protection of the host by AMPs through a range of mechanisms: chemotactic activity, attracting leukocytes; modulation of host-cell responsiveness to TLR ligands; stimulation of angiogenesis; enhancement of leukocyte/monocyte activation and differentiation; and modulation of the expression of proinflammatory cytokines/chemokines [56]. While some AMPs promote host defense by modulating host cellular immunity, overproduction of AMPs can also generate inflammatory diseases such as psoriasis and rosacea. Although several limitations remain, overuse of conventional antibiotics has stimulated interest in the development of AMPs as the next generation anti-infectives and as methods to more selectively combat pathogens; though mechanistic understanding of the expression of these AMPs. Control of endogenous AMP production may represent the next major archetype for the treatment of various infections as an alternative to antibiotics [56].

Nanotechnology plays a major role in dosage form preparation for AMPs. Passive nanoparticles and active nanoparticles with surface functionalization have been used. Cyclosporine loaded Chitosan and Polylactic-co-glycolide-co-caprolactone nanoparticles, Nisin loaded liposomes, polycaprolactone nanoparticles, polyvinylalcohol nanofibers, Vancomycin loaded PLGA nanoparticles, polycaprolactone microparticles, PLGA microparticles and nanofibers, and solid lipid nanoparticles, Polymixin loaded solid lipid nanoparticles and other synthetic peptide-loaded polymer nanoparticles are among nanoparticle-based AMPs [58].

Gene Editing Technologies

In addition to nanoengineered drug delivery systems and antimicrobial peptides, targeting SOS response which is the bacterial response to DNA damage and gene transfer can also be potential therapeutic options. Antibiotic resistance is acquired in response to antibiotic therapy by activation of SOS-mediated DNA repair, mutagenesis and horizontal gene transfer pathways. SOS response inhibitors can be the key to potentiate the activity of antibiotics from different classes including B-lactams, aminoglycosides and fluoroquinolones. Phthalocyanine tetrasulfonic acid is one for the example of SOS response blocker [59]. Construction of recombinant bacteriophage –derived enzymes such as endolysins and other peptidoglycan hydrolases, and their conjugation to nanoparticles is also an emerging novel delivery strategy. These lytic enzymes represent a potential alternative to conventional therapies by providing a high degree of host specificity. For example Lysk is one of the best characterized endolysin against multiple *staphylococcal* species [60].

The latest technology that researchers are exploring for antimicrobial resistance is the genome editing to be able to change the organism's DNA. Specifically, clustered regularly interspaced short palindromic repeats (CRISPR) and protein 9 associated with it (Cas9) have generated a lot of excitement among the scientific community. In this technology, a small piece of RNA with a defined sequence is used to alter the genome of microorganisms and disable their antimicrobial-resistant genes. Three types of CRISPR-Cas9 systems include type I cleave and degrade DNA, type II cleave DNA and type III, cleave DNA and RNA. Reprogramming the microbial genome to eradicate the resistant strains through CRISPR- Cas9 shows a possible method to aid in the treatment of MDROs [61, 62]. Some of the examples of research studies conducted include the delivery of phagemids encoded spacers to *S. Aureus* to target antibiotic-resistant genes, conjugative plasmid carried by *E.coli* to target host organisms and target the sequence responsible for resistance in extended-spectrum β-lactamase producing *E.Coli.* The goal of this research was to restore the sensitivity of antibiotics in these bacteria [61, 63 - 65]. Although some results have proven more efficient than antibiotics, there are some limitations to this technology. The challenges include delivery *invivo*, large size and negative charge of plasmids, permeability through the membranes and low serum levels. Additionally, the low delivery efficiency of non-viral vector and the production of vectors at large scale also present great challenges. Although CRISPR currently has limitations, it shows a great potential to remove the resistant genes from microorganisms [61].

SUMMARY

Antimicrobial resistance is the phenomenon adapted by microorganisms to survive against antibiotics. Microbial resistance to one or more antibiotics despite advances in modern medicines threatens our ability to treat common infectious diseases. This endangers effective antimicrobial treatment in several therapies and surgical procedures for example, organ replacement and transplantation, c-sections, and increase the overall health care cost in addition to a global threat. Therefore understanding the mechanisms of microbial resistance against conventional antibiotics and its utilization for the development of next-generation antimicrobial agents is the pressing need. Apart from recently emerging gene-editing techniques that require further research, the use of nanotechnology and novel hybrids with conventional antibiotics and antimicrobial peptides emerges as the promising path forward in our fight against microbial resistance. In addition, the association of the new drug delivery systems discussed in this chapter can prove to be efficient in controlling MDR. *E.g.* nanosystems can be designed to facilitate the delivery of CRISPRs. As the resistance to current antibiotics increases and there is a lack of research in the area of developing new antibiotics, the drug delivery systems discussed in this chapter can prove to be efficient in treating infections against MDR organisms.

Although there is a plethora of *in vitro* evidence for the efficacy of nanomaterials and these new technologies, research in the area of safety, toxicity and *in vivo* efficacy are much needed to obtain meaningful commercial applications approved by drug regulatory authorities. Therefore as targeted synergistic modifications to drug delivery approaches are gaining traction, more research, development, and evaluation, worldwide, is required to prove the much needed scientific breakthroughs in disease control.

CONSENT FOR PUBLICATION

Not applicable.

CONFLICT OF INTEREST

The authors confirm that the contents of this chapter have no conflict of interest.

ACKNOWLEDGEMENTS

Declared none.

REFERENCES

[1]   Munita JM, Arias CA. Mechanisms of Antibiotic Resistance. Microbiol Spectr 2016; 4(2).
        [http://dx.doi.org/10.1128/microbiolspec.VMBF-0016-2015] [PMID: 27227291]

[2]   Mohammad IS, He W, Yin L. Understanding of human ATP binding cassette superfamily and novel
        multidrug resistance modulators to overcome MDR. Biomed Pharmacother 2018; 100: 335-48.
        [http://dx.doi.org/10.1016/j.biopha.2018.02.038] [PMID: 29453043]

[3]   Poulsen BE, Deber CM. Drug efflux by a small multidrug resistance protein is inhibited by a
        transmembrane peptide. Antimicrob Agents Chemother 2012; 56(7): 3911-6.
        [http://dx.doi.org/10.1128/AAC.00158-12] [PMID: 22526304]

[4]   Scutti S. CDC Reports 1 in 7 Hospital-Acquired Infections Now Caused By Antibiotic-Resistant Super
        Bugs: Medical Daily. 2016. Available from: https://www.medicaldaily.com/cdc-hospital-acquir-
        d-infections-super-bugs-antibiotics-376410

[5]   Fisch J, Lansing B, Wang L, *et al.* New acquisition of antibiotic-resistant organisms in skilled nursing
        facilities. J Clin Microbiol 2012; 50(5): 1698-703.
        [http://dx.doi.org/10.1128/JCM.06469-11] [PMID: 22378900]

[6]   McKinnell JA, Miller LG, Singh R, *et al.* Prevalence of and factors associated with multidrug resistant
        organism (MDRO) colonization in 3 nursing homes. Infect Control Hosp Epidemiol 2016; 37(12):
        1485-8.
        [http://dx.doi.org/10.1017/ice.2016.215] [PMID: 27671022]

[7]   Crnich CJ, Duster M, Hess T, Zimmerman DR, Drinka P. Antibiotic resistance in non-major
        metropolitan skilled nursing facilities: prevalence and interfacility variation. Infect Control Hosp
        Epidemiol 2012; 33(11): 1172-4.
        [http://dx.doi.org/10.1086/668018] [PMID: 23041821]

[8]   Maslow JN, Lee B, Lautenbach E. Fluoroquinolone-resistant *Escherichia coli* carriage in long-term
        care facility. Emerg Infect Dis 2005; 11(6): 889-94.
        [http://dx.doi.org/10.3201/eid1106.041335] [PMID: 15963284]

[9]   Viray M, Linkin D, Maslow JN, *et al.* Longitudinal trends in antimicrobial susceptibilities across long-
        term-care facilities: emergence of fluoroquinolone resistance. Infect Control Hosp Epidemiol 2005;
        26(1): 56-62.
        [http://dx.doi.org/10.1086/502487] [PMID: 15693409]

[10]   Braykov NP, Eber MR, Klein EY, Morgan DJ, Laxminarayan R. Trends in resistance to carbapenems
        and third-generation cephalosporins among clinical isolates of *Klebsiella pneumoniae* in the United
        States, 1999-2010. Infect Control Hosp Epidemiol 2013; 34(3): 259-68.
        [http://dx.doi.org/10.1086/669523] [PMID: 23388360]

[11]   WHO publishes list of bacteria for which new antibiotics are urgently needed [press release]. 02-2-
        -2017

[12]   Pradeepa, Vidya SM, Mutalik S, Udaya Bhat K, Huilgol P, Avadhani K. Preparation of Gold
        Nanoparticles by Novel Bacterial Exopolysaccharide for Antibiotic Delivery. Life Sci 2016; 153: 171-
        9.
        [http://dx.doi.org/10.1016/j.lfs.2016.04.022]

[13]   Wang L, Hu C, Shao L. The antimicrobial activity of nanoparticles: present situation and prospects for the future. Int J Nanomed 2017; 12: 1227-49.
[http://dx.doi.org/10.2147/IJN.S121956] [PMID: 28243086]

[14]   Aung MS, Zi H, Nwe KM, *et al.* Drug resistance and genetic characteristics of clinical isolates of staphylococci in Myanmar: high prevalence of PVL among methicillin-susceptible *Staphylococcus aureus* belonging to various sequence types. New Microbes New Infect 2016; 10: 58-65.
[http://dx.doi.org/10.1016/j.nmni.2015.12.007] [PMID: 27257489]

[15]   Coetzee J, Corcoran C, Prentice E, *et al.* Emergence of plasmid-mediated colistin resistance (MCR-1) among *Escherichia coli* isolated from South African patients. S Afr Med J 2016; 106(5): 35-6.
[http://dx.doi.org/10.7196/SAMJ.2016.v106i5.10710] [PMID: 27138657]

[16]   Liu Y-Y, Wang Y, Walsh TR, *et al.* Emergence of plasmid-mediated colistin resistance mechanism MCR-1 in animals and human beings in China: a microbiological and molecular biological study. Lancet Infect Dis 2016; 16(2): 161-8.
[http://dx.doi.org/10.1016/S1473-3099(15)00424-7] [PMID: 26603172]

[17]   Tsutsui M, Kawakubo H, Hayashida T, *et al.* Comprehensive screening of genes resistant to an anticancer drug in esophageal squamous cell carcinoma. Int J Oncol 2015; 47(3): 867-74.
[http://dx.doi.org/10.3892/ijo.2015.3085] [PMID: 26202837]

[18]   Mehdipour Moghaddam MJ, Mirbagheri AA, Salehi Z, Habibzade SM. Prevalence of class 1 integrons and extended spectrum beta lactamases among multi-drug resistant*Escherichia coli* isolates from North of Iran. Iran Biomed J 2015; 19(4): 233-9.
[PMID: 26220727]

[19]   Mavu D, Nowaseb S, Haakuria V, Kibuule D. A Review of Rise of Modern Pharmaceutical Biotechnology in Antibiotic Drug Discovery and Development from Natural Sources and Future Implications. 15th Asia-Pacific Biotechnology Congress. July 20-22, 2017; Melbourne, Australia. 2017.

[20]   Daeihamed M, Dadashzadeh S, Haeri A, Akhlaghi MF. Potential of liposomes for enhancement of oral drug absorption. Curr Drug Deliv 2017; 14(2): 289-303.
[PMID: 26768542]

[21]   Naseri N, Valizadeh H, Zakeri-Milani P. Solid lipid nanoparticles and nanostructured lipid carriers: structure, preparation and application. Adv Pharm Bull 2015; 5(3): 305-13.
[http://dx.doi.org/10.15171/apb.2015.043] [PMID: 26504751]

[22]   Thukral DK, Dumoga S, Mishra AK. Solid lipid nanoparticles: promising therapeutic nanocarriers for drug delivery. Curr Drug Deliv 2014; 11(6): 771-91.
[http://dx.doi.org/10.2174/156720181106141202122335] [PMID: 25469779]

[23]   Abed N, Couvreur P. Nanocarriers for antibiotics: a promising solution to treat intracellular bacterial infections. Int J Antimicrob Agents 2014; 43(6): 485-96.
[http://dx.doi.org/10.1016/j.ijantimicag.2014.02.009] [PMID: 24721232]

[24]   Liu Y, Tee JK, Chiu GN. Dendrimers in oral drug delivery application: current explorations, toxicity issues and strategies for improvement. Curr Pharm Des 2015; 21(19): 2629-42.
[http://dx.doi.org/10.2174/1381612821666150416102058] [PMID: 25876918]

[25]   Erdem A, Metzler D, Cha DK, Huang CP. The short-term toxic effects of TiO_2nanoparticles toward bacteria through viability, cellular respiration, and lipid peroxidation. Environ Sci Pollut Res Int 2015; 22(22): 17917-24.
[http://dx.doi.org/10.1007/s11356-015-5018-1] [PMID: 26165996]

[26]   Sondi I, Salopek-Sondi B. Silver nanoparticles as antimicrobial agent: a case study on *E. coli* as a model for Gram-negative bacteria. J Colloid Interface Sci 2004; 275(1): 177-82.
[http://dx.doi.org/10.1016/j.jcis.2004.02.012] [PMID: 15158396]

[27]   Nataraj N, Anjusree GS, Madhavan AA, *et al.* Synthesis and anti-staphylococcal activity of TiO2

nanoparticles and nanowires in *ex vivo* porcine skin model. J Biomed Nanotechnol 2014; 10(5): 864-70.
[http://dx.doi.org/10.1166/jbn.2014.1756] [PMID: 24734539]

[28] Li H, Chen Q, Zhao J, Urmila K. Enhancing the antimicrobial activity of natural extraction using the synthetic ultrasmall metal nanoparticles. Sci Rep 2015; 5(1): 11033.
[http://dx.doi.org/10.1038/srep11033] [PMID: 26046938]

[29] Armentano I, Arciola CR, Fortunati E, *et al.* The Interaction of Bacteria with Engineered Nanostructured Polymeric Materials: A Review. Article, ID: The Scientific World Journal 2014; p. 410423.

[30] Gao W, Thamphiwatana S, Angsantikul P, Zhang L. Nanoparticle approaches against bacterial infections. Wiley Interdiscip Rev Nanomed Nanobiotechnol 2014; 6(6): 532-47.
[http://dx.doi.org/10.1002/wnan.1282] [PMID: 25044325]

[31] Luan B, Huynh T, Zhou R. Complete wetting of graphene by biological lipids. Nanoscale 2016; 8(10): 5750-4.
[http://dx.doi.org/10.1039/C6NR00202A] [PMID: 26910517]

[32] Noinaj N, Kuszak AJ, Gumbart JC, *et al.* Structural insight into the biogenesis of β-barrel membrane proteins. Nature 2013; 501(7467): 385-90.
[http://dx.doi.org/10.1038/nature12521] [PMID: 23995689]

[33] Mu H, Tang J, Liu Q, Sun C, Wang T, Duan J. Potent antibacterial nanoparticles against biofilm and intracellular bacteria. Sci Rep 2016; 6(1): 18877.
[http://dx.doi.org/10.1038/srep18877] [PMID: 26728712]

[34] Wu B, Zhuang W-Q, Sahu M, Biswas P, Tang YJ. Cu-doped TiO(2) nanoparticles enhance survival of Shewanella oneidensis MR-1 under ultraviolet light (UV) exposure. Sci Total Environ 2011; 409(21): 4635-9.
[http://dx.doi.org/10.1016/j.scitotenv.2011.07.037] [PMID: 21855961]

[35] Masri A, Anwar A, Khan NA, Siddiqui R. The use of nanomedicine for targeted therapy against bacterial infections. Antibiotics (Basel) 2019; 8(4): 260.
[http://dx.doi.org/10.3390/antibiotics8040260] [PMID: 31835647]

[36] Ruddaraju LK, Pammi SVN, Guntuku Gs, Padavala VS, Kolapalli VRM. A review on anti-bacterials to combat resistance from ancient era of plants and metals to present and future perspectives of green nano technological combinations. Asian J Pharm Sci 2019; 15(1): 42-59.

[37] Kunrath MF, Leal BF, Hubler R, de Oliveira SD, Teixeira ER. Antibacterial potential associated with drug-delivery built TiO$_2$ nanotubes in biomedical implants. AMB Express 2019; 9(1): 51.
[http://dx.doi.org/10.1186/s13568-019-0777-6] [PMID: 30993485]

[38] Padmavathy N, Vijayaraghavan R. Interaction of ZnO nanoparticles with microbes-a physio and biochemical assay. J Biomed Nanotechnol 2011; 7(6): 813-22.
[http://dx.doi.org/10.1166/jbn.2011.1343] [PMID: 22416581]

[39] Yamanaka M, Hara K, Kudo J. Bactericidal actions of a silver ion solution on *Escherichia coli*, studied by energy-filtering transmission electron microscopy and proteomic analysis. Appl Environ Microbiol 2005; 71(11): 7589-93.
[http://dx.doi.org/10.1128/AEM.71.11.7589-7593.2005] [PMID: 16269810]

[40] Shrivastava S, Bera T, Roy A, Singh G, Ramachandrarao P, Dash D. Characterization of enhanced antibacterial effects of novel silver nanoparticles. Nanotechnology 2007; 18(22): 225103.
[http://dx.doi.org/10.1088/0957-4484/18/22/225103]

[41] Cui Y, Zhao Y, Tian Y, Zhang W, Lü X, Jiang X. The molecular mechanism of action of bactericidal gold nanoparticles on *Escherichia coli*. Biomaterials 2012; 33(7): 2327-33.
[http://dx.doi.org/10.1016/j.biomaterials.2011.11.057] [PMID: 22182745]

[42] Zhukova LV. Evidence for Compression of *Escherichia coli* K12 Cells under the Effect of TiO$_2$

Nanoparticles. ACS Appl Mater Interfaces 2015; 7(49): 27197-205.
[http://dx.doi.org/10.1021/acsami.5b08042] [PMID: 26584239]

[43]	Iram NE, Khan MS, Jolly R, *et al.* Interaction mode of polycarbazole-titanium dioxide nanocomposite with DNA: Molecular docking simulation and *in-vitro* antimicrobial study. J Photochem Photobiol B 2015; 153: 20-32.
[http://dx.doi.org/10.1016/j.jphotobiol.2015.09.001] [PMID: 26386641]

[44]	Su G, Zhang X, Giesy JP, *et al.* Comparison on the molecular response profiles between nano zinc oxide (ZnO) particles and free zinc ion using a genome-wide toxicogenomics approach. Environ Sci Pollut Res Int 2015; 22(22): 17434-42.
[http://dx.doi.org/10.1007/s11356-015-4507-6] [PMID: 25940466]

[45]	Qi G, Li L, Yu F, Wang H. Vancomycin-modified mesoporous silica nanoparticles for selective recognition and killing of pathogenic gram-positive bacteria over macrophage-like cells. ACS Appl Mater Interfaces 2013; 5(21): 10874-81.
[http://dx.doi.org/10.1021/am403940d] [PMID: 24131516]

[46]	Baptista PV, McCusker MP, Carvalho A, *et al.* Nano-strategies to fight multidrug resistant bacteria-"a battle of the titans". Front Microbiol 2018; 9(1441): 1441.
[http://dx.doi.org/10.3389/fmicb.2018.01441] [PMID: 30013539]

[47]	Wang Z, Dong K, Liu Z, *et al.* Activation of biologically relevant levels of reactive oxygen species by Au/g-C$_3$N$_4$ hybrid nanozyme for bacteria killing and wound disinfection. Biomaterials 2017; 113: 145-57.
[http://dx.doi.org/10.1016/j.biomaterials.2016.10.041] [PMID: 27815998]

[48]	Katva S, Das S, Moti HS, Jyoti A, Kaushik S. Antibacterial synergy of silver nanoparticles with gentamicin and chloramphenicol against *Enterococcus faecalis.* Pharmacogn Mag 2018; 13 (Suppl. 4): S828-33.
[PMID: 29491640]

[49]	Hemeg HA. Nanomaterials for alternative antibacterial therapy. Int J Nanomed 2017; 12: 8211-25.
[http://dx.doi.org/10.2147/IJN.S132163] [PMID: 29184409]

[50]	Pallela PNVK, Ummey S, Ruddaraju LK, *et al.* Antibacterial efficacy of green synthesized α-Fe$_2$O$_3$ nanoparticles using *Sida cordifolia* plant extract. Heliyon 2019; 5(11): e02765.
[http://dx.doi.org/10.1016/j.heliyon.2019.e02765] [PMID: 31799458]

[51]	de Oliveira JFA, Saito Â, Bido AT, Kobarg J, Stassen HK, Cardoso MB. Defeating bacterial resistance and preventing mammalian cells toxicity through rational design of antibiotic-functionalized nanoparticles. Sci Rep 2017; 7(1): 1326.
[http://dx.doi.org/10.1038/s41598-017-01209-1] [PMID: 28465530]

[52]	Marín-Menéndez A, Montis C, Díaz-Calvo T, *et al.* Antimicrobial nanoplexes meet model bacterial membranes: the key role of cardiolipin. Sci Rep 2017; 7(1): 41242.
[http://dx.doi.org/10.1038/srep41242] [PMID: 28120892]

[53]	Marquardt RR, Li S. Antimicrobial resistance in livestock: advances and alternatives to antibiotics. Anim Front 2018; 8(2): 30-7.
[http://dx.doi.org/10.1093/af/vfy001] [PMID: 32002216]

[54]	Li J, Koh J-J, Liu S, Lakshminarayanan R, Verma CS, Beuerman RW. Membrane active antimicrobial peptides: translating mechanistic insights to design. Front Neurosci 2017; 11(73): 73.
[http://dx.doi.org/10.3389/fnins.2017.00073] [PMID: 28261050]

[55]	Pachón-Ibáñez ME, Smani Y, Pachón J, Sánchez-Céspedes J. Perspectives for clinical use of engineered human host defense antimicrobial peptides. FEMS Microbiol Rev 2017; 41(3): 323-42.
[http://dx.doi.org/10.1093/femsre/fux012] [PMID: 28521337]

[56]	Zhang LJ, Gallo RL. Antimicrobial peptides. Curr Biol 2016; 26(1): R14-9.
[http://dx.doi.org/10.1016/j.cub.2015.11.017] [PMID: 26766224]

[57]   The antimicrobial peptide database. University of Nebraska Medical Center. 2020. Available from: http://aps.unmc.edu/AP/main.php

[58]   Biswaro LS, da Costa Sousa MG, Rezende TMB, Dias SC, Franco OL. Antimicrobial Peptides and Nanotechnology, Recent Advances and Challenges. Front Microbiol 2018; 9(855): 855.
[http://dx.doi.org/10.3389/fmicb.2018.00855] [PMID: 29867793]

[59]   Alam MK, Alhhazmi A, DeCoteau JF, Luo Y, Geyer CR, Rec A. RecA inhibitors potentiate antibiotic activity and block evolution of antibiotic resistance. Cell Chem Biol 2016; 23(3): 381-91.
[http://dx.doi.org/10.1016/j.chembiol.2016.02.010] [PMID: 26991103]

[60]   Haddad Kashani H, Schmelcher M, Sabzalipoor H, Seyed Hosseini E, Moniri R. Recombinant endolysins as potential therapeutics against antibiotic-resistant *Staphylococcus aureus*: Current Status of Research and Novel Delivery Strategies. Clin Microbiol Rev 2017; 31(1): e00071-17.
[http://dx.doi.org/10.1128/CMR.00071-17] [PMID: 29187396]

[61]   Ali J, Rafiq QA, Ratcliffe E. Antimicrobial resistance mechanisms and potential synthetic treatments. Future Sci OA 2018; 4(4): FSO290.
[http://dx.doi.org/10.4155/fsoa-2017-0109] [PMID: 29682325]

[62]   Hsu PD, Lander ES, Zhang F. Development and applications of CRISPR-Cas9 for genome engineering. Cell 2014; 157(6): 1262-78.
[http://dx.doi.org/10.1016/j.cell.2014.05.010] [PMID: 24906146]

[63]   Bikard D, Euler CW, Jiang W, *et al.* Exploiting CRISPR-Cas nucleases to produce sequence-specific antimicrobials. Nat Biotechnol 2014; 32(11): 1146-50.
[http://dx.doi.org/10.1038/nbt.3043] [PMID: 25282355]

[64]   Citorik RJ, Mimee M, Lu TK. Sequence-specific antimicrobials using efficiently delivered RNA-guided nucleases. Nat Biotechnol 2014; 32(11): 1141-5.
[http://dx.doi.org/10.1038/nbt.3011] [PMID: 25240928]

[65]   Kim J-S, Cho D-H, Park M, *et al.* CRISPR/Cas9-Mediated Re-Sensitization of Antibiotic-Resistant *Escherichia coli* Harboring Extended-Spectrum β-Lactamases. J Microbiol Biotechnol 2016; 26(2): 394-401.
[http://dx.doi.org/10.4014/jmb.1508.08080] [PMID: 26502735]

CHAPTER 3

Alternative   Routes   of   Antimicrobial Administration

Michael J. Cawley[*]

Philadelphia College of Pharmacy, University of the Sciences, Philadelphia, PA, USA

Abstract: Antimicrobial administration requires drug therapy to target the site of infection. Traditionally, commercial oral and intravenous agents are the first route of administration for systemic infections. The use of alternative routes of administration is often required to optimize both pharmacokinetic and pharmacodynamic properties of antimicrobials that may not be achieved with oral or intravenous products. Optimizing both pharmacokinetic and pharmacodynamic properties help achieve adequate penetration of the target drug into the site of infection by maintaining antibiotic serum concentration in a time or concentration-dependent manner. The result is the achievement of drug concentrations above the minimum inhibitory concentration of a targeted organism resulting in both clinical and microbiological cure. In addition, pharmaceutically compounded antimicrobials must also be an option to target infections that may not be achieved with commercial antibiotics. A description of the various routes of antimicrobial administration is presented in this chapter including current evidence, guidelines for use and new and novel administrative methods.

Keywords: Aerosol, Bone, Compounded Antimicrobials, Intramuscular, Intraventricular, Minimum Inhibitory Concentration, Ophthalmic, Pharmacodynamics, Pharmacokinetics, Rectal, Routes of Administration, Topical.

INTRODUCTION

The systemic delivery of pharmacological agents is an ever-evolving science. Pharmaceutical companies must address the technological challenges to adapt new molecular entities to optimize treatments for human disease. These new molecular entities must undergo a full regulatory review to address many drug-related endpoints including pharmacokinetic and pharmacodynamic modeling, biopharmaceutical endpoints (osmolality, stability, solubility, and bioavailability), drug efficacy, safety and ultimately result in the improvement of human disease. These requirements are particularly important to the antimicrobial class of drug therapy.

[*] **Corresponding author Michael J. Cawley:** Philadelphia College of Pharmacy, University of the Sciences, Philadelphia, PA, USA; E-mail: m.cawley@usciences.edu

Islam M. Ghazi & Michael J. Cawley (Eds.)

Traditionally, antimicrobials are administered *via* the oral and IV route. Both routes of administration combined with proper dosing generally achieve the desired bacteriostatic or bactericidal efficacy to optimize pharmacodynamic endpoints. However, other delivery methods may be required when traditional methods fail to achieve clinical and microbiological success. This chapter will discuss alternative routes of antimicrobial administration including current evidence, guidelines for use and novel administrative methods to assist the clinician in achieving infection eradication.

BASIC OVERVIEW OF PHARMACOKINETIC AND PHARMACODYNAMIC PRINCIPLES

Clinicians utilizing alternative routes of antimicrobial administration must be familiar with pharmacokinetic and pharmacodynamic principles of antimicrobial drug delivery. Pharmacokinetics of a drug is simply its rate of change as it passes through a biological system determined by four essential processes including absorption, distribution, metabolism and excretion [1]. In addition, other parameters including drug plasma concentration (peak and trough), volume of distribution (Vd), drug solubility, protein binding and renal elimination all are variables that must be considered to achieve adequate penetration of the target drug into the site of infection. Increases or decreases in these pharmacokinetic parameters may require a dosing change to optimize drug concentrations at various sites of action including blood, lung, skin, soft tissue, bone and central nervous system.

Pharmacodynamics is the study of the biological effects that result from the interaction between drugs and biological systems [2]. Antibiotics demonstrate their effectiveness by a number of pharmacodynamic principles including a concentration-dependent concentration above the minimum inhibitory concentration (Cmax/MIC), time-dependent concentration above the MIC (T > MIC), area under the concentration-time curve over the MIC (AUC/MIC) and post-antibiotic effect (PAE). PAE is simply maintaining suppression of bacterial growth after a brief exposure to an antimicrobial agent [3]. Antibiotics may be assessed for microbiological success by one pharmacodynamic endpoint while others may have several. Examples include aminoglycosides (Cmax/MIC, AUC/MIC and PAE), β-lactams (T > MIC and PAE) and glycopeptides (AUC/MIC) [1, 4]. Many antimicrobials demonstrate a variety of pharmacodynamic parameters that correlate with *in vivo* efficacy (Fig. **1**).

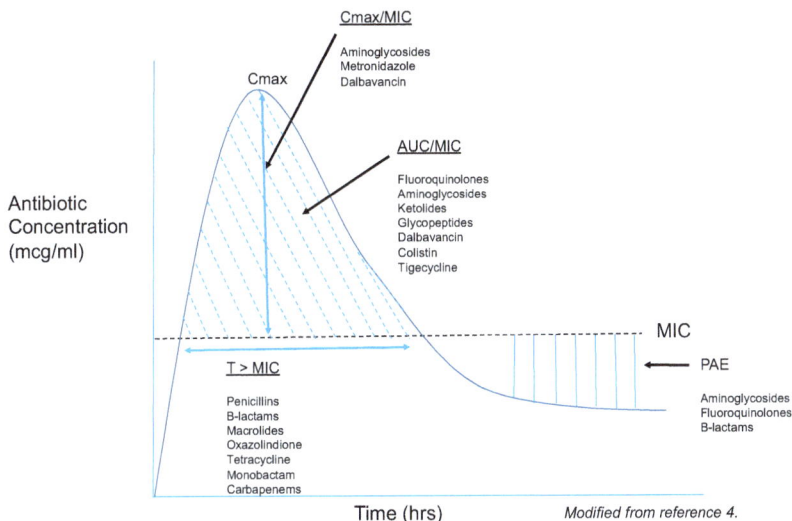

Fig. (1). Pharmacodynamics of Common Antimicrobials.

ROUTES OF ANTIMICROBIAL ADMINISTRATION

Aerosol

Aerosol therapy has been a mainstay of treatment for patients with respiratory disease for decades. Aerosol therapy is routinely used in spontaneously breathing patients and patients receiving mechanical ventilation. Aerosol administration requires a variety of respiratory delivery devices including nebulizers (small-volume (SVN) and large-volume (LVN), pressurized metered-dosed inhalers (pMDIs), and dry powder inhalers (DPIs). Currently, nebulizer administration provides the most versatile method for aerosol delivery of a variety of drug formulations. Drug formulations include bronchodilators, anticholinergics, corticosteroids, antiretrovirals, vasodilators, antiprotozoals and antimicrobials. Aerosol antibiotics do have a number of pharmacokinetic and pharmacodynamic advantages to assist in drug effectiveness including the concentration-dependent effect (high concentration in the airway to maximize bactericidal activity), the drug ability to penetrate infected airway secretion and limited systemic absorption to limit adverse effects [5]. In addition, other factors include the inspiratory flow rate, aerosol delivery system selected and aerodynamic size of droplets produced or mass median aerodynamic diameter (MMAD) [5]. An MMAD of 10-15 μm deposit in the upper airways, 5-10 μm deposit in the conducting airways and large bronchi and 1-5 μm penetrates the lower airways and lung periphery [6]. Medical aerosol delivery systems generally produce MMAD between 1-5 μm to optimize pulmonary drug delivery.

Aerosol delivery systems for nebulizer administration have evolved to include greater enhancement of electronic technology to optimize drug delivery. Nebulizer classification includes pneumatic jet, ultrasonic and mesh technology.

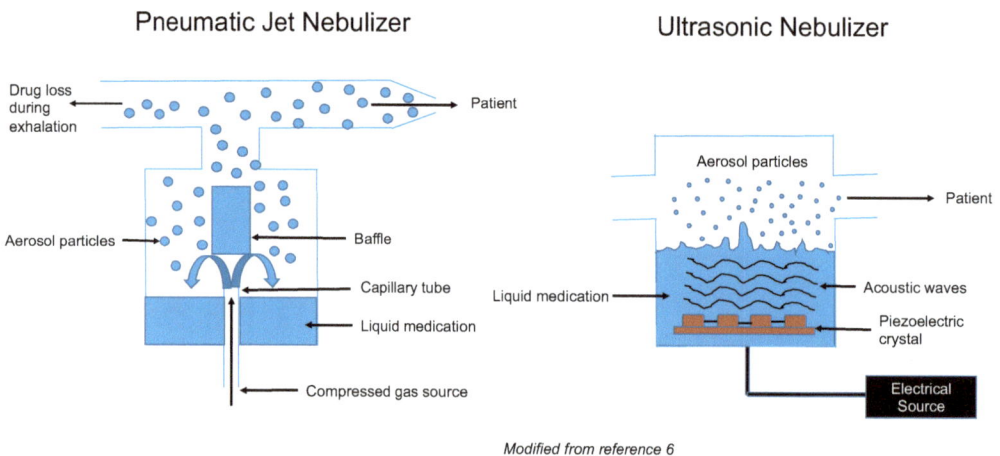

Modified from reference 6

Fig. (2). Aerosol Delivery System.

Pneumatic jet nebulizers are the most common aerosol delivery system used in clinical practice; however, they are also the least efficient [7]. Pneumatic jet devices utilize compressed gas, which powers the device. The liquid medication forms droplets which are then placed in the stream of a baffle. The result is shearing forces that create the aerosol particles. Ultrasonic nebulizers use a piezoelectric crystal vibrating at high frequencies (1-3 MHz) [8]. The vibrations transfer to the surface of the solution creating the aerosol (Fig. **2**). Due to the heat generated by high-frequency vibrations, viscous solutions, suspension or protein based products may degrade and are not recommended [8]. Mesh nebulizers are the newest technology classified into two categories: active mesh and passive mesh. Active mesh nebulizers utilize a piezoelectric crystal that vibrates at approximately 128 KHz. In addition, some devices use a "micropump" system, which results in the upward and downward movement of the mesh by a few micrometers. The result is liquid moved through an aperture plate or mesh with 1,000-4,000 holes determining the size of the aerosol particle [6, 9]. Passive mesh uses a transducer horn that pushes fluid through a mesh with 6,000 tapered holes to produce an aerosol [6] (Fig. **3**). Mesh and ultrasonic nebulizers demonstrate similar drug delivery; however, mesh nebulizers are more efficient than pneumatic jet nebulizers [8]. In addition, software incorporated with these aerosol delivery systems include SmartCard electronic controls, Adaptive Aerosol Delivery (AAD) and others. The software is designed to optimize aerosol MMAD, drug delivery time, and the timing of patient inspiration with aerosol device output [10, 11].

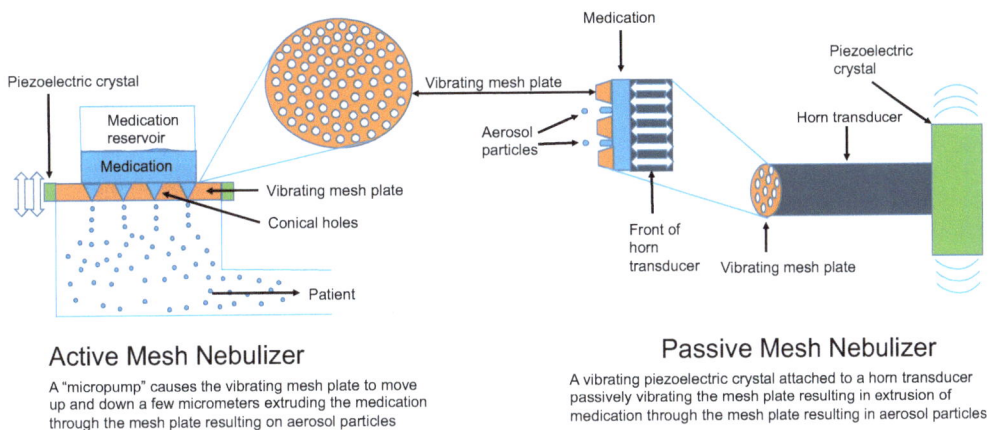

Active Mesh Nebulizer

A "micropump" causes the vibrating mesh plate to move up and down a few micrometers extruding the medication through the mesh plate resulting on aerosol particles

Passive Mesh Nebulizer

A vibrating piezoelectric crystal attached to a horn transducer passively vibrating the mesh plate resulting in extrusion of medication through the mesh plate resulting in aerosol particles

Modified from reference 9 and 10

Fig. (3). Aerosol Delivery System.

Aerosol antimicrobial administration by nebulizer has been well established for the treatment of patients with *Pseudomonas* infections including: cystic fibrosis, non-cystic fibrosis bronchiectasis, difficult to treat hospital-acquired pneumonia (HAP), ventilator-associated pneumonia (VAP) and in combination with systemic antibiotics for patients with multidrug-resistant (MDR) pathogens [12 - 15].

Multiple studies have documented the utility of aerosol delivery of antimicrobials for patients with pulmonary infections. 520 cystic fibrosis patients were randomly assigned to receive 300 mg inhaled tobramycin or placebo twice weekly for four weeks followed by four weeks of study drug. Patients receiving inhaled tobramycin demonstrated increases in FEV1 of 10% at week 20 compared to a decline in FEV1 by 2 percent ($p<0.001$), decline in *P. aeruginosa* sputum density by an average of 0.8 log10 colony-forming units (CFU) from week 0 to 20 compared to an increase of 0.3 log10 CFU in the placebo group ($p<0.001$). Patients in the tobramycin group were 26% less likely to be hospitalized compared to the placebo group [12].

A retrospective cohort study of patients with VAP compared IV colistin to IV colistin plus aerosolized colistin. Seventy-eight patients received IV colistin plus aerosolized colistin compared to forty-three patients receiving IV colistin alone. Clinical cure rate was 62/78 (79.5%) who received IV colistin plus aerosolized colistin *vs* 26/43 (60.5%) who received IV colistin alone (0.025); all cause in-house mortality was 31/78 (39.7%) *vs* 19/43 (44.2%), p=0.63. The use of inhaled colistin was associated with the cure for VAP in a multivariable analysis (OR 2.53, 95% CI 1.11 – 5.76). The outcome of VAP was better for patients receiving IV colistin plus aerosolized colistin than those receiving IV alone [16].

Guidelines for the management of adult patients with HAP and VAP recommend for gram-negative bacilli infections only susceptible to aminoglycosides or polymyxins, both inhaled and systemic antibiotics, rather than systemic antibiotics alone should be recommended (weak recommendation, very low-quality evidence) [14]. However, it is reasonable to consider adjunctive inhaled antibiotics as a last resort in patients not responding to IV antibiotics alone, whether the organism is or is not MDR [14]. Despite more than 30 years of use, there has not been any well-designed clinical trials demonstrating antibiotic aerosol efficacy in mechanically ventilated patients [17].

Due to advances in aerosol delivery, other methods besides nebulizer delivery are showing promise. Data has shown that tobramycin delivered *via* a (DPI) device achieved improved lung deposition, faster delivery and convenience of administration compared to traditional pneumatic jet nebulized formulations [18]. Also, both DPI and liposomal formulations of ciprofloxacin demonstrated reduction in bacterial load and delayed time to first exacerbation. However, data discrepancies from two phase III clinical trials (ORBIT-3 and ORBIT-4) resulted in an FDA advisory panel voting against recommending the drug for approval in patients with non-cystic fibrosis bronchiectasis [19, 20]. The following antimicrobials have been administered as an aerosol in patients with pulmonary infections (cystic fibrosis, non-cystic fibrosis and bronchiectasis), patients with an artificial airway (endotracheal or tracheostomy) and patients receiving mechanical ventilation (Table **1**).

Intramuscular

Intramuscular (IM) is the delivery method for immunizations but also has utility for a number of antimicrobials. IM administration is the first route of choice for patients unable to tolerate oral medications due to emesis, inability to swallow or to verify medication compliance [37]. Pharmacokinetic studies for various antimicrobials have shown complete absorption administered *via* IM route and that IV and IM can be used interchangeability [38, 39]. IM administration is considered safe; however, complications can occur including pain, sterile abscess, cellulitis and nerve injury [40, 41]. Relative contraindications include known bleeding disorders or thrombocytopenia [42].

Table 1. Antimicrobials Administered as an Aerosol in Patients with Pulmonary Infections [21 - 36].

Drug Class	Drug	Mechanical Ventilation	Absence of [A] Mechanical Ventilation	Dosing Strategies
Aminoglycosides	Tobramycin	X	X	300mg BID (28 days)
	Amikacin	X	X	400mg BID (7-14 days)
	Liposomal Amikacin		X	590mg daily (84 -168 days)
	Gentamycin	X	X	80mg Q8hrs (14-21 days)
B-lactams	Ceftazidime	X		250mg Q12hrs (up to 7 days)
Carbapenems	Imipenem/cilastatin	X		1500mg x 2 doses
Glycopeptides	Vancomycin	X		120mg Q8hrs (up to 14 days)
Monobactams	Aztreonam		X	75mg TID (28 days)
Fluoroquinolones	Ciprofloxacin		X	32.5mg BID (14 or 28 days)
	Liposomal Ciprofloxacin		X	150mg daily x 28 days (3 cycles)
	Levofloxacin		X	180mg daily/240mg daily (7days)
Polymyxins	Colistin/polymyxin B	X	X	80mg Q8hrs (7 days)
Phosphonic acid	Fosfomycin	X	X	40-240mg Q22-26hrs (3 doses)
Antifungals	Amphotericin B	X	X	20mg (3 times weekly)
	Liposomal Amphotericin B	X	X	50mg (2 times weekly) [B]
Retrovirals	Pentamidine	X	X	300mg Q4 weeks x 6 months
	Ribavirin	X	X	20mg/1ml x12-18hrs (3-7 days)

[A]Absence of mechanical ventilation includes patients with cystic fibrosis, non-cystic fibrosis bronchiectasis, artificial airway (endotracheal or tracheostomy tube).

[B] Duration of treatment unknown.

IM administration has been compared to oral medications in adults and children for a number of disorders including urinary tract infections, otitis media, and prevention of meningitis [43 - 45]. Specific indications where IM administration is preferred or can be recommended as an alternative to oral administration include *Neisseria gonorrhoeae, Treponema pallidum,* group A beta-hemolytic streptococcal pharyngitis, pelvic inflammatory disease and epididymitis [46 - 49]. The following agents can be administered *via* IM injection (Table **2**).

Table 2. Common Antimicrobials Administered *via* the Intramuscular Route [50].

Drug	Drug Class	Infections
Penicillin G sodium	Natural Penicillin	Meningitis, syphilis, tetanus, endocarditis
Penicillin G benzathine	Natural Penicillin	Respiratory tract, syphilis, prevention of rheumatic fever
Ampicillin	Aminopenicillin	Respiratory tract, meningitis, endocarditis
Piperacillin	Ureidopenicillin	Respiratory tract, gonorrhea, uncomplicated UTI
Oxacillin	β-lactamase resistant penicillin	Bacteremia, skin structure, bone and joint
Nafcillin	β-lactamase resistant penicillin	Bacteremia, skin structures, bone and joint
Cefazolin	Cephalosporin	Respiratory tract, skin structure, bone and joint
Cefotetan	Cephalosporin	Skin structure, urinary tract
Ceftazidime	Cephalosporin	Respiratory tract, urinary tract, endocarditis
Cefamandole	Cephalosporin	Respiratory tract, skin and soft tissue, urinary tract
Cefotaxime	Cephalosporin	Respiratory tract, skin and soft tissue, urinary tract
Ceftizoxime	Cephalosporin	Otitis media, gonorrhea, chlamydia, pelvic inflammatory disease
Cefuroxime	Cephalosporin	Respiratory tract, skin and skin structure, urinary tract
Cefepime	Cephalosporin	Respiratory tract, skin and skin structure, urinary tract
Ceftriaxone	Cephalosporin	Respiratory tract, skin and skin structure, urinary tract
Aztreonam	Monobactam	Respiratory tract, skin and skin structure, urinary tract
Amikacin	Aminoglycoside	Respiratory tract, *mycobacterium* avium complex, bacteremia
Gentamicin	Aminoglycoside	Respiratory tract, skin and skin structure, endocarditis,

(Table 2) cont.....

Tobramycin	Aminoglycoside	Respiratory tract, skin and skin structure, urinary tract
Streptomycin	Aminoglycoside	Respiratory tract, meningitis, tularemia, endocarditis
Ertapenem	Carbapenem	Respiratory tract, skin and skin structure, intra-abdominal, urinary tract
Imipenem/cilastatin	Carbapenem	Respiratory tract, skin and skin structure, intra-abdominal, urinary tract
Clindamycin	Lincosamide	Respiratory tract, skin and skin structure, diabetic foot, intra-abdominal
Lincomycin	Lincosamide	Respiratory tract, bacteremia
Colistimethate	Polymyxin	Respiratory tract, meningitis, ventriculitis

IM needle injections are delivered by a healthcare provider to a number of anatomical locations including the upper deltoid muscle, vastus lateralis, rectus femoris, dorsogluteal and ventrogluteal muscles [51]. Large-volume injections are considered 3ml or greater. Maximum volumes that have been proposed is 5ml in adults with lower volumes in patients with less muscle mass [51]. Antibiotics are administered by large volume injections. The deltoid is used for immunizations since the volume is less than 1ml. The dorsogluteal and ventrogluteal muscles are the general accepted areas for large-volume administration based upon nursing education practice and clinical practice guidelines [52, 53].

Needle systems are the delivery method used most often in clinical practice, however, needle free systems are also available. These systems use unique energy sources for delivery including spring powered and gas propelled, unfortunately, these systems are limited to a maximum volume up to 1ml [54]. Since antibiotic administration requires a large-volume injections, the needle free systems have limited utility for antibiotic administration at this time.

Intracerebroventricular

Delivery of drugs into the central nervous system (CNS) is challenging due to physiological anatomy including the blood brain barrier and blood-cerebrospinal fluid barrier. In addition, neurosurgical interventions including external ventricular drains and lumbar drains also contribute to challenges in treating patients with CNS infections. Intracerebroventricular administration of drugs into the CNS include direct installation into brain ventricles, intrathecal (IT) or intraventricular (IVT) routes. However, due to pathophysiological challenges each method poses unique challenges. Since elimination of many antimicrobials from the cerebral spinal fluid (CSF) is based upon CSF outflow and active transport systems, administering by ventricular installation may lead to increased drug elimination before the next dosing interval leading to subtherapeutic antimicrobial serum concentrations [55]. In addition, dosing *via* the IT route also is less than desirable due to frequent lumbar punctures or possibility of infectious risk due to catheter placement [55]. Infections within the CNS requiring a non-traditional administration technique involve serious life-threatening infections including meningitis and ventriculitis. Typical pathogens include gram positive cocci (*Staphylococcus* and *S. aureus)* and gram-negative organisms developing MDR including gram negative bacilli (*Klebsiella pneumonia* and *Pseudomonas aeruginosa*) and gram-negative coccobacilli (*Acinetobacter spp)* [56, 57]. These pathogens often develop MDR to common antimicrobials and often pose a challenge for successful treatment. Many factors have an impact on the success of antimicrobial treatment including MIC of the antimicrobial to identified pathogen, meningeal inflammation, and drug related parameters including lipophilicity, molecular size, plasma protein binding, active transport and metabolism in the CNS [58].

Dosing strategies for treatment of meningitis or ventriculitis have differed within the literature. Clinicians traditionally initiate IV antibiotics alone with conventional dosing when CSF cultures are positive. Infectious Diseases Society of America (IDSA) treatment guidelines recommend that IVT antimicrobial agents may be an option for patients with healthcare-associated ventriculitis and meningitis not responding to systemic antimicrobials alone [59]. Others recommend if CSF cultures remain positive or MIC values demonstrate MDR organisms, more aggressive IV dosing with extended treatment durations have been used with success with no adverse effects [60]. Other strategies have suggested if IV antibiotics are ineffective despite 5 days of therapy or if the first CSF analysis identified pus, both IV and IVT may be used together [61]. Aggressive IV dosing for extended treatment durations, IVT administration alone or IVT administered with high-dose IV therapy are all strategies to maximize pharmacodynamic response in an attempt to sterilize the CSF.

Wang *et al.* studied 127 patients for postsurgical gram-negative meningitis or ventriculitis and administered IVT gentamicin, amikacin or colistin. Antibiotic treatment required an average of 13.3 days which resulted in a 73.3% cure rate and mean time for CSF sterilization was 6.6 days [62].

Remes *et al.* treated 34 patients with meningitis and ventriculitis. Patients received a variety of antibiotics including gentamycin (N=16), vancomycin (N=15), colistin (N=5), meropenem (N=1) and netilimicin (N=1). A combination of two antibiotics were used in four patients. CSF cultures became negative 24 hrs after IVT/IT administration in 50% of patients with a CSF sterilization achieved in 2.2 days [63].

Khan *et al.* evaluated 21 patients with MDR meningitis and ventriculitis. Patients received amikacin, polymyxin B and colisitin for treatment of *Acinetobacter spp, P. aeruginosa. K. pneumonia and Enterobacter cloacae.* Mean duration of IVT/IT therapy was 15 (9-25) days, resulting in 95% sterility of the CSF from 2 to 16 days [61]. Both IVT/IT methods are effective when used together since it may be impossible to achieve optimum bactericidal eradication with IV alone [64].

The IVT route is an option for CNS infections, however, efficacy and safety of this route of administration has not been proven in clinical trials [59]. Also, since there is great variation in regards to the published literature there is limited consensus on their use [59]. The following intraventricular dosing recommendations are available for a limited number of antimicrobial agents including aminoglycosides, glycopeptides, polymyxin B, colistin, lipopeptides, and streptogramins (Table **3**).

Table 3. Antimicrobial Agents Administered by the Intraventricular Route for Adults [58 - 59].

Drug Class	Drug	Adult Dose/Duration [A]
Aminoglycosides	Amikacin Gentamycin Tobramycin	30mg Q24 hours 4-8mg Q24 hours [B] 5-20mg Q24 hours
Glycopeptides	Vancomycin	5-20mg Q24 hours
Polymyxins	Polymyxin B Colistin (colistimethate)	5mg Q24 hours 10mg Q24 hours
Lipopeptides	Daptomycin	5-10mg Q72 hours
Streptogramins	Streptogramins	2-5mg Q24 hours
Antifungal	Amphotericin B	0.01 - 0.5mg Q24 hours

[A] Duration of therapy range from 10-14 days for gram + infections and 21 days for gram-negative bacilli. In patients with repeated positive CSF cultures, treatment should continue for 10-14 days after the last positive culture.

[B] Recommended frequency of administration (Q24, Q48 and Q72 hours) is based upon external ventricular drain output over 24 hours.

Ophthalmic

Eye infections are traditionally considered a "minor infection" however, in some instances these infections can be vision-threatening. Common infections include bacterial conjunctivitis, keratitis and blepharitis that often require topical antimicrobial treatment. However, more invasive infections including endophthalmitis may require more aggressive antibiotic administration. Bacteria associated with these infections can vary widely including *Staphylococcus aureus,* coagulase-negative *Staphylococcus, Streptococcal pneumoniae, Haemophilus influenza, Pseudomonas aeruginosa and Klebsiella pneumonia* [65].

Common first-line commercial antibiotics for minor infections that can be administered as eye drops or ointments include aminoglycosides, macrolides, polymyxin B combinations, trimethoprim and fluoroquinolones [66]. All antibiotic classes achieve adequate concentrations in both formulations. Antimicrobial activity of antibiotics such as azithromycin achieve high concentrations in ocular tissues in both ophthalmic drop and ointment formulations. In addition, added benefit of macrolides exhibit anti-inflammatory activity by decreasing production of proinflammatory cytokines and neutrophils [66].

Intravitreal administration of various drugs including corticosteroids and anti-vascular endothelial growth factor have been used for patients with age-related macular degeneration and other forms of retinal venous occlusive disease. Serious infections including endophthalmitis can be treated with topical, systemic and intravitreal antibiotics. However, there are limitations in delivery methods. Topical antibiotics may fail to reach desired MIC level in the vitreous cavity. Systemic antibiotics can achieve concentrations above MIC of most organisms, however, may take 2-3 days. Intravitreal administration has achieved 10-100-fold serum concentrations in vitreous, thus, is considered the standard of care for patients with infectious endophthalmitis [67].

Gan *et al.* treated 11 patients with postoperative endophthalmitis. Bacterial cultures identified coagulase-negative *staphylococci*. Patients were administered intravitreal vancomycin 0.2mg followed by 0.05mg gentamicin followed by a repeated intravitreal vancomycin injection of 0.2mg after 3 or 4 days. Intravitreal vancomycin serum levels varied between 2.6 and 18 mcg/ml (mean 10.3mcg/ml) after 3 days and between 3.1 and 16.6 mcg/ml (mean 7.5mcg/ml) after 4 days. The authors concluded that this dosing regimen resulted in intravitreal serum concentrations well above the MIC of most organisms, intravitreal serum levels were maintained over a week which resulted in negative repeat cultures [68].

In addition to intravitreal administration, studies have advocated for the use of intracamerol delivery. Antibiotics commonly administered include cefuroxime and moxifloxacin. Intracamerol cefuroxime and moxifloxacin has been administered at the end of cataract surgery to prevent postoperative endophthalmitis [69, 70]. However, although the use of intrecamerol injection use has increased in the United States, this mode of delivery has not received Food and Drug Administration (FDA) approval at this time. In addition, a recent review has identified that the routine use of intracamerol antibiotics use has increased around the world, but data from multicenter, randomized prospective trials is needed to better provide guidance for use [71].

Topical

Topical antibiotic use has included a variety of products including creams, ointments, antibiotic powders and antibiotic-containing lavage solutions. Other creative methods may include antibiotic impregnated fleeces and beads to prevent surgical site infections. Many large reviews and meta-analysis have been done on this topic over the past 60 years of study and the data has summarized that there is insufficient evidence to support the use of topical application of antibiotics for infected wounds [72]. In addition, a recent systematic review also supported this evidence by identifying limited and low-quality evidence on the use of topical antibiotics for infected wounds [73]. Also based upon the risk of their use in the surgical environment, topical antibiotic use should be targeted by antibiotic stewardship programs as another mechanism to limit their use [72].

Antibiotic-containing solutions have been used for direct installation into a surgical wound at the site of a surgical procedures in the hopes of limiting bacterial contamination or infection. Common procedures in which antibiotic-containing irrigation solutions have been used include appendectomy, colorectal surgery, peritoneal lavage, blunt abdominal trauma, mediastinitis, thoracic empyema, peritonitis, urinary bladder infection and prosthetic joint infection [74]. The intent of utilizing these solutions is to limit bacterial contamination, however, other adverse effects of their use need to be considered. Some potential risks associated with their use include contact time between organism and antibiotic solution, systemic absorption of antibiotic, antibiotic resistance and adverse reactions [72].

The use of antibiotic containing solutions are still used in general surgical procedures. A 2008 survey of 168 surgeons reported that 46% reported the regular use of an antibiotic irrigation solution during surgery and a 2017 survey of 164 infection prevention practitioners reported 33% that topical antibiotic powders were used during surgery in their facility [75, 76]. Authors have suggested some support for antibiotic irrigation solutions for treatment of empyema following lobectomy, pneumonectomy and pyocytis [74]. However, other evidence does not support this practice. Organizations including the American Society of Health System Pharmacists (ASHP), IDSA, and Society for Healthcare Epidemiology of America (SHEA) do not support the use of topical antimicrobial irrigation solutions due to limited evidence [77]. Also, The World Health Organization (WHO) surgical site infection panel strongly protests the use of antibiotic irrigation solutions before closure to prevent surgical site infections [78].

Topical antibiotic therapy has the greatest utility in burn wound infections. Topical products reduce the microbial load on the burn wound surface and reduce the risk of infection [79]. Many options are available for treatment of the burn patient including mafenide, bacitracin, mupirocin, neosporin, polymyxin b, nitrofurazone, nyastatin, and topical silver and iodine preparations [80]. Data has demonstrated efficacy of each agent for the treatment of burn wound infections, however, there is limited data on a comprehensive systematic review or meta-analysis assessing these agents for treatment or prophylaxis.

Barajas-Neva *et al.* performed a comprehensive review of 36 Randomized Controlled Trials (RCT), (2117) participants which included twenty-six (76%) received topical antibiotics for prophylaxis of burn wound infections. Eleven trials (645 participants) evaluated topical silver sulfadiazine were pooled in the analysis. Results determined that there was a statically significant increase in burn wound infections associated with silver sulfadiazine compared to dressings/skin substitutes (OR=1.87, 95% CI: 1.09 to 3.19) and longer length of stay (MD=2.11 days; 95% CI: 1.93 to 2.28). The authors concluded that many of the studies evaluated were small and of poor quality and no reliable conclusions can be made [81].

Bone

Osteomyelitis is an inflammatory process of the bone associated with infection. Pathogens common to this infection include both *methicillin-resistant Staphylococcus aureus* (MRSA) and non-MRSA, *Enterococcus sp.*, including vancomycin-resistant *Enterococcus* (VRE), β-hemolytic *Streptococcus* and gram-negative bacilli including *Pseudomonas aeruginosa* [82]. Antimicrobial initiation may include vancomycin, daptomycin, linezolid, quinupristin/dalfopristin, penicillin, nafcillin, ceftriaxone, cefepime, and ciprofloxacin. Treatment durations are traditionally 4-6 weeks in duration. Treatment duration may be increased to > 6 weeks followed by oral therapy for 3 months or longer in patients at high risk for failure (MRSA) [82]. Although these agents have demonstrated their effectiveness administered as IV or oral regimens, there is virtually no data on the administration of these agents by alternative delivery methods including bone cement, antibiotic-impregnated hip and knee spacers, stabilizers and other advanced methods.

Evolving treatments for osteomyelitis require a product to have limited adverse effects and have localized effectiveness. Bone cements are non-biodegradable materials that are designed to promote osteocyte binding, provide useful antibiotic release over time and promote bone regeneration [83]. Desirable characteristics of an antibiotic to be incorporated as bone cement include: availability as a powder form, bactericidal at low concentrations, using <1 gram antibiotic(s)/40 grams polymethylmethacrylate (PMMA) in high concentrations for prolonged periods, heat stability, limited risk of allergic or delayed hypersensitivity, low influence on the mechanical properties of the cement and has low serum protein binding [84]. Pharmacokinetic studies have evaluated the use of vancomycin, gentamicin, tobramycin and aztreonam loaded spacers. Masri *et al.* measured intraarticular antibiotic concentrations. Peak concentrations from wound drainage were 107 mcg/ml for tobramycin and 19 mcg/ml for vancomycin on day 1 of insertion. The concentrations achieved between a 10-30 higher concentration than the MIC of the infecting organism [85]. Also, data has shown that concentrations of gentamicin and vancomycin can be maintained over time.

Hsieh *et al.* shown that vancomycin peak concentrations achieved on day 1 were 1,538 mcg/ml and dropped to a mean value of 519 mcg/ml after 7 days. The high concentrations were based upon the high dosing incorporated in the cement 4 grams vancomycin/4 grams aztreonam/40 grams bone cement [86]. Glycopeptides and aminoglycosides are known for their nephrotoxicity. However, when either of these agents are used alone within a bone cement delivery method they do not always induce systemic side effects, but when combined with an intravenous antibiotic with nephrotoxic properties, nephrotoxic injury is more likely to occur [84].

Technology incorporating stabilizers such as antibiotic infused cement coated rods, polymer injections and use of other material that have been associated with antibacterial properties continues to grow with very promising results [83].

New technologies including polylactide-co-glycolic acid (PLGA), silver, gold and diamond nanoparticles, nitric and zinc oxide, bioactive glass particles and mesoporous silica nanospheres have all demonstrated some success as new delivery methods for the delivery of antibiotics to the bone [83]. Until more rigorous prospective randomized trials are completed on these products it is difficult to determine microbiological and clinical cure including the true impact on quality of life of patients with osteomyelitis.

Rectal

The need to administer medications *via* the rectal route may be used when oral or parenteral administration is not possible or to optimize drug delivery to target specific infections within the gastrointestinal tract such as *clostridium difficile*. Rectal administration may come in the form of suppositories, rectal capsules and enemas. Rectal absorption of antibiotics is primarily based upon passive transport. This process is the result of a multitude of factors including chemical properties of these agents (molecular weight, liposolubility, and drug molecule ionization and host factors (variations of mucous layer, volume of rectal fluid and basal cell membrane) [87]. Thus, the pharmaceutical formulations would play a major role in the rectal absorption and systemic delivery of the antibiotic. Pharmaceutical formulations including fatty acid salts (sodium capronate and sodium caprylate), glyceride and triglyceride compounds have been used successfully in administering β-lactam and aminoglycoside agents. These agents assist antimicrobial delivery by increasing improving mucosal permeability [87].

Approximately eight different classes of antibiotics that have been studied by rectal administration in humans, however, three classes have received the most attention of researchers [87]. The three classes include β-lactams (ampicillin), macrolides (erythromycin) and imidazoles (metronidazole).

Ampicillin administered by suppositories in children demonstrated serum concentrations of 5.9mg/L (range 4.8 to 7.0 mg/L) and 8.5mg/L (6.0 to 11 mg/L) with doses of 125 and 250mg (25-50mg/kg), respectively. The authors did determine the serum concentrations exceeded all MICs of all pathogens associated with acute otitis media [88]. Iwai *et al.* also administered rectal ampicillin in children with respiratory tract infections. Serum concentrations of 250mg dose (11.4 – 17.7mg/kg) achieved serum levels from 6.4 mcg/ml at 1/4 hr after administration to 0.7 mcg/ml after 2 hours. Bacteriologically, 100% eradication was achieved including 5 strains of *S. pyogenes,* 4 strains of *S. pneumoniae* and 3 strains of *H. influenza*. The authors concluded that ampicillin administered as a rectal suppository is an effective treatment for children with respiratory tract infections [89].

Erythromycin serum concentrations also achieved adequate serum concentrations after administered *via* the rectal route. Erythromycin suppository of 125 and 250mg administered in children achieved serum concentrations ranging from 0.35mg/L-0.49mg/L between 2-4 hours after administration [90]. Also, data has demonstrated adequate AUC concentrations achieved in children and infants. Dosing of 15mg/kg bid suppositories achieved a serum AUC concentration from 9.7 – 16.2 mg/hr.L [91].

Metronidazole has also been studied comparing suppository, oral and IV formulations. Doses of 500mg and 1000mg suppository doses achieved similar serum concentrations (5.5 and 9.5 mg/L) compared to oral (9.8 and 11.8 mg/L) and 1000mg IV (9.4 mg/L) [92, 93]. The results determined that metronidazole suppositories achieved adequate absorption and achieved similar serum concentrations to oral and IV administration.

Compounded Antimicrobial Agents

Compounded agents offer another potential option of antimicrobial administration for a limited number of clinical conditions. Many compounded pharmacies offer services for compounding antimicrobial agents for infections associated with skin, ophthalmic, vaginal, gastrointestinal and pulmonary infections including chronic sinusitis. Products can be customized to meet the needs of the patient that may not be possible with commercial antimicrobial agents. Many challenges face compounding pharmacies including physician understanding of compounded products, greater oversight of products covered by third-party reimbursement and out-of-pocket costs associated with this service [94 - 96]. Other challenges include societal mistrust and new legislative changes based upon the landmark New England Compounding Center meningitis outbreak in 2012 resulting in injuries to at least 753 patients including 64 deaths [97]. Since this tragedy, some clinicians have had greater challenges in acquiring compounded pharmaceutical products. Recently the American Society of Retina Specialists (ASRS) submitted comments to the FDA regarding the need for specialty compounded antibiotics for treatment of emergency infections including endophthalmitis. Currently 503A and 503B compounders are limited to what products can be produced. Examples of 503A products include acyclovir, amikacin, amphotericin, clindamycin, foscarnet, gancyclivir, and vorconizole compared to vancomycin and ceftazidime which are only available through 503B facilities. ASRS requested for patients in immediate need or an emergency such as fungal endophthalmitis to allow office use of compounded products from a 503A facility when such drugs can't be procured from a 503B facility. If 503A antibiotics for ophthalmic use in the setting of limited options from 503B retina doctors may return to "do-it-yourself" mixing of antibiotics in the office setting [98]. If this was to occur the potential risk of infections and associated toxicities may increase due to the lack or absence of quality control measures to maintain the purest pharmaceutical product.

CONCLUSION

Antimicrobial agent administration requires various routes of administration to achieve microbiological and clinical cure. Clinicians must continue to stay current in understanding the many options available in the delivery of antimicrobials including specialty compounded pharmaceutical products. In addition to the antimicrobial agent route of administration, technical advances in antimicrobial administration methods must be continuously assessed to determine the most optimum delivery technology. Future practitioners would need to be able to assess the best evidence available and choose the best route of administration utilizing the best technology to optimize pharmaceutical care and ultimately improve the patient's quality of life.

CLINICAL CASE SCENARIOS

Case 1

A 57-year-old female is admitted to the MICU due to exacerbation of COPD requiring intubation and mechanical ventilation. A long-complicated course ensued including a tracheostomy. bacterial sepsis, pulmonary embolism, upper gastrointestinal hemorrhage and resolving acute kidney injury (AKI). On day 24 the patient experiencing a fever of 102.8F, respiratory decompensation (worsening hypoxemia), and copious sputum production. CXR is indicative of LLL pneumonia. Piperacillin 3.375 (3g piperacillin/ 0.375g tazobactam) IV every eight hours and vancomycin 1g every eight hours are initiated empirically. Bronchoalveolar lavage (BAL) identified *Pseudomonas aeruginosa*. Susceptibilities are limited to piperacillin/tazobactam, tobramycin and meropenem (MIC 32 mcg/ml, 4 mcg/ml and 4 mcg/ml, respectively).

1. Based upon the data presented do you agree with the antibiotic choice and dosing regimen for piperacillin/tazobactam? Please provide rationale

> *Based upon BAL results identifying Pseudomonas aeruginosa only 3 antibiotics demonstrate efficacy to treat this infection. Although IV tobramycin may be an option it would not be the most optimum since the patient has resolving AKI. Restarting the drug IV may potentiate and exacerbate the AKI. Meropenem and piperacillin/tazobactam would be alternative options and both would be acceptable. However, more aggressive dosing of piperacillin/tazobactam (4.5 grams IV every 6 hours) should be considered based upon VAP IDSA guideline recommendation and also to optimize pharmacodynamic antimicrobial effects.*

2. If the patient was experiencing septic shock requiring vasopressor treatment to maintain an acceptable MAP how would of that changed your INITIAL antibiotic choice(s) for gram-negative bacilli coverage?

> *Since the patient was experiencing septic shock or at a high risk of death, and MDR P. aeruginosa, combination therapy would have been the best therapeutic approach. An IV aminoglycoside or IV carbapenem would have been added to piperacillin/tazobactam. Either choice would be acceptable.*

3. Ten days of antimicrobial therapy repeat sputum cultures continue to grow *Pseudomonas aeruginosa* demonstrate MDR resistance with only susceptibility to piperacillin/tazobactam and tobramycin (MIC 64 mcg/ml and 4 mcg/ml). The patient is now experiencing AKI. What antibiotic change would you consider at this time? Would aerosolized agent be appropriate at this time? What are potential advantages of this therapeutic decision?

Based upon MIC data, piperacillin/tazobactam would be an appropriate initial choice. However, higher doses would be required to achieve adequate bactericidal effect. Some clinicians would lower the dose due to patient's AKI, but lowering the dose may worsen the infectious process. Yes, aerosolized therapy would be an appropriate add on option at this time. Tobramycin still demonstrates effectiveness based upon susceptibility profile. Administering *via* the IV route would potentially worsen the patient's AKI. Administering tobramycin by aerosol in combination with IV piperacillin/tazobactam would be appropriate based upon a number of pharmacokinetic and pharmacodynamic properties to assist in drug effectiveness including: concentration-dependent effect (high concentration in the airway to maximize bactericidal activity), the drug ability to penetrate infected airway secretion and limited systemic absorption to limit adverse effects.

Case 2

A 49-year old female is admitted to the SICU the victim of a MVA. The patient experienced acute head trauma associated with impact to her car's windshield. Upon admission the patient is intubated and hemodynamically stabilized. A CT scan demonstrates intracranial hemorrhage of the frontal skull region. After emergency surgery an intraventricular catheter is required for control of post-operative intracranial hypertension. After 48 hours the patient experiences a fever of 103.6F and need of increasing doses of vasopressors in maintaining adequate MAP. Cerebrospinal fluid identified WBC 2,200 cells/mm3, protein 473mg/dl, glucose 23 mg/dL. Microscopic examination identified gram negative coccobacilli.

1. Which organism identified as gram negative coccobacilli would you consider the cause of the CSF infection?

> *Preliminary identification of gram-negative coccobacilli would determine the species to be either Haemophilus or Acinetobacter spp. Acinetobacter spp. accounts for approximately 80% of reported infections.*

2. Which antibiotic category would you consider for empiric treatment at this time?

   A number of antibiotics can be chosen for treatment of gram-negative coccobacilli including carbapenems, β-lactams, aminoglycosides or colistin.

Acinetobacter baumanii is identified. The pathogen is sensitive to ampicillin/sulbactam and colistin (MIC 16mcg/ml and 0.5 mcg/ml, respectively) and resistant to amikacin and imipenem/cilastatin (MIC 64 mcg/ml and 8 mcg/ml, respectively). Ampicillin/sulbactam is initiated at 3g (2 grams ampicillin/1 g sulbactam) IV every six hours. Approximately 96 hours later the patient continues with a persistent fever of 102F and continued detection of *A. baumanii* within the CSF.

3. What are three potential antibiotic strategies for treatment of this persistent infection? Please provide rationale.
   ○ *Strategies include increasing the IV dosing frequency of ampicillin/sulbactam to more aggressive dosing strategy (i.e every 3 hours).*
   ○ *Continue the ampicillin/sulbactam at present IV dose and then add IVT ampicillin/sulbactam*
   ○ *Consider switching patient to IV colistin only or add IVT colistin to IV therapy.*

   All three strategies would optimize drug concentrations and maximize pharmacodynamic response by maintaining drug concentrations above the MIC in an attempt to sterilize the CSF.

Case 3

A 61-year-old male is admitted to the SICU after surgery to repair a broken right hip due to a fall at his home. The patient required a total hip replacement utilizing an acetabular reconstruction. Approximately 48 hours later the patient demonstrates a fever of 102.7F and noticeable pain at the surgical site. Blood cultures x 2 identified MRSA. MRSA demonstrates sensitivity to vancomycin and daptomycin (MIC vancomycin 1 mcg/ml, daptomycin 0.5 mcg/ml). Vancomycin is initiated at 1g IV every eight hours. Trough levels are 18 mcg/ml on day 4 and 20 mcg/ml on day 7. After 7 days the patient continues to demonstrate positive blood cultures for MRSA. (Susceptibilities identify vancomycin MIC 2mcg/ml, daptomycin 0.5mcg/ml).

1. What antibiotic strategy would you recommend at this time including drug and dose?

> The patient has been on vancomycin for 10 days and has achieved adequate vancomycin trough levels x 2. In addition, MIC data regarding vancomycin has shown an increase from 1 mcg/ml to 2 mcg/ml (MIC drift) suggesting greater resistance. Vancomycin would be discontinue and changed to daptomycin. Although 6mg/kg would be the approved FDA dose many clinicians may opt for 8mg/kg dosing to maximize the pharmacodynamic response due to potential development of osteomyelitis.

After 5 days of the new antibiotic that was selected above the patient continues to demonstrate a fever and blood cultures remained MRSA positive. Surgery is consulted for concern of hip hardware infection. Surgery is scheduled for debridement of the surgical site and potential antimicrobial strategies for the local hip infection.

2. What is a potential antibiotic strategies for treatment of this difficult deep-seated bone infection?

> Based upon this deep seated infection surgery would determine to remove or replace any infected hardware. In addition, antibiotic bone cement utilizing vancomycin can be utilized in spacers, rods or other hardware deemed appropriate by the attending surgeon. Adding vancomycin to the site of infection has demonstrated 10-30 times higher concentration than the MIC of the infecting organism.

CONSENT FOR PUBLICATION

Not applicable.

CONFLICT OF INTEREST

The authors confirm that the contents of this chapter have no conflict of interest.

ACKNOWLEDGEMENTS

Declared none.

REFERENCES

[1] Onufrak NJ, Forrest A, Gonzalez D. Pharmacokinetic and pharmacodynamic principles of anti-infective dosing. Clin Ther 2016; 38(9): 1930-47.
[http://dx.doi.org/10.1016/j.clinthera.2016.06.015] [PMID: 27449411]

[2] Evans WE, Schentag JJ, Jusko WJ. Applied pharmacokinetics: Principles of therapeutic drug monitoring. 3rd ed., New York, NY: Applied Therapeutics 1996.

[3] Burgess DS. Pharmacodynamic principles of antimicrobial therapy in the prevention of resistance. Chest 1999; 115(3) (Suppl.): 19S-23S.
[http://dx.doi.org/10.1378/chest.115.suppl_1.19S] [PMID: 10084455]

[4] Rybak MJ. Pharmacodynamics: relation to antimicrobial resistance. Am J Infect Control 2006; 34(5) (Suppl. 1): S38-45.
[http://dx.doi.org/10.1016/j.ajic.2006.05.227] [PMID: 16813981]

[5] Restrepo MI, Keyt H, Reyes LF. Aerosolized Antibiotics. Respir Care 2015; 60(6): 762-1.
[http://dx.doi.org/10.4187/respcare.04208] [PMID: 26070573]

[6] Gardenhire DS, Burnett D, Strickland S, Myers TR. American Association for Respiratory Care A guide to aerosol delivery devices for respiratory therapists. 4th ed., American Association for Respiratory Care 2017.

[7] Harvey CJ, O'Doherty MJ, Page CJ, Thomas SH, Nunan TO, Treacher DF. Comparison of jet and ultrasonic nebulizer pulmonary aerosol deposition during mechanical ventilation. Eur Respir J 1997; 10(4): 905-9.
[PMID: 9150333]

[8] Ari A. Jet, ultrasonic and mesh nebulizers: An evaluation of nebulizers for better clinical outcomes. Eurasian J Pulmonol 2014; 16: 1-7.
[http://dx.doi.org/10.5152/ejp.2014.00087]

[9] Ghazanfari T, Elhissi AMA, Ding Z, Taylor KMG. The influence of fluid physicochemical properties on vibrating-mesh nebulization. Int J Pharm 2007; 339(1-2): 103-11.
[http://dx.doi.org/10.1016/j.ijpharm.2007.02.035] [PMID: 17451896]

[10] Kleinstreuer C, Feng Y, Childress E. Drug-targeting methodologies with applications: A review. World J Clin Cases 2014; 2(12): 742-56.
[http://dx.doi.org/10.12998/wjcc.v2.i12.742] [PMID: 25516850]

[11] Chan JGY, Wong J, Zhou QT, Leung SSY, Chan HK. Advances in device and formulation technologies for pulmonary drug delivery. AAPS PharmSciTech 2014; 15(4): 882-97.
[http://dx.doi.org/10.1208/s12249-014-0114-y] [PMID: 24728868]

[12] Ramsey BW, Pepe MS, Quan JM, *et al.* Cystic Fibrosis Inhaled Tobramycin Study Group. Intermittent administration of inhaled tobramycin in patients with cystic fibrosis. N Engl J Med 1999; 340(1): 23-30.
[http://dx.doi.org/10.1056/NEJM199901073400104] [PMID: 9878641]

[13] Nadig TR, Flume PA. Aerosolized antibiotics for patients with bronchiectasis. Am J Respir Crit Care Med 2016; 193(7): 808-10.
[http://dx.doi.org/10.1164/rccm.201507-1449LE] [PMID: 27035784]

[14] Kalil AC, Metersky ML, Klompas M, *et al.* Management of adults with hospital-acquired and ventilator-associated pneumonia: 2016 clinical practice guidelines by the Infectious Disease Society of America and the American Thoracic Society. Clin Infect Dis 2016; 63(5): e61-e111.

[http://dx.doi.org/10.1093/cid/ciw353] [PMID: 27418577]

[15]   Arnold HM, Sawyer AM, Kollef MH. Use of adjunctive aerosolized antimicrobial therapy in the treatment of *Pseudomonas aeruginosa* and *Acinetobacter baumannii* ventilator-associated pneumonia. Respir Care 2012; 57(8): 1226-33.
[http://dx.doi.org/10.4187/respcare.01556] [PMID: 22349038]

[16]   Korbila IP, Michalopoulos A, Rafailidis PI, Nikita D, Samonis G, Falagas ME. Inhaled colistin as adjunctive therapy to intravenous colistin for the treatment of microbiologically documented ventilator-associated pneumonia: a comparative cohort study. Clin Microbiol Infect 2010; 16(8): 1230-6.
[http://dx.doi.org/10.1111/j.1469-0691.2009.03040.x] [PMID: 19732088]

[17]   Kollef MH, Hamilton CW, Montgomery BA. Aerosolized antibiotics: do they add to the treatment of pneumonia. Curr Opion Infect Dis 3013 26(6): 538-44.

[18]   Geller DE, Weers J, Heuerding S. Development of an inhaled dry-powder formulation of tobramycin using PulmoSphere™ technology. J Aerosol Med Pulm Drug Deliv 2011; 24(4): 175-82.
[http://dx.doi.org/10.1089/jamp.2010.0855] [PMID: 21395432]

[19]   O'Donnell A, Bilton D, Serisier D, *et al.*

[20]   Food and Drug Administration. FDA briefing document 2018. https://www.fda.gov/ downloads/AdvisoryCommittees/CommitteesMeetingMaterials/Drugs/Anti-InfectiveDrugsAdvisory Committee/UCM591746.pdf

[21]   Olivier KN, Griffith DE, Eagle G, *et al.* Randomized trial of liposomal amikacin for inhalation in nontuberculous mycobacterial lung disease. Am J Respir Crit Care Med 2017; 195(6): 814-23.
[http://dx.doi.org/10.1164/rccm.201604-0700OC] [PMID: 27748623]

[22]   Palmer LB, Smaldone GC, Chen JJ, *et al.* Aerosolized antibiotics and ventilator-associated tracheobronchitis in the intensive care unit. Crit Care Med 2008; 36(7): 2008-13.
[http://dx.doi.org/10.1097/CCM.0b013e31817c0f9e] [PMID: 18552684]

[23]   Serisier DJ, Bilton D, De Soyza A, *et al.* ORBIT-2 investigators. Inhaled, dual release liposomal ciprofloxacin in non-cystic fibrosis bronchiectasis (ORBIT-2): a randomised, double-blind, placebo-controlled trial. Thorax 2013; 68(9): 812-7.
[http://dx.doi.org/10.1136/thoraxjnl-2013-203207] [PMID: 23681906]

[24]   Leoung GS, Feigal DW Jr, Montgomery AB, *et al.* Aerosolized pentamidine for prophylaxis against Pneumocystis carinii pneumonia. The San Francisco community prophylaxis trial. N Engl J Med 1990; 323(12): 769-75.
[http://dx.doi.org/10.1056/NEJM199009203231201] [PMID: 1975426]

[25]   Geller DE, Flume PA, Staab D, Fischer R, Loutit JS, Conrad DJ. Mpex 204 Study Group. Levofloxacin inhalation solution (MP-376) in patients with cystic fibrosis with Pseudomonas aeruginosa. Am J Respir Crit Care Med 2011; 183(11): 1510-6.
[http://dx.doi.org/10.1164/rccm.201008-1293OC] [PMID: 21471106]

[26]   Proesmans M, Vermeulen F, Vreys M, De Boeck K. Use of nebulized amphotericin B in the treatment of allergic bronchopulmonary aspergillosis in cystic fibrosis. Int J Pediatr 2010; 2010: 376287.
[http://dx.doi.org/10.1155/2010/376287] [PMID: 21234103]

[27]   Prescribing information. 2002. https://redbook.streamliners.co.nz/6608.pdf

[28]   Athanassa ZE, Markantonis SL, Fousteri MZ, *et al.* Pharmacokinetics of inhaled colistimethate sodium (CMS) in mechanically ventilated critically ill patients. Intensive Care Med 2012; 38(11): 1779-86.
[http://dx.doi.org/10.1007/s00134-012-2628-7] [PMID: 22810779]

[29]   Badia JR, Soy D, Adrover M, *et al.* Disposition of instilled *Versus* nebulized tobramycin and imipenem in ventilated intensive care unit (ICU) patients. J Antimicrob Chemother 2004; 54(2): 508-14.
[http://dx.doi.org/10.1093/jac/dkh326] [PMID: 15215224]

[30] Luyt CE, Clavel M, Guntupalli K, *et al.* Pharmacokinetics and lung delivery of PDDS-aerosolized amikacin (NKTR-061) in intubated and mechanically ventilated patients with nosocomial pneumonia. Crit Care 2009; 13(6): R200.
[http://dx.doi.org/10.1186/cc8206] [PMID: 20003269]

[31] Montgomery AB, Vallance S, Abuan T, Tservistas M, Davies A. A randomized double-blind placebo-controlled dose-escalation phase 1 study of aerosolized amikacin and fosfomycin delivered *via* the PARI investigational eFlow® inline nebulizer system in mechanically ventilated patients. J Aerosol Med Pulm Drug Deliv 2014; 27(6): 441-8.
[http://dx.doi.org/10.1089/jamp.2013.1100] [PMID: 24383962]

[32] Palmer LB, Smaldone GC, Simon SR, O'Riordan TG, Cuccia A. Aerosolized antibiotics in mechanically ventilated patients: delivery and response. Crit Care Med 1998; 26(1): 31-9.
[http://dx.doi.org/10.1097/00003246-199801000-00013] [PMID: 9428540]

[33] Wood GC, Boucher BA, Croce MA, Hanes SD, Herring VL, Fabian TC. Aerosolized ceftazidime for prevention of ventilator-associated pneumonia and drug effects on the proinflammatory response in critically ill trauma patients. Pharmacotherapy 2002; 22(8): 972-82.
[http://dx.doi.org/10.1592/phco.22.12.972.33596] [PMID: 12173800]

[34] Geller DE, Pitlick WH, Nardella PA, Tracewell WG, Ramsey BW. Pharmacokinetics and bioavailability of aerosolized tobramycin in cystic fibrosis. Chest 2002; 122(1): 219-26.
[http://dx.doi.org/10.1378/chest.122.1.219] [PMID: 12114362]

[35] Prescribing information. 2012. https://www.accessdata.fda.gov/drugsatfda_docs/label/2012/050814 s007lbl.pdf

[36] Quittner A, Quittner A, De Soyza A, Aksamit TR, *et al.* Effects of ciprofloxacin dry powder for inhalation (ciprofloxacin DPI) on health-related quality of life in patients with non-cystic fibrosis bronchiectasis (ncfb): Results from the phase III RESPIRE 1 study. Am J Respir Crit Care Med 2017; 195: A7303.

[37] Shatsky M. Evidence for the use of intramuscular injections in outpatient practice. Am Fam Physician 2009; 79(4): 297-300.
[PMID: 19235496]

[38] Antony KK, Lewis EW, Kenny MT, *et al.* Pharmacokinetics and bioavailability of a new formulation of teicoplanin following intravenous and intramuscular administration to humans. J Pharm Sci 1991; 80(6): 605-7.
[http://dx.doi.org/10.1002/jps.2600800621] [PMID: 1834827]

[39] Goonetilleke AK, Dev D, Aziz I, Hughes C, Smith MJ, Basran GS. A comparative analysis of pharmacokinetics of ceftriaxone in serum and pleural fluid in humans: a study of once daily administration by intramuscular and intravenous routes. J Antimicrob Chemother 1996; 38(6): 969-76.
[http://dx.doi.org/10.1093/jac/38.6.969] [PMID: 9023644]

[40] Hunter J. Intramuscular injection techniques. Nurs Stand 2008; 22(24): 35-40.
[http://dx.doi.org/10.7748/ns2008.02.22.24.35.c6413] [PMID: 18318317]

[41] Ogston-Tuck S. Intramuscular injection technique: an evidence-based approach. Nurs Stand 2014; 29(4): 52-9.
[http://dx.doi.org/10.7748/ns.29.4.52.e9183] [PMID: 25249123]

[42] Hanson DJ. Intramuscular injection injuries and complications. Am J Nurs 1963; 63(4): 99-101.

[43] Green SM, Rothrock SG. Single-dose intramuscular ceftriaxone for acute otitis media in children. Pediatrics 1993; 91(1): 23-30.
[PMID: 8416502]

[44] Fleisher GR, Rosenberg N, Vinci R, *et al.* Intramuscular *Versus* oral antibiotic therapy for the prevention of meningitis and other bacterial sequelae in young, febrile children at risk for occult bacteremia. J Pediatr 1994; 124(4): 504-12.

[http://dx.doi.org/10.1016/S0022-3476(05)83126-9] [PMID: 8151462]

[45] Baker PC, Nelson DS, Schunk JE. The addition of ceftriaxone to oral therapy does not improve outcome in febrile children with urinary tract infections. Arch Pediatr Adolesc Med 2001; 155(2): 135-9.
[http://dx.doi.org/10.1001/archpedi.155.2.135] [PMID: 11177086]

[46] Centers for Disease Control. MMWR weekly report 2015. https://www.cdc.gov/std/tg2015/tg-201--print.pdf

[47] Bignell C, Unemo M. European STI Guidelines Editorial Board. 2012 European guideline on the diagnosis and treatment of gonorrhoea in adults. Int J STD AIDS 2013; 24(2): 85-92.
[http://dx.doi.org/10.1177/0956462412472837] [PMID: 24400344]

[48] Shulman ST, Bisno AL, Clegg HW, *et al.* Infectious Diseases Society of America. Clinical practice guideline for the diagnosis and management of group A streptococcal pharyngitis: 2012 update by the Infectious Diseases Society of America. Clin Infect Dis 2012; 55(10): e86-e102.
[http://dx.doi.org/10.1093/cid/cis629] [PMID: 22965026]

[49] Centers for Disease Control and Prevention. Sexually transmitted diseases treatment guidelines 2015. https://www.cdc.gov/std/tg2015/pid.htm

[50] Lexi-Drugs. http://online.lexi.com

[51] Hopkins U. Large-volume IM injection. A review of best practices. Oncol Nurse Advis 2013; 32-7.

[52] Wynaden D, Landsborough I, Chapman R, McGowan S, Lapsley J, Finn M. Establishing best practice guidelines for administration of intra muscular injections in the adult: a systematic review of the literature. Contemp Nurse 2005; 20(2): 267-77.
[http://dx.doi.org/10.5172/conu.20.2.267] [PMID: 16393108]

[53] Nicoll LH, Hesby A. Intramuscular injection: an integrative research review and guideline for evidence-based practice. Appl Nurs Res 2002; 15(3): 149-62.
[http://dx.doi.org/10.1053/apnr.2002.34142] [PMID: 12173166]

[54] Ravi AD, Sadhna D, Nagpaal D, Chawla L. Needle free injection technology: A complete insight. Int J Pharm Investig 2015; 5(4): 192-9.
[http://dx.doi.org/10.4103/2230-973X.167662] [PMID: 26682189]

[55] Cook AM, Mieure KD, Owen RD, Pesaturo AB, Hatton J. Intracerebroventricular administration of drugs. Pharmacotherapy 2009; 29(7): 832-45.
[http://dx.doi.org/10.1592/phco.29.7.832] [PMID: 19558257]

[56] Srihawan C, Castelblanco RL, Salazar L, *et al.* Clinical characteristics and predictors of adverse outcome in adult and pediatric patients with healthcare-associated ventriculitis and meningitis. Open Forum Infect Dis 2016; 3(2): ofw077.
[http://dx.doi.org/10.1093/ofid/ofw077] [PMID: 27419154]

[57] Rodríguez Guardado A, Blanco A, Asensi V, *et al.* Multidrug-resistant *Acinetobacter* meningitis in neurosurgical patients with intraventricular catheters: assessment of different treatments. J Antimicrob Chemother 2008; 61(4): 908-13.
[http://dx.doi.org/10.1093/jac/dkn018] [PMID: 18281693]

[58] Nau R, Sörgel F, Eiffert H. Penetration of drugs through the blood-cerebrospinal fluid/blood-brain barrier for treatment of central nervous system infections. Clin Microbiol Rev 2010; 23(4): 858-83.
[http://dx.doi.org/10.1128/CMR.00007-10] [PMID: 20930076]

[59] Tunkel AR, Hasbun R, Bhimraj A, *et al.* 2017 Infectious Diseases Society of America's clinical practice guidelines for healthcare-associated ventriculitis and meningitis. Clin Infect Dis 2017; 64(6): e34-65.
[http://dx.doi.org/10.1093/cid/ciw861] [PMID: 28203777]

[60] Cawley MJ, Suh C, Lee S, Ackerman BH. Nontraditional dosing of ampicillin-sulbactam for

multidrug-resistant *Acinetobacter baumannii* meningitis. Pharmacotherapy 2002; 22(4): 527-32.
[http://dx.doi.org/10.1592/phco.22.7.527.33676] [PMID: 11939689]

[61]   Khan SA, Waqas M, Siddiqui UT, *et al.* Intrathecal and intraventricular antibiotics for postoperative
       Gram-negative meningitis and ventriculitis. Surg Neurol Int 2017; 8: 226.
       [http://dx.doi.org/10.4103/sni.sni_81_17] [PMID: 29026662]

[62]   Wang JH, Lin PC, Chou CH, *et al.* Intraventricular antimicrobial therapy in postneurosurgical Gram-
       negative bacillary meningitis or ventriculitis: a hospital-based retrospective study. J Microbiol
       Immunol Infect 2014; 47(3): 204-10.
       [http://dx.doi.org/10.1016/j.jmii.2012.08.028] [PMID: 23201321]

[63]   Remeš F, Tomáš R, Jindrák V, Vaniš V, Setlík M. Intraventricular and lumbar intrathecal
       administration of antibiotics in postneurosurgical patients with meningitis and/or ventriculitis in a
       serious clinical state. J Neurosurg 2013; 119(6): 1596-602.
       [http://dx.doi.org/10.3171/2013.6.JNS122126] [PMID: 23952688]

[64]   Wirt TC, McGee ZA, Oldfield EH, Meacham WF. Intraventricular administration of amikacin for
       complicated Gram-negative meningitis and ventriculitis. J Neurosurg 1979; 50(1): 95-9.
       [http://dx.doi.org/10.3171/jns.1979.50.1.0095] [PMID: 363982]

[65]   Teweldemedhin M, Gebreyesus H, Atsbaha AH, Asgedom SW, Saravanan M. Bacterial profile of
       ocular infections: a systematic review. BMC Ophthalmol 2017; 17(1): 212.
       [http://dx.doi.org/10.1186/s12886-017-0612-2] [PMID: 29178851]

[66]   Bremond-Gignac D, Chiambaretta F, Milazzo S. A European perspective on topical ophthalmic
       antibiotics: current and evolving options. Ophthalmol Eye Dis 2011; 3: 29-43.
       [http://dx.doi.org/10.4137/OED.S4866] [PMID: 23861622]

[67]   Hegde S, Pathengay A. Intravitreal antibiotics.Endophthalmitis A guide to diagnosis and management.
       Singapore: Springer Singapore 2011; pp. 239-51.

[68]   Gan IM, van Dissel JT, Beekhuis WH, Swart W, van Meurs JC. Intravitreal vancomycin and
       gentamicin concentrations in patients with postoperative endophthalmitis. Br J Ophthalmol 2001;
       85(11): 1289-93.
       [http://dx.doi.org/10.1136/bjo.85.11.1289] [PMID: 11673290]

[69]   Daien V, Papinaud L, Gillies MC, *et al.* Effectiveness and safety of an intracameral injection of
       cefuroxime for the prevention of endophthalmitis after cataract surgery with or without perioperative
       capsular rupture. JAMA Ophthalmol 2016; 134(7): 810-6.
       [http://dx.doi.org/10.1001/jamaophthalmol.2016.1351] [PMID: 27136069]

[70]   Haripriya A, Chang DF, Namburar S, Smita A, Ravindran RD. Efficacy of intracameral moxifloxacin
       endophthalmitis prophylaxis at Aravind Eye Hospital. Ophthalmology 2016; 123(2): 302-8.
       [http://dx.doi.org/10.1016/j.ophtha.2015.09.037] [PMID: 26522705]

[71]   George NK, Stewart MW. The routine use of intracameral antibiotics to treat endophthalmitis after
       cataract surgery: How good is the evidence? Ophthalmol Ther 2018; 7(2): 233-45.
       [http://dx.doi.org/10.1007/s40123-018-0138-6] [PMID: 29974362]

[72]   Edmiston CE Jr, Leaper D, Spencer M, *et al.* Considering a new domain for antimicrobial stewardship:
       Topical antibiotics in the open surgical wound. Am J Infect Control 2017; 45(11): 1259-66.
       [http://dx.doi.org/10.1016/j.ajic.2017.04.012] [PMID: 28596018]

[73]   Cowling T, Jones S. https://www.cadth.ca/sites/default/files/pdf/htis/2017/RC0853%20Topical%20
       Antibiotics%20for%20Infected%20Wounds%20Final.pdf

[74]   Falagas ME, Vergidis PI. Irrigation with antibiotic-containing solutions for the prevention and
       treatment of infections. Clin Microbiol Infect 2005; 11(11): 862-7.
       [http://dx.doi.org/10.1111/j.1469-0691.2005.01201.x] [PMID: 16216099]

[75]   Tejwani NC, Immerman I. Myths and legends in orthopaedic practice: are we all guilty? Clin Orthop
       Relat Res 2008; 466(11): 2861-72.

[http://dx.doi.org/10.1007/s11999-008-0458-2] [PMID: 18726654]

[76]   Survey Monkey Inc. Antibiotic stewardship survey. https://www.surveymonkey.com/results/SM-8FST8KPF/

[77]   Bratzler DW, Dellinger EP, Olsen KM, *et al*. American Society of Health-System Pharmacists; Infectious Disease Society of America; Surgical Infection Society; Society for Healthcare Epidemiology of America. Clinical practice guidelines for antimicrobial prophylaxis in surgery. Am J Health Syst Pharm 2013; 70(3): 195-283.
[http://dx.doi.org/10.2146/ajhp120568] [PMID: 23327981]

[78]   World Health Organization. Prevention and management of wound infections. http://www.who.int/hac/techguidance/tools/guidelines_prevention_and_management_wound_infection .pdf

[79]   Church D, Elsayed S, Reid O, Winston B, Lindsay R. Burn wound infections. Clin Microbiol Rev 2006; 19(2): 403-34.
[http://dx.doi.org/10.1128/CMR.19.2.403-434.2006] [PMID: 16614255]

[80]   Dai T, Huang YY, Sharma SK, Hashmi JT, Kurup DB, Hamblin MR. Topical antimicrobials for burn wound infections. Recent Pat Antiinfect Drug Discov 2010; 5(2): 124-51.
[http://dx.doi.org/10.2174/157489110791233522] [PMID: 20429870]

[81]   Barajas-Nava DA. Lopez-Alcalde, Roque I Figuls M, Sola I, Bonfill CX. Antibiotic prophylaxis for preventing burn wound infections. Cochrane Database Syst Rev 2013; 6: 1-177.

[82]   Berbari EF, Kanj SS, Kowalski TJ, *et al*. Infectious Diseases Society of America. 2015 Infectious Disease Society of America (IDSA) clinical practice guidelines for the diagnosis and treatment of native vertebral osteomyelitis in adults. Clin Infect Dis 2015; 61(6): e26-46.
[http://dx.doi.org/10.1093/cid/civ482] [PMID: 26229122]

[83]   Snoddy B, Jayasuriya AC. The use of nanomaterials to treat bone infections. Mater Sci Eng C 2016; 67: 822-33.
[http://dx.doi.org/10.1016/j.msec.2016.04.062] [PMID: 27287180]

[84]   Anagnostakos K. Therapeutic use of antibiotic-loaded bone cement in the treatment of hip and knee joint infections. J Bone Jt Infect 2017; 2(1): 29-37.
[http://dx.doi.org/10.7150/jbji.16067] [PMID: 28529862]

[85]   Masri BA, Duncan CP, Beauchamp CP, Paris NJ, Arntorp J. Tobramycin and vancomycin elution from bone cement. An *in vivo* and *in vitro* study. Orthop Trans 1994; 18: 130.

[86]   Hsieh PH, Chang YH, Chen SH, Ueng SW, Shih CH. High concentration and bioactivity of vancomycin and aztreonam eluted from Simplex cement spacers in two-stage revision of infected hip implants: a study of 46 patients at an average follow-up of 107 days. J Orthop Res 2006; 24(8): 1615-21.
[http://dx.doi.org/10.1002/jor.20214] [PMID: 16788986]

[87]   Bergogne-Bérézin E, Bryskier A. The suppository form of antibiotic administration: pharmacokinetics and clinical application. J Antimicrob Chemother 1999; 43(2): 177-85.
[http://dx.doi.org/10.1093/jac/43.2.177] [PMID: 11252322]

[88]   Bergström BK, Bertilson SO, Movin G. Clinical evaluation of rectally administered ampicillin in acute otitis media. J Int Med Res 1988; 16(5): 376-85.
[http://dx.doi.org/10.1177/030006058801600507] [PMID: 3197915]

[89]   Iwai N, Sasaki A, Taneda Y, Mizoguchi F, Nakamura H. [Clinical evaluation of an ampicillin suppository (KS-R1) in respiratory tract infections in children]. Jpn J Antibiot 1983; 36(7): 1851-62.
[PMID: 6655814]

[90]   Acerbi L, De La Pierre L, Periette L, Coppi G. Bioavailability studies of erythromycin administered by rectal route in paediatric patients. Chemoterapia 1983; 2: 200-2.

[91] Stratchunsky LS, Nazarov AD, Firsov AA, Petrachenkova NA. Age dependence of erythromycin rectal bioavailability in children. Eur J Drug Metab Pharmacokinet 1991; 3(Spec No 3): 321-3. [PMID: 1820902]

[92] Luke DR, Foulds G, Going PC, Melnik G, Lawrence V. Rectal azithromycin in healthy subjects. In: Zinner SH, Ed. Expanding indications of the New Macrolides, Azalides, and Streptogramins. New York: Marcel Dekker 1997; pp. 474-7.

[93] Bergan T, Arnold E. Pharmacokinetics of metronidazole in healthy adult volunteers after tablets and suppositories. Chemotherapy 1980; 26(4): 231-41. [http://dx.doi.org/10.1159/000237911] [PMID: 7389423]

[94] Sellers S, Utian WH. Pharmacy compounding primer for physicians: prescriber beware. Drugs 2012; 72(16): 2043-50. [http://dx.doi.org/10.2165/11640850-000000000-00000] [PMID: 23039281]

[95] Department of Health and Human Services. https://oig.hhs.gov/oei/reports/oei-03-13-00270.pdf

[96] McPherson T, Fontane P, Iyengar R, Henderson R. Utilizations and costs of compounded medications for commercially insured patients. 2012-2013. J Manag Care Spec Pharm 2016; 22(2): 172-81. [http://dx.doi.org/10.18553/jmcp.2016.22.2.172] [PMID: 27015256]

[97] Center of Disease Control. https://www.cdc.gov/hai/outbreaks/meningitis-map-large.html

[98] American Society of Retinal Specialists. Compounding listening session. https://www.asrs.org/content/documents/asrsfdalisteningsession2016.pdf

CHAPTER 4

Molecular Basis of Resistance I

Adebowale O. Adeluola[1,*] and **Kolawole S. Oyedeji**[2]

[1] *Department of Pharmaceutical Microbiology and Biotechnology, Faculty of Pharmacy, College of Medicine campus, University of Lagos. Lagos, Nigeria*

[2] *Department of Medical Laboratory Science, College of Medicine, University of Lagos, Lagos, Nigeria*

Abstract: This section of the treatise discussed the molecular basis of bacteria resistance exhibited phenotypically as a result of an inherent genotypic makeup of the bacterial cell (intrinsic). It could also result from mutational changes of the bacterial genes or through a process by which resistance genes are acquired through transfer from one bacterial cell to another (acquired). Some of the mechanisms of resistance discussed result from the encoding genes of the enzymes responsible for the enzymatic destruction of antibiotics. For example, virginiamycin acetyltransferases (VATs), which inactivate the type A streptogramins; aminoglycoside phosphotransferases (APHs), also known as aminoglycoside kinases, which inactivate aminoglycosides and the thioltransferases, a fosfomycin resistance enzyme (mediated by fos B). All of these have been located in some Gram-positive pathogens. Bacteria resistance due to alteration of binding sites is evident in penicillin-binding proteins (PBP), which is mediated by the mecA gene of methicillin-resistant *S. aureus* (MRSA). This gives elevated resistance levels against methicillin amongst other β-lactam antibiotics. Similarly, in vancomycin-resistant enterococci (VRE), the gene clusters of VanA and VanB are responsible for encoding the enzymes which catalyze the production of the modified peptidoglycan precursor in *Enterococcus faecium* and *Enterococcus faecalis*. Fluoroquinolone antibiotic resistance results from a situation whereby two enzymes are inhibited in the process of synthesis of bacterial DNA. These are DNA gyrase with 2 subunits encoded in the gyrA and gyrB genes and the Topoisomerase IV with subunits encoded in the parC and parE genes. The macrolide, lincosamide and streptogramin B resistance are observed following a transcriptional modification of the 23S rRNA portion of the 50S ribosomal subunit of the resistant organism. Meanwhile, trimethoprim resistance, due to mutation in the dhfr gene, is known in Gram-positive bacteria. Resistance in *Staphylococcus aureus* strains is known to be due to mutations to varying levels in Isoleucyl-tRNA synthetase genes, mupA and ileS. The resistance to fusidic acid through point mutations has been identified in the fusA gene, which is chromosomally located in clinical isolates and laboratory selected resistant isolates of Gram-positive organisms.

* **Corresponding author Adebowale O. Adeluola**: Department of Pharmaceutical Microbiology and Biotechnology, Faculty of Pharmacy, College of Medicine campus, University of Lagos. Lagos, Nigeria. E-mail:aadeluola@unilag.edu.ng

Islam M. Ghazi & Michael J. Cawley (Eds.)

The other form of resistance observed in Gram-positive and some other bacteria is due to the activities of bacterial antibiotic efflux transporters. These are categorized into five different groups otherwise known as families: The small multidrug resistance (SMR) family, the major facilitator superfamily (MFS), the adenosine triphosphate (ATP)-binding cassette (ABC) superfamily, the resistance-nodulation-cell division (RND) superfamily and the Multidrug and toxic compound extrusion (MATE) family. Concisely, having a good knowledge of the efflux pump inhibitors (EPI) is important in the development of combination drugs, which can improve the activity of otherwise ineffective antibiotics. Therefore, based on the above discourse, this chapter will be discussing the molecular basis of resistant Gram-positive bacteria to antibiotics based on drug inactivation and modifications and how this constitutes a great challenge to the control of infectious diseases by these organisms.

Keywords: Antibiotics resistant genes, Efflux transporters, Gram-positive bacteria, Molecular antimicrobial resistance, Resistance inducing enzymes.

MEANS OF BACTERIAL PROPAGATION

The ability of Bacterial species to develop resistance to existing antibiotics at a much faster rate as compared to new antibiotic drug molecules is being developed. This is a continued challenge to clinicians in their effort to treat bacterial infections in patients. Bacterial resistance to antibiotics may be due to the inherent phenotypic or genotypic make-up of the bacterial cell. In this case, it is referred to as "Intrinsic". On the other hand, it may be "acquired" through mutation of the genes of the bacterial cell or by the acquisition of resistance genes through horizontal transfer of genes from one bacterial cell to another. Mostly, acquired resistance is inferred when a previously sensitive bacterium becomes resistant to the same antibiotic.

The mutation has been described as a genetic alteration that could occur on the spur-of-the-moment, even in the absence of the antibiotic. Any such bacterial organism bearing this kind of mutation will produce a resistant subpopulation while other cells which continue to be susceptible are swiftly being eliminated by the antibacterial agent [1]. Gene mutations are of two types. It could be a spontaneous mutation, and it could be a mutation at the level of the chromosome. These mutations may be as a result of mistakes during the process of replication or due to an error during the repair of damaged DNA. Mutations at the level of the chromosomes are rare but often translates to resistance to structurally related compounds. Horizontal gene transfer occurs between bacterial strains, which may or may not be of the same species. It may also occur between bacterial cells irrespective of species or genera [2].

The propagation of bacteria occurs through various means. One is the simple binary fission in which there is a division of the chromosome into two identical circles. Each of these segregates at the ends of the cell, directly opposite to each other. The cell wall grows inwards through the middle of the cell. With these, two new identical cells are formed, each having a separate cell wall and nucleus. These two cells so formed are exact copies of the old mother cell without the loss of any genetic material and no formation of any new genetic material [3].

Another means of bacterial propagation is genetic exchange, a process that may arise between adjacent cells giving rise to some form of sexual reproduction. The genetic exchange can occur *via* the following processes:

a. Transformation
b. Conjugation and
c. Transduction

Transformation

Before DNA and its role in genetic coding and bacterial genetics was known, Griffith in 1928 found that certain strains of capsule deficient *Streptococcus pneumonia* could be converted to normal capsule producing *Streptococcus pneumonia* cells by merely adding a filtered culture (cell-free), from which cells with normal capsules were previously grown. The material in the cell filtrate, which made this possible, was later shown to be DNA. Transformation is a process whereby a cell takes up "naked" DNA released by lyses of other cells. This process is now being used to introduce plasmid DNA material from one bacterial population to another. The recipient cell must be in the early log phase of growth. The extraneous DNA material can be integrated into the host genetic apparatus while replacing a part of the original genome through a process called genetic recombination. However, transformation occurs in only a few bacterial genera.

Conjugation

Through a natural process, certain bacterial genera are involved in the active exchange of genetic material between contiguously placed cells *via* the F-pili (sex-Pili). This process, discovered in 1946, did not make it possible to designate male and female bacteria, in spite of its resemblance to the complex generation exchange found in leukocytes. However, bacteria capable of effective transfer either in part or in whole contain a fertility factor in their genetic make-up. This is designated as F+ strains, while those who received them are designated F- strains.

Conjugation may therefore be considered as a natural process, which represents the early stages of a true sexually reproductive process.

There is a pairing between F+ and the F- strains during which a conjugation bridge is built between them through the F-pili. Once pairing is completed, the F-plasmid is replicated and one copy passes over to the F- strain. F-plasmid is also capable of being integrated into the chromosome to produce Hfr (High frequency of recombination) male. When Hfr+ are mixed together with F- strain, conjugation occurs as in the case of F+ strain and F- strain. Chromosomal replication begins in the Hfr cell and one of the replicates is transferred to the F-strain starting with a position of the F-plasmid [4]. There are certain mobile components in bacterial cells known as conjugative transposons, plasmids, and insertion sequences. These act as carriers of many antibiotic resistance genes. With these, transfer of DNA across genera and species is enabled by conjugation of plasmids that host a wide range of resistance genes. This is not so in the case of Transformation and Transduction, which are usually more restricted to the same species [5]. Usually, conjugation among Gram-positive bacteria begins with the production of a Conjugation Bridge (sex pheromones), built through the F-pili between the mating pair. This enables the exchange of DNA through the enhanced clumping of donor and recipient cells. Plasmids are in the form of circular pieces of DNA that are capable of self-replication. Plasmids are smaller in size than the bacterial genome, which encodes their transfer through replication into other bacterial strains or species. Plasmids are capable of carrying and transferring multiple resistance genes located at the segment of DNA that are capable of relocating from one plasmid to another plasmid, to the genome or a transposon (jumping gene). Transposons possess the significant ability to spread resistance genes through a wide range of bacterial cells. This is quite unlike for the plasmids, which have limited capability to spread resistance across the cell.

Transduction

This is common with the group of viruses called bacteriophages. Bacteriophage is a group of viruses which can attack bacterial cell. Viral DNA injected into the bacterial cells then proceeds to make new viral particles which later destroy the cell. There are some of these viral particles which are known as temperate viruses. These can pass on the genetic material from one cell to another without destroying their host cell [6].

MECHANISMS/BASIS OF ANTIMICROBIAL RESISTANCE

In antibiotic resistance, four major biochemical mechanisms are of significance.

Antibiotic Modification

Antibiotic modification is the best-known mechanism for antimicrobial resistance. The same sensitive target site present in antibiotic sensitive strains is still present in the resistant bacteria, but the antibiotic is rendered ineffective and unable to act on it in its modified form. A good example is a case with the β lactamases. The four-membered β-lactam ring is cleaved by the β-lactamase enzyme, which renders the antibiotic inactive. Most of the β-lactamase enzymes that have been described in the literature act against both the penicillins and cephalosporins to varying degrees. Examples are the cephalosporinases, mediated by the AmpC gene, which have been detected in *Enterobacter spp* and the penicillinases found in the *Staphylococcus aureus*. B-lactamases occur widely amid both Gram-positive and Gram-negative bacterial species. They are inhibited to varying degrees by β lactamase inhibitors, *e.g.,* clavulanic acid [7].

Alterations in The Primary Site of Action

Due to the structural changes in the molecular structure of the target site of action, the antibiotic may penetrate the cytoplasm of the cell and reach the target site, but it may not be able to inhibit the biochemical activity of the cell at the target site. For example, the enterococci are considered to be inherently resistant to the class of cephalosporins. This is because the cell wall transpeptidase (CWT) enzymes, which is responsible for the production of the polymer, peptidoglycan in the course of the synthesis of its cell wall, is also the substrate for the antibiotic and sometimes referred to as penicillin-binding proteins (PBPs). The modified forms are less attracted to the cephalosporins and consequently not inhibited.

The majority of *Streptococcus pneumoniae* strains are very much susceptible to penicillins and cephalosporins. However, with their ability to acquire DNA from other bacteria, there can be alterations in the peptidoglycan forming enzyme to the extent that they become resistant to inhibition by the penicillins. As a result, a lower affinity for penicillins is thereby developed [8].

Reduction in Drug Accumulation in Bacterial Cells

The targets of antibiotic action are protected by retarding the access of the antibiotic into the cell or by extrusion of the antibiotic out of the cell at a faster rate than it can flow into the cell.

Production of Alternative Target

Self-preservation by bacteria from antibacterial agents may be as a result of a fourth biochemical mechanism. This could be in the form of the concurrent production of an alternative enzyme substrate as a substitute target. This alternative target is not subjected to inhibition by the antibiotic despite the continued production of the original sensitive target. The alternative penicillin-binding protein (PBP) 2a is a very good example of this mechanism. PBP 2a is produced alongside the "normal" penicillin-binding proteins (PBPs) produced by methicillin-resistant *Staphylococcus aureus* (MRSA). Since, PBP2a is not inhibited by some β-lactam antibiotics, *e.g.*, flucloxacillin, the cell continues to manufacture peptidoglycan, resulting in the production of a cell wall with a strong structure [9]. In the case of vancomycin sensitive enterococci (VSE), a cell wall precursor which contains a penta-peptide with a D-alanine-D-alanine ending, which may bind onto the vancomycin, is the normal target of vancomycin. This binding thus prevents the continued synthesis of the cell wall. Vancomycin-resistant enterococci (VRE) discovered about three decades ago, is known to have a variant of the target which can produce the substitute cell wall precursor with a D-alanine-D-lactate ending that has little or no affinity for vancomycin [10]. This has generated much interest because of the possibility of a genetic transfer to *S. aureus*, and theoretically, this can bring about the production of vancomycin resistance in MRSA.

MOLECULAR BASIS OF RESISTANCE

Drug Inactivation or Modification: Enzymatic Degradation of Antibiotics

Streptogramin Acetyltransferases

Streptogramin acetyltransferases, also known as VATs (virginiamycin acetyltransferase), can bring about the inactivation of the type A streptogramins. This occurs at position 14 of the chemical structure of type A streptogramins, when the free hydroxyl groups are acetylated. The genes encoding the five known VAT enzymes have been detected in some Gram-positive pathogens, including the staphylococci and enterococci [11].

Phosphotransferases Kinases

The Phosphotransferases Kinases are enzymes that act by catalyzing the transfer of the phosphate group from ATP (adenosine triphosphate) to different types of substrates. Among them are the *O*-phosphotransferases such as Ser, Thr, and Tyr kinases. Some others are the sugar kinases, such as the hexokinase, and the amino acid kinases (*e.g.* aspartate kinase). The *O*-phosphotransferases are antibiotic kinases that are well known for their involvement in the resistance.

Aminoglycoside Kinases

Aminoglycoside kinases are also termed as aminoglycoside phosphotransferases (APHs). They are very common with pathogenic bacteria. The dramatic effect on the ability of the antibiotics to bind to their target on the A-site of the ribosome is due to the phosphorylation of the antibiotics [12]. Multi-drug resistant integrons, transposons, and R plasmids are often the carriers of the genes encoding these enzymes. Therefore, even in the absence of wide usage of aminoglycosides in a particular environment, the genes coding for its resistance may still be present in the bacterial population in that environment [12]. Among the aminoglycoside kinases are APH (3") encoded by the gene, *StrA* and APH (6) encoded by the gene, *StrB*. Both of which modify streptomycin and APH (9) (the enzyme capable of modifying spectinomycin) [13]. The four APH (2") enzymes are encoded by 4 genes, *aph (2")* – *Ia to Id*. They are highly problematic in the clinic conferring various levels of resistance against most of the clinically used aminoglycosides such as kanamycin, gentamicin and tobramycin [12, 13]. The bifunctional enzyme, AAC (6') – APH (2"), which is encoded by the *aph (2")* – *Ia* gene, is widely dispersed among pathogenic bacteria and bestows a high level of resistance to most aminoglycosides except streptomycin and spectinomycin. The AAC (6') domain also gives resistance to fortimicin antibiotics. This AAC is also unusual by the fact that it has some measures of *O*-acetyltransferase activity. It can, therefore, modify aminoglycosides like paromomycin [12, 13].

Macrolide Kinases

Resistance to antibiotics like macrolides, *e.g.*, erythromycin and peptide antibiotics like viomycin, has been achieved through the molecular strategy of covalent modification by phosphate. Certain macrolide kinases, MPHs and viomycin kinase (Vph) have been cloned and well defined. The MPHs have been detected in *S. aureus* [14, 15]. Modification of the macrolide occurs on the hydroxyl group at position 23 of its structure and is thought to interfere with its binding to RNA polymerase. Thioltransferases, the reactive epoxides of fosfomycin, make fosfomycin vulnerable to nucleophilic ring-opening reactions. The fosfomycin resistance enzyme fosB is usually detected on resistance plasmids present in Gram-positive bacteria, such as staphylococci, and also on the chromosome of *Bacillus subtilis* [14, 15]. A modification of the inactivation method becomes necessary as a result of the absence of glutathione in these

Gram-positive bacteria thus making FosB an efficient fosfomycin Cys transferase.

Nucleotidyltransferases

The two major classes of nucleotidyltransferases include the ANTs (which can modify aminoglycosides) and the Lin proteins (that render the lincosaminide antibiotics such as lincomycin and its semi-synthetic derivative-clindamycin ineffective). The NMP portion of NTPs are moved by these enzymes to a receptive hydroxyl group on the antibiotic. The three-dimensional structure of ANT (4', 4") from *S. aureus* is well known. Three known and characterized lincosaminide nucleotidyl transferase genes include linA from *Staphylococcus haemoliticus*, linAV from *Staphylococcus aureus*, and linB from *Enterococcus faecium* [16, 15]. LinA and LinAV are known to transform clindamycin structure at position 4 while linB act by modifying lincomycin at position 3.

Glycosyltransferases

To a large extent, glycosyltransfer is not commonly regarded as a mechanism of antibiotic resistance. However, it plays a role in self-preservation in organisms that produce antibiotics. Glycosylation of the macrolide structure in *Streptomyces lividans* from the product of the mtg gene is a typical example from this class [17, 18]. The enzyme from the mtg gene catalyzes glycosylation of erythromycin and other macrolides at position 2' of the hexosamine sugar. UDP glucose is used as the glucose donor. Rifampim glycosylation at position 23 by *Nocardia* species has been reported as well, although the characterization of the enzymes has not been reported [17].

DNA Gyrase and Topoisomerase IV

In the process of bacterial DNA synthesis, inhibition of DNA gyrase and Topoisomerase IV enzymes are the main targets of the Fluoroquinolone antibiotics [19, 20]. There are 4 DNA gyrase subunits consisting of 2 each of GyrA and GyrB, each of which is encoded by *gyrA* and *gyrB* genes, respectively. The DNA replication is disrupted during the formation of the DNA double helix by DNA gyrase enzyme. It occurs by introducing negative superhelical twists before the replication fork. At the end of each round of replication, the unlinking or decatenation of interlinked daughter chromosomes is the responsibility of the Topoisomerase IV enzyme. The Topoisomerase IV enzyme, like the DNA gyrase has 4 sub-units of 2 ParC (GrlA in *Staphylococcus aureus*), encoded by the *parC* gene and 2 ParE subunits (GrlB in *Staphylococcus aureus*) encoded by the parE gene. These two enzymes are of utmost importance in the separation of daughter chromosomes in the course of replication. The complexes created between DNA and the DNA gyrase or topoisomerase IV enzymes act as the point of interaction with Fluoroquinolones. This disrupts the normal conformation resulting in the inhibition of normal enzyme activity. By binding to the enzyme–DNA complex, they bring about stability of the DNA strand breaks created by DNA gyrase and topoisomerase IV. The three-fold complexes of drug, enzyme and DNA hinder the progress of the replication fork. The activity of fluoroquinolone is a result of the conversion of the topoisomerase–quinolone–DNA complex to an irreversible form and the generation of double-strand breaks in DNA through the denaturation of the topoisomerase. Resistance to fluoroquinolones can therefore be a result of mutations at the level of the chromosomes in both the DNA gyrase and topoisomerase IV target enzymes [20, 21].

Mutations in the GyrA subunit occur in the quinolone resistance-determining region of the gyrA gene which encodes the portion of the GyrA subunit that is bound to DNA during enzyme activity. Resistance resulting from decreased drug affinity for the altered gyrase–DNA complex is brought about by the most common genetic alterations in this region [20, 22]. GyrB mutations are not as common as the gyrA mutations. Rather, they are clustered in a corresponding quinolone resistance-determining region or domain but their effect on drug binding is still unclear. The levels of resistance produced by GyrB mutations are lower than that produced by mutations in *gyrA* gene. Changes in Topoisomerase IV resulting from mutations in ParC or ParE also occur in Gram-negative bacteria but do not seem to be of much importance. This is so because resistance to fluoroquinolone will only take place when there are concomitant mutations present in the DNA gyrase.

In the case of Gram-positive bacteria, the situation is the reverse. Here, the Topoisomerase IV is the primary target while the DNA gyrase serves as a secondary target. Thus, the occurrence in DNA gyrase mutations are less frequent than in topoisomerase IV. For Gram-positive bacteria which are fluoroquinolone-resistant, mutations in Topoisomerase IV may occur in subunit especially in *S. aureus* and *S. pneumoniae*. Although genetic alterations in ParC (GrlA in *S. aureus*) occur more frequently than in ParE (GrlB in *S. aureus*), they are assumed to be of greater significance in their role in resistance [20, 23]. The ParC subunit has a similar region domain that determines quinolone resistance and this resistance is assumed to be a result of lower attraction to the drug [20].

The macrolide, lincosamide and streptogramin B group of antibiotics are able to hinder protein synthesis in bacteria through the process of binding to the 50S ribosomal subunit. The resistance to this group of antibiotic is referred to as the

MLS(B) type resistance which occurs widely among Gram-positive and Gram-negative bacteria. The MLS(B) type resistance is consequent upon a modification of the 23S rRNA, component of the 50S ribosomal subunit following the process of transcription, a process which involves either the methylation or demethylation of vital adenine bases in the peptidyl transferase functional domain. Macrolide-resistant *Streptococcus pneumoniae* has exhibited alterations in the L4 and L22 proteins of the 50S subunit in furtherance to manifold mutations taking place in the 23S rRNA. Telithromycin which is a ketolide maintains activity against bacterial isolates which develop their resistance characteristics from these mechanisms. As for the oxazolidinones, such as linezolid, their mechanism of action involves multiple stages in protein synthesis. Whereas, they bind to the 50S subunit, yet interfere with translocation of peptidyl-tRNA, from the A site to the P site and with inhibition of the formation of the initiation complex form part of the effects [20, 24]. Mutations in the 23S rRNA leading to the reduced affinity for binding have been linked to resistance which has been reported in a number of organisms [20, 25]. G to U substitutions are involved in most mutations at position 2576 in the peptidyl transferase region of 23S rRNA, which is a part of the P site. Increased resistance of VRE bacteraemia isolates to linezolid due to which this mutation has been detected within a six-month period of use [20, 26].

Other Mechanisms of Resistance

There are some other examples of mechanisms of resistance that are based on enzymatic reactions that have not been commonly exploited by pathogenic bacteria. These include Redox enzymes Oxidation. This Redox enzyme oxidation is a mechanism for the detoxification of xenobiotics in mammals which occurs mainly through a unit of membrane-bound cytochrome P-450s with a wide-ranging substrate specificity that brings about the hydroxylation of xenobiotics, thus facilitating their excretion. A good example of some of the best-studied cases includes the activity of TetX enzyme through its oxidation of tetracycline antibiotics [15, 17]. The gene that encodes for TetX detected in the obligate anaerobe *Bacteroides fragilis,* was found located on conjugative transposons. The monohydroxylation of tetracycline antibiotics by TetX is catalyzed at position 11a. This leads to the disruption of the Mg^{2+}-binding site of the antibiotic which is a key requirement for its antibacterial activity. A non-enzymatic rearrangement of the antibiotic into unstable products that polymerize into a black product after several hours comes into effect after the TetX-catalyzed hydroxylation [15].

In one example of redox-mediated resistance, another predicted monooxygenase with the ability to inactivate antibiotic is cloned from *Rhodococcus equi, a* rifampin-resistant microorganism. Some other examples include *Streptomyces virginiae*, a producer of the type A streptogramin antibiotic, virginiamycin M1. It produces an inactive compound by bringing about the reduction of a critical ketone group to alcohol at position 16, and thus protects itself from its own antibiotic. This reduction generates the (14S, 16R)-dihydrovirginiamycin M1 isomer entirely with the aid of NADPH and it is also specific [15]. The type B streptogramin resistance which stems from the antibiotic resistance lyase, Vgb, has been extensively studied. Vgb is known to be cloned from streptogramin B-resistant staphylococci. Earlier studies reported it to be a lactonase with hydrolytic properties which is connected with the opening of the ring of the antibiotic around the susceptible ester bond [15, 17].

Examples of inhibitors of the bacterial enoyl reductase, encoded by *fabI* are the antibacterial agents namely, triclosan and hexachlorophene. This enzyme catalyzes the reduction of β-unsaturated fatty acids esterified to the acyl carrier protein (ACP), which is an important phase in the biosynthetic cycle of the fatty acid. The *FabI* enzymes from *S. aureus* use NADPH as cofactor.

In *S. aureus,* mupirocin resistance is a result of alterations in isoleucyl-tRNA synthetase which is also the target enzyme. High-level resistance with about 512 µg/ml MIC levels is recognized to be plasmid-mediated. It is also known to involve the acquisition of a second gene, the mupA which codes for the mupirocin-resistant isoleucyl-tRNA synthetase enzyme. Low-level resistance in the range of 8 to 256 µg/ml MIC levels in clinical isolates and in strains trained *in vitro* to attain high resistance levels, results from point mutations of isoleucyl-tRNA synthetase gene, *ileS* present in the chromosome [20]. Val-to-Phe changes at either residue 588 (V588F) or residue 631 (V631F) of the synthetase produced by point mutations have been identified in resistant *S. aureus strains* [20, 27].

Due to the interference with the function of elongation factor G (EF-G), Fusidic acid is able to block bacterial protein synthesis in staphylococci [20]. *Staphylococcus aureus* resistance to fusidic acid comes as a result of modifications in the target appearing in natural mutants and which are harbored at low rates in the normal populations of staphylococci. Among clinical and laboratory selected fusidic acid-resistant isolates, point mutations in *fusA* gene which encode for EF-G within the chromosome have been identified [20, 28]. Moreover, L461K, P406L, and H457Y alterations in EF-G created by mutagenesis at specific sites have been revealed to bring about increased MIC of fusidic acid among sensitive laboratory bacterial strains to those levels observed in resistant clinical isolates [20, 28]. Table **1** highlights the biochemical homologues exhibited by antibiotic-producing organisms [29].

Table 1. Resistance determinants with biochemical homologues in antibiotic-producing organisms [29].

Antibiotic	Resistance Mechanisms
Penicillins, Cephalosporins	β-lactamases, penicillin-binding proteins
Aminoglycosides	Acetyltransferases, phosphotransferases adenyltransferases
Chloramphenicol	Acetyltransferases
Tetracyclines	efflux system ribosomal protection
Macrolides Streptogramins, Lincosamides	ribosomal RNA methylation esterases, phosphotransferases acetyltransferases
Phosphonates	phosphorylation glutathionylation
Bleomycin	acetyltransferase immunity protein
Vancomycin	D-Ala-D-Lac ligase

Alteration of Target/Binding Sites - Penicillin Binding Proteins (PBP)

Phenotypic expression of the mecA gene in MRSA results in the high-level of resistance exhibited towards β-lactam antibiotics and methicillin [20, 30]. The penicillin-binding protein 2a, which is also referred to as PBP2' is encoded by the mecA gene. PBP2a is one of the biosynthetic enzymes which catalyze the formation of the peptidoglycan linkages in the course of the construction of cell wall in bacteria. This gene is borne on a large genetic element referred to as 'the staphylococcal cassette chromosome mec' (SCCmec). It is incorporated into the chromosomes of MRSA close to the source of replication [20, 30]. A coagulase-negative *Staphylococcus species, Staphylococcus sciuri* which is a known animal pathogen is believed to be the source of SCCmec through genetic transfer. Types I to V and a few known variants of SCCmec are currently recognized in literature [31]. The β-lactam antibiotics and a PBP form a reversible non-covalent complex. At the active site of the enzyme, an oxygen atom of a serine residue then initiates a nucleophilic attack on the side chain of the β-lactam ring. A relatively stable covalent complex in which the serine is acylated by the hydrolysed β-lactam is then formed [20, 30]. A number of new agents such as β-lactam antibiotics that retain activity against PBP2a and MRSA have been reported in literature. These are currently in various stages of development. Among them are modified cephalosporins, carbapenems and a trinem [20, 30].

Formation of a mosaic of PBPs with decreased attraction for β-lactam antibiotics is accountable for resistance to β-lactam antibiotics in *Streptococcus pneumoniae*. The existence of changed forms of PBP1a and 2a are responsible for resistance to the third-generation cephalosporins while penicillin resistance is a result of alterations in PBP2b [20, 30]. Five PBPs with naturally low affinity and having low susceptibility to β-lactams are present in *Enterococcus faecalis* while six can be detected in *Enterococcus faecium*. The PBPs 3 and 4 of *Enterococcus faecalis* and PBPs 4 and 5 of *Enterococcus faecium are the* target enzymes to the β-lactam antibiotics [20, 30]. The highly resistant strains of *E. faecium* overproduce the PBP 5 with low level affinity, unlike the PBP 5 with lower penicillin-binding capacity present in moderately resistant strains. Resistance to β-Lactams without the production of β-lactamase in *Haemophilus influenzae* has been reported in Japan. Multiple mutations are known in the ftsI gene which encodes PBP 3.

Investigation into the PBPs of a strain of *Listeria monocytogenes,* having diminished susceptibility to imipenem and penicillin G showing higher susceptibility to cefotaxime, gives the notion that the modification of PBP 3 might be the cause of the diminished susceptibility to penicillin and imipenem. It also gives one impression that PBP 3 may be a crucial target of β-lactam antibiotics in *L. monocytogenes* [20, 30].

Vancomycin and teicoplanin are the glycopeptide antibiotics which bind non-covalently to the peptidyl-d-alanyl-d-alanine (d-Ala-d-Ala) terminal of peptidoglycan N- precursors. Through the activity of the transglycosylase, they are able to block their integration into the cell wall and thereby obstruct the synthesis of bacterial cell wall [20]. Vancomycin resistant S. *aureus* (VRSA) exhibit some changes in their cell wall metabolism when compared with vancomycin susceptible *Staphylococcus aureus* (VSSA) control strains. Their cell wall thickness increases 2-fold the ratio of peptidoglycan stem peptides which contains the non-amidated glutamine residues increased with a resultant reduction in peptidoglycan cross-linking [20, 31]. The development of intermediate level of vancomycin resistance through an affinity trapping mechanism may have been caused by these factors. The many binding sites for vancomycin present on the thicker cell wall have been shown to be capable of trapping the antibiotic molecules. This results in a reduction in the amount of vancomycin molecules that may get to the cytoplasmic membrane, which is the location of the targets of the transglycosylase [20, 31].

The presence of either of the two related gene clusters, termed VanA and VanB often results in the alteration of the peptidoglycan precursors thereby causing resistance to the glycopeptide antibiotics in *E. faecium* and *E. faecalis*. The *VanA* and *VanB* gene clusters are responsible for encoding the enzymes that produce the altered forms of the peptidoglycan precursor, which ends in d-Alanyl-d-Lactate (d-Ala-dLac) instead of d-Ala-d-Ala. The glycopeptides bind to d-Ala-d-Lac with much-reduced affinity than to d-Ala-d-Ala [20, 31]. *VanA* and *VanB* gene clusters responsible for conferring resistance traits are located on transposable elements. The spreading of these resistance genes to other bacterial species such as enterococci is done by both transposition and plasmid transfer.

VanD in *E. faecium*; *VanE* and *VanG* in *E. faecalis* are other uncommon types of the acquired resistance gene clusters [20, 31]. Manifold alterations in peptidoglycan composition manifest as a result of the occurrence of two different antibiotic resistance mechanisms in the same strain, which are encoded by *SCCmecA* in the chromosome on the one hand, and the *VanA* cluster on a plasmid on the other hand. The assemblage of modified peptidoglycan results from the use of different sets of enzymes which are encoded by the two gene clusters [20].

Reduced Drug Accumulation and Increasing Active Efflux

Reduced drug accumulation within the cell cytoplasm results from decreasing drug permeability through the cell membrane and/or increasing active efflux (pumping out) of the drugs from the cell cytoplasm across the cell surface.

Proteins of the Outer Membrane Porins

There are special proteins which possess genetic codes for *ompF*, *ompC*, and *phoE* genes in *E. coli K-12*. These are called 'Porins'. These porins are able to produce relatively nonspecific pores or channels which allow small hydrophilic molecules to move across the outer membrane of the *E. coli K-12* cell. The physiological capability of porins to selectively allow the diffusion of certain nutrients, antibiotics, and/or inhibitors across an outer membrane barrier has been demonstrated by using mutants having no porins [32 - 35]. Other strains of enteric bacteria, such as *S. typhimurium* LT2 at times, produce additional porins like the *OmpD* porin [36], the prophage-coded protein 2 or Lc of *E. coli* [37, 38], and protein K, found among encapsulated strains of *E. coli* [39 - 41]. A modification of the outer membrane porin may restrict the passage of antibiotics through them into the cell cytoplasm thus compounding the problem of antibiotic resistance.

Efflux Pump Activity

The drug efflux transporters of bacteria belong to five known families as shown below. The known families include the:

Major Facilitator Superfamily (MFS)

MFS transporters commonly work as single-component pumps as in *NorA* of *Staphylococcus aureus* [42, 43]. They are involved in the movement of sugars, metabolites, anions and drugs. There are three subfamilies of the MFS proteins that influence drug efflux. These include drug/H+ antiporter (DHA) 1 (*e.g., Bmr* of Bacillus subtilis), DHA2 (*e.g.*, *QacA* of *S. aureus* and DHA3 (*e.g.*, *MefA* of *Streptococcus pyogenes*). Members of the DHA3 subfamily which are present only in the prokaryotes are known to efflux macrolides and tetracycline, amongst other antibiotics. Although most of them confer resistance to tetracycline, they are ineffective against minocycline or glycylcyclines [44, 45].

The adenosine triphosphate (ATP)-binding cassette (ABC) superfamily

This is made up of both uptake and efflux transport systems. Members of the ABC superfamily utilize energy obtained from the hydrolytic process on ATP to transport various substances such as sugars, polysaccharides, ions, amino acids, drugs and proteins. Drug efflux pumps of the ABC-superfamily are not so common in bacteria. The LmrA pump of *Lactococcus lactis* is perhaps the best-known example of this family [44, 45].

Small Multidrug Resistance (SMR) Family

The transporters of the SMR family are made up of about 110 amino acid residues containing 4 TMS. They utilize energy generated by the proton-motive force. The pump in this family, which has been well studied, such as the Smr pump of *S. aureus* [45] is capable of effluxing drugs, dyes, and cations.

Resistance-Nodulation-Cell Division (RND) Superfamily

The RND drug transporters were originally known to be encoded by genes of chromosomal origin. However, RND drug transporter, which is encoded by plasmid, has been recorded recently. RND pumps are known to feature prominently the acquired and intrinsic resistance of Gram-negative bacteria to diverse antimicrobial agents. All RND pumps that have been studied to date are known to be multidrug transporters [44].

Multidrug and Toxic Compound Extrusion (MATE) Family

NorM of *Vibrio parahaemolyticus* is a good example of proteins of this family [44]. The length of these proteins is about 450 amino acid residues. They also contain 12 transmembrane domains. The proteins that are members of this family utilize the Na^+ gradient as their source of energy to carry out its efflux activity on fluoroquinolones and cationic dyes [44].

The ABC and MFS families are the very large families compared with the other three smaller families. Further classification of the efflux transporters gives the single-component and multi-component pumps. Substrates of the single component pumps are transported across the cytoplasmic membrane of the bacterial cells. The multicomponent pumps, which are usually located in Gram-negative organisms, work closely with an outer membrane protein (OMP) component and also with a periplasmic membrane fusion protein (MFP) component. They usually extrude their substrates out of the cytoplasm of the cell through the cell envelope.

Gram-positive bacteria possess efflux pumps which have cell envelope with a relatively simple structure. They have only a single component and are situated in the cytoplasmic membrane. Even without an outer membrane diffusion blockade, drug-specific efflux pump and multidrug efflux pumps have been found in Gram-positive bacteria. Some of these have featured prominently the macrolide and fluoroquinolone efflux. Efflux pumps that have been characterized in *S. aureus,* which is a major cause of hospital-acquired infections, include *QacA* (MFS family), *Smr* (SMR family) and *NorA* (MFS family) [46]. *QacA* and *Smr* are plasmid-encoded efflux pumps while *NorA* is encoded on the chromosome. *QacA* are known to efflux acriflavine, crystal violet, diamidines, ethidium bromide, and quaternary ammonium compounds [46]. Moderate fluoroquinolone resistance of *S. aureus* has been revealed to be mediated by the *NorA* efflux pump due to a *norA* gene that is not so strongly expressed. This pump is accountable for the resistance of *S. aureus* to only hydrophilic substrates of which fluoroquinolones but it is not able to extrude lipophilic substrates [46]. Respiratory tract infections are majorly caused by some isolates of *Streptococcus pneumonia, many of* which are known to be resistant to a broad selection of antibiotics, including macrolides, β-lactams, quinolones and tetracycline [47]. It has been demonstrated through target mutations that quinolone resistance of isolates of *Streptococcus pneumonia* is influenced by efflux mechanisms. A 24% similarity between the *NorA* pump of *S. aureus* and the *PmrA* pump of *S. pneumoniae* has been detected [46]. Expression of the PmrA pump results in higher levels of resistance to several fluoroquinolones results in about 2- to 4-fold increase. There are reasons to suggest that the wild-type strains of *S. pneumoniae* do not express the *PmrA* pump. The *Mef E* pump of the MFS family confers resistance in *S. pneumoniae* to macrolides. This *Mef E* pump of the MFS family shares 90% similarity with MefA of *S. pyogenes*. Together both are often denoted as *Mef(A)*. Both have also been revealed to have the capability to efflux both 14- and 15-member structured macrolides. *Mef(A)* is known to be responsible for about 70% of *S. pneumoniae* resistance to macrolides which have been detected around the United States of America [47]. The *mef(A)* gene of *S. pneumoniae* is transferable by transformation *via* mobile elements.

Bmr and *Blt* are two different MFS-type efflux pumps which have been recognized and described in *B. subtilis* [44]. Although *B. subtilis* organism is not of much clinical importance, the two Bmr and Blt MFS efflux pumps found in it offer archetypal systems for mechanistic studies of MFS-type multidrug efflux systems with ethidium bromide, fluoroquinolones and energy inhibitors as substrates [48].

Alteration of Metabolic Pathway

The production of single amino acid substitution in the dihydrofolate reductase target enzyme through mutation in the dhfr gene brings about trimethoprim resistance in *S. aureus* and *S. pneumonia* [20]. Mutations in the promoter region and the coding region of the *dhfr* gene have been detected in resistant *H. influenzae* strains. Mobile *dhfr* genes conferring resistance to trimethoprim have also been detected in Gram-positive bacteria [20, 15]. Another example of metabolic pathway alteration is found in some bacteria which are resistant to sulfonamide that does not have much use for para-amino benzoic acid (PABA), a vital precursor for the synthesis of folic acid and nucleic acids in bacteria which are inhibited by sulfonamides. As in mammalian cells, they resort to utilize pre-formed folic acid [49].

MITIGATING BACTERIAL MOLECULAR RESISTANCE MECHANISM

Efflux pumps are considered as veritable drug targets and making it imperative in the development of drug combination therapies [50]. Inhibition of these pumps at different levels is usually by reducing the binding of drug to the inner membrane pumps, thus hindering the interactions of different components of a multi-component pump, targeting the energy source of pumps and / or the regulatory networks that regulate efflux pump expression.

Efflux Pump Inhibitors have been recognized for various bacteria from various sources. For example, efflux pump inhibition is able to potentiate the efficacy of chloramphenicol, norfloxacin, tetracycline and cefepime by lowering MICs up to 8-fold [51]. The TetB efflux pump is known to be inhibited by a number of tetracycline derivatives [52]. Among the doxycycline derivatives, 13-cyclopentylthio-5-OH tetracycline (13-CPTC) is considered the most potent. 13-CPTC, in combination with doxycycline is able to bring about a drop in MIC values for doxycycline by 4- to 10-fold [50]. Efflux Pump Inhibitors (EPIs) extracted from plant origin, which showed no antibacterial activity of their own, are known to be able to increase the antibacterial activity of norfloxacin against *S. aureus* by impeding the NorA pump [50]. EPIs exhibit a potential for developing antibacterial formulations with antibacterial agents which are currently in use to restore their antibacterial activity against multidrug-resistant bacteria [53]. The alternative to EPIs may be the bypass of the efflux pump. This could be accomplished by developing newer drugs that possess a lower affinity for these pumps. It appears that some of the more recently developed fluoroquinolones are poor substrates for some pumps located in Gram-positive bacteria [53]. However, it is uncertain whether the increased activity is a result of a higher affinity for the target or due to lower affinity for these pumps [52]. It has been noted that an alternate pump may be induced in response to an introduction to an antibiotic that is a poor substrate for a certain pump. An example of such a substrate that is a poorer substrate for Tet pumps is glycylcycline tigecycline (GRA-936) [54].

As observed in MRSA and VRE, antibiotic resistance due to alterations of the target structure constitutes a great challenge to the control of infectious diseases. Continued development of newer antibiotic drug molecules, *e.g.*, the ketolides, azalides, oxazolidinones, streptogramins and glycylcyclines is of paramount importance to keep overcoming the continuously occurring cases of antibiotic resistance development. Good knowledge of the mechanisms of action of the existing antibiotics is an advantage in identifying new targets [55]. A re-assessment of the capabilities of existing agents is also necessary. Discovery of novel classes of inhibitory agents, such as the peptide deformylase (PDF) inhibitors, may bring about a useful impact on the uncontrolled emergence of drug-resistant organisms. It is however, clear that mutational changes in the essential defB deformylase gene can lead to the occurrence of resistance [56]. Despite the promise which genome-driven drug discovery offers, the observed effects of catechins of plant origin are able to restore MRSA back to being methicillin-sensitive, also evidently provide significant opportunities [57]. DK-507k and WCK 771 are among new experimental quinolones which have been found to maintain efficient inhibitory action against penicillin-resistant *S. pneumoniae* and MRSA despite the occurrence of mutational changes in the targets and the activity of efflux pumps [57].

Finally, many semi-synthetic glycopeptides with activity against VRE and MRSA are showing better-quality pharmacokinetic and pharmacodynamic properties. They are currently in various stages of assessment and clinical development [58]. Others are Oritavancin, a derivative of chloroemomycin; also an analogue to vancomycin possesses activity against VRE, penicillin-resistant *S. pneumoniae*, MRSA and Vancomycin intermediate *S. aureus* (VISA) strains.

CONCLUSION

It has been postulated that the biggest current threat to global health is the rising occurrence of drug-resistant bacteria, caused by the spreading antibiotic resistance amongst them. It is in a bid to curtail this trend that scientists unraveled the molecular basis of this major antibiotic resistance transfer mechanism. However, there is a need for more research on the molecular structure of resistance transfer mechanisms and future applications. That is why this chapter is focused on the better understanding and elucidation of the molecular basis of resistance and the transfer mechanisms, including all the enzymes involved in the action.

CONSENT FOR PUBLICATION

Not applicable.

CONFLICT OF INTEREST

The authors confirm that the contents of this chapter have no conflict of interest.

ACKNOWLEDGEMENTS

Declared none.

REFERENCES

[1]   Pena-Miller R, Laehnemann D, Jansen G, *et al.* When the most potent combination of antibiotics selects for the greatest bacterial load: the smile-frown transition. PLoS Biol 2013; 11(4): e1001540.
       [http://dx.doi.org/10.1371/journal.pbio.1001540] [PMID: 23630452]

[2]   Winstel V, Liang C, Sanchez-Carballo P, *et al.* Wall teichoic acid structure governs horizontal gene transfer between major bacterial pathogens. Nat Commun 2013; 4(1): 2345.
       [http://dx.doi.org/10.1038/ncomms3345] [PMID: 23965785]

[3]   Gao J, Shi LZ, Zhao H, *et al.* Loss of IFN-γ pathway genes in tumor cells as a mechanism of resistance to anti-CTLA-4 therapy. Cell 2016; 167(2): 397-404.e9.
       [http://dx.doi.org/10.1016/j.cell.2016.08.069] [PMID: 27667683]

[4]   Arutyunov D, Frost LS. F conjugation: back to the beginning. Plasmid 2013; 70(1): 18-32.
       [http://dx.doi.org/10.1016/j.plasmid.2013.03.010] [PMID: 23632276]

[5]   Smillie C, Garcillán-Barcia MP, Francia MV, Rocha EP, de la Cruz F. Mobility of plasmids. Microbiol Mol Biol Rev 2010; 74(3): 434-52.
       [http://dx.doi.org/10.1128/MMBR.00020-10] [PMID: 20805406]

[6]   Jassim SA, Limoges RG. Natural solution to antibiotic resistance: bacteriophages 'The Living Drugs'. World J Microbiol Biotechnol 2014; 30(8): 2153-70.
       [http://dx.doi.org/10.1007/s11274-014-1655-7] [PMID: 24781265]

[7]   Drawz SM, Papp-Wallace KM, Bonomo RA. New β-lactamase inhibitors: a therapeutic renaissance in an MDR world. Antimicrob Agents Chemother 2014; 58(4): 1835-46.
       [http://dx.doi.org/10.1128/AAC.00826-13] [PMID: 24379206]

[8]   Berg KH, Stamsås GA, Straume D, Håvarstein LS. Effects of low PBP2b levels on cell morphology and peptidoglycan composition in *Streptococcus pneumoniae* R6. J Bacteriol 2013; 195(19): 4342-54.

[http://dx.doi.org/10.1128/JB.00184-13] [PMID: 23873916]

[9] Jaiswal S, Pandey R, Sharma B, Kaski N. Reduction of antibiotic resistance in bacteria: a review. Int J Pharm Sci Res 2012; 3(1): 695-9.

[10] Bakry M A, Hakim AS, Nagwa S. Role played by Gene Factor in Initiation of Bacterial Antibiotic Resistance. Life Sci J 2014; 11(6).

[11] Jensen LB, Garcia-Migura L, Valenzuela AJS, Løhr M, Hasman H, Aarestrup FM. A classification system for plasmids from enterococci and other Gram-positive bacteria. J Microbiol Methods 2010; 80(1): 25-43.
[http://dx.doi.org/10.1016/j.mimet.2009.10.012] [PMID: 19879906]

[12] Zhanel GG, Lawson CD, Zelenitsky S, *et al.* Comparison of the next-generation aminoglycoside plazomicin to gentamicin, tobramycin and amikacin. Expert Rev Anti Infect Ther 2012; 10(4): 459-73.
[http://dx.doi.org/10.1586/eri.12.25] [PMID: 22512755]

[13] Vakulenko SB, Mobashery S. Versatility of aminoglycosides and prospects for their future. Clin Microbiol Rev 2003; 16(3): 430-50.
[http://dx.doi.org/10.1128/CMR.16.3.430-450.2003] [PMID: 12857776]

[14] Falagas ME, Athanasaki F, Voulgaris GL, Triarides NA, Vardakas KZ. Resistance to fosfomycin: mechanisms, frequency and clinical consequences. Int J Antimicrob Agents 2019; 53(1): 22-8.
[http://dx.doi.org/10.1016/j.ijantimicag.2018.09.013] [PMID: 30268576]

[15] Wright GD. Bacterial resistance to antibiotics: enzymatic degradation and modification. Adv Drug Deliv Rev 2005; 57(10): 1451-70.
[http://dx.doi.org/10.1016/j.addr.2005.04.002] [PMID: 15950313]

[16] Puglia AM, Gualerzi CO. Antibiotic resistance: Mechanisms and impact. Kirk Othmer Encyclopedia of Chemical Technology. 2000; pp. 1-41.

[17] Gallo G, Puglia AM. Antibiotics and Resistance: a fatal Attraction. In: Claudio OG, Brandi L, Fabbretti A, Pon CL, Pon CL, Eds. Antibiotics: Targets, Mechanisms and Resistance. KGaA: Wiley-VCH Verlag GmbH & Co. 2014; pp. 73-108.

[18] Heinsch SC, Hsu SY, Otto-Hanson L, Kinkel L, Smanski MJ. Complete genome sequences of Streptomyces spp. isolated from disease-suppressive soils. BMC Genomics 2019; 20(1): 994.
[http://dx.doi.org/10.1186/s12864-019-6279-8] [PMID: 31856709]

[19] Bansal S, Tandon V. Contribution of mutations in DNA gyrase and topoisomerase IV genes to ciprofloxacin resistance in *Escherichia coli* clinical isolates. Int J Antimicrob Agents 2011; 37(3): 253-5.
[http://dx.doi.org/10.1016/j.ijantimicag.2010.11.022] [PMID: 21236644]

[20] Lambert PA. Bacterial resistance to antibiotics: modified target sites. Adv Drug Deliv Rev 2005; 57(10): 1471-85.
[http://dx.doi.org/10.1016/j.addr.2005.04.003] [PMID: 15964098]

[21] Hooper DC, Jacoby GA. Topoisomerase inhibitors: fluoroquinolone mechanisms of action and resistance. Cold Spring Harb Perspect Med 2016; 6(9): a025320.
[http://dx.doi.org/10.1101/cshperspect.a025320] [PMID: 27449972]

[22] Aldred KJ, Kerns RJ, Osheroff N. Mechanism of quinolone action and resistance. Biochemistry 2014; 53(10): 1565-74.
[http://dx.doi.org/10.1021/bi5000564] [PMID: 24576155]

[23] McCurdy S, Lawrence L, Quintas M, *et al.* In vitro activity of delafloxacin and microbiological response against fluoroquinolone-susceptible and nonsusceptible Staphylococcus aureus isolates from two phase 3 studies of acute bacterial skin and skin structure infections. Antimicrob Agents Chemother 2017; 61(9): e00772-17.
[http://dx.doi.org/10.1128/AAC.00772-17] [PMID: 28630189]

[24]   Wilson DN. Ribosome-targeting antibiotics and mechanisms of bacterial resistance. Nat Rev Microbiol 2014; 12(1): 35-48.
[http://dx.doi.org/10.1038/nrmicro3155] [PMID: 24336183]

[25]   O'Driscoll T, Crank CW. Vancomycin-resistant enterococcal infections: epidemiology, clinical manifestations, and optimal management. Infect Drug Resist 2015; 8: 217-30.
[PMID: 26244026]

[26]   Ntokou E, Vester B. Resistance to linezolid 22. Antimicrobial Drug Resistance: Mechanisms of Drug Resistance 2017; 1: 319.
[http://dx.doi.org/10.1007/978-3-319-46718-4_22]

[27]   Van Duijkeren E, Schink A K, Roberts M C, Wang Y, Schwarz S. Mechanisms of bacterial resistance to antimicrobial agents. Antimicrobial Resistance in Bacteria from Livestock and Companion Animals 2018; 51-82.

[28]   Liu X, Deng S, Huang J, *et al.* Dissemination of macrolides, fusidic acid and mupirocin resistance among *Staphylococcus aureus* clinical isolates. Oncotarget 2017; 8(35): 58086-97.
[http://dx.doi.org/10.18632/oncotarget.19491] [PMID: 28938539]

[29]   Didier M, Julian D. Antibiotic resistance – the big picture. In: Nathan B, Cohen Irun R, David K, Bary P. Rosen, Shahriar M, Eds. Advances in Experimental Medicine and Biology. Springer science business media, LLC 1998.

[30]   Paterson GK, Harrison EM, Holmes MA. The emergence of mecC methicillin-resistant Staphylococcus aureus. Trends Microbiol 2014; 22(1): 42-7.
[http://dx.doi.org/10.1016/j.tim.2013.11.003] [PMID: 24331435]

[31]   Utaida S. Gene expression in Staphylococcus aureus induced by cell wall-active antibiotic stress. Illinois State University 2005.

[32]   Nikaido H, Vaara M. Molecular basis of bacterial outer membrane permeability. Microbiol Rev 1985; 49(1): 1-32.
[http://dx.doi.org/10.1128/MMBR.49.1.1-32.1985] [PMID: 2580220]

[33]   Bavoil P, Nikaido H, von Meyenburg K. Pleiotropic transport mutants of *Escherichia coli* lack porin, a major outer membrane protein. Mol Gen Genet 1977; 158(1): 23-33.
[http://dx.doi.org/10.1007/BF00455116] [PMID: 342907]

[34]   Beacham IR, Haas D, Yagil E. Mutants of *Escherichia coli* "cryptic" for certain periplasmic enzymes: evidence for an alteration of the outer membrane. J Bacteriol 1977; 129(2): 1034-44.
[http://dx.doi.org/10.1128/JB.129.2.1034-1044.1977] [PMID: 320175]

[35]   Lutkenhaus JF. Role of a major outer membrane protein in *Escherichia coli* . J Bacteriol 1977; 131(2): 631-7.
[http://dx.doi.org/10.1128/JB.131.2.631-637.1977] [PMID: 328491]

[36]   Nurminen M, Lounatmaa K, Sarvas M, Mäkelä PH, Nakae T. Bacteriophage-resistant mutants of Salmonella typhimurium deficient in two major outer membrane proteins. J Bacteriol 1976; 127(2): 941-55.
[http://dx.doi.org/10.1128/JB.127.2.941-955.1976] [PMID: 783123]

[37]   Pugsley AP, Schnaitman CA. Outer membrane proteins of *Escherichia coli* . VII. Evidence that bacteriophage-directed protein 2 functions as a pore. J Bacteriol 1978; 133(3): 1181-9.
[http://dx.doi.org/10.1128/JB.133.3.1181-1189.1978] [PMID: 346560]

[38]   Schnaitman CA. Outer membrane proteins of *Escherichia coli* . IV. Differences in outer membrane proteins due to strain and cultural differences. J Bacteriol 1974; 118(2): 454-64.
[http://dx.doi.org/10.1128/JB.118.2.454-464.1974] [PMID: 4597444]

[39]   Paakkanen J, Gotschlich EC, Mäkelä PH. Protein K: a new major outer membrane protein found in encapsulated *Escherichia coli* . J Bacteriol 1979; 139(3): 835-41.

[http://dx.doi.org/10.1128/JB.139.3.835-841.1979] [PMID: 383695]

[40]   Sutcliffe J, Blumenthal R, Walter A, Foulds J. *Escherichia coli* outer membrane protein K is a porin. J Bacteriol 1983; 156(2): 867-72.
[http://dx.doi.org/10.1128/JB.156.2.867-872.1983] [PMID: 6313620]

[41]   Whitfield C, Hancock REW, Costerton JW. Outer membrane protein K of *Escherichia coli* : purification and pore-forming properties in lipid bilayer membranes. J Bacteriol 1983; 156(2): 873-9.
[http://dx.doi.org/10.1128/JB.156.2.873-879.1983] [PMID: 6313621]

[42]   Chen S, Wang H, Katzianer DS, Zhong Z, Zhu J. LysR family activator-regulated major facilitator superfamily transporters are involved in *Vibrio cholerae* antimicrobial compound resistance and intestinal colonisation. Int J Antimicrob Agents 2013; 41(2): 188-92.
[http://dx.doi.org/10.1016/j.ijantimicag.2012.10.008] [PMID: 23201336]

[43]   Soto SM. Role of efflux pumps in the antibiotic resistance of bacteria embedded in a biofilm. Virulence 2013; 4(3): 223-9.
[http://dx.doi.org/10.4161/viru.23724] [PMID: 23380871]

[44]   Li XZ, Nikaido H. Efflux-mediated drug resistance in bacteria. Drugs 2004; 64(2): 159-204.
[http://dx.doi.org/10.2165/00003495-200464020-00004] [PMID: 14717618]

[45]   Poole K. Efflux-mediated antimicrobial resistance. J Antimicrob Chemother 2005; 56(1): 20-51.
[http://dx.doi.org/10.1093/jac/dki171] [PMID: 15914491]

[46]   Costa SS, Viveiros M, Amaral L, Couto I. Multidrug efflux pumps in *Staphylococcus aureus*: an update. Open Microbiol J 2013; 7: 59-71.
[http://dx.doi.org/10.2174/1874285801307010059] [PMID: 23569469]

[47]   Cherazard R, Epstein M, Doan TL, Salim T, Bharti S, Smith MA. Antimicrobial resistant *Streptococcus pneumoniae* : prevalence, mechanisms, and clinical implications. Am J Ther 2017; 24(3): e361-9.
[http://dx.doi.org/10.1097/MJT.0000000000000551] [PMID: 28430673]

[48]   Sun J, Deng Z, Yan A. Bacterial multidrug efflux pumps: mechanisms, physiology and pharmacological exploitations. Biochem Biophys Res Commun 2014; 453(2): 254-67.
[http://dx.doi.org/10.1016/j.bbrc.2014.05.090] [PMID: 24878531]

[49]   Fernández-Villa D, Aguilar MR, Rojo L. Folic acid antagonists: antimicrobial and immunomodulating mechanisms and applications. Int J Mol Sci 2019; 20(20): 4996.
[http://dx.doi.org/10.3390/ijms20204996] [PMID: 31601031]

[50]   Staudinger JL. Clinical applications of small molecule inhibitors of Pregnane X receptor. Mol Cell Endocrinol 2019; 485: 61-71.
[http://dx.doi.org/10.1016/j.mce.2019.02.002] [PMID: 30726709]

[51]   Douafer H, Andrieu V, Phanstiel O IV, Brunel JM. Antibiotic adjuvants: make antibiotics great again! J Med Chem 2019; 62(19): 8665-81.
[http://dx.doi.org/10.1021/acs.jmedchem.8b01781] [PMID: 31063379]

[52]   Dwivedi GR, Tiwari N, Singh A, *et al.* Gallic acid-based indanone derivative interacts synergistically with tetracycline by inhibiting efflux pump in multidrug resistant E. coli. Appl Microbiol Biotechnol 2016; 100(5): 2311-25.
[http://dx.doi.org/10.1007/s00253-015-7152-6] [PMID: 26658982]

[53]   Docquier JD, Mangani S. An update on β-lactamase inhibitor discovery and development. Drug Resist Updat 2018; 36: 13-29.
[http://dx.doi.org/10.1016/j.drup.2017.11.002] [PMID: 29499835]

[54]   Kumar A, Schweizer HP. Bacterial resistance to antibiotics: active efflux and reduced uptake. Adv Drug Deliv Rev 2005; 57(10): 1486-513.
[http://dx.doi.org/10.1016/j.addr.2005.04.004] [PMID: 15939505]

[55] Brown ED, Wright GD. Antibacterial drug discovery in the resistance era. Nature 2016; 529(7586): 336-43.
[http://dx.doi.org/10.1038/nature17042] [PMID: 26791724]

[56] Martínez JL, Coque TM, Baquero F. What is a resistance gene? Ranking risk in resistomes. Nat Rev Microbiol 2015; 13(2): 116-23.
[http://dx.doi.org/10.1038/nrmicro3399] [PMID: 25534811]

[57] Reed P, Atilano ML, Alves R, *et al.* Staphylococcus aureus survives with a minimal peptidoglycan synthesis machine but sacrifices virulence and antibiotic resistance. PLoS Pathog 2015; 11(5): e1004891.
[http://dx.doi.org/10.1371/journal.ppat.1004891] [PMID: 25951442]

[58] Abbas M, Paul M, Huttner A. New and improved? A review of novel antibiotics for Gram-positive bacteria. Clin Microbiol Infect 2017; 23(10): 697-703.
[http://dx.doi.org/10.1016/j.cmi.2017.06.010] [PMID: 28642145]

CHAPTER 5

Molecular Basis of Resistance II

Diaa Alrahmany[1] and **Islam M. Ghazi**[2,*]

[1] Inpatient Pharmacy, Sohar Hospital, Sultanate of Oman

[2] Phialdelphia College of Pharmacy, Univeristy of the Sciences, Philadelphia, USA

Abstract: Evolution of microbial resistance, particularly in Gram-negative bacteria, became a nightmare for the healthcare professionals and contributed effectively to high treatment failures as well as infection-related mortality rates. Understanding the diverse mechanisms by which the organisms acquire and transmit these resistance trends is a key determining step in any research endeavors aiming to develop either new drug molecules or treatment guidelines.

Gram-negative bacteria develop resistance through several mechanisms that render it less susceptible or even absolutely resistant to clinically relevant antibiotics. Enzymatic deactivation is the most common bacterial defense mechanism, in addition to other molecular mechanisms like decreased cell wall permeability through down-regulation of its porins, or over-expression of efflux pumps responsible for the decreased intracellular minimum inhibitory concentration of antibiotics, biofilm construction which is a protective barrier against threatening from bacterial surroundings, and antibiotic-specific target modification that leads to impaired drug-target fitting resulting inferior or prohibited clinical response.

Keywords: Antibiotic-specific target, Down-regulation, Efflux pumps, Evolution, Gram-negative bacteria, Molecular basis, Resistance.

INTRODUCTION

The irrational use of antimicrobials has led to an increase in resistance acquired by pathogenic bacteria at an alarming rate, if this trend continues without effective interventions initiated by health care professionals, policymakers, governmental authorities and drug developers, it will lead to catastrophic consequences.

Microbiological resistance can be defined as the enhanced ability of the microorganisms to counteract the lethal or static effects of antimicrobials through adaptation of specific biological mechanisms that render them absolutely resistant or less susceptible to antimicrobials than other members of the same species,

* **Corresponding author Islam M. Ghazi:** Phialdelphia College of Pharmacy, Univeristy of the Sciences, Philadelphia, USA; Tel: +1 (215) 596-7121; Fax: +1 (215) 596-8585; E-mail: i.ghazi@usciences.edu

whether this *in vitro* resistance is correlated to clinical outcomes or not. Clinically, bacterial resistance can be addressed with properly selected antibiotic/antibiotic combinations, adequate dose regimens, and tailored treatment duration to ameliorate clinical outcomes.

Diverse molecular and genetic mechanisms (Fig. **1**), enzymatic degradation of antimicrobials, modifying the antibiotic target site, modified porins, augmented efflux of antibiotics and biofilm formation can be developed by bacteria to evade the action of antibiotics. Identification of these resistance modalities and understanding of their mode of action, inducing factors and the possibility of transmission inter genera or species are pivotal components in guiding the drug development research and clinical practice.

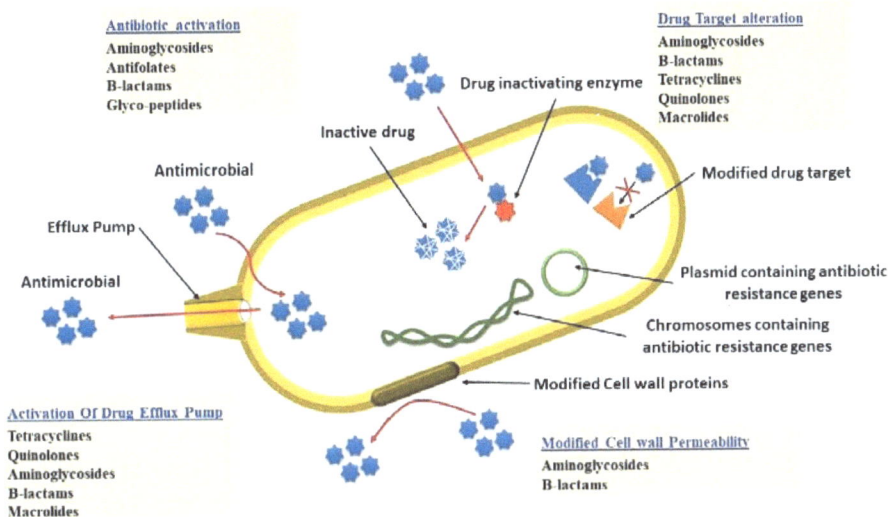

Fig. (1). Mechanisms of bacterial resistance.

On the basis of Gram stain, bacteria can be Gram-negative, which is distinguished by a thin peptidoglycan layer and an outer lipid membrane, or Gram-positive that possesses a thick peptidoglycan layer and no outer lipid membrane. The Gram-negative structure is unable to retain the crystal violet stain, colored only by the red color of the safranin counterstain. On the contrary, Gram-positive appears with a distinctively purple colour when observed under a light microscope following Gram staining. This is due to the retention of the purple crystal violet stain in the thick peptidoglycan layer of the cell wall. This unique, complicated bacterial cell wall structure of Gram-negative bacteria (Fig. **2**) predisposes to higher resistance capabilities and hinders the ability for certain antimicrobials to penetrate [1].

This chapter will discuss the prominent mechanisms utilized by which Gram-negative bacteria to combat antimicrobial action, how genetic and molecular resistance determinants manifest as specific phenotypes, and finally, how resistance impacts the clinical selection of antimicrobials.

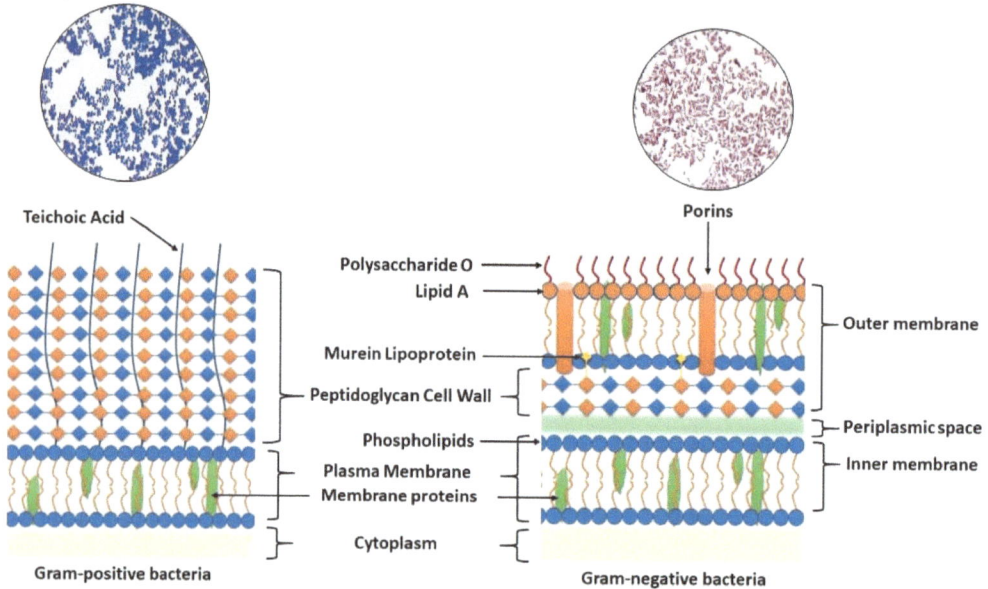

Fig. (2). Gram-negative *Vs* Gram-positive cell wall composition and Gram stain.

DEVELOPMENT OF RESISTANCE

Bacterial resistance can be classified into i) Intrinsic resistance (naturally existent), which is due to inherent characteristics of the bacteria that confer resistance to certain antibiotics. Examples are lack of antibiotic target or transfer mechanism. Gram-negative bacteria are resistant to vancomycin due to the inability to penetrate the cell wall. The same principle applies in atypical bacteria, which are wall-less (*Mycoplasma* species), which are naturally resistant to antimicrobials that exert its action through inhibition of bacterial cell wall synthesis [2, 3]. ii) Extrinsic (acquired) resistance arises as a result of mutational changes of the default genetic material of the organism leading to the acquisition of resistance to certain antibiotics that were not previously detectable and not manifested by the species.

Mutations usually occur due to chromosomal or extrachromosomal (plasmid- or transposon-mediated) changes. Spontaneous emergence of chromosomal mutations occurs in response to physical or chemical stimuli resulting in a structural change like modified antibiotic targets or decreased bacterial cell wall permeability or increased efflux, which finally lead to partial to absolute resistance to the specific antimicrobial drug [3]. Extra-chromosomal-mediated acquired resistance occurs due to external transferrable mobile genetic elements like plasmids, transposons and integrons from other bacteria. Plasmids are independently replicant DNA fragments, usually harboring the genetic determinants controlling the production of antibiotic-resistance mechanisms. A transposon is a DNA sequence that can change its position within the genome, as well as their mobility to exchange genetic material from bacterial chromosomes to plasmid and vice versa. Integrons are immobile carriers of genetic elements responsible for antimicrobial resistance. They rely on transposons to migrate between microbial cells, which could be the same species, intraspecies or even different genera [4].

This process of genetic material exchange is known as horizontal gene transfer (HGT) and can be carried out through different pathways; i) Transformation process is performed through the uptake of snippets of free DNA carrying resistant determinants of the ruptured cell from surroundings through the cell wall to the recipient cell, in which, it is incorporated into the new host cell's chromosome resulting in the genetic alteration of the recipient cell (Fig. **3**).

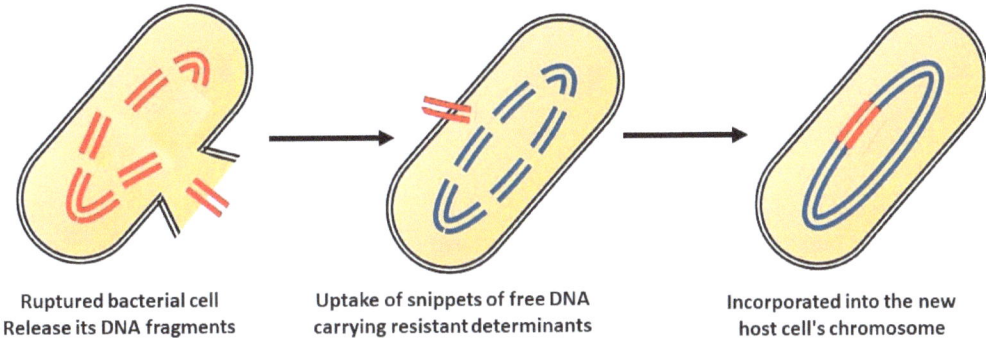

| Ruptured bacterial cell | Uptake of snippets of free DNA | Incorporated into the new |
| Release its DNA fragments | carrying resistant determinants | host cell's chromosome |

Fig. (3). Genetic determinants exchange process through transformation.

ii) Transduction is done through bacteriophages, able to transmit genetic material from one organism to another. As the virus replicates inside the host bacterial cell, the newly formed viral DNA or RNA will be polluted by genetic material from the host bacteria DNA, which becomes available to surroundings after rupture or lysis of host cell and can easily migrate and uptaken by other bacteria to be incorporated in the cell DNA *via* DNA binding protein called competence factor, iii) Conjugation, unlike transformation and transduction, is a process in which the genetic material migrates between cells through cell-to-cell contact or by a bridge-like connection between two cells. It is a kind of sexual process in which the donor cell provides a mobilizable genetic element in the form of a plasmid or transposon that can be transferred to the acceptor cell. Both cells become interconnected with each other and plasmid is located near the start of specific units of integration called integrons. Later, both cells synthesize a complementary strand to produce a double-stranded circular plasmid and they become viable donors or F-factor [5] (Fig. **4**).

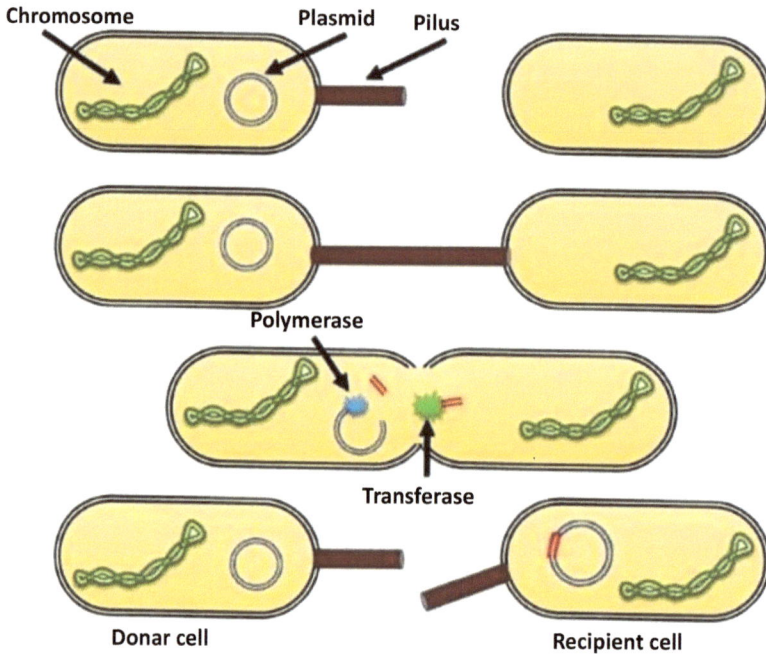

Fig. (4). Genetic exchange through conjugation.

Cross-resistance is a term that describes the ability of an organism to resist different classes of antibiotics that exert their action through similar mechanism or possess structural similarities, cross-resistance between members of β-lactam antibiotics class (penicillin, cephalosporins, monobactams, and carbapenems) is attributed to the common core structure and inhibition of cell synthesis mode of action. However, the cross-resistance between two chemically unrelated drugs can occur, like in the case of erythromycin-lincomycin. Although Gram-negative bacteria are generally resistant to both antibiotics, with few exceptions (*i.e.*, *Bordetella pertussis, Campylobacter, Chlamydia, Helicobacter,* and *Legionella* species). This cross-resistance is clearly identified in Gram-positive organisms. The induced expression of an *ermA ermC* genes has been reported in *Streptococcus pneumoniae* which leads to methylation of rRNA (target modification) that confer cross-resistance to macrolides, lincosamide, and streptogramin B (MLS$_B$) and form one MLS$_B$, resistance group [6].

Multiple-drug resistance (MDR) is defined as resistance to three or more classes of antimicrobials, primarily in response to antimicrobial injudicious selection or overuse pressure, resulting in the selection of resistant phenotypes, or due to over-expression of multiple genes that encode a variety of resistance determinants. If the organism is resistant to all but one or two antibiotic groups, they are considered as extensively-drug-resistant (XDR), while pan-resistance organisms are resistant to all available antibiotics [2]. See Table **1**.

Table 1. Examples of resistance mechanisms related to specific types of antimicrobials.

Antibiotics	Resistance Mechanism	References
β-lactams	Synthesis of β-lactamase enzymes.	[7]
	Loss of specific porins.	[8,9]
	Efflux pump over-expression.	[10]
	Altered penicillin-binding proteins.	[11]
Aminoglycosides	Decreased uptake.	[12]
	Aminoglycosides modifying enzymes.	
	Phospho-transferase, Adenyl-transferase, Acetyl-transferase.	
Glycopeptides	Target modification. D-Ala-D-Ala to D-Ala-D-Lac	[13,14]
	Target over-expression.	
Oxazolidinones	Target modification Ribosomal methylation, Ribosomal DNA mutation.	[15]
Quinolones	Sequestration. Quinolone resistant protein	[16], 17
	Efflux pump over-expression.	
	Enzymatic deactivation. Aminoglycosides acetyltransferase.	
Lincosamide	Target modification Ribosomal methylation	[18]
Chloramphenicol	Efflux pump over-expression.	[19]
	Enzymatic deactivation. Chloramphenicol acetyltransferase.	
Macrolides	Efflux pump over-expression.	[20]
	Target modification Ribosomal methylation.	
Sulfonamides and Trimethoprim	Production of the low-affinity target (DHFR), Dihydrofolate reductase	[21]
	Target over-expression.	
Polymyxins (Colistin)	Target modification, lipopolysaccharide modifications	[22]
Glycylcycline (Tigecycline)	Efflux pump over-expression.	[23]
	Ribosome protection	

MECHANISMS OF RESISTANCE

Decreased Antimicrobial Uptake (Porins-mediated Resistance)

Selective permeability of the bacterial membranes effectively offers protection from harmful compounds and harsh conditions in the extracellular environment while providing sufficient access to the required nutrients for bacterial cell vitality [24]. The uptake process throughout the cell membranes is performed through porins, protein specialized structures, located in the outer cell membrane [25] (Fig. **5**). General porins, which are determining the permeability characters of the cell membranes, are found side by side to more specific porins that enable the uptake of specific substrates. Porins represent gate openings in the cytoplasmic membrane through which antimicrobial agents can gain entry.

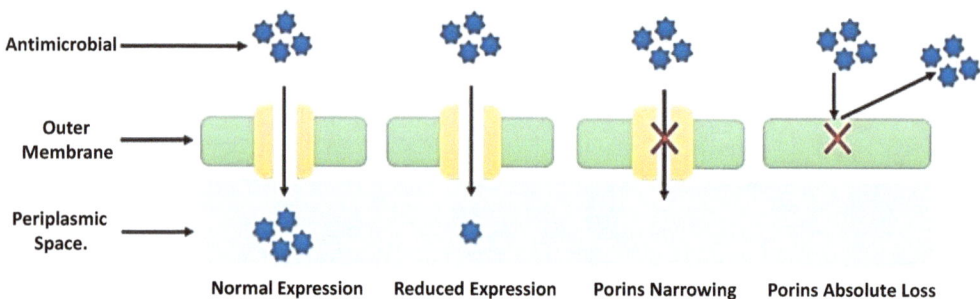

Fig. (5). Examples of different mechanisms of acquisition of mutational resistance associated with porins.

Crystallographic imaging of outer-membrane porins demonstrates a structure that consists of transmembrane antiparallel strands with alternating outwards directed hydrophobic amino acids and inward-directed hydrophilic amino acids, assembled into distinctive barrels rather than hydrophobic helices, which are more often found in proteins located in the cytoplasmic membrane. Several classes of porins were identified; general porins with a hydrophobic protein surface and a polar interior that possess a high tolerance against mutational alterations [26]. The outer membrane protein A (OmpA) occurs at about 100 000 copies per cell [27], that serves as a natural physical linkage between the outer membrane and underlying peptidoglycan layer, which determines the permeability characteristics of the cell membrane [24, 28].

The general diffusion porins allow the diffusion of hydrophilic molecules (< 600 Da) and show no specificity towards specific substrates, although it shows diffusion selectivity according to the substrate either electric charge or particle size, with some preference for molecules with charges opposite to those of the amino acids lining the channels. The charge cloud on each porin contributes to the formation of a specific electrical field, giving each porin its unique properties, and the trans-membranous potential determines whether the porin become open or closed. This potential is affected by several parameters, such as pH, ionic strength, osmotic pressure, presence of polysaccharides, membrane-derived oligosaccharides or polycations [29]. Transportation through general porins is a passive diffusion process, diffusion across the porins aqueous channels is only dependent on the compatibility between the substrate and the porins physicochemical properties, (polarity, particle size, and concentration gradient across the cell membrane). Thus, its more probable that small, hydrophilic antibiotics such as tetracycline, fluoroquinolones, and β-lactams can gain access to the bacterial cell through these porins [30]. The lack or reduced number of such porins is one of the means of antimicrobial resistance (Fig. **5**).

On the other hand, substrate-specific porins (Table **2**) have surface-located stereospecific binding sites for their substrates, only substrates of matching structural properties can cross it. For example; (OmpX) a three-dimensional small β-barrel membrane protein porin, they are responsible for organism virulence by neutralizing the host defense mechanisms [31]. The fishing rod-like structure has been proposed to function in cell adhesion and invasion as well as in the inhibition of the complement system by binding to one of its essential proteins [32]. Phospholipase A (OMPLA) is more or less with a similar structure of (OmpA) and (OmpX). It demonstrates a functional role in the hydrolysis of phospholipids (OmpF) which is a diffusion porins for ions and small molecules, malto-oligosaccharide- specific malto-porin (LamB) involved in the uptake of maltose and maltodextrins. These OMPs are most pertinent to the issue of antibacterial susceptibility and resistance.

Gated porins (TonB-dependent receptors) are another large molecules-specific porins. It is blocked by a globular domain "plug". The substrate is introduced into the gates in conjugation with an energy source "TonB energy transducing protein" leading a conformational change in the plug ends with the substrate release and the revelation of a translocation pathway [33, 34]. As an example, ferric enterochelin channel (FebA) responsible for iron-siderophore and vitamin B_{12} transportation, large molecular weight antibiotics like bacitracin and vancomycin find its way to the bacterial cells through such porins [35]. It is now clear that the level of expression of the porins not only controls the permeability of the outer nutrients but also differentially regulates the concentration of certain antibiotics in the surrounding environment, an example been demonstrated in *Escherichia coli*; the over-expression of OmpX (responsible for cell wall stabilization) leads to a decrease in the expression of OmpC and OmpF porins and a decreased susceptibility to beta-lactams and other antibiotics [36]. Decreased expression of porins increases the minimum inhibitory concentration (MIC) of relevant antibiotics leading to decreased susceptibility, while the complete disappearance of porins leads to absolute resistance. Table **2** summarizes some porin mediated antibiotic resistance in Gram-negative bacteria.

Table 2. Examples of porins related to antibiotic resistance in different Gram-negative bacteria.

Organism	Antibiotic	Porin	References
Acinetobacter baumannii	β-Lactams	CarO	[8, 9]
Klebsiella pneumoniae	β-Lactams Fluoroquinolones	OmpK35, OmpK36	[37, 38] 37
Klebsiella oxytoca	Carbapenems	OmpK36	[39, 40]
Escherichia coli	β-Lactams	OmpC, OmpF	[41, 42]
Pseudomonas aeruginosa	Carbapenems	OprD	[43, 44]
Serratia marcescens	β-Lactams Quinolones	OmpC, OmpF Omp1	[45] [45]
Neisseria gonorrhoeae:	β-lactams Tetracycline	penB penB2	[46] [47]
Salmonella typhi	Fluoroquinolones	OmpF	[48]
Yersinia pestis	Phagocytosis resistance	OmpR	[49]

Efflux Pumps Mediated Resistance

Efflux pumps are an energy-mediated pumping system responsible for the cell excretion job; it prevents the accumulation of waste products and toxic compounds inside the cytoplasm. This process does not involve any chemical alteration or degradation of the expelled compounds. Research has revealed the relationship between the overexpression of the substrate-specific efflux pump and the acquired clinical resistance of Gram-negative bacteria towards antimicrobials [50]. Mutations of chromosomal or plasmid-encoded genes may cause amino acid changes leading to either the overexpression of efflux pumps or increased extrusion ability related to a specific substrate, resulting in the acquisition of resistance to this molecule.

Five major classes of efflux pumps have been identified; ATP-binding cassette (ABC), the major facilitator superfamily (MFS), the multidrug and toxic compound extrusion (MATE), the small multidrug resistance (SMR) and the resistance-nodulation cell division (RND) class [51].

The most recently discovered class – (RND) – includes the efflux pumps contributing to *in vivo* broad-range antimicrobial resistance in Gram-negative bacteria [50, 52] (Table **2**). RND group members are structurally composed of an inner membrane (IM) transporter, a periplasmic adapter protein and an outer membrane (OM) protein. Whole-genome sequencing of *Stenotrophomonas maltophilia* exposed to high concentrations of ceftazidime showed mutation of SmeH, the transporter protein of the SmeGH RND efflux pump, which led to cephalosporin resistance, and cross-resistance to other β-lactams [53]. Moreover, the mutant cytoplasmic exporter protein MexB of MexAB-OprM efflux pump of *Pseudomonas aeruginosa* was a marker for fluoroquinolones and β-lactams resistance [54] and AcrAB-TolC efflux pump from *Escherichia coli* that is constitutively expressed and has a broad substrate profile which includes fluoroquinolones, β-lactams, and tetracyclines [50]. See Table **3** for more examples about Efflux pump-related antibiotic resistance in different Gram-negative bacteria.

Table 3. Efflux pump-related antibiotic resistance in different Gram-negative bacteria.

Organism	Antibiotic(s)	Pump	References
Pseudomonas aeruginosa	Fluoroquinolones, Aminoglycosides and β-lactams	Mex efflux pumps (MexA, MexC and MexE)	[55, 56] [10]
Pseudomonas aeruginosa	Fluoroquinolones	MexB-OprM	[54, 57]
Escherichia coli	Fluoroquinolones	AcrAB	[58]
Escherichia coli	Fluoroquinolones	QepA2	[59]
Klebsiella pneumoniae	Fluoroquinolones	AcrAB	[58]
Vibrio spp	1st and 3rd generation cephalosporins	VexD and VexC	[60]
Burkholderia pseudomallei	Meropenem, Doxycycline Trimethoprim-Sulfamethoxazole.	AmrAB-OprA, BpeAB-OprB and BpeEF-OprC	[61]
Neisseria gonorrhoeae	β-lactams		[62]
Salmonella typhimurium	Fluoroquinolones and β-lactams	AcrD, MdtABC, EmrAB, MdtK, and MacAB	[63]
Mycobacterium smegmatis	Fluoroquinolones and β-lactams	LfrA and LfrX	[64]
Mycobacterium tuberculosis	Erythromycin	EfpA	[64]
Mycobacterium fortuitum	Tetracyclines		[65]
Stenotrophomonas maltophilia	Cephalosporins	SmeGH	[53]

Reduced intracellular concentration of aminoglycosides in *Pseudomonas* spp. through over-expression of (MexA, MexC and MexE) efflux pump system is one of the leading resistance mechanisms for a variety of aminoglycosides (streptomycin, gentamicin, neomycin, kanamycin, and amikacin) [66], potentiate the value designing of new efflux assembly inhibitors as a promising strategy in future plans for the research and development of novel antimicrobials and substantiating of the action of already existing molecules [67].

Target Modification/Bypass/Protection

Antimicrobials act through attacking specific targets of the cell components. These targets can be the cell wall peptides, ribosomes or nuclear DNA. They exert action through binding to specific receptors on these targets. Bacterial mutations that lead to alterations of the antimicrobial-binding sites hinder the ability of antimicrobials to fit the corresponding receptors and thus mitigate the biologic action; in other words the organism becomes resistant to this antimicrobial. Diversity of resistance levels can be developed against certain types of antibiotics through the alteration of its specific target receptors, increased acquisition of an additional low-affinity Penicillin-Binding Proteins (PBPs), and the overexpression of an endogenous low-affinity PBP (Fig. **6**). Target site alteration often occurs due to either spontaneous genetic mutation or selection in the presence of the antimicrobial [68]. PBPs are enzymes with molecular weights ranging from 40,000 to 120,000 responsible for the assembly of bacterial cell wall outer membrane peptidoglycan layer which gives the bacterial cell its well-defined characteristic shape, as PBP is catalyzing the glycan strands polymerization (trans-glycosylation) and the formation of cross-links between these glycan strands (transpeptidation).

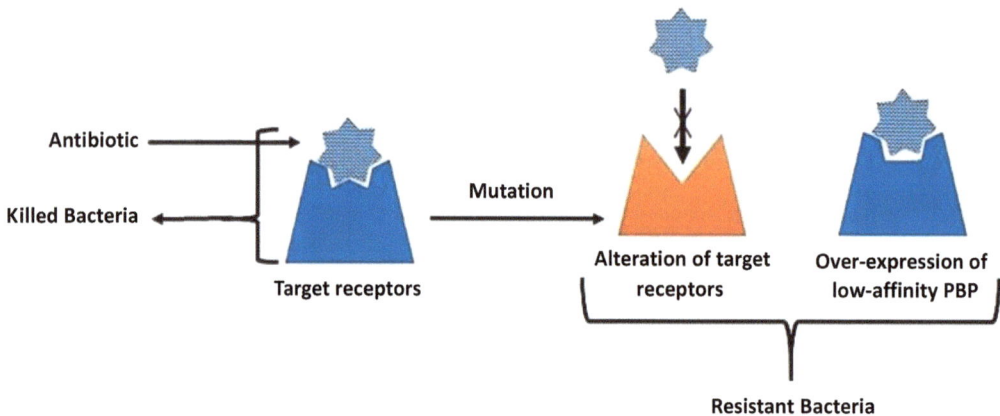

Fig. (6). Modification mechanisms of PBP.

Acylation of the active serine site of the chromosomally encoded (PBP's) allows penicillin and other β-lactam antibiotics to exert its action [69]. Due to the structural similarity between penicillin and (D-Ala-D-Ala) substrate, the former is able to form a long-lived acyl-enzyme that impairs their peptidoglycan cross-linking capability [70].

Several classes of bacterial PBPs have been identified in different bacterial species. They are broadly classified based on their molecular weight into high molecular mass (HMM-PBPs) and low molecular mass (LMM-PBPs). (HMM-PBPs) are responsible for peptidoglycan polymerization and insertion into pre-existing cell wall [71], while (LMM-PBPs) are involved in cell separation, peptidoglycan maturation, or recycling [72]. Further structural and action-based classification into classes A, B, C, where A and B classes belong mainly to (HMM-PBPs) and C class belongs mainly to (LMM-PBPs). Fig. (7) shows the classification of PBPs in Gram-negative bacteria based on amino acid sequence.

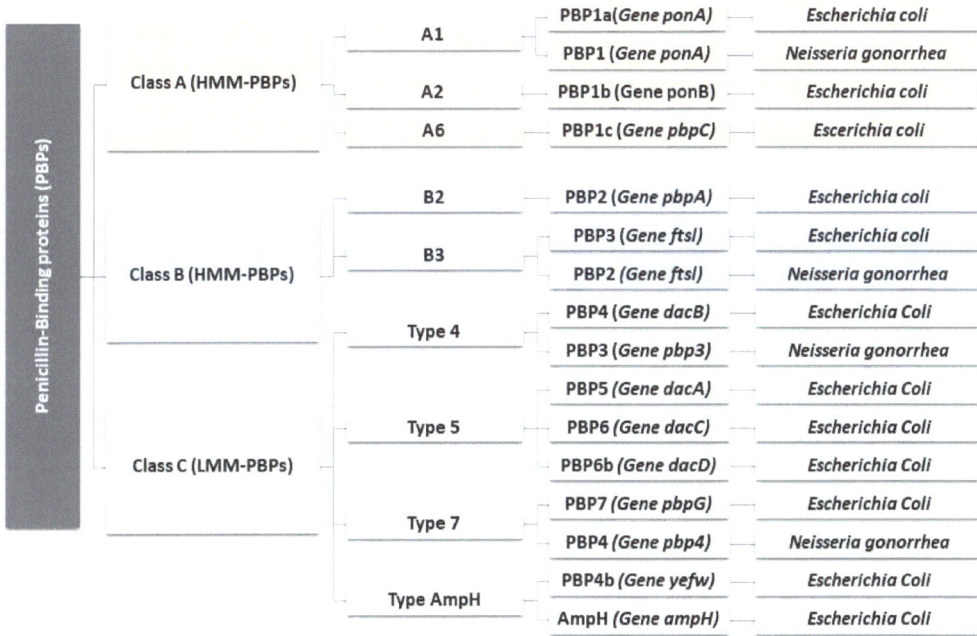

Penicillin-Binding proteins (PBPs)	Class	Subclass	PBP (Gene)	Species
	Class A (HMM-PBPs)	A1	PBP1a (Gene *ponA*)	*Escherichia coli*
		A1	PBP1 (Gene *ponA*)	*Neisseria gonorrhea*
		A2	PBP1b (Gene *ponB*)	*Escherichia coli*
		A6	PBP1c (Gene *pbpC*)	*Escerichia coli*
	Class B (HMM-PBPs)	B2	PBP2 (Gene *pbpA*)	*Escherichia coli*
		B3	PBP3 (Gene *ftsI*)	*Escherichia coli*
		B3	PBP2 (Gene *ftsI*)	*Neisseria gonorrhea*
	Class C (LMM-PBPs)	Type 4	PBP4 (Gene *dacB*)	*Escherichia Coli*
		Type 4	PBP3 (Gene *pbp3*)	*Neisseria gonorrhea*
		Type 5	PBP5 (Gene *dacA*)	*Escherichia Coli*
		Type 5	PBP6 (Gene *dacC*)	*Escherichia Coli*
		Type 5	PBP6b (Gene *dacD*)	*Escherichia Coli*
		Type 7	PBP7 (Gene *pbpG*)	*Escherichia Coli*
		Type 7	PBP4 (Gene *pbp4*)	*Neisseria gonorrhea*
		Type AmpH	PBP4b (Gene *yefw*)	*Escherichia Coli*
		Type AmpH	AmpH (Gene *ampH*)	*Escherichia Coli*

Fig. (7). Classification of PBPs in Gram-negative bacteria based on amino acid sequence.

The N-terminal domain in class A is responsible for their glycosyltransferase activity, catalyzing the elongation of uncross-linked glycan chains, while the N-terminal domain in class B is believed to play a role in cell morphogenesis by interacting with other proteins involved in the cell cycle [73]. Generally, class A is classified into 7 subclasses, but only subclasses A1, A2 and A6 belong to Gram-negative PBPs, whereas; the remaining classes belong to Gram-positive

PBPs [71]. Class A PBPs are necessary for cell growth in Gram-negative bacteria, in *Escherichia coli*; concomitant loss of (PBP1a) and (PBP1b) is lethal to the bacterial cell [74], while *Escherichia coli* strains lacking one or more D,D-carboxypeptidases (D,D-CPases) or D,D-endopeptidases (D,D-EPases) (LMM-PBPs) is subjected to morphological irregularities [75], while the loss of (PBP1) in *Neisseria gonorrhea* led the cell to lose its viability [11].

Mutations in the genes encoding the bacterial target will essentially lead to impaired antibiotic-target interaction which leads to resistance development (Table **4**), for instance; in Gram-positive species, the change in the peptidoglycan precursor from (D-Ala-D-Ala) to (D-Ala-D-Lac) or (D-Ala-D-Ser), causes 1000 folds reduction in affinity for the vancomycin [76], while the di-methylation of 23S rRNA at residue A-2058 of 50S ribosomal subunit by 23S rRNA methyltransferases will cause high-level resistance to macrolide and lincosamide antibiotics [77]. Rifampin resistance in many bacterial pathogens results in mutation of the 81-bp region of *rpoB* genes encoding the DNA-dependent RNA polymerase β subunit, the target of rifampin [78]. Acquisition of resistance to ceftazidime and the treatment failure of *Burkholderia pseudomallei* (Gram-negative bacilli) was due to the deletion of a gene encoding PBP3 [79], while developed resistance towards the same antibiotic and other β-lactam antibiotics in *Escherichia coli* and *Pseudomonas aeruginosa* species was mainly due to the mutation of genes encoding PBP3 (primary target), PBP1a and PBP1b (secondary targets) [80].

Table 4. Examples of PBP modification mediated resistance in Gram-negative bacteria.

PBP	Gene	Organism	Antibiotic	References
Nonessential PBP4	*dacB*	*Pseudomonas aeruginosa*	β-lactams	[81]
PBP 3	*gyrA*	*Enterobacteriaceae*	Fluoroquinolones	[82]
PBP1	*ponA*	*Neisseria gonorrhea*	β-Lactams	[11]
PBP3	*FtsI*	*Escherichia coli*	Cephalosporins	[83]
PBP3	*FtsI*	*Burkholderia pseudomallei*	Cephalosporins	[79]
PBP2	*pbpA*	*Escherichia coli*	Carbapenems	[84]

While the mutations in *pmrB* gene are the main chromosomal target for induction of colistin and polymyxin B resistance in *Klebsiella pneumoniae* and *Escherichia coli* [85, 86], the substitution of leucine at position 10 of *pmrB* with other amino acids (glycine and glutamine), resulting in 32-64 folds increased MIC values for both antimicrobials [86, 87].

Fluoroquinolones resistance is recognized through mutation of the bacterial enzymes' DNA gyrase encoded by the genes *gyrA* and *gyrB* and DNA topoisomerase IV; the main target of quinolones. Both enzymes play a main role in the replication, transcription, recombination, and repair of DNA through facilitating the separation of strands of the double-stranded DNA, and, in an ATP-dependent reaction, pass a second DNA double helix through the break, which is then resealed [88]. Fluoroquinolones act through complexation with both enzymes to form a drug-enzyme-DNA complex, with subsequent release of lethal double-stranded DNA breaks [89]. Mutations involving amino acid substitutions of the quinolone-resistance–determining region of GyrA enzyme leads to the reduced binding affinity of quinolones to the enzyme-DNA complex.

Biofilm Production

Biofilm is a thick, slimy, extracellular barrier consists of exopolysaccharides (EPS), extracellular DNA (e-DNA), proteins, amyloidogenic proteins, and enzymes in which the bacteria are embedded [90]. These biofilms can be attached to a living or non-living surface like surgical devices, vascular or urinary catheters [91], endotracheal tubes, internal implants and sutures.

The biofilm construction process rate-determining step is the organism adhesion to the surface of the device by the aid of the surface adsorption properties and the presence of biological proteins available on theses surfaces (Fig. **8**), for example; the epithelial cells lacking fibronectin promotes the adhesion of Gram-negative species (*Escherichia coli* or *Pseudomonas aeruginosa*) in the oral cavity, while fibronectin rich cells promote adhesion of Gram-positive *Staphylococcus aureus* [92]. Bacterial adhesion to the surface is followed by the release of extracellular polymeric substances (EPS), which ends with colony formation and biofilm maturation. The mature formed biofilm possesses a metabolic activity as compared to the planktonic cells, such as increased rates of EPS production, activation or inhibition of particular genes associated with biofilm formation and decreased growth rate [93]. Biofilm provides protection to its members against pH changes, osmolarity, nutrients scarcity, mechanical and shear forces, as well as being an effective barrier against antibiotics and host's immune cells invasion, which lead to the emergence of serious infections caused by MDR, XDR and pan-resistant bacteria.

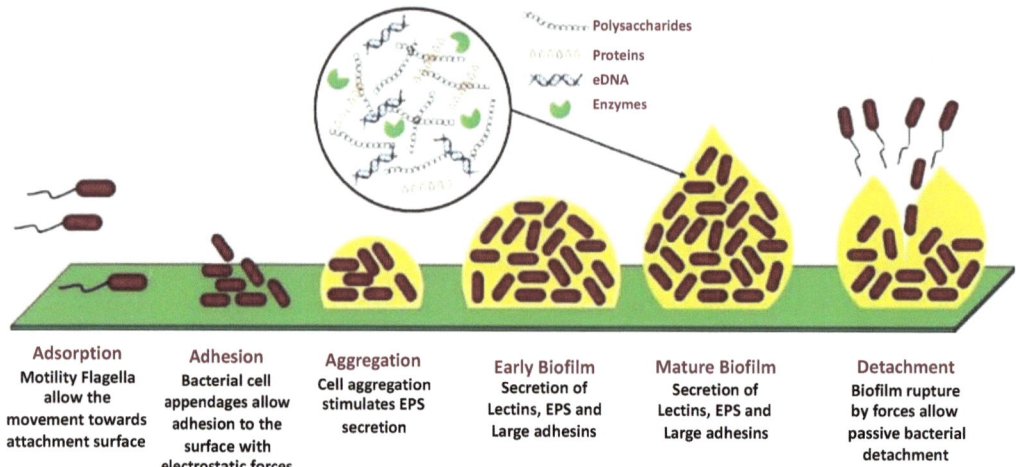

Fig. (8). Biofilm construction and detachment.

Biofilms are currently recognized as one of the most relevant drivers of persistent infections. A relationship between biofilm formation and antimicrobial resistance in Gram-negative bacteria is verified in many species. Gentamicin and ceftazidime resistance was related to biofilm formation in *Escherichia coli*, piperacillin/tazobactam, and colistin in *Klebsiella pneumoniae*, and ciprofloxacin in *Pseudomonas aeruginosa* [94]. There is a significant relationship between biofilm formation abilities and occurrences of advanced resistance mechanisms on Gram-negative bacteria like been demonstrated in biofilm positive *Escherichia coli*, *Acinetobacter* spp., *Klebsiella* spp., and *Pseudomonas* spp., (26.75%) and (16.24%) were confirmed as extended-spectrum β-lactamase (ESBL) and metallo-β-lactamases (MBL) producers, respectively. Most of the biofilm and MBL producing strains were multi-drug resistant [95]. Biofilm-associated *Escherichia coli* needed 500 folds of the MIC to provide a 3-log reduction [96].

Biofilm formation promotes microbial resistance in Gram-negative bacteria through different mechanisms, hindered antimicrobial diffusion through the matrix of the biofilm (extracellular polymeric substances EPSs) or by chemical inactivation of the antimicrobial, like been demonstrated with biofilm-associated *Pseudomonas aeruginosa* that showed 15 folds increase in MIC values towards tobramycin compared to free isolates [97]. Furthermore, the harsh conditions of nutrients and oxygen within the biofilm matrix greatly affect the growth and division rates of enclosed bacteria, which in turn affects the antimicrobial kinetics and susceptibility towards biofilm-associated bacteria, oxygen-deprived *Escherichia coli* demonstrated a decreased susceptibility to aminoglycoside antibiotics [98]. While the increased plasmid conjugation transfer rates were higher in biofilm-associated bacteria compared to free one due to higher conjugation probability [99].

Based on the fact that the concentrations of antimicrobial agents required to inactivate biofilm-associated organisms are much higher than that required for free organisms, and difficulty of achieving MIC values of antimicrobials within the biofilm, it is advisable to use antibiotics known to be more effective against biofilm-producing organisms, for example, ciprofloxacin and tobramycin at normal MICs were more effective against biofilms of *Pseudomonas aeruginosa* than were a number of other antibiotics which needed 100-1000 folds normal MICs, such as piperacillin, imipenem, and ceftazidime [100, 101]. Recent endeavors in microbiological nanotechnology are directed towards developing nanotechnology-based antimicrobials for the control of biofilm-infection [102].

Genetic Elements of Biofilm

Biofilm formation and dispersal are tightly controlled processes with the complex interaction between a variety of genes and response to external factors. In the literature, a number of studies illustrated genes involved in *E. coli* biofilm formation. When comparing differential expression of biofilm-forming to planktonic cells, about 79 genes (1.84% of the whole genome) were altered. Examples are; genes encoding structural proteins; OmpC, OmpF, OmpT (encoding membrane porins), lpxC (encoding protein associated with lipid A biosynthesis) and slp (encoding an outer membrane lipoprotein) [103]. Genes encoding motility cyaA and crp (encoding flagella biosynthesis), fimA and fimB (encoding Type I fimbriae) [104]. Genes encoding surface sensing and adhesion cpxR (encoding two-component signaling transduction pathway) and nleP (encoding outer membrane protein [105].

Stenotrophomonas maltophilia is another pathogen known for its ability to form complex biofilms, augmenting its virulence. Studying biofilm forming clinical isolates revealed that the presence of *spgM* gene (as well as *rpfF*, *rmlA*) encoding an enzyme with both PGM and phosphormannomutase activities contributed to biofilm formation [106]. Other studies have identified structural genes encoding the proteins involved in lipopolysaccharide/exopolysaccharide-coupled biosynthesis of cell wall components (*rmlA*, *rmlC*, and *xanB*) and the pump-encoding genes *macABCsm* and *smeYZ*have as required for biofilm formation [107, 108]. Genes encoding three transcription regulators (*fleQ*, *fsnR*, and *bfmA*) controlling flagellar gene expression and assembly also play a role in biofilm formation [109, 110].

The orchestration of biofilm formation in *Pseudomonas aeruginosa* -an etiological agent of significant nosocomial infections- was extensively studied

[111 - 113]. Three major systems control biofilm development; quorum sensing (QS), c-di-GMP and small molecules sRNA. QS control system incorporates genes lasR (encoding sensor regulator), rhlR (encoding transcriptional regulator), lasL and rhlL (encoding autoinducers), ultimately regulating the synthesis of rhamnolipids that maintain oxygen and nutrient channels in sessile biofilm colonies [114]. Hitherward, c-di-CMP stimulates the production of adhesins and matrix polysaccharides, leading to biofilm formation. The level of c-di-GMP is gauged by signal receptors (WspA, YfiB, and RocS1), diguanylate cyclases (WspR, YfiN, SadC, RoeA, and SiaD) and phosphodiesterases (BifA, DipA, RocR, MucR, and NbdA) encoded by their respective genes [115]. The sRNA system encoded by genes rsmY and rsmZ, increased expression ameliorates initial attachment to abiotic surfaces, but continued high level of these sRNAs embeds later steps of biofilm development [116, 117].

Enzymatic Inactivation of Antibiotics

Since the discovery of penicillin in the early 20th century, antibiotics have been one of the most influential therapeutic classes treating previously incurable infections and saving lives. Unfortunately, shortly after that with the characterization of resistance to penicillin, scientists began to realize that microorganisms can acquire the skills and tools required to survive and combat the antibiotics. Not only that, but they can also educate each other and transfer their skills and resistance trends among members of the same species or even members of different species. A number of bacterial resistance mechanisms were discussed in the previous lines, among which enzymatic inactivation of antimicrobials is the most efficient and most widely studied, several antibiotic molecules are rendered inactive through this mode of microbial resistance, macrolides, aminoglycoside antibiotics (gentamycin, and streptomycin), chloramphenicol, and β-lactams.

Macrolides antibiotics group members (erythromycin, roxithromycin, azithromycin, and clarithromycin) share the same characteristic lactone ring that differs in the size of the ring, and the substitutions at various positions, they possess differential activity against Gram-positives (*Streptococcus pneumoniae, Streptococcus pyogenes, Staphylococcus aureus*), some Gram-negative *(Hemophilus influenzae, Bordetella* spp.*, Legionella* spp.*, and Chlamydia* spp.*)*, as well as atypical pathogens *(Mycoplasma pneumoniae, Chlamydia trachomatis, Treponema pallidum)*. Macrolides share a similar antimicrobial spectrum activity with penicillins. Thus, they can be used as alternatives in the treatment of respiratory tract infections, community-acquired pneumonias, skin, soft tissue, and sexually transmitted diseases in people with a history of penicillin allergy or intolerance [118].

Macrolides are either bactericidal or bacteriostatic, depending on the concentration and the bacterial species. They act through inhibition of synthesis and elongation of bacterial proteins by reversible binding to the 23S rRNA. They bind in the peptide exit tunnel of the large ribosomal subunit, immediately adjacent to the peptidyl transferase center. They block the lumen of the tunnel preventing an elongating polypeptide chain to pass through it [119]. Structural modification of the prototype erythromycin yielded more pharmacokinetically and pharmacologically efficient semi-synthetic molecules with increased stability against hydrolytic enzymes and enhanced antimicrobial effect against specific species of Gram-negative isolates (roxithromycin, azithromycin, telithromycin and clarithromycin).

Lately, macrolides resistance has reached alarming levels. On the cellular level, macrolides resistance can be achieved through multiple pathways. Target modification through erythromycin ribosome methylase *erm* plasmid-encode--genes for methyltransferase enzymes able for methylation of the ribosome at key adenine positions on 23S rRNA, or even substitution of alanine with cytosine hinder erythromycin from binding its target [120, 121]. Meanwhile, over-expression of porins and energy-dependent efflux pumps through *msr, erp, mer, mre* mutation genes [122] and drug modification through phosphorylation and glycosylation makes it unavailable in effective state and concentrations at the site of action [123].

Plasmid-mediated genes encoding macrolides inactivating enzyme erythromycin ribosome esterase (Ere) have been found in a variety of bacterial species. Four erythromycin esterases (EreA from *Providencia stuartii*, EreB from *Escherichia coli*, and two Ere's from *Saccharopolyspora erythraea* and *Bacillus cereus*) were identified [124] (Table **5**). The fact that these genes are attached to mobile genetic elements (plasmid-mediated) increases the possibility that this mechanism will become more prevalent in the future.

Enzymatic modification of macrolides, macrolide phosphotransferases (MPHs) and macrolide esterases (Eres) diminish their capability to bind effectively to the 50S ribosome (Fig. **9**) and are thus become unable to exert an antibiotic effect. Macrolide 2'-phosphotransferases (MPHs) is capable of phosphorylating the hydroxyl group located at the 20 positions of the C5 linked desosamine moiety of erythromycin. This phosphorylation makes a variety of Gram-negative organisms resistant to macrolides (*Escherichia coli, Pseudomonas aeruginosa, Klebsiella pneumoniae, Serratia marcescens*) [125]. Plasmid-encoded macrolide esterases EreA methylate A2058 of the 23S rRNA, leading to hydrolysis of the ester bonds formed during the synthesis of macrolides cyclic lactone. This eventually leads to the linearization of the macrolide molecule, rendering it unable to bind to the ribosomal site of action [126]. Among this group, EreA2 is the most widely spread clinically relevant variant, it is isolated in the mobile genetic elements of *Pseudomonas* spp., *Salmonella Indiana*, *Klebsiella pneumoniae* and *Escherichia coli*. Next-generation macrolides should be designed on the basis of the ability to acquire differential affinity towards target ribosomes and inactivating enzymes. It should be resistant to hydrolytic enzymes with retained or maximized affinity toward target ribosomes.

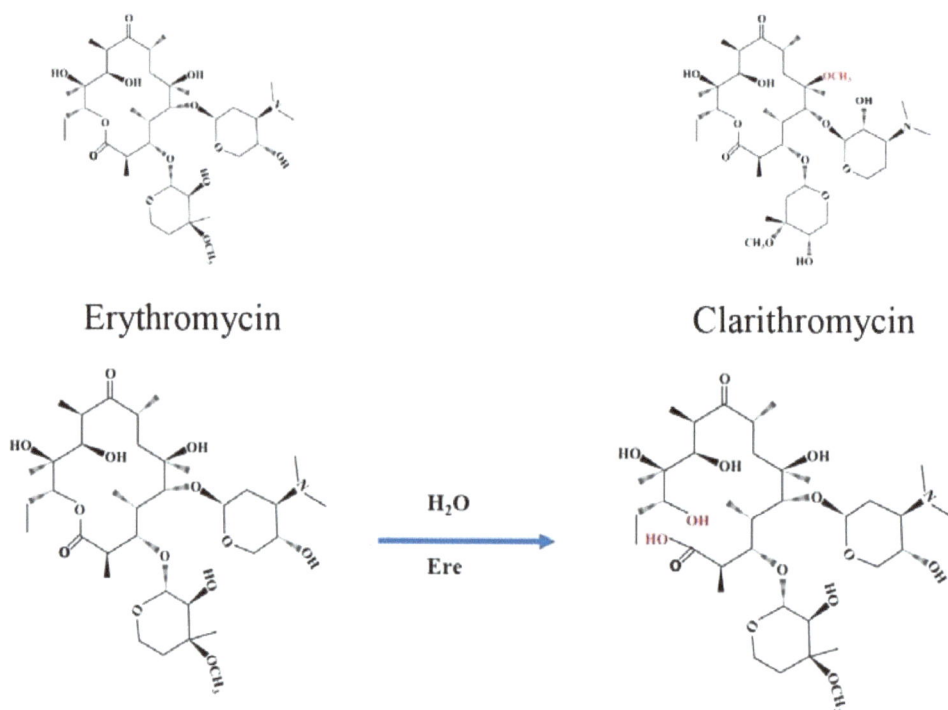

Erythromycin   Clarithromycin

Fig. (9). Hydrolysis of lactone ring of erythromycin.

Table 5. Macrolides resistance employed by Gram-negative species.

Organism	Enzyme	Source	Class	Reference
Escherichia coli	MPH(A), (B), and (C)	Plasmid	Phosphotransferase	[121]
Escherichia coli	EreA, EreB	Plasmid	Esterases	[127]
Providencia stuortii	EreB	Plasmid	Esterases	[77]
Klebsiella pneumoniae	EreC	Plasmid	Esterases	[125]
Pseudomonas aeruginosa	APH (3′)	Plasmid	Phosphotransferase	[125]
Serratia marcescens	EreA	Plasmid	Esterases	[77]
Vibrio cholerae	EreA2	Plasmid	Esterases	[128]

Aminoglycosides are potent antibiotics widely used against Gram-negative bacteria. They disrupt the bacterial cell membrane integrity *via* binding to 16S rRNA that leads to inhibition of cell wall protein synthesis. Early aminoglycosides faced the impact of microbial resistance, which led to the invention of semi-synthetic aminoglycosides (amikacin, netilmicin) in the early seventies. Several mechanisms contribute to the growing resistance to aminoglycosides; among which enzymatic deactivation is the most predominant and effective resistance pathway (Table **6**). Aminoglycosides-modifying enzymes can cause drug acetylation *via* aminoglycoside acetyltransferase (AAC), adenylation *via* aminoglycoside nucleotidyl-transferase (ANT) or phosphorylation *via* aminoglycoside phosphotransferase (APH) [129]. This structural modification causes impaired binding to the ribosomes and thus fails to trigger energy-dependent phase II.

Table 6. Examples of enzyme-related Aminoglycosides resistance.

Class	Enzyme	Substrate
Acetyltransferases	AAC (3)-I - IV	Gentamicin, Tobramycin, Kanamycin
	AAC (2')	Gentamicin, Tobramycin, Netilmicin, Neomycin
	AAC (6')-I - IV	Kanamycin, Gentamicin, Neomycin, Tobramycin, Netilmicin, Amikacin
Adenyl-transferases	ANT (6)	Streptomycin
	ANT (9)	Spectinomycin
	ANT (4')	Kanamycin, Tobramycin, Neomycin, Amikacin
	ANT (2")	Gentamicin, Tobramycin, Kanamycin
	ANT (3")	Streptomycin
Phosphotransferases	APH (2")$^{-I}$	Kanamycin, Gentamicin, Tobramycin, Dibekacin, Sisomicin, Netilmicin, Amikacin, Isepamicin, Neomycin, Ribostamycin, Paromomycin, Lividomycin, Butirosin
	APH (2")$^{-II}$	Kanamycin, Gentamicin, Tobramycin, Dibekacin, Sisomicin, Netilimicin, Amikacin, Isepamicin, Arbekacin
	APH (2")$^{-III}$	Kanamycin, Gentamicin, Tobramycin, Dibekacin, Sisomicin, Netilimicin

The family of β-lactams, including penicillins, cephalosporins, monobactams and carbapenems, is the most widely used antibiotics. They all exert their antibacterial effect through inactivation of the penicillin-binding proteins (PBPs) responsible for the building of the bacterial cell wall [130].

Carbapenems are the most potent β-lactams with broad antibacterial spectrum against both Gram-negative and -positive bacteria, owing to the chemical structure that contains both carbapenem and β-lactam rings. They manifest a maximized stability against the microbially produced inactivation enzymes. They are considered as the most reliable option for highly resistant microbial infections, especially infections caused by Gram-negative strains, carbapenems remain the last-resort option in the treatment of community-acquired infections to severe life-threatening nosocomial infections.

Carbapenem-resistant *Enterobacteriaceae* (CRE) has been included in the priority pathogens list issued by the World health organization (WHO) May 2017 as a priority 1 pathogen associated with high mortality rates and morbidities [131]. The dramatic increase and spread of carbapenem-resistant caused infections over the past decade were reported from many countries with variable prevalence and impact on healthcare systems [132 - 136].

Risk factors predisposing to the spread of infections caused by CRE strains are mainly the prior-exposure to an antibiotic for long durations [137, 138], prolonged hospitalization [139], admission to critical care areas [140, 141], mechanical ventilation and catheterization [142], advanced ages with multiple co-morbidities [138], solid organs transplantation [143] and immune-compromising.

Some species are intrinsically resistant to β-lactams like in the case of *Stenotrophomonas maltophilia*, as it produces two chromosomal β-lactamases: a clavulanic acid-sensitive class A (L2) and tetrameric carbapenemases (L1 or BlaS) [144]. While Gram-positive bacteria become β-lactams resistant through mutation-derived changes of their PBPs, Gram-negative bacteria acquire the resistance by mutational events or gene acquisition *via* horizontal gene transfer. CRE employs resistance to carbapenems through the production of carbapenemases, enzymes able for antimicrobial degradation, as well as, the previously discussed mechanisms, over-expression of efflux pumps, and decreased outer membrane permeability *via* porin mutations.

Reports of β-lactamases production (considered the major mechanism of acquired resistance in Gram-negative pathogens) began to ensue in the early 70's. β-lactamases were classified according to either to functional capacity or molecular structure. The functional classification of β-lactamases was first presented in 1995 by Bush into 4 main groups with multiple sub-groups according to the group-specific substrate or inhibition profiles. Group 1 includes specific inhibitory effect against cephalosporins and monobactams more than penicillins. They are chromosomally encoded enzymes that belong to molecular class C, and found mainly in family *Enterobacteriaceae*, which are not inhibited by clavulanic acid, tazobactam or EDTA [145]. Group 2; cephalosporinases, penicillinases and broad-spectrum β-lactamases that are generally inhibited by active site-directed β-lactamase inhibitors generally belong to structural groups A and D. Group 3; metallo-β-lactamases that are poorly inhibited by all classical β-lactamase inhibitors except EDTA and *p*-chloromercuribenzoate (pCMB), and Group 4; penicillinases that are not inhibited by clavulanic acid [146].

Clinically-relevant β-lactamases are divided structurally on the basis of their amino acid sequences and catalytic mechanisms, into 4 molecular classes (Ambler class). Classes A, C and D contain active-site serine β-lactamases (SBLs) whose reaction pathways involve acyl-enzyme adducts while class B contains metallo--lactamases (MBLs), which do not form such intermediates [147].

Class A β-lactamases are able to deactivate all β-lactam antibiotics through attacking the serine active site at position 70 of the enzyme with a higher affinity toward cephalosporins and monobactams compared to penicillins and carbapenems, class A combines β-lactamases that demonstrate broad-spectrum (Temoneira TEM and sulfhydryl variable SHV), extended-spectrum (ESBLs - cefotaxime hydrolyzing capabilities CTX-M-15), and carbapenemases activity (*Klebsiella pneumoniae* carbapenamase KPC, GES), β-lactamases like IMI-1, NMC, SME, PenA are usually chromosomally encoded; thus they are weakly contributing for the spread-out of carbapenems resistance, while KPC, GES and IMI-2 are plasmid-encoded, so they granted different levels of microbial carbapenem resistance ranging from a reduced susceptibility to absolute resistance.

Klebsiella pneumoniae carbapenemases (KPC) β-lactamases (23 variants) are the most commonly occurring among class A β-lactamases. It stands behind the tremendous ability of *Klebsiella pneumonia* to deactivate extended-spectrum cephalosporins and carbapenems. They are not necessarily confined to *Klebsiella pneumoniae* as they can also be found as plasmid-encoded bla_{KPC} gene in *Escherichia coli*, *Klebsiella oxytoca*, Salmonella enterica, *Pseudomonas aeruginosa*, Citrobacter freundii, Proteus mirabilis, *Serratia marcescens* and *Enterobacter cloacae*. They show variant susceptibility to clavulanic acid and tazobactam [4, 148]. Novel β-lactamase inhibitors combinations like ceftazidime-avibactam, meropenem-vaborbactam, and imipenem-relebactam increases the susceptibility of the combined antibiotics from almost 0% to 85% [149].

Serratia marcescens enzyme SME is restricted to *Serratia marcescens*. They comprise 5 chromosomally-encoded variants in contrast to plasmid-encoded KPC enzymes, although SME are infrequently isolated; nowadays, increasing identification of *Serratia marcescens* harboring bla_{SME} gene has been reported in the USA [150].

Imipenemase IMI and Imipenemase/non-metallocarbapenemase IMI-NMC are chromosomally-encoded bla_{IMI-1} gene and Plasmid-encoded bla_{IMI-2} found in *Enterobacter cloacae* strains. They are known to be potent hydrolyzer to carbapenems but remain susceptible to expanded spectrum cephalosporins and can be inhibited by clavulanic acid and tazobactam [151, 152].

TEM β-lactamases is the most commonly-encountered antibiotics degradation in Gram-negative bacteria. There are almost 213 variants of this enzymatic class different in protein sequencing, found in a wide range of Gram-negative bacteria (*Hemophilus influenzae, Neisseria gonorrhoeae, Escherichia coli* and *Klebsiella pneumonia, Klebsiella oxytoca, Proteus mirabilis*, and *Citrobacter freundi*) (Table 7). Although they are not extended-spectrum β-lactamases ESBLs, the amino acid substitutions of the enzyme active sites change its configuration into ESBLs derivatives. TEM β-lactamases are resistant to clavulanic acid and sulbactam with partial susceptibility to tazobactam [153].

SHV β-lactamases (almost 191 variants) are structurally similar to TEM, commonly responsible for plasmid-mediated resistance to cephalosporins, extended-spectrum cephalosporins and carbapenems in ESBL producers *Klebsiella pneumoniae, Escherichia coli* and *Klebsiella oxytoca* [154].

Guiana extended-spectrum β-lactamases GES is another category (29 variants) of Class A β-lactamases. They are found on transferable plasmids in both *Pseudomonas aeruginosa* and *Klebsiella pneumonia*. It possesses high activity against early cephalosporins, extended-spectrum cephalosporins and carbapenems. Thus they are classified as (ESBLs) and contributed to highly resistant phenotypes of *Klebsiella pneumonia, Escherichia coli* and *Pseudomonas aeruginosa* [155].

Table 7. Examples of Class A β-lactamases.

Molecular Class	Bush Class	Enzyme	Production	Host	Hydrolysis Profile					Inhibited by			Ref.
					PEN	Early Ceph.	ESCP	MBM	CARB	CLA	TAZ	EDTA	
A	2a	PC1	Chr.	*Staphylococcus aureus*	++	+	+	+	-	+	+	-	[156]
	2b	TEM-1	Chr.	*Klebsiella oxytoca*	+	++	+	+	±	+	+	-	[157]
		TEM-2	Chr.	*Escherichia coli*	+	+	+	+	±	±	+	-	[158]
		SHV-1	Pla.	*Escherichia coli*	+	+	+	+	+	+	+	-	[159]
	2be	TEM-3	Pla.	*Klebsiella pneumoniae*	+	+	+	+	+	+	+	-	[160]
		SHV-2	Pla.	*Klebsiella pneumoniae*	+	+	+	+	-	+	+	-	[161]
		CTX-M-14	Chr.	*Escherichia coli*	+	+	+	+	-	-	-	-	[162]
		CTX-M-15	Chr.	*Klebsiella pneumoniae*	+	+	+	+	-	-	-	-	[162]

(Table 7) cont.....

Molecular Class	Bush Class	Enzyme	Production	Host	Hydrolysis Profile					Inhibited by			Ref.
					PEN	Early Ceph.	ESCP	MBM	CARB	CLA	TAZ	EDTA	
		PER-1	Pla.	*Pseudomonas aeruginosa*	+	+	+	+	+	+	+	-	[163]
		VEB-1	Pla.	*Pseudomonas aeruginosa*	+	+	+	+	+	+	+	-	[163]
	2br	TEM-30	Pla.	*Escherichia coli*	+	+	+	+	+	-	±	-	[164]
		TEM-32	Pla.	*Escherichia coli*	+	+	+	+	+	-	±	-	[164]
		TEM-34	Pla.	*Escherichia coli*	+	+	+	+	+	-	±	-	[164]
		SHV-10	Pla.	*Escherichia coli*	+	+	+	+	+	-	-	-	[165]
		SHV-46	Pla.	*Klebsiella oxytoca*	+	+	+	+	+	-	-	-	[157]
	2ber	TEM-50	Pla.	*Escherichia coli*	+	+	+	+	+	-	-	-	[166]
	2c	PSE-1	Pla.	*Pseudomonas aeruginosa*	+	+	+	+	++	+	+	-	[167]
		CARB-3	Pla.	*Pseudomonas aeruginosa*	+	+	+	+	+	+	+	-	[168]
	2ce	RTG-4	Pla.	*Acinetobacter baumannii*	+	+	+	+	+	+	+	-	[169]
	2e	CepA	Chr.	*Bacteroides fragilis*	+	+	+	±	±	+	-	-	[170]
	2f	IMI-1	Chr.	*Enterobacter cloacae*	+	+	+	+	+	+	+	-	[152]
		IMI-2	Pla.	*Enterobacter cloacae*	+	+	+	+	+	+	+	-	[151]
		KPC-1	Pla.	*Klebsiella pneumoniae*	+	+	+	+	+	+	+	-	[171]
		KPC-2	Pla.	*Klebsiella pneumoniae*	+	+	+	+	±	±	NR	-	[172]
			Pla. /Chr.	*Pseudomonas aeruginosa*	+	+	+	+	+	±	NR	-	[173]
			Pla.	C. freundii	+	+	+	+	+	±	NR	-	[173]
			Pla.	*Escherichia coli*	+	+	+	+	+	±	+	-	[174]
			Pla.	*Klebsiella oxytoca*	+	+	+	+	+	±	+	-	[157]
			Pla.	Enterobacter spp.	+	+	+	+	+	±	NR	-	[175]
		KPC-3	Pla.	*Klebsiella pneumoniae*	+	+	+	+	+	+	NR	-	[176]
			Pla.	*Enterobacter cloacae*	+	+	+	+	+		NR	-	[177]
		KPC-4	Pla.	*Enterobacter cloacae*	+	+	+	+	+	±	+	-	[4]
		KPC-5	Pla.	*Pseudomonas aeruginosa*	+	+	+	+	++	+	NR	-	[148]
		SME-1	Chr.	*Serratia marcescens*	+	+	±	+	+	+	++	-	[178]
		SME-2	Chr.	*Serratia marcescens*	+	+	±	+	+	+	NR	-	[179]
		SME-3	Chr.	*Serratia marcescens*	+	+	±	+	+	+	NR	-	[180]
		NMC-A	Chr.	*Enterobacteriaceae*	+	+	+	+	+	+	+	-	[181]
		GES-1	Pla.	*Klebsiella pneumoniae*	+	+	+	+	-	+	+	-	[182]

(Table 7) cont.....

Molecular Class	Bush Class	Enzyme	Production	Host	Hydrolysis Profile					Inhibited by			Ref.
					PEN	Early Ceph.	ESCP	MBM	CARB	CLA	TAZ	EDTA	
		GES-2	Pla. /Chr.	*Pseudomonas aeruginosa*	+	+	+	+	+	±	±	-	[155]
		GES-4	Pla.	*Klebsiella pneumoniae*	+	+	+	-	±	+	±	-	[155]
		GES-5	Pla. /Chr.	*Klebsiella pneumoniae*	+	+	+	+	+	±	±	-	[155]
		GES-6	Pla. /Chr.	*Klebsiella pneumoniae*	+	+	+	+	+	±	±	-	[183]

Pen: Penicillin, **Ceph**.: Cephalosporins, **ESCP**: Extended-spectrum cephalosporins, **MBM**: Monobactam, **CARB**: Carbapenem, **CLA**: Clavulanic acid, **TAZ**: Tazobactam, **Chr**.: Chromosomal, **Pla**: Plasmid, **NR**: Not reported.

Class B β-lactamases (Metallo-β-lactamases) (MBLs) utilize zinc ions Zn^{+2} as an essential cofactor in cleaving the β-lactam ring. They hydrolyze all β-lactams except monobactams. Although they are resistant to the inhibitory effect of tazobactam, clavulanic acid, and even novel carbapenemases inhibitors like avibactam, they preserve their susceptibility to metal chelating agents like EDTA, which inhibits the enzymatic action through Zn^{+2} sequestration. However, MBLs demonstrated good susceptibility to the combination aztreonam/avibactam and newly introduced cephalosporin; cefiderocol [184], but their occurrence is noxious to practitioners due to their broad-spectrum hydrolytic effect, the high probability for horizontal gene transfer, and the fact that β-lactams resistance due to MBLs is usually associated with high rates of concomitant resistance to other antibiotics categories like fluoroquinolones and aminoglycosides (multiple drug resistance).

On the basis of amino acid sequence and the structural characteristics of the active site, it can be classified into 3 subclasses B1, B2 and B3, MBLs from B1 and B3 subclasses use two zinc ions within their active sites and have a much broader resistance spectrum compared to subclass B2, which uses only one zinc ion and only shows activity against carbapenems [185], subclass B1 comprises the most abundant MBLs; IMP, VIM, CcrA, GIM, SIM and NDM enzymes (Table **8**).

The chromosomally encoded gene of CcrA enzyme is found in *Bacteroides fragilis* isolates, this metalloenzymes deactivates cephalosporins and carbapenems, it resists the effect of clavulanic acid and sulbactam with concentration-dependent susceptibility to tazobactam (>10I1/4m) [186]. The plasmid-mediated IMP-type MBLs (26 variants) were first discovered in the early 90s on the transferable plasmid of *Enterobacteriaceae*, *Pseudomonas* and *Acinetobacter* species. They are able to hydrolyze all β-lactams except monobactams and resistant to all β-lactamase inhibitors [187]. A few years later, Verona integron-encoded metallo-β-lactamases VIM-type is discovered (>40 variants) integrated as a gene cassette located in a class I integron of *Escherichia coli* and *Klebsiella pneumoniae*, more variants of VIM is reported in a *Pseudomonas aeruginosa* clinical isolate in many European countries [187]. New Delhi metallo-β-lactamases NDM are identified on bacterial chromosomes and plasmids of *Escherichia coli* capable of hydrolyzing all penicillins, cephalosporins and carbapenem group of antimicrobials, with some variants, such as NDM-4, NDM -5 and NDM -7, present higher efficiencies of carbapenem hydrolysis [188], and it is now one of the most common carbapenemases in all *Enterobacteriaceae* and in *Acinetobacter baumannii*. Frequently, plasmids carrying bla_{NDM} co-harbor multiple genetic determinants contributing resistance not only to β-lactamases but extend to quinolone, and 16S rRNA methylases that confer resistance to all aminoglycosides.

Table 8. Examples of Class B β-lactamases found in Gram-negative bacteria.

Molecular Class	Bush Class	Enzyme	Production	Host	Hydrolysis Profile					Inhibited by			Ref.
					PEN	Early Ceph.	ESCP	MBM	CARB	CLA	TAZ	EDTA	
B1	3a	IMP-1	Pla.	*Pseudomonas aeruginosa*	+	+	+	-	+	-	-	+	[189]
		VIM-1	Pla. / Chr.	*Klebsiella pneumoniae*	+	+	+	-	+	-	-	+	[187]
		CcrA	Chr.	*Bacteroides fragilis*	+	+	+	-	+	-	±	+	[186]
		NDM-1	Pla. / Chr.	*Escherichia coli*	+	+	+	+	+	-	-	+	[188]
B2	3b	CphA	Pla. / Chr.	*Aeromonas hydrophilia*	±	±	±	±	++	-	-	+	[190]
		Sfh-1	Pla. / Chr.	*Serratia fonticola*	±	±	±	±	++	-	-	+	[191]
B3	-	L1 proteins		*Stenotrophomonas maltophilia*	+	+	+	-	+	-	-	+	[184]
		GOB proteins		*Chryseobacterium meningosepticum*	+	+	+	-	+	-	-	+	[184]
		FEZ-1		*Legionella gormanii*	+	+	+	-	+	-	±	+	[184]
		THIN-B		*Janthinobacterium lividum*	+	+	+	+	+	-	-	+	[184]

Pen: Penicillin, **Ceph.**: Cephalosporins, **ESCP**: Extended-spectrum cephalosporins, **MBM**: Monobactam, **CARB**: Carbapenem, **CLA**: Clavulanic acid, **TAZ**: Tazobactam, **Chr.**: Chromosomal, **Pla**: Plasmid, **NR**: Not reported.

Less clinically relevant enzymes posing low tendency for dissemination like Seoul Imipenemase SIM-**1** and German Imipenemase GIM-1s have not spread beyond the original organisms where they were first discovered; *Pseudomonas* and *Acinetobacter* spp., São Paulo metallo-β-lactamases SPM-1s possess a broad hydrolyzing profile against penicillins, cephalosporins and carbapenems.

Type CphA and Sfh belong to Ambler sub-class B2 metallo-β-lactamases; both groups possess high hydrolytic specificity with a narrow spectrum activity against carbapenems, CphA is originally isolated from *Aeromonas hydrophilia* and *Aeromonas veronii* [190], while Sft is isolated from *Serratia fonticola* [191]. Finally, subclass B3 includes the L1 proteins from *Stenotrophomonas maltophilia*, GOB proteins from *Chryseobacterium meningosepticum,* the FEZ-1 enzyme from *Legionella gormanii*, and the THIN-B β-lactamase produced by *Janthinobacterium lividum* [184, 192].

Table 9. Examples of Class C β-lactamases found in Gram-negative bacteria.

Molecular Class	Bush Class	Enzyme	Production	Host	Hydrolysis Profile					Inhibited by			Ref.
					PEN	Early Ceph.	ESCP	MBM	CARB	CLA	TAZ	EDTA	
C	1	*E. coli* AmpC1	Pla. /Chr	*Escherichia coli*	+	++	++	++	+	-	-	-	[194]
		ACT-1	Chr.	*Klebsiella pneumoniae*	+	+	+	++	+	-	-	-	[195]
		DHA-1	Chr.	*Klebsiella pneumoniae*	+	+	+	++	+	-	-	-	[195]
		CMY-2	Pla.	*Klebsiella pneumoniae*	+	+	+	++	±	-	-	-	[196]
		FOX-1	Pla.	*Escherichia coli*	+	+	++	++	±	-	-	-	[197]
		MIR-1	Pla.	*Klebsiella pneumoniae*	+	+	++	++	±	-	-	-	[198]

Pen: Penicillin, **Ceph.**: Cephalosporins, **ESCP**: Extended spectrum cephalosporins, **MBM**: Monobactam, **CARB**: Carbapenem, **CLA**: Clavulanic acid, **TAZ**: Tazobactam, **Chr.**: Chromosomal, **Pla**: Plasmid, **NR**: Not reported.

In Class C β-lactamases (AmpC beta-lactamases), although this class of β-lactamases is typically chromosomally encoded in many Gram-negative bacteria, including *Citrobacter, Serratia, Enterobacter* species, and *Pseudomonas aeruginosa* where its expression is usually inducible, it could also be plasmid-encoded in some species. In contrast to ESBLs, AmpC beta-lactamases are capable of hydrolyzing broad/extended-spectrum cephalosporins, with special variants like CMY-2, CMY-10, ACT-1 and DHA-1 have a potent inhibitory effect against carbapenems [193], and they are resistant to β-lactamases inhibitors like clavulanic acid and tazobactam (Table **9**).

ACT β-lactamases are chromosomally encoded class C β-lactamases. They are inducible by the presence of cephalosporins, recently they are found as plasmid-encoded genes in *Escherichia coli* and *Klebsiella pneumoniae* that can be expressed under high pressure of β-lactam antibiotics [195]. Recently added member to this class is the chromosomally encoded Acinetobacter derived cephalosporinase ADC-68 [193].

Class D β-lactamases (Oxacillinases) (Table **10**) are relatively less prevalent among all classes. They are also known as OXA β-lactamases for their oxacillin, related anti-staphylococcal penicillins hydrolytic abilities, weak affinity to carbapenems and the fact that they are poorly inhibited by classical inhibitors, and some became able to confer resistance to cephalosporins. The serine β-lactamases from class D can be either most probably plasmid-encoded or, to a lesser extent, chromosomally-encoded [199]. Although OXA β-lactamases were first discovered in *Acinetobacter* spp [200], it demonstrated the potentiality to spread out among *Enterobacteriaceae* and other Gram-negative bacteria.

Based on amino acid sequence several subgroups belonging to the oxacillinase family were identified; plasmid-encoded subgroups (OXA-23-like), (OXA-2--like), (OXA-51-like), and (OXA-58) are mainly identified in *Acinetobacter* species [201], whereas; many variants of OXA-48 enzyme has been identified in *Klebsiella pneumoniae*, *Escherichia coli*, Citrobacter freundii, and *Enterobacter cloacae*. They are much selective for penicillins compared to carbapenems with minimal effect against cephalosporins [202].

The OXA-23-like group was first identified in imipenem resistant *Acinetobacter baumannii* in the United Kingdom in the mid-eighties of the 20th century, later on, several alleles of the transferable plasmid-encoded bla_{OXA-23}-like gene have been identified on the chromosomes of *Acinetobacter* spp. (bla_{OXA-23}, $bla_{OXA-102}$, $bla_{OXA-103}$, $bla_{OXA-105}$, $bla_{OXA-133}$, and $bla_{OXA-134}$) responsible for expression of many variants of OXA-23 like expression (OXA-23, OXA-27, OXA-49, OXA-73, OXA-102, OXA-103, OXA-105, OXA-133, OXA-134, OXA-146, OXA-165, OXA-171, OXA-225, OXA-239) [199, 203]. These enzymes exert its hydrolytic effect against oxyiminocephalosporins, aminopenicillins, piperacillin, oxacillin, and aztreonam in addition to higher turnover rate for imipenem than for meropenem, ertapenem, or doripenem, with a confined expanded hydrolytic spectrum of only OXA-146 that includes ceftazidime [186].

In Spain 10 years later, plasmid-encoded genes of the OXA-40 group were identified in the natural source of the OXA group; - *Acinetobacter* spp.-, which spread out later to other groups of *Enterobacteriaceae* like *Pseudomonas aeruginosa* and *Klebsiella pneumoniae* [204]. OXA-40 group is generally highly specific against penicillins with inferior activity against cephalosporins and carbapenems.

Table 10. Examples of Class D β-lactamases found in Gram-negative bacteria.

Molecular Class	Bush Class	Enzyme	Production	Host	Hydrolysis Profile					Inhibited by			Ref
					PEN	Early Ceph.	ESCP	MBM	CARB	CLA	TAZ	EDTA	
D	2d	OXA-1	Pla.	*Pseudomonas aeruginosa*	+	±	±	+	±	±	±	-	[163]
		OXA-10	Pla.	*Acinetobacter baumannii*	+	±	±	+	±	±	±	-	[200]
	2de	OXA-11	Pla.	*Pseudomonas aeruginosa*	+	±	±	+	±	±	±	-	[207]
		OXA-15	Pla.	*Pseudomonas aeruginosa*	+	±	±	+	±	±	±	-	[208]
	2df	OXA-23	Pla.	*Acinetobacter baumannii*	+	±	±	+	±	±	±	-	[201]
		OXA-48	Pla.	*Klebsiella pneumoniae*	+	±	±	+	±	±	±	-	[202]

Pen: Penicillin, **Ceph**.: Cephalosporins, **ESCP**: Extended-spectrum cephalosporins, **MBM**: Monobactam, **CARB**: Carbapenem, **CLA**: Clavulanic acid, **TAZ**: Tazobactam, **Chr**.: Chromosomal, **Pla**: Plasmid, **NR**: Not reported.

OXA-51-like β-lactamases are naturally found on the chromosome of *Acinetobacter* spp., this is the most widely distributed group among class D with a large number of variants. It shows weak hydrolytic activity against carbapenems when compared to cephalosporins with favorable activity against oxacillin [205].

OXA-134a were identified from a carbapenem sensitive *Acinetobacter lwoffii* isolate, although it induced reduced susceptibility to the carbapenems, cephalosporins and penicillins when cloned into *Escherichia coli*. [206] While OXA-143 β-lactamases isolated from *Acinetobacter baumannii and Acinetobacter pittii* were showing hydrolytic effect to almost all β-lactam antibiotics.

CONCLUSION

As discussed above, Gram-negative bacteria possess a tremendous ability to evolve and survive the lethal action of antibiotics through a diverse array of molecular and genetic mechanisms that supersedes our research and drug development capacity. Knowledge of such resistance mechanisms is essential for clinicians to guide the judicious utilization of antibiotics, for industry scientists to inform drug discovery pathways and for academic researchers to enhance the design of scientific experiments. In the end, we hope that our efforts have succeeded in providing the reader with information that is readily comprehensible and, at the same time, valuable to their field of interest.

CONSENT FOR PUBLICATION

Not applicable.

CONFLICT OF INTEREST

The authors confirm that the contents of this chapter have no conflict of interest.

ACKNOWLEDGEMENTS

Declared none.

REFERENCES

[1]   Schulz GE. The structure of bacterial outer membrane proteins. Biochim Biophys Acta 2002; 1565(2): 308-17.
        [http://dx.doi.org/10.1016/S0005-2736(02)00577-1] [PMID: 12409203]

[2]   Nikaido H. Multidrug resistance in bacteria. Annu Rev Biochem 2009; 78: 119-46.
        [http://dx.doi.org/10.1146/annurev.biochem.78.082907.145923] [PMID: 19231985]

[3]   Al-Kobaisi MF. Jawetz, Melnick & Adelberg's Medical Microbiology: 24(th) Edition. Sultan Qaboos Univ Med J 2007; 7(3): 273-5.

[4]   Bryant KA, Van Schooneveld TC, Thapa I, *et al.* KPC-4 Is encoded within a truncated Tn4401 in an IncL/M plasmid, pNE1280, isolated from *Enterobacter cloacae* and *Serratia marcescens*. Antimicrob Agents Chemother 2013; 57(1): 37-41.
        [http://dx.doi.org/10.1128/AAC.01062-12] [PMID: 23070154]

[5]   Mayer KH, Opal SM, Medeiros AA. Mechanisms of antibiotic resistance. In: Mandell GL, Bennett JB, Dolin R, Eds. Mandell, Douglas and Bennett's Principles and Practice of Infectious Diseases. 4th edn. New York, NY: Churchill Livingstone Inc 1995; pp. 212-5.

[6]   Jawetz E, Melnick JL, Adelberg EA. Medical Microbiology. East Norwalk, CT: Appleton & Lange 1995; pp. 137-67.

[7]   Brakhage AA, Al-Abdallah Q, TA1/4ncher A, SprAte P. Evolution of beta-lactam biosynthesis genes and recruitment of trans-acting factors. Phytochemistry 2005; 66(11): 1200-10.
        [http://dx.doi.org/10.1016/j.phytochem.2005.02.030] [PMID: 15950251]

[8]   Limansky AS, Mussi MA, Viale AM. Loss of a 29-kilodalton outer membrane protein in *Acinetobacter baumannii* is associated with imipenem resistance. J Clin Microbiol 2002; 40(12): 4776-8.
        [http://dx.doi.org/10.1128/JCM.40.12.4776-4778.2002] [PMID: 12454194]

[9]   Bratu S, Landman D, Martin DA, Georgescu C, Quale J. Correlation of antimicrobial resistance with beta-lactamases, the OmpA-like porin, and efflux pumps in clinical isolates of *Acinetobacter baumannii* endemic to New York City. Antimicrob Agents Chemother 2008; 52(9): 2999-3005.
        [http://dx.doi.org/10.1128/AAC.01684-07] [PMID: 18591275]

[10]   Poole K, Tetro K, Zhao Q, Neshat S, Heinrichs DE, Bianco N. Expression of the multidrug resistance operon mexA-mexB-oprM in *Pseudomonas aeruginosa*: mexR encodes a regulator of operon expression. Antimicrob Agents Chemother 1996; 40(9): 2021-8.
        [http://dx.doi.org/10.1128/AAC.40.9.2021] [PMID: 8878574]

[11]   Ropp PA, Hu M, Olesky M, Nicholas RA. Mutations in ponA, the gene encoding penicillin-binding protein 1, and a novel locus, penC, are required for high-level chromosomally mediated penicillin resistance in *Neisseria gonorrhoeae*. Antimicrob Agents Chemother 2002; 46(3): 769-77.
        [http://dx.doi.org/10.1128/AAC.46.3.769-777.2002] [PMID: 11850260]

[12]   Touati A. Aminoglycoside resistance mechanism inference algorithm: Implication for underlying resistance mechanisms to aminoglycosides. EBioMedicine 2019; 46: 8.
[http://dx.doi.org/10.1016/j.ebiom.2019.07.045] [PMID: 31350220]

[13]   Gladstone BP, Cona A, Shamsrizi P, *et al.* Antimicrobial resistance rates in gram-positive bacteria do not drive glycopeptides use. PLoS One 2017; 12(7): e0181358.
[http://dx.doi.org/10.1371/journal.pone.0181358] [PMID: 28727741]

[14]   Chen CJ, Huang YC, Chiu CH. Multiple pathways of cross-resistance to glycopeptides and daptomycin in persistent MRSA bacteraemia. J Antimicrob Chemother 2015; 70(11): 2965-72.
[http://dx.doi.org/10.1093/jac/dkv225] [PMID: 26216581]

[15]   Schuster S, Vavra M, Kern WV. Efflux-Mediated Resistance to New Oxazolidinones and Pleuromutilin Derivatives in *Escherichia coli* with Class Specificities in the Resistance-Nodulatio- -Cell Division-Type Drug Transport Pathways. Antimicrob Agents Chemother 2019; 63(9): e01041- 19.
[http://dx.doi.org/10.1128/AAC.01041-19] [PMID: 31209014]

[16]   Niero G, Bortolaia V, Vanni M, Intorre L, Guardabassi L, Piccirillo A. High diversity of genes and plasmids encoding resistance to third-generation cephalosporins and quinolones in clinical *Escherichia coli* from commercial poultry flocks in Italy. Vet Microbiol 2018; 216: 93-8.
[http://dx.doi.org/10.1016/j.vetmic.2018.02.012] [PMID: 29519532]

[17]   Yan M, Xu C, Huang Y, Nie H, Wang J. Tetracyclines, sulfonamides and quinolones and their corresponding resistance genes in the Three Gorges Reservoir, China. Sci Total Environ 2018; 631- 632: 840-8.
[http://dx.doi.org/10.1016/j.scitotenv.2018.03.085] [PMID: 29727994]

[18]   Marosevic D, Kaevska M, Jaglic Z. Resistance to the tetracyclines and macrolide-lincosamid- -streptogramin group of antibiotics and its genetic linkage - a review. Ann Agric Environ Med 2017; 24(2): 338-44.
[http://dx.doi.org/10.26444/aaem/74718] [PMID: 28664720]

[19]   Yang YJ, Singh RP, Lan X, Zhang CS, Sheng DH, Li YQ. Whole transcriptome analysis and gene deletion to understand the chloramphenicol resistance mechanism and develop a screening method for homologous recombination in Myxococcus xanthus. Microb Cell Fact 2019; 18(1): 123.
[http://dx.doi.org/10.1186/s12934-019-1172-3] [PMID: 31291955]

[20]   Fu P, Wang C, Tian H, Kang Z, Zeng M. Bordetella pertussis Infection in Infants and Young Children in Shanghai, China, 2016-2017: Clinical Features, Genotype Variations of Antigenic Genes and Macrolides Resistance. Pediatr Infect Dis J 2019; 38(4): 370-6.
[http://dx.doi.org/10.1097/INF.0000000000002160] [PMID: 30882726]

[21]   Sun H, Chen R, Jiang W, Chen X, Lin Z. QSAR-based investigation on antibiotics facilitating emergence and dissemination of antibiotic resistance genes: A case study of sulfonamides against mutation and conjugative transfer in *Escherichia coli*. Environ Res 2019; 173: 87-96.
[http://dx.doi.org/10.1016/j.envres.2019.03.020] [PMID: 30903818]

[22]   Poirel L, Jayol A, Bontron S, *et al.* The mgrB gene as a key target for acquired resistance to colistin in *Klebsiella pneumoniae*. J Antimicrob Chemother 2015; 70(1): 75-80.
[http://dx.doi.org/10.1093/jac/dku323] [PMID: 25190723]

[23]   Sun J, Chen C, Cui CY, *et al.* Plasmid-encoded tet(X) genes that confer high-level tigecycline resistance in *Escherichia coli*. Nat Microbiol 2019; 4(9): 1457-64.
[http://dx.doi.org/10.1038/s41564-019-0496-4] [PMID: 31235960]

[24]   Koebnik R, Locher KP, Van Gelder P. Structure and function of bacterial outer membrane proteins: barrels in a nutshell. Mol Microbiol 2000; 37(2): 239-53.
[http://dx.doi.org/10.1046/j.1365-2958.2000.01983.x] [PMID: 10931321]

[25]   Nakae T. Identification of the outer membrane protein of *E. coli* that produces transmembrane

channels in reconstituted vesicle membranes. Biochem Biophys Res Commun 1976; 71(3): 877-84.
[http://dx.doi.org/10.1016/0006-291X(76)90913-X] [PMID: 786294]

[26]   Freudl R. Insertion of peptides into cell-surface-exposed areas of the *Escherichia coli* OmpA protein does not interfere with export and membrane assembly. Gene 1989; 82(2): 229-36.
[http://dx.doi.org/10.1016/0378-1119(89)90048-6] [PMID: 2684781]

[27]   Achouak W, Heulin T, Pagès JM. Multiple facets of bacterial porins. FEMS Microbiol Lett 2001; 199(1): 1-7.
[http://dx.doi.org/10.1111/j.1574-6968.2001.tb10642.x] [PMID: 11356559]

[28]   Sonntag I, Schwarz H, Hirota Y, Henning U. Cell envelope and shape of *Escherichia coli*: multiple mutants missing the outer membrane lipoprotein and other major outer membrane proteins. J Bacteriol 1978; 136(1): 280-5.
[http://dx.doi.org/10.1128/JB.136.1.280-285.1978] [PMID: 361695]

[29]   Delcour AH. Function and modulation of bacterial porins: insights from electrophysiology. FEMS Microbiol Lett 1997; 151(2): 115-23.
[http://dx.doi.org/10.1111/j.1574-6968.1997.tb12558.x] [PMID: 9228742]

[30]   Hernández-Allés S, Conejo Md, Pascual A, Tomás JM, BenedA- VJ, Martínez-Martínez L. Relationship between outer membrane alterations and susceptibility to antimicrobial agents in isogenic strains of *Klebsiella pneumoniae*. J Antimicrob Chemother 2000; 46(2): 273-7.
[http://dx.doi.org/10.1093/jac/46.2.273] [PMID: 10933652]

[31]   Heffernan EJ, Wu L, Louie J, Okamoto S, Fierer J, Guiney DG. Specificity of the complement resistance and cell association phenotypes encoded by the outer membrane protein genes rck from *Salmonella typhimurium* and ail from Yersinia enterocolitica. Infect Immun 1994; 62(11): 5183-6.
[http://dx.doi.org/10.1128/IAI.62.11.5183-5186.1994] [PMID: 7927803]

[32]   Vogt J, Schulz GE. The structure of the outer membrane protein OmpX from *Escherichia coli* reveals possible mechanisms of virulence. Structure 1999; 7(10): 1301-9.
[http://dx.doi.org/10.1016/S0969-2126(00)80063-5] [PMID: 10545325]

[33]   Ferguson AD, Hofmann E, Coulton JW, Diederichs K, Welte W. Siderophore-mediated iron transport: crystal structure of FhuA with bound lipopolysaccharide. Science 1998; 282(5397): 2215-20.
[http://dx.doi.org/10.1126/science.282.5397.2215] [PMID: 9856937]

[34]   Locher KP, Rees B, Koebnik R, *et al.* Transmembrane signaling across the ligand-gated FhuA receptor: crystal structures of free and ferrichrome-bound states reveal allosteric changes. Cell 1998; 95(6): 771-8.
[http://dx.doi.org/10.1016/S0092-8674(00)81700-6] [PMID: 9865695]

[35]   Braun M, Killmann H, Braun V. The beta-barrel domain of FhuADelta5-160 is sufficient for TonB-dependent FhuA activities of *Escherichia coli*. Mol Microbiol 1999; 33(5): 1037-49.
[http://dx.doi.org/10.1046/j.1365-2958.1999.01546.x] [PMID: 10476037]

[36]   Viveiros M, Dupont M, Rodrigues L, *et al.* Antibiotic stress, genetic response and altered permeability of *E. coli*. PLoS One 2007; 2(4): e365.
[http://dx.doi.org/10.1371/journal.pone.0000365] [PMID: 17426813]

[37]   Wong JLC, Romano M, Kerry LE, *et al.* OmpK36-mediated Carbapenem resistance attenuates ST258 *Klebsiella pneumoniae in vivo*. Nat Commun 2019; 10(1): 3957.
[http://dx.doi.org/10.1038/s41467-019-11756-y] [PMID: 31477712]

[38]   Lee CH, Chu C, Liu JW, Chen YS, Chiu CJ, Su LH. Collateral damage of flomoxef therapy: *in vivo* development of porin deficiency and acquisition of blaDHA-1 leading to ertapenem resistance in a clinical isolate of *Klebsiella pneumoniae* producing CTX-M-3 and SHV-5 beta-lactamases. J Antimicrob Chemother 2007; 60(2): 410-3.
[http://dx.doi.org/10.1093/jac/dkm215] [PMID: 17576696]

[39]   Cai JC, Hu YY, Zhang R, Zhou HW, Chen G-X. Detection of OmpK36 porin loss in Klebsiella spp.

by matrix-assisted laser desorption ionization-time of flight mass spectrometry. J Clin Microbiol 2012; 50(6): 2179-82.
[http://dx.doi.org/10.1128/JCM.00503-12] [PMID: 22493329]

[40]   Chen LR, Zhou HW, Cai JC, Zhang R, Chen GX. Combination of IMP-4 metallo-beta-lactamase production and porin deficiency causes carbapenem resistance in a *Klebsiella oxytoca* clinical isolate. Diagn Microbiol Infect Dis 2009; 65(2): 163-7.
[http://dx.doi.org/10.1016/j.diagmicrobio.2009.07.002] [PMID: 19748427]

[41]   Sugawara E, Kojima S, Nikaido H. *Klebsiella pneumoniae* Major Porins OmpK35 and OmpK36 Allow More Efficient Diffusion of β-Lactams than Their *Escherichia coli* Homologs OmpF and OmpC. J Bacteriol 2016; 198(23): 3200-8.
[http://dx.doi.org/10.1128/JB.00590-16] [PMID: 27645385]

[42]   Curtis NA, Eisenstadt RL, Turner KA, White AJ. Porin-mediated cephalosporin resistance in *Escherichia coli* K-12. J Antimicrob Chemother 1985; 15(5): 642-4.
[http://dx.doi.org/10.1093/jac/15.5.642] [PMID: 3891712]

[43]   Pang Z, Raudonis R, Glick BR, Lin T-J, Cheng Z. Antibiotic resistance in *Pseudomonas aeruginosa*: mechanisms and alternative therapeutic strategies. Biotechnol Adv 2019; 37(1): 177-92.
[http://dx.doi.org/10.1016/j.biotechadv.2018.11.013] [PMID: 30500353]

[44]   Agah Terzi H, Kulah C, Riza Atasoy A, Hakki Ciftci I. Investigation of OprD Porin Protein Levels in Carbapenem-Resistant *Pseudomonas aeruginosa* Isolates. Jundishapur J Microbiol 2015; 8(12): e25952.
[http://dx.doi.org/10.5812/jjm.25952] [PMID: 26865937]

[45]   Ruiz N, Montero T, Hernandez-Borrell J, Viñas M. The role of *Serratia marcescens* porins in antibiotic resistance. Microb Drug Resist 2003; 9(3): 257-64.
[http://dx.doi.org/10.1089/107662903322286463] [PMID: 12959404]

[46]   Olesky M, Zhao S, Rosenberg RL, Nicholas RA. Porin-mediated antibiotic resistance in *Neisseria gonorrhoeae*: ion, solute, and antibiotic permeation through PIB proteins with penB mutations. J Bacteriol 2006; 188(7): 2300-8.
[http://dx.doi.org/10.1128/JB.188.7.2300-2308.2006] [PMID: 16547016]

[47]   Olesky M, Hobbs M, Nicholas RA. Identification and analysis of amino acid mutations in porin IB that mediate intermediate-level resistance to penicillin and tetracycline in *Neisseria gonorrhoeae*. Antimicrob Agents Chemother 2002; 46(9): 2811-20.
[http://dx.doi.org/10.1128/AAC.46.9.2811-2820.2002] [PMID: 12183233]

[48]   Vidovic S, An R, Rendahl A. Molecular and physiological characterization of fluoroquinolone-highly resistant *Salmonella* Enteritidis strains. Front Microbiol 2019; 10: 729.
[http://dx.doi.org/10.3389/fmicb.2019.00729] [PMID: 31024504]

[49]   Gao H, Zhang Y, Han Y, *et al.* Phenotypic and transcriptional analysis of the osmotic regulator OmpR in Yersinia pestis. BMC Microbiol 2011; 11: 39.
[http://dx.doi.org/10.1186/1471-2180-11-39] [PMID: 21345178]

[50]   Nikaido H, PagA"s JM. Broad-specificity efflux pumps and their role in multidrug resistance of Gram-negative bacteria. FEMS Microbiol Rev 2012; 36(2): 340-63.
[http://dx.doi.org/10.1111/j.1574-6976.2011.00290.x] [PMID: 21707670]

[51]   Piddock LJ. Multidrug-resistance efflux pumps - not just for resistance. Nat Rev Microbiol 2006; 4(8): 629-36.
[http://dx.doi.org/10.1038/nrmicro1464] [PMID: 16845433]

[52]   Bohnert JA, Schuster S, FAhnrich E, Trittler R, Kern WV. Altered spectrum of multidrug resistance associated with a single point mutation in the *Escherichia coli* RND-type MDR efflux pump YhiV (MdtF). J Antimicrob Chemother 2007; 59(6): 1216-22.
[http://dx.doi.org/10.1093/jac/dkl426] [PMID: 17062614]

[53]   Blanco P, Corona F, MartA-nez JL. Involvement of the RND efflux pump transporter SmeH in the acquisition of resistance to ceftazidime in *Stenotrophomonas maltophilia*. Sci Rep 2019; 9(1): 4917.
[http://dx.doi.org/10.1038/s41598-019-41308-9] [PMID: 30894628]

[54]   Choudhury D, Talukdar AD, Chetia P, Bhattacharjee A, Choudhury MD. Screening of natural products and derivatives for the identification of RND efflux pump inhibitors. Comb Chem High Throughput Screen 2016; 19(9): 705-13.
[http://dx.doi.org/10.2174/1386207319666160720101502] [PMID: 27450181]

[55]   Lin W, Wan K, Zeng J, Li J, Li X, Yu X. Low nutrient levels as drinking water conditions can reduce the fitness cost of efflux pump-mediated ciprofloxacin resistance in *Pseudomonas aeruginosa*. J Environ Sci (China) 2019; 83: 123-32.
[http://dx.doi.org/10.1016/j.jes.2019.03.022] [PMID: 31221375]

[56]   Adabi M, Talebi-Taher M, Arbabi L, *et al.* Spread of efflux pump overexpressing-mediated fluoroquinolone resistance and multidrug resistance in *Pseudomonas aeruginosa* by using an efflux pump inhibitor. Infect Chemother 2015; 47(2): 98-104.
[http://dx.doi.org/10.3947/ic.2015.47.2.98] [PMID: 26157587]

[57]   Hirai K, Suzue S, Irikura T, Iyobe S, Mitsuhashi S. Mutations producing resistance to norfloxacin in *Pseudomonas aeruginosa*. Antimicrob Agents Chemother 1987; 31(4): 582-6.
[http://dx.doi.org/10.1128/AAC.31.4.582] [PMID: 3111356]

[58]   Aono R, Tsukagoshi N, Yamamoto M. Involvement of outer membrane protein TolC, a possible member of the mar-sox regulon, in maintenance and improvement of organic solvent tolerance of *Escherichia coli* K-12. J Bacteriol 1998; 180(4): 938-44.
[http://dx.doi.org/10.1128/JB.180.4.938-944.1998] [PMID: 9473050]

[59]   Atac N, Kurt-Azap O, Dolapci I, *et al.* The Role of AcrAB-TolC Efflux Pumps on Quinolone Resistance of *E. coli* ST131. Curr Microbiol 2018; 75(12): 1661-6.
[http://dx.doi.org/10.1007/s00284-018-1577-y] [PMID: 30283991]

[60]   Lloyd NA, Nazaret S, Barkay T. Genome-facilitated discovery of RND efflux pump-mediated resistance to cephalosporins in Vibrio spp. isolated from the mummichog fish gut. J Glob Antimicrob Resist 2019; 19: 294-300.
[http://dx.doi.org/10.1016/j.jgar.2019.05.006] [PMID: 31100504]

[61]   Webb JR, Price EP, Somprasong N, *et al.* Development and validation of a triplex quantitative real-time PCR assay to detect efflux pump-mediated antibiotic resistance in *Burkholderia pseudomallei*. Future Microbiol 2018; 13: 1403-18.
[http://dx.doi.org/10.2217/fmb-2018-0155] [PMID: 30256166]

[62]   Veal WL, Nicholas RA, Shafer WM. Overexpression of the MtrC-MtrD-MtrE efflux pump due to an mtrR mutation is required for chromosomally mediated penicillin resistance in *Neisseria gonorrhoeae*. J Bacteriol 2002; 184(20): 5619-24.
[http://dx.doi.org/10.1128/JB.184.20.5619-5624.2002] [PMID: 12270819]

[63]   Uddin MJ, Ahn J. Characterization of β-lactamase- and efflux pump-mediated multiple antibiotic resistance in *Salmonella typhimurium*. Food Sci Biotechnol 2018; 27(3): 921-8.
[http://dx.doi.org/10.1007/s10068-018-0317-1] [PMID: 30263820]

[64]   Li XZ, Zhang L, Nikaido H. Efflux pump-mediated intrinsic drug resistance in *Mycobacterium smegmatis*. Antimicrob Agents Chemother 2004; 48(7): 2415-23.
[http://dx.doi.org/10.1128/AAC.48.7.2415-2423.2004] [PMID: 15215089]

[65]   Ramón-García S, Martín C, Aínsa JA, De Rossi E. Characterization of tetracycline resistance mediated by the efflux pump Tap from *Mycobacterium fortuitum*. J Antimicrob Chemother 2006; 57(2): 252-9.
[http://dx.doi.org/10.1093/jac/dki436] [PMID: 16373429]

[66]   Gad GF, Mohamed HA, Ashour HM. Aminoglycoside resistance rates, phenotypes, and mechanisms of Gram-negative bacteria from infected patients in upper Egypt. PLoS One 2011; 6(2): e17224-4.

[http://dx.doi.org/10.1371/journal.pone.0017224] [PMID: 21359143]

[67]   Hart EM, Mitchell AM, Konovalova A, *et al.* A small-molecule inhibitor of BamA impervious to efflux and the outer membrane permeability barrier. Proc Natl Acad Sci USA 2019; 116(43): 21748-57.
[http://dx.doi.org/10.1073/pnas.1912345116] [PMID: 31591200]

[68]   Zapun A, Contreras-Martel C, Vernet T. Penicillin-binding proteins and beta-lactam resistance. FEMS Microbiol Rev 2008; 32(2): 361-85.
[http://dx.doi.org/10.1111/j.1574-6976.2007.00095.x] [PMID: 18248419]

[69]   Yeats C, Finn RD, Bateman A. The PASTA domain: a beta-lactam-binding domain. Trends Biochem Sci 2002; 27(9): 438-40.
[http://dx.doi.org/10.1016/S0968-0004(02)02164-3] [PMID: 12217513]

[70]   Tipper DJ, Strominger JL. Mechanism of action of penicillins: a proposal based on their structural similarity to acyl-D-alanyl-D-alanine. Proc Natl Acad Sci USA 1965; 54(4): 1133-41.
[http://dx.doi.org/10.1073/pnas.54.4.1133] [PMID: 5219821]

[71]   Goffin C, Ghuysen JM. Multimodular penicillin-binding proteins: an enigmatic family of orthologs and paralogs. Microbiol Mol Biol Rev 1998; 62(4): 1079-93.
[http://dx.doi.org/10.1128/MMBR.62.4.1079-1093.1998] [PMID: 9841666]

[72]   Sauvage E, Kerff F, Terrak M, Ayala JA, Charlier P. The penicillin-binding proteins: structure and role in peptidoglycan biosynthesis. FEMS Microbiol Rev 2008; 32(2): 234-58.
[http://dx.doi.org/10.1111/j.1574-6976.2008.00105.x] [PMID: 18266856]

[73]   den Blaauwen T, de Pedro MA, Nguyen-DistA"che M, Ayala JA. Morphogenesis of rod-shaped sacculi. FEMS Microbiol Rev 2008; 32(2): 321-44.
[http://dx.doi.org/10.1111/j.1574-6976.2007.00090.x] [PMID: 18291013]

[74]   Denome SA, Elf PK, Henderson TA, Nelson DE, Young KD. *Escherichia coli* mutants lacking all possible combinations of eight penicillin binding proteins: viability, characteristics, and implications for peptidoglycan synthesis. J Bacteriol 1999; 181(13): 3981-93.
[http://dx.doi.org/10.1128/JB.181.13.3981-3993.1999] [PMID: 10383966]

[75]   Potluri L-P, de Pedro MA, Young KD. *Escherichia coli* low-molecular-weight penicillin-binding proteins help orient septal FtsZ, and their absence leads to asymmetric cell division and branching. Mol Microbiol 2012; 84(2): 203-24.
[http://dx.doi.org/10.1111/j.1365-2958.2012.08023.x] [PMID: 22390731]

[76]   Bugg TD, Wright GD, Dutka-Malen S, Arthur M, Courvalin P, Walsh CT. Molecular basis for vancomycin resistance in *Enterococcus faecium* BM4147: biosynthesis of a depsipeptide peptidoglycan precursor by vancomycin resistance proteins VanH and VanA. Biochemistry 1991; 30(43): 10408-15.
[http://dx.doi.org/10.1021/bi00107a007] [PMID: 1931965]

[77]   Fyfe C, Grossman TH, Kerstein K, Sutcliffe J. Resistance to macrolide antibiotics in public health pathogens. Cold Spring Harb Perspect Med 2016; 6(10): a025395.
[http://dx.doi.org/10.1101/cshperspect.a025395] [PMID: 27527699]

[78]   Musser JM. Antimicrobial agent resistance in mycobacteria: molecular genetic insights. Clin Microbiol Rev 1995; 8(4): 496-514.
[http://dx.doi.org/10.1128/CMR.8.4.496] [PMID: 8665467]

[79]   TArAk ME, Chantratita N, Peacock SJ. Bacterial gene loss as a mechanism for gain of antimicrobial resistance. Curr Opin Microbiol 2012; 15(5): 583-7.
[http://dx.doi.org/10.1016/j.mib.2012.07.008] [PMID: 23022568]

[80]   Hayes MV, Orr DC. Mode of action of ceftazidime: affinity for the penicillin-binding proteins of *Escherichia coli* K12, *Pseudomonas aeruginosa* and *Staphylococcus aureus*. J Antimicrob Chemother 1983; 12(2): 119-26.

[http://dx.doi.org/10.1093/jac/12.2.119] [PMID: 6413485]

[81] Moya B, DAtsch A, Juan C, *et al.* Beta-lactam resistance response triggered by inactivation of a nonessential penicillin-binding protein. PLoS Pathog 2009; 5(3): e1000353.
[http://dx.doi.org/10.1371/journal.ppat.1000353] [PMID: 19325877]

[82] Bryskier A. Fluoroquinolones: mechanisms of action and resistance. Int J Antimicrob Agents 1993; 2(3): 151-83.
[http://dx.doi.org/10.1016/0924-8579(93)90052-7] [PMID: 18611533]

[83] Guzman LM, Barondess JJ, Beckwith J. FtsL, an essential cytoplasmic membrane protein involved in cell division in *Escherichia coli*. J Bacteriol 1992; 174(23): 7716-28.
[http://dx.doi.org/10.1128/JB.174.23.7717-7728.1992] [PMID: 1332942]

[84] Yamachika S, Sugihara C, Kamai Y, Yamashita M. Correlation between penicillin-binding protein 2 mutations and carbapenem resistance in *Escherichia coli*. J Med Microbiol 2013; 62(Pt 3): 429-36.
[http://dx.doi.org/10.1099/jmm.0.051631-0] [PMID: 23222859]

[85] Rodrigues ACS, Santos ICO, Campos CC, *et al.* Non-clonal occurrence of pmrB mutations associated with polymyxin resistance in carbapenem-resistant *Klebsiella pneumoniae* in Brazil. Mem Inst Oswaldo Cruz 2019; 114: e180555.
[http://dx.doi.org/10.1590/0074-02760180555] [PMID: 31116243]

[86] Phan MD, Nhu NTK, Achard MES, *et al.* Modifications in the pmrB gene are the primary mechanism for the development of chromosomally encoded resistance to polymyxins in uropathogenic *Escherichia coli*. J Antimicrob Chemother 2017; 72(10): 2729-36.
[http://dx.doi.org/10.1093/jac/dkx204] [PMID: 29091192]

[87] Cannatelli A, Giani T, Aiezza N, *et al.* An allelic variant of the PmrB sensor kinase responsible for colistin resistance in an *Escherichia coli* strain of clinical origin. Sci Rep 2017; 7(1): 5071.
[http://dx.doi.org/10.1038/s41598-017-05167-6] [PMID: 28698568]

[88] Kampranis SC, Bates AD, Maxwell A. A model for the mechanism of strand passage by DNA gyrase. Proc Natl Acad Sci USA 1999; 96(15): 8414-9.
[http://dx.doi.org/10.1073/pnas.96.15.8414] [PMID: 10411889]

[89] Hiasa H, Shea ME. DNA gyrase-mediated wrapping of the DNA strand is required for the replication fork arrest by the DNA gyrase-quinolone-DNA ternary complex. J Biol Chem 2000; 275(44): 34780-6.
[http://dx.doi.org/10.1074/jbc.M001608200] [PMID: 11053451]

[90] Whitchurch CB, Tolker-Nielsen T, Ragas PC, Mattick JS. Extracellular DNA required for bacterial biofilm formation. Science 2002; 295(5559): 1487.
[http://dx.doi.org/10.1126/science.295.5559.1487] [PMID: 11859186]

[91] Raad II, Sabbagh MF, Rand KH, Sherertz RJ. Quantitative tip culture methods and the diagnosis of central venous catheter-related infections. Diagn Microbiol Infect Dis 1992; 15(1): 13-20.
[http://dx.doi.org/10.1016/0732-8893(92)90052-U] [PMID: 1730183]

[92] Abraham SN, Beachey EH, Simpson WA. Adherence of S*treptococcus pyogenes, Escherichia coli,* and *Pseudomonas aeruginosa* to fibronectin-coated and uncoated epithelial cells. Infect Immun 1983; 41(3): 1261-8.
[http://dx.doi.org/10.1128/IAI.41.3.1261-1268.1983] [PMID: 6411621]

[93] Flemming H-C, Neu TR, Wozniak DJ. The EPS Matrix: The "House of Biofilm Cells". J Bacteriol 2007; 189(22): 7945-7.
[http://dx.doi.org/10.1128/JB.00858-07] [PMID: 17675377]

[94] Cepas V, López Y, Muñoz E, *et al.* Relationship between biofilm formation and antimicrobial resistance in gram-negative bacteria. Microb Drug Resist 2019; 25(1): 72-9.
[http://dx.doi.org/10.1089/mdr.2018.0027] [PMID: 30142035]

[95] Dumaru R, Baral R, Shrestha LB. Study of biofilm formation and antibiotic resistance pattern of

gram-negative Bacilli among the clinical isolates at BPKIHS, Dharan. BMC Res Notes 2019; 12(1): 38-8.
[http://dx.doi.org/10.1186/s13104-019-4084-8] [PMID: 30658694]

[96]   Williams I, Venables WA, Lloyd D, Paul F, Critchley I. The effects of adherence to silicone surfaces on antibiotic susceptibility in *Staphylococcus aureus*. Microbiology 1997; 143(Pt 7): 2407-13.
[http://dx.doi.org/10.1099/00221287-143-7-2407] [PMID: 9245822]

[97]   Hoyle BD, Wong CK, Costerton JW. Disparate efficacy of tobramycin on Ca(2+)-, Mg(2+)-, and HEPES-treated *Pseudomonas aeruginosa* biofilms. Can J Microbiol 1992; 38(11): 1214-8.
[http://dx.doi.org/10.1139/m92-201] [PMID: 1477794]

[98]   Tresse O, Jouenne T, Junter GA. The role of oxygen limitation in the resistance of agar-entrapped, sessile-like *Escherichia coli* to aminoglycoside and beta-lactam antibiotics. J Antimicrob Chemother 1995; 36(3): 521-6.
[http://dx.doi.org/10.1093/jac/36.3.521] [PMID: 8830016]

[99]   Hausner M, Wuertz S. High rates of conjugation in bacterial biofilms as determined by quantitative in situ analysis. Appl Environ Microbiol 1999; 65(8): 3710-3.
[http://dx.doi.org/10.1128/AEM.65.8.3710-3713.1999] [PMID: 10427070]

[100] Ceri H, Olson ME, Stremick C, Read RR, Morck D, Buret A. The Calgary Biofilm Device: new technology for rapid determination of antibiotic susceptibilities of bacterial biofilms. J Clin Microbiol 1999; 37(6): 1771-6.
[http://dx.doi.org/10.1128/JCM.37.6.1771-1776.1999] [PMID: 10325322]

[101] Tanwar J, Das S, Fatima Z, Hameed S. Multidrug resistance: an emerging crisis. Interdiscip Perspect Infect Dis 2014; 2014: 541340.
[http://dx.doi.org/10.1155/2014/541340] [PMID: 25140175]

[102] Liu Y, Shi L, Su L, *et al.* Nanotechnology-based antimicrobials and delivery systems for biofilm-infection control. Chem Soc Rev 2019; 48(2): 428-46.
[http://dx.doi.org/10.1039/C7CS00807D] [PMID: 30601473]

[103] Prigent-Combaret C, Vidal O, Dorel C, Lejeune P. Abiotic surface sensing and biofilm-dependent regulation of gene expression in *Escherichia coli*. J Bacteriol 1999; 181(19): 5993-6002.
[http://dx.doi.org/10.1128/JB.181.19.5993-6002.1999] [PMID: 10498711]

[104] Niba ET, Naka Y, Nagase M, Mori H, Kitakawa M. A genome-wide approach to identify the genes involved in biofilm formation in *E. coli*. DNA Res 2007; 14(6): 237-46.
[http://dx.doi.org/10.1093/dnares/dsm024] [PMID: 18180259]

[105] Otto K, Silhavy TJ. Surface sensing and adhesion of *Escherichia coli* controlled by the Cpx-signaling pathway. Proc Natl Acad Sci USA 2002; 99(4): 2287-92.
[http://dx.doi.org/10.1073/pnas.042521699] [PMID: 11830644]

[106] Zhuo C, Zhao QY, Xiao SN. The impact of spgM, rpfF, rmlA gene distribution on biofilm formation in *Stenotrophomonas maltophilia*. PLoS One 2014; 9(10): e108409.
[http://dx.doi.org/10.1371/journal.pone.0108409] [PMID: 25285537]

[107] Huang TP, Somers EB, Wong AC. Differential biofilm formation and motility associated with lipopolysaccharide/exopolysaccharide-coupled biosynthetic genes in *Stenotrophomonas maltophilia*. J Bacteriol 2006; 188(8): 3116-20.
[http://dx.doi.org/10.1128/JB.188.8.3116-3120.2006] [PMID: 16585771]

[108] Lin YT, Huang YW, Chen SJ, Chang CW, Yang TC. The SmeYZ efflux pump of *Stenotrophomonas maltophilia* contributes to drug resistance, virulence-related characteristics, and virulence in mice. Antimicrob Agents Chemother 2015; 59(7): 4067-73.
[http://dx.doi.org/10.1128/AAC.00372-15] [PMID: 25918140]

[109] Kang XM, Wang FF, Zhang H, Zhang Q, Qiana W. Genome-wide identification of genes necessary for biofilm formation by nosocomial pathogen *Stenotrophomonas maltophilia* reveals that orphan

response regulator FsnR is a critical modulator. Appl Environ Microbiol 2015; 81(4): 1200-9.
[http://dx.doi.org/10.1128/AEM.03408-14] [PMID: 25480754]

[110] Yang JG, Shih MS, Kuo WT, Chin KH, Shen GH, Chou SH. Crystallization of the N-terminal regulatory domain of the enhancer-binding protein FleQ from *Stenotrophomonas maltophilia*. Acta Crystallogr F Struct Biol Commun 2014; 70(Pt 3): 326-30.
[http://dx.doi.org/10.1107/S2053230X14001514] [PMID: 24598919]

[111] Boukerb AM, Simon M, Pernet E, *et al.* Draft genome sequences of four *Pseudomonas aeruginosa* clinical strains with various biofilm phenotypes. 2020.
[http://dx.doi.org/10.1128/MRA.01286-19]

[112] Çankirili NK, Kart D, Çelebi-Saltik B. Evaluation of the biofilm formation of *Staphylococcus aureus* and *Pseudomonas aeruginosa* on human umbilical cord CD146+ stem cells and stem cell-based decellularized matrix. Cell Tissue Bank 2020.
[http://dx.doi.org/10.1007/s10561-020-09815-6] [PMID: 32020424]

[113] Gao XY, Liu Y, Miao LL, Liu ZP. Pseudomonas sp. AOB-7 utilizes PHA granules as a sustained-release carbon source and biofilm carrier for aerobic denitrification of aquaculture water. Appl Microbiol Biotechnol 2020; 104(7): 3183-92.
[http://dx.doi.org/10.1007/s00253-020-10452-y] [PMID: 32055912]

[114] Ahmed T, Pattnaik S, Khan MB, Ampasala DR, Busi S, Sarma VV. Inhibition of quorum sensing-associated virulence factors and biofilm formation in *Pseudomonas aeruginosa* PAO1 by *Mycoleptodiscus indicus* PUTY1. Braz J Microbiol 2020; 51(2): 467-87.
[http://dx.doi.org/10.1007/s42770-020-00235-y] [PMID: 32086747]

[115] Karballaei Mirzahosseini H, Hadadi-Fishani M, Morshedi K, Khaledi A. Meta-analysis of biofilm formation, antibiotic resistance pattern, and biofilm-related genes in *Pseudomonas aeruginosa* isolated from clinical samples. Microb Drug Resist 2020; 26(7).
[http://dx.doi.org/10.1089/mdr.2019.0274] [PMID: 31976811]

[116] Li Y, Xia H, Bai F, *et al.* PA5001 gene involves in swimming motility and biofilm formation in *Pseudomonas aeruginosa*. Microb Pathog 2020; 144: 103982.
[http://dx.doi.org/10.1016/j.micpath.2020.103982] [PMID: 32105802]

[117] Zhu Y, Li JJ, Reng J, Wang S, Zhang R, Wang B. Global trends of *Pseudomonas aeruginosa* biofilm research in the past two decades: A bibliometric study. MicrobiologyOpen 2020; 9(1) .
[http://dx.doi.org/10.1002/mbo3.1021] [PMID: 32120451]

[118] Zhanel GG, Dueck M, Hoban DJ, *et al.* Review of macrolides and ketolides: focus on respiratory tract infections. Drugs 2001; 61(4): 443-98.
[http://dx.doi.org/10.2165/00003495-200161040-00003] [PMID: 11324679]

[119] Svetlov MS, Vázquez-Laslop N, Mankin AS. Kinetics of drug-ribosome interactions defines the cidality of macrolide antibiotics. Proc Natl Acad Sci USA 2017; 114(52): 13673-8.
[http://dx.doi.org/10.1073/pnas.1717168115] [PMID: 29229833]

[120] Zhong P, Cao Z, Hammond R, *et al.* Induction of ribosome methylation in MLS-resistant Streptococcus pneumoniae by macrolides and ketolides. Microb Drug Resist 1999; 5(3): 183-8.
[http://dx.doi.org/10.1089/mdr.1999.5.183] [PMID: 10566867]

[121] Zaman S, Fitzpatrick M, Lindahl L, Zengel J. Novel mutations in ribosomal proteins L4 and L22 that confer erythromycin resistance in *Escherichia coli*. Mol Microbiol 2007; 66(4): 1039-50.
[http://dx.doi.org/10.1111/j.1365-2958.2007.05975.x] [PMID: 17956547]

[122] Ojo KK, Striplin MJ, Ulep CC, *et al.* Staphylococcus efflux msr(A) gene characterized in Streptococcus, Enterococcus, Corynebacterium, and Pseudomonas isolates. Antimicrob Agents Chemother 2006; 50(3): 1089-91.
[http://dx.doi.org/10.1128/AAC.50.3.1089-1091.2006] [PMID: 16495276]

[123] Pernodet JL, Fish S, Blondelet-Rouault MH, Cundliffe E. The macrolide-lincosamide-streptogramin B

resistance phenotypes characterized by using a specifically deleted, antibiotic-sensitive strain of *Streptomyces lividans*. Antimicrob Agents Chemother 1996; 40(3): 581-5.
[http://dx.doi.org/10.1128/AAC.40.3.581] [PMID: 8851574]

[124] Noguchi N, Emura A, Matsuyama H, O'Hara K, Sasatsu M, Kono M. Nucleotide sequence and characterization of erythromycin resistance determinant that encodes macrolide 2-phosphotransferase I in *Escherichia coli*. Antimicrob Agents Chemother 1995; 39(10): 2359-63.
[http://dx.doi.org/10.1128/AAC.39.10.2359] [PMID: 8619599]

[125] Golkar T, Zieliński M, Berghuis AM. Look and outlook on enzyme-mediated macrolide resistance. Front Microbiol 2018; 9: 1942-2.
[http://dx.doi.org/10.3389/fmicb.2018.01942] [PMID: 30177927]

[126] Barthelemy CR, Nakayama DA, Carrera GF, Lightfoot RW Jr, Wortmann RL. Gouty arthritis: a prospective radiographic evaluation of sixty patients. Skeletal Radiol 1984; 11(1): 1-8.
[http://dx.doi.org/10.1007/BF00361124] [PMID: 6710175]

[127] Ounissi H, Courvalin P. Nucleotide sequence of the gene ereA encoding the erythromycin esterase in *Escherichia coli*. Gene 1985; 35(3): 271-8.
[http://dx.doi.org/10.1016/0378-1119(85)90005-8] [PMID: 3899861]

[128] Thungapathra M, Amita , Sinha KK, *et al*. Occurrence of antibiotic resistance gene cassettes aac(6′)-Ib, dfrA5, dfrA12, and ereA2 in class I integrons in non-O1, non-O139 *Vibrio cholerae* strains in India. Antimicrob Agents Chemother 2002; 46(9): 2948-55.
[http://dx.doi.org/10.1128/AAC.46.9.2948-2955.2002] [PMID: 12183252]

[129] Shakil S, Khan R, Zarrilli R, Khan AU. Aminoglycosides versus bacteria--a description of the action, resistance mechanism, and nosocomial battleground. J Biomed Sci 2008; 15(1): 5-14.
[http://dx.doi.org/10.1007/s11373-007-9194-y] [PMID: 17657587]

[130] Veinberg G, Vorona M, Shestakova I, Kanepe I, Lukevics E. Design of beta-lactams with mechanism based nonantibacterial activities. Curr Med Chem 2003; 10(17): 1741-57.
[http://dx.doi.org/10.2174/0929867033457089] [PMID: 12871119]

[131] Global Priority List of Antibiotic-Resistant Bacteria to Guide Research, Discovery, and Development of New Antibiotics. Geneva, Switzerland: WHO 2017.

[132] Magiorakos AP, Suetens C, Monnet DL, Gagliotti C, Heuer OE. The rise of carbapenem resistance in Europe: just the tip of the iceberg? Antimicrob Resist Infect Control 2013; 2(1): 6.
[http://dx.doi.org/10.1186/2047-2994-2-6] [PMID: 23410479]

[133] Xu A, Zheng B, Xu YC, Huang ZG, Zhong NS, Zhuo C. National epidemiology of carbapenem-resistant and extensively drug-resistant Gram-negative bacteria isolated from blood samples in China in 2013. Clin Microbiol Infect 2016; 22 (Suppl. 1): S1-8.
[http://dx.doi.org/10.1016/j.cmi.2015.09.015] [PMID: 26846351]

[134] van Duin D, Doi Y. The global epidemiology of carbapenemase-producing *Enterobacteriaceae*. Virulence 2017; 8(4): 460-9.
[http://dx.doi.org/10.1080/21505594.2016.1222343] [PMID: 27593176]

[135] Meletis G, Chatzidimitriou D, Malisiovas N. Double- and multi-carbapenemase-producers: the excessively armored bacilli of the current decade. Eur J Clin Microbiol Infect Dis 2015; 34(8): 1487-93.
[http://dx.doi.org/10.1007/s10096-015-2379-9] [PMID: 25894987]

[136] Castanheira M, Deshpande LM, Mendes RE, Canton R, Sader HS, Jones RN. Variations in the Occurrence of Resistance Phenotypes and Carbapenemase Genes Among *Enterobacteriaceae* Isolates in 20 Years of the SENTRY Antimicrobial Surveillance Program. Open Forum Infect Dis 2019; 6 (Suppl. 1): S23-33.
[http://dx.doi.org/10.1093/ofid/ofy347] [PMID: 30895212]

[137] Lautenbach E, Patel JB, Bilker WB, Edelstein PH, Fishman NO. Extended-spectrum beta-lactamas-

-producing *Escherichia coli* and *Klebsiella pneumoniae*: risk factors for infection and impact of resistance on outcomes. Clin Infect Dis 2001; 32(8): 1162-71.
[http://dx.doi.org/10.1086/319757] [PMID: 11283805]

[138] Gasink LB, Edelstein PH, Lautenbach E, Synnestvedt M, Fishman NO. Risk factors and clinical impact of *Klebsiella pneumoniae* carbapenemase-producing *K. pneumoniae*. Infect Control Hosp Epidemiol 2009; 30(12): 1180-5.
[http://dx.doi.org/10.1086/648451] [PMID: 19860564]

[139] Alvim ALS, Couto BRGM, Gazzinelli A. Epidemiological profile of healthcare-associated infections caused by Carbapenemase-producing *Enterobacteriaceae*. Rev Esc Enferm USP 2019; 53: e03474.
[http://dx.doi.org/10.1590/s1980-220x2018001903474] [PMID: 31291394]

[140] Ghaith DM, Mohamed ZK, Farahat MG, Aboulkasem Shahin W, Mohamed HO. Colonization of intestinal microbiota with carbapenemase-producing *Enterobacteriaceae* in paediatric intensive care units in Cairo, Egypt. Arab J Gastroenterol 2019; 20(1): 19-22.
[http://dx.doi.org/10.1016/j.ajg.2019.01.002] [PMID: 30733176]

[141] Fernando SA, Phan T, Parker C, Cai T, Gottlieb T. Increased detection of carbapenemase-producing *Enterobacteriaceae* on post-clean sampling of a burns unit's wet surfaces. J Hosp Infect 2019; 101(2): 179-82.
[http://dx.doi.org/10.1016/j.jhin.2018.10.002] [PMID: 30321628]

[142] Chiotos K, Tamma PD, Flett KB, *et al.* Multicenter study of the risk factors for colonization or infection with carbapenem-resistant *Enterobacteriaceae* in children. Antimicrob Agents Chemother 2017; 61(12): e01440-17.
[http://dx.doi.org/10.1128/AAC.01440-17] [PMID: 28971864]

[143] Errico G, Gagliotti C, Monaco M, *et al.* Colonization and infection due to carbapenemase-producing *Enterobacteriaceae* in liver and lung transplant recipients and donor-derived transmission: a prospective cohort study conducted in Italy. Clin Microbiol Infect 2019; 25(2): 203-9.
[http://dx.doi.org/10.1016/j.cmi.2018.05.003] [PMID: 29800674]

[144] Mercuri PS, Ishii Y, Ma L, *et al.* Clonal diversity and metallo-beta-lactamase production in clinical isolates of *Stenotrophomonas maltophilia*. Microb Drug Resist 2002; 8(3): 193-200.
[http://dx.doi.org/10.1089/107662902760326904] [PMID: 12363008]

[145] Jacoby GA. AmpC beta-lactamases. Clin Microbiol Rev 2009; 22(1): 161-82. [Table of Contents.].
[http://dx.doi.org/10.1128/CMR.00036-08] [PMID: 19136439]

[146] Bush K, Jacoby GA, Medeiros AA. A functional classification scheme for beta-lactamases and its correlation with molecular structure. Antimicrob Agents Chemother 1995; 39(6): 1211-33.
[http://dx.doi.org/10.1128/AAC.39.6.1211] [PMID: 7574506]

[147] Poirel L, Pitout JD, Nordmann P. Carbapenemases: molecular diversity and clinical consequences. Future Microbiol 2007; 2(5): 501-12.
[http://dx.doi.org/10.2217/17460913.2.5.501] [PMID: 17927473]

[148] Wolter DJ, Kurpiel PM, Woodford N, Palepou MF, Goering RV, Hanson ND. Phenotypic and enzymatic comparative analysis of the novel KPC variant KPC-5 and its evolutionary variants, KPC-2 and KPC-4. Antimicrob Agents Chemother 2009; 53(2): 557-62.
[http://dx.doi.org/10.1128/AAC.00734-08] [PMID: 19015357]

[149] Haidar G, Clancy CJ, Chen L, *et al.* Identifying spectra of activity and therapeutic niches for ceftazidime-avibactam and imipenem-relebactam against carbapenem-resistant *Enterobacteriaceae*. Antimicrob Agents Chemother 2017; 61(9): e00642-17.
[http://dx.doi.org/10.1128/AAC.00642-17] [PMID: 28630202]

[150] Bush K, Pannell M, Lock JL, *et al.* Detection systems for carbapenemase gene identification should include the SME serine carbapenemase. Int J Antimicrob Agents 2013; 41(1): 1-4.
[http://dx.doi.org/10.1016/j.ijantimicag.2012.08.008] [PMID: 23219246]

[151]   Yu YS, Du XX, Zhou ZH, Chen YG, Li LJ. First isolation of blaIMI-2 in an *Enterobacter cloacae* clinical isolate from China. Antimicrob Agents Chemother 2006; 50(4): 1610-1.
[http://dx.doi.org/10.1128/AAC.50.4.1610-1611.2006] [PMID: 16569898]

[152]   Rasmussen BA, Bush K, Keeney D, *et al.* Characterization of IMI-1 beta-lactamase, a class A carbapenem-hydrolyzing enzyme from *Enterobacter cloacae.* Antimicrob Agents Chemother 1996; 40(9): 2080-6.
[http://dx.doi.org/10.1128/AAC.40.9.2080] [PMID: 8878585]

[153]   Bradford PA. Extended-spectrum beta-lactamases in the 21st century: characterization, epidemiology, and detection of this important resistance threat. Clin Microbiol Rev 2001; 14(4): 933-51. [table of contents.].
[http://dx.doi.org/10.1128/CMR.14.4.933-951.2001] [PMID: 11585791]

[154]   Paterson DL, Hujer KM, Hujer AM, *et al.* Extended-spectrum beta-lactamases in *Klebsiella pneumoniae* bloodstream isolates from seven countries: dominance and widespread prevalence of SHV- and CTX-M-type beta-lactamases. Antimicrob Agents Chemother 2003; 47(11): 3554-60.
[http://dx.doi.org/10.1128/AAC.47.11.3554-3560.2003] [PMID: 14576117]

[155]   Queenan AM, Bush K. Carbapenemases: the versatile beta-lactamases. Clin Microbiol Rev 2007; 20(3): 440-58. [table of contents.].
[http://dx.doi.org/10.1128/CMR.00001-07] [PMID: 17630334]

[156]   Herzberg O, Moult J. Bacterial resistance to beta-lactam antibiotics: crystal structure of beta-lactamase from *Staphylococcus aureus* PC1 at 2.5 A resolution. Science 1987; 236(4802): 694-701.
[http://dx.doi.org/10.1126/science.3107125] [PMID: 3107125]

[157]   Yigit H, Queenan AM, Rasheed JK, *et al.* Carbapenem-resistant strain of *Klebsiella oxytoca* harboring carbapenem-hydrolyzing beta-lactamase KPC-2. Antimicrob Agents Chemother 2003; 47(12): 3881-9.
[http://dx.doi.org/10.1128/AAC.47.12.3881-3889.2003] [PMID: 14638498]

[158]   Brown RP, Aplin RT, Schofield CJ. Inhibition of TEM-2 beta-lactamase from *Escherichia coli* by clavulanic acid: observation of intermediates by electrospray ionization mass spectrometry. Biochemistry 1996; 35(38): 12421-32.
[http://dx.doi.org/10.1021/bi961044g] [PMID: 8823177]

[159]   Shaokat S, Ouellette M, Sirot D, Joly B, Cluzel R. Spread of SHV-1 beta-lactamase in *Escherichia coli* isolated from fecal samples in Africa. Antimicrob Agents Chemother 1987; 31(6): 943-5.
[http://dx.doi.org/10.1128/AAC.31.6.943] [PMID: 3304158]

[160]   Petit A, Gerbaud G, Sirot D, Courvalin P, Sirot J. Molecular epidemiology of TEM-3 (CTX-1) beta-lactamase. Antimicrob Agents Chemother 1990; 34(2): 219-24.
[http://dx.doi.org/10.1128/AAC.34.2.219] [PMID: 2327769]

[161]   Ben Yaghlane H, Ben Redjeb S, Boujenah A, Philippon A, Labia R. Obtainment of SHV-2 beta-lactamase overproducing mutants from *Escherichia coli* and *Klebsiella pneumoniae* clinical isolates. J Chemother 1989; 1(4) (Suppl.): 326.
[PMID: 16312423]

[162]   Ogbolu DO, Alli OAT, Webber MA, Oluremi AS, Oloyede OM. CTX-M-15 is established in most multidrug-resistant uropathogenic *Enterobacteriaceae* and Pseudomonaceae from hospitals in Nigeria. Eur J Microbiol Immunol (Bp) 2018; 8(1): 20-4.
[http://dx.doi.org/10.1556/1886.2017.00012] [PMID: 29760961]

[163]   Amirkamali S, Naserpour-Farivar T, Azarhoosh K, Peymani A. Distribution of the bla OXA, bla VEB-1, and bla GES-1 genes and resistance patterns of ESBL-producing *Pseudomonas aeruginosa* isolated from hospitals in Tehran and Qazvin, Iran. Rev Soc Bras Med Trop 2017; 50(3): 315-20.
[http://dx.doi.org/10.1590/0037-8682-0478-2016] [PMID: 28700048]

[164]   Wang X, Minasov G, Shoichet BK. The structural bases of antibiotic resistance in the clinically derived mutant beta-lactamases TEM-30, TEM-32, and TEM-34. J Biol Chem 2002; 277(35): 32149-

56.
[http://dx.doi.org/10.1074/jbc.M204212200] [PMID: 12058046]

[165] Prinarakis EE, Miriagou V, Tzelepi E, Gazouli M, Tzouvelekis LS. Emergence of an inhibitor-resistant beta-lactamase (SHV-10) derived from an SHV-5 variant. Antimicrob Agents Chemother 1997; 41(4): 838-40.
[http://dx.doi.org/10.1128/AAC.41.4.838] [PMID: 9087500]

[166] Sirot D, Recule C, Chaibi EB, *et al.* A complex mutant of TEM-1 beta-lactamase with mutations encountered in both IRT-4 and extended-spectrum TEM-15, produced by an *Escherichia coli* clinical isolate. Antimicrob Agents Chemother 1997; 41(6): 1322-5.
[http://dx.doi.org/10.1128/AAC.41.6.1322] [PMID: 9174192]

[167] Huovinen P, Jacoby GA. Sequence of the PSE-1 beta-lactamase gene. Antimicrob Agents Chemother 1991; 35(11): 2428-30.
[http://dx.doi.org/10.1128/AAC.35.11.2428] [PMID: 1804019]

[168] Lachapelle J, Dufresne J, Levesque RC. Characterization of the blaCARB-3 gene encoding the carbenicillinase-3 beta-lactamase of *Pseudomonas aeruginosa.* Gene 1991; 102(1): 7-12.
[http://dx.doi.org/10.1016/0378-1119(91)90530-O] [PMID: 1650733]

[169] Potron A, Poirel L, CroizA(c) J, Chanteperdrix V, Nordmann P. Genetic and biochemical characterization of the first extended-spectrum CARB-type beta-lactamase, RTG-4, from *Acinetobacter baumannii.* Antimicrob Agents Chemother 2009; 53(7): 3010-6.
[http://dx.doi.org/10.1128/AAC.01164-08] [PMID: 19380596]

[170] Rogers MB, Parker AC, Smith CJ. Cloning and characterization of the endogenous cephalosporinase gene, cepA, from *Bacteroides fragilis* reveals a new subgroup of Ambler class A beta-lactamases. Antimicrob Agents Chemother 1993; 37(11): 2391-400.
[http://dx.doi.org/10.1128/AAC.37.11.2391] [PMID: 8285623]

[171] Yigit H, Queenan AM, Anderson GJ, *et al.* Novel carbapenem-hydrolyzing beta-lactamase, KPC-1, from a carbapenem-resistant strain of *Klebsiella pneumoniae.* Antimicrob Agents Chemother 2001; 45(4): 1151-61.
[http://dx.doi.org/10.1128/AAC.45.4.1151-1161.2001] [PMID: 11257029]

[172] Smith Moland E, Hanson ND, Herrera VL, *et al.* Plasmid-mediated, carbapenem-hydrolysing beta-lactamase, KPC-2, in *Klebsiella pneumoniae* isolates. J Antimicrob Chemother 2003; 51(3): 711-4.
[http://dx.doi.org/10.1093/jac/dkg124] [PMID: 12615876]

[173] Villegas MV, Lolans K, Correa A, Kattan JN, Lopez JA, Quinn JP. First identification of *Pseudomonas aeruginosa* isolates producing a KPC-type carbapenem-hydrolyzing beta-lactamase. Antimicrob Agents Chemother 2007; 51(4): 1553-5.
[http://dx.doi.org/10.1128/AAC.01405-06] [PMID: 17261621]

[174] Navon-Venezia S, Chmelnitsky I, Leavitt A, Schwaber MJ, Schwartz D, Carmeli Y. Plasmid-mediated imipenem-hydrolyzing enzyme KPC-2 among multiple carbapenem-resistant *Escherichia coli* clones in Israel. Antimicrob Agents Chemother 2006; 50(9): 3098-101.
[http://dx.doi.org/10.1128/AAC.00438-06] [PMID: 16940107]

[175] Hossain A, Ferraro MJ, Pino RM, *et al.* Plasmid-mediated carbapenem-hydrolyzing enzyme KPC-2 in an Enterobacter sp. Antimicrob Agents Chemother 2004; 48(11): 4438-40.
[http://dx.doi.org/10.1128/AAC.48.11.4438-4440.2004] [PMID: 15504876]

[176] Alba J, Ishii Y, Thomson K, Moland ES, Yamaguchi K. Kinetics study of KPC-3, a plasmid-encoded class A carbapenem-hydrolyzing beta-lactamase. Antimicrob Agents Chemother 2005; 49(11): 4760-2.
[http://dx.doi.org/10.1128/AAC.49.11.4760-4762.2005] [PMID: 16251324]

[177] Kanamori H, Parobek CM, Juliano JJ, *et al.* A Prolonged Outbreak of KPC-3-Producing *Enterobacter cloacae* and *Klebsiella pneumoniae* Driven by Multiple Mechanisms of Resistance Transmission at a Large Academic Burn Center. Antimicrob Agents Chemother 2017; 61(2): e01516-16.

[http://dx.doi.org/10.1128/AAC.01516-16] [PMID: 27919898]

[178] Queenan AM, Torres-Viera C, Gold HS, *et al.* SME-type carbapenem-hydrolyzing class A beta-lactamases from geographically diverse *Serratia marcescens* strains. Antimicrob Agents Chemother 2000; 44(11): 3035-9.
[http://dx.doi.org/10.1128/AAC.44.11.3035-3039.2000] [PMID: 11036019]

[179] CarrA"r A, Poirel L, Pitout JD, Church D, Nordmann P. Occurrence of an SME-2-producing *Serratia marcescens* isolate in Canada. Int J Antimicrob Agents 2008; 31(2): 181-2.
[http://dx.doi.org/10.1016/j.ijantimicag.2007.10.007] [PMID: 18083009]

[180] Queenan AM, Shang W, Schreckenberger P, Lolans K, Bush K, Quinn J. SME-3, a novel member of the *Serratia marcescens* SME family of carbapenem-hydrolyzing beta-lactamases. Antimicrob Agents Chemother 2006; 50(10): 3485-7.
[http://dx.doi.org/10.1128/AAC.00363-06] [PMID: 17005839]

[181] Mariotte-Boyer S, Nicolas-Chanoine MH, Labia R. A kinetic study of NMC-A beta-lactamase, an Ambler class A carbapenemase also hydrolyzing cephamycins. FEMS Microbiol Lett 1996; 143(1): 29-33.
[PMID: 8807798]

[182] Poirel L, Le Thomas I, Naas T, Karim A, Nordmann P. Biochemical sequence analyses of GES-1, a novel class A extended-spectrum beta-lactamase, and the class 1 integron In52 from *Klebsiella pneumoniae*. Antimicrob Agents Chemother 2000; 44(3): 622-32.
[http://dx.doi.org/10.1128/AAC.44.3.622-632.2000] [PMID: 10681329]

[183] Vourli S, Giakkoupi P, Miriagou V, Tzelepi E, Vatopoulos AC, Tzouvelekis LS. Novel GES/IBC extended-spectrum beta-lactamase variants with carbapenemase activity in clinical enterobacteria. FEMS Microbiol Lett 2004; 234(2): 209-13.
[PMID: 15135524]

[184] Wang X, Zhang F, Zhao C, *et al. In vitro* activities of ceftazidime-avibactam and aztreonam-avibactam against 372 Gram-negative bacilli collected in 2011 and 2012 from 11 teaching hospitals in China. Antimicrob Agents Chemother 2014; 58(3): 1774-8.
[http://dx.doi.org/10.1128/AAC.02123-13] [PMID: 24342639]

[185] Palzkill T. Metallo-β-lactamase structure and function. Ann N Y Acad Sci 2013; 1277: 91-104.
[http://dx.doi.org/10.1111/j.1749-6632.2012.06796.x] [PMID: 23163348]

[186] Yang Y, Rasmussen BA, Bush K. Biochemical characterization of the metallo-beta-lactamase CcrA from *Bacteroides fragilis* TAL3636. Antimicrob Agents Chemother 1992; 36(5): 1155-7.
[http://dx.doi.org/10.1128/AAC.36.5.1155] [PMID: 1510410]

[187] Oelschlaeger P, Ai N, Duprez KT, Welsh WJ, Toney JH. Evolving carbapenemases: can medicinal chemists advance one step ahead of the coming storm? J Med Chem 2010; 53(8): 3013-27.
[http://dx.doi.org/10.1021/jm9012938] [PMID: 20121112]

[188] Grover SS, Doda A, Gupta N, *et al.* New Delhi metallo-β-lactamase - type carbapenemases producing *Escherichia coli* isolates from hospitalized patients: A pilot study. Indian J Med Res 2017; 146(1): 105-10.
[http://dx.doi.org/10.4103/ijmr.IJMR_594_15] [PMID: 29168466]

[189] Walsh TR, Toleman MA, Poirel L, Nordmann P. Metallo-beta-lactamases: the quiet before the storm? Clin Microbiol Rev 2005; 18(2): 306-25.
[http://dx.doi.org/10.1128/CMR.18.2.306-325.2005] [PMID: 15831827]

[190] LiA(c)nard BM, Garau G, Horsfall L, *et al.* Structural basis for the broad-spectrum inhibition of metallo-beta-lactamases by thiols. Org Biomol Chem 2008; 6(13): 2282-94.
[http://dx.doi.org/10.1039/b802311e] [PMID: 18563261]

[191] Fonseca F, Arthur CJ, Bromley EHC, *et al.* Biochemical characterization of Sfh-I, a Subclass B2 Metallo-β-Lactamase from *Serratia fonticola* UTAD54. Antimicrob Agents Chemother 2011; 55(11):

5392.
[http://dx.doi.org/10.1128/AAC.00429-11] [PMID: 21876065]

[192] Hall BG, Barlow M. Revised Ambler classification of β-lactamases. J Antimicrob Chemother 2005;
       55(6): 1050-1.
       [http://dx.doi.org/10.1093/jac/dki130] [PMID: 15872044]

[193] Jeon JH, Hong M-K, Lee JH, *et al.* Structure of ADC-68, a novel carbapenem-hydrolyzing class C
       extended-spectrum β-lactamase isolated from *Acinetobacter baumannii.* Acta Crystallogr D Biol
       Crystallogr 2014; 70(Pt 11): 2924-36.
       [http://dx.doi.org/10.1107/S1399004714019543] [PMID: 25372683]

[194] Liu X, Liu Y. Detection of plasmid-mediated AmpC β-lactamase in *Escherichia coli.* Biomed Rep
       2016; 4(6): 687-90.
       [http://dx.doi.org/10.3892/br.2016.661] [PMID: 27284407]

[195] Barguigua A, El Otmani F, Talmi M, *et al.* Prevalence and genotypic analysis of plasmid-mediated β-
       lactamases among urinary *Klebsiella pneumoniae* isolates in Moroccan community. J Antibiot (Tokyo)
       2013; 66(1): 11-6.
       [http://dx.doi.org/10.1038/ja.2012.91] [PMID: 23093031]

[196] Bauernfeind A, Stemplinger I, Jungwirth R, Giamarellou H. Characterization of the plasmidic beta-
       lactamase CMY-2, which is responsible for cephamycin resistance. Antimicrob Agents Chemother
       1996; 40(1): 221-4.
       [http://dx.doi.org/10.1128/AAC.40.1.221] [PMID: 8787910]

[197] Chika E, Charles E, Ifeanyichukwu I, Michael A. First Detection of FOX-1 AmpC β-lactamase Gene
       Expression Among *Escherichia coli* Isolated from Abattoir Samples in Abakaliki, Nigeria. Oman Med
       J 2018; 33(3): 243-9.
       [http://dx.doi.org/10.5001/omj.2018.44] [PMID: 29896333]

[198] Papanicolaou GA, Medeiros AA, Jacoby GA. Novel plasmid-mediated beta-lactamase (MIR-1)
       conferring resistance to oxyimino- and alpha-methoxy beta-lactams in clinical isolates of *Klebsiella
       pneumoniae.* Antimicrob Agents Chemother 1990; 34(11): 2200-9.
       [http://dx.doi.org/10.1128/AAC.34.11.2200] [PMID: 1963529]

[199] Evans BA, Amyes SGB. OXA β-lactamases. Clin Microbiol Rev 2014; 27(2): 241-63.
       [http://dx.doi.org/10.1128/CMR.00117-13] [PMID: 24696435]

[200] Maurya AP, Dhar D, Basumatary MK, *et al.* Expansion of highly stable bla $_{OXA-10}$ β-lactamase family
       within diverse host range among nosocomial isolates of Gram-negative bacilli within a tertiary referral
       hospital of Northeast India. BMC Res Notes 2017; 10(1): 145.
       [http://dx.doi.org/10.1186/s13104-017-2467-2] [PMID: 28376860]

[201] Yang Y, Xu Q, Li T, Fu Y, Shi Y, Lan P, *et al.* OXA-23 Is a Prevalent Mechanism Contributing to
       Sulbactam Resistance in Diverse *Acinetobacter baumannii* Clinical Strains. Antimicrob Agents
       Chemother 2019; 63(1): e01676-18.
       [PMID: 30348663]

[202] Balkan II, AygA1/4n G, Aydn S, *et al.* Blood stream infections due to OXA-48-like carbapenemase-
       producing *Enterobacteriaceae*: treatment and survival. Int J Infect Dis 2014; 26: 51-6.
       [http://dx.doi.org/10.1016/j.ijid.2014.05.012] [PMID: 24998423]

[203] Boo TW, Crowley B. Detection of blaOXA-58 and blaOXA-23-like genes in carbapenem-susceptible
       Acinetobacter clinical isolates: should we be concerned? J Med Microbiol 2009; 58(Pt 6): 839-41.
       [http://dx.doi.org/10.1099/jmm.0.008904-0] [PMID: 19429765]

[204] Bou G, Oliver A, MartA-nez-BeltrAn J. OXA-24, a novel class D beta-lactamase with carbapenemase
       activity in an *Acinetobacter baumannii* clinical strain. Antimicrob Agents Chemother 2000; 44(6):
       1556-61.
       [http://dx.doi.org/10.1128/AAC.44.6.1556-1561.2000] [PMID: 10817708]

[205] Tiwari V, Nagpal I, Subbarao N, Moganty RR. In-silico modeling of a novel OXA-51 from β-lacta-
-resistant *Acinetobacter baumannii* and its interaction with various antibiotics. J Mol Model 2012;
18(7): 3351-61.
[http://dx.doi.org/10.1007/s00894-011-1346-3] [PMID: 22271096]

[206] Figueiredo S, Poirel L, Seifert H, Mugnier P, Benhamou D, Nordmann P. OXA-134, a naturally
occurring carbapenem-hydrolyzing class D beta-lactamase from Acinetobacter lwoffii. Antimicrob
Agents Chemother 2010; 54(12): 5372-5.
[http://dx.doi.org/10.1128/AAC.00629-10] [PMID: 20837764]

[207] Hall LM, Livermore DM, Gur D, Akova M, Akalin HE. OXA-11, an extended-spectrum variant of
OXA-10 (PSE-2) beta-lactamase from *Pseudomonas aeruginosa*. Antimicrob Agents Chemother
1993; 37(8): 1637-44.
[http://dx.doi.org/10.1128/AAC.37.8.1637] [PMID: 8215276]

[208] Danel F, Hall LM, Gur D, Livermore DM. OXA-15, an extended-spectrum variant of OXA-2 beta-
lactamase, isolated from a *Pseudomonas aeruginosa* strain. Antimicrob Agents Chemother 1997;
41(4): 785-90.
[http://dx.doi.org/10.1128/AAC.41.4.785] [PMID: 9087490]

CHAPTER 6

Molecular Basis of Resistance III

Islam M. Ghazi[1,*]**, Diaa Alrahmany**[2] **and Wasim S. El Nekidy**[3]

[1] Phialdelphia College of Pharmacy, Univeristy of the Sciences, Philadelphia, USA

[2] Inpatient Pharmacy, Sohar Hospital, Sultanate of Oman

[3] Department of Pharmacy, Cleveland Clinic Abu Dhabi, Abu Dhabi, UAE

Abstract: The rapid evolvement of fungal resistance to therapeutic agents merits a thorough understanding of the molecular and genetic basis of this deleterious phenomenon. Accumulating efforts expanded our understanding of potential resistance mechanisms that fungi utilize to combat Antifungal therapy like modification of biological targets, gene overexpression, efflux pumps, and regulation of transcriptional factors in response to stress and biofilm formation. The tremendous genomic plasticity of fungi added to the involvement of a multitude of molecular resistance determinants and the paucity of novel targets for therapy mandate utilizing innovative approaches to therapy in parallel to relentless research to develop effective antifungal agents surmounting rapidly increasing resistance. In this chapter, we illustrate a myriad of resistance mechanisms along with other relevant topics like the mechanism of action of antifungal classes, laboratory methods for detecting resistance, clinical susceptibility testing and future insights.

Keywords: Allylamines, Antifungal agents, Azoles, Echinocandins, Fungal resistance, Nucleoside Analogues, Polyenes.

INTRODUCTION

Microbial resistance has been observed shortly after the introduction of penicillin (known as the first discovered compound with antimicrobial activity) to clinical use [1]. The ability of pathogens to halt the effects of therapeutic agents represents a health care challenge and culminates in grave consequences on patient outcomes raising mortality, and morbidity in addition to augmenting the financial burden. Considerable attention has been devoted to characterize bacterial resistance determinants owing to numerous infections, the existence of diverse classes of antibiotics and the availability of established methods for genetic manipulation [2]. Millions of fungi exist naturally in our environment;

---

* **Corresponding author Islam M. Ghazi:** Phialdelphia College of Pharmacy, Univeristy of the Sciences, Philadelphia, USA; Tel: +1 (215) 596-7121; Fax: +1 (215) 596-8585; E-mail: i.ghazi@usciences.edu they may be found in soil, on plant surfaces, or even attached to many indoor surfaces and human skin. Among these fungi, only hundreds are considered clinically relevant and may contribute to infections in almost a billion human beings yearly.

Respiratory fungal infections, fungal meningitis, fungal bloodstream infections, in addition to the frequently occurring fungal skin infections are symptomatically similar to infections caused by other organisms, but; these can be even more serious, which necessitates a prompt and targeted antifungal treatment. Understanding the mechanism of action of available antifungals and the molecular resistance tactics of fungi will be a success-determining step in achieving proper antifungal selection and guiding research endeavors to develop novel molecules.

Fungal infections' invasion to internal organs and dissemination to the bloodstream may occur during major surgeries, excessive burns, prolonged hospitalization especially in critical care areas and excessive unwarranted exposure to antimicrobials [3]. Advances in cancer chemotherapy, the introduction of antiretroviral therapy and availability of immunosuppressive medications for organ transplant have resulted in increased survival of patients with the compromised immune system; furthermore, the injudicious prescription of broad-spectrum antibiotics and widespread use of indwelling intravenous devices, all are factors that have led fungi to surface as significant pathogens causing serious infections [4]. Prolonged prophylactic use of antifungal therapy, particularly fluconazole is probably the major contributor to the development of fungal resistance, coupled with the availability of a limited number of systemic antifungal classes has stimulated the interest to study fungal resistance that was previously not considered as a priority [5]. The dearth of antifungal agents is probably partially attributed to the close evolutionary relatedness of eukaryotic fungal cells to the host human cells, narrowing the spectrum of biological targets that could be utilized therapeutically.

A variety of fungal species could cause human infections (mycosis) ranging from superficial to life-threatening invasive infections; commonly *Candida albicans*, "a commensal of the oral cavity, gastrointestinal and genitourinary tract" [6], with an increasing geographically-dependent incidence of multi-drug resistant (MDR) non-albicans species (*C. glabrata, C. krusie, C. tropicalis, C. lusitanae, C. parapsilosis and recently C. auris)* which own high propensity of nosocomial transmission and cause serious 90% of treatment-challenging invasive infections. Among non-albicans species, MDR *Candida auris* is one of the most virulent organisms. It possesses high resistance rates towards amphotericin B, fluconazole, voriconazole and to some extent toward micafungin and anidulafungin [7].

Aspergillus is a ubiquitous saprophytic fungus that causes invasive infections (*A. niger, A. fumigatus and A. flavus*). *Cryptococcus neoformans* causing AIDS-defining infections and *C. gattii* capable of infecting immunocompetent host. *Histoplasma capsulatum* and other emerging fungal infections *Fusarium, Trichosporon, Murcor, Rhizopus* are etiological pathogens causing disseminated infections in neutropenic patients associated with high morbidity and mortality [8, 9].

Detection of resistance *in vitro* (antifungal susceptibility testing) is performed by reference methods established by the Clinical Laboratory Standards Institute (CLSI) in the United States and European Committee for Antimicrobial Susceptibility Testing (EUCAST). These methods generate reliable data with intra/interlaboratory reproducibility that will establish breakpoints and guide clinicians in selecting the optimal therapy for patients considering another immune status, drug dosing, and site of infection among other factors contributing to therapeutic outcomes [10, 11].

Pathogenic fungi do not only impact human health but also instigate unfavorable environmental consequences perishing wild animal species leading to their extinction and perturbing biodiversity [12]. Fungi devastate crops and damage stored grain contaminating nutritious sources with toxins and carcinogens, thus intimidating food security that creates economic and political turbulence [13].

Understanding how fungi resist the action of therapeutic agents will assist in optimizing the use of existing agents and developing new agents that are safe, effective and capable of eluding development of resistance. This chapter will discuss how fungal cells resist the action of antifungal agents and explain genetic and biomolecular level issues with susceptibility testing and selection of an optimal agent. Finally, we briefly elucidate the clinical impact of fungal resistance and provide some future insights.

ANTIFUNGAL AGENTS' MODE OF ACTION

Proper understanding of fungal resistance necessitates a mechanistic knowledge of how antifungals exert their action on fungal cells, below is a brief description of the mechanism of action of major antifungal drug classes (Fig. **1**).

Azoles

Azoles are clinically the most widely used antifungal drug class. This class comprises a multitude of compounds, for example, miconazole, econazole, ketoconazole (mainly used topically) in addition to fluconazole, voriconazole, posaconazole and the most recent is isavuconazole. They act intracellularly by binding to and inhibiting one of the principle enzymes in the ergosterol synthesis pathway; lanosterol 14- α- demethylase (ERG11 in yeasts or CYP 51A/CYP51B in molds) that belongs to the cytochrome P450 family of enzymes, additionally, in specific fungal species they are capable of inhibiting Δ 22 desaturase that catalyzes a further step down the same synthesis pathway [14, 15]. The targeted enzyme exhibits P450 mono-oxygenase activity that excises 14- α- methyl group. Azole antifungals bind to the iron atom in the protoporphyrin component on the active site *via* a nitrogen atom located in the imidazole (2 nitrogen atoms) or triazole (3 nitrogen atoms) of the molecule five-membered azole ring. Moreover, the other part of the azole molecule binds to the apoprotein in a structure-specific fashion and the nature of interaction determines the antifungal inhibitory activity [16]. Ergosterol functions as membrane stabilizer preserving its fluidity, asymmetry and consequentially its integrity; thus, modification of sterol structure leads to increased stress and growth inhibition. The altered membrane integrity induced by azoles also leads to the inactivation of vacuolar ATPases (V-ATPase) [17] and inhibition of hyphal development [18]. Membrane integrity is maintained by sterols that lack C-4-methyl groups, thus inhibition of 14-α- demethylase culminates in accumulation of 14-methylated sterol precursors (lanosterol, 4,14-dimethylzymosterol and 24-methylenedihydrolanosterol) producing structurally and functionally defective membranes.

Echinocandins

Echinocandins (caspofungin, micafungin and anidulafungin) are lipoprotein compounds possessing a three-dimensional structure composed of hexapeptide core, and a lipid side chain 'gun-barrel-like'. They exhibit concentration-dependent fungicidal activity by inhibiting the synthesis of a major cell wall component; β,1,3 glucans through interfering with the membrane subunits of β-1,3-glucan synthetase (FKS1). Complete mechanistic detail of glucan synthesis inhibition remains to be revealed, including the exact location of the binding site relative to the cell membrane and the precise role of FKS1 as a catalytic subunit [19]. In the representative example of *Sarccomyces cerevisiae*, the protein complex is composed of two proteins Fks1p and Fks2p that are regulated by the components of the calcineurin pathway in addition to a GTP-binding Rho1p peptide [20]. Undoubtedly, echinocandins mechanistically bind to Fksp1 but the non-competitive inhibition of glucan synthesis does circumstantiate that Fksp1 is the catalytic subunit, furthermore, the exact location of echinocandins-Fksp1 binding site relative to the cell membrane side (interior or exterior) remains undetermined. Of note, the mode of action may explain their effect on Candida biofilms where β,1,3 glucans are the primary constituents of extracellular matrix

Polyenes

Polyenes (amphotericin B, nystatin and natamycin) act by forming a complex with ergosterol in the cell membrane resulting in instability and pore formation, the altered fungal cell wall permeability eventually leads to leakage of cell components and consequently to cell death. Polyenes are the broadest spectrum fungicidal drugs when compared to other classes especially to azoles which are mainly of fungistatic action [21]. The precise mechanism of this physical binding still needs to be elucidated. The relative selectivity of amphotericin B to fungal ergosterol over mammalian cholesterol could be attributed to the three-dimensional conformational dissimilitude (the former being cylindrical and the latter being sigmoid in shape) and elevated ergosterol to phospholipid ratio in the fungal counterpart. The process of amphotericin B-membrane binding disturbs the balance between the hydrophobic and hydrophilic moieties of the amphoteric molecule which necessitates alignment of the hydrophilic faces of the compound-membrane complex creating a local tension perturbing the membrane function. The non-specific mode of action insinuates a broad spectrum of activity and in the meantime the mammalian toxicity, specifically nephrotoxicity [22]. Formulation of amphotericin B with lipid combinations (encapsulation in liposomes or attachment to ribbon-like and disc-like complexes) reduces the rate of delivery to the kidneys and consequently nephrotoxicity [23].

Nucleoside Analogues

Flucytosine (5- fluorocytosine) is a fluorinated derivative of cytosine "an essential amino acid component of DNA"; the flucytosine conversion pathway to its antifungal activity requires cytosine permease to influx the molecule intercellularly then cytosine deaminase to catalyze its conversion to 4-fluorouracil that subsequently becomes converted to a substrate for nucleic acid synthesis by the action of uracil phosphoribosyl transferase to 5-fluorodeoxyuridine monophosphate. Flucytosine is integrated into RNA promoting premature chain termination and inhibits thymidylate synthetase halting DNA synthesis and consequently cell division. The set of enzymes moderating flucytosine action exists in yeasts, while the majority of filamentous fungi are destitute of such metabolic machinery which explains the selective efficacy of these compounds [24].

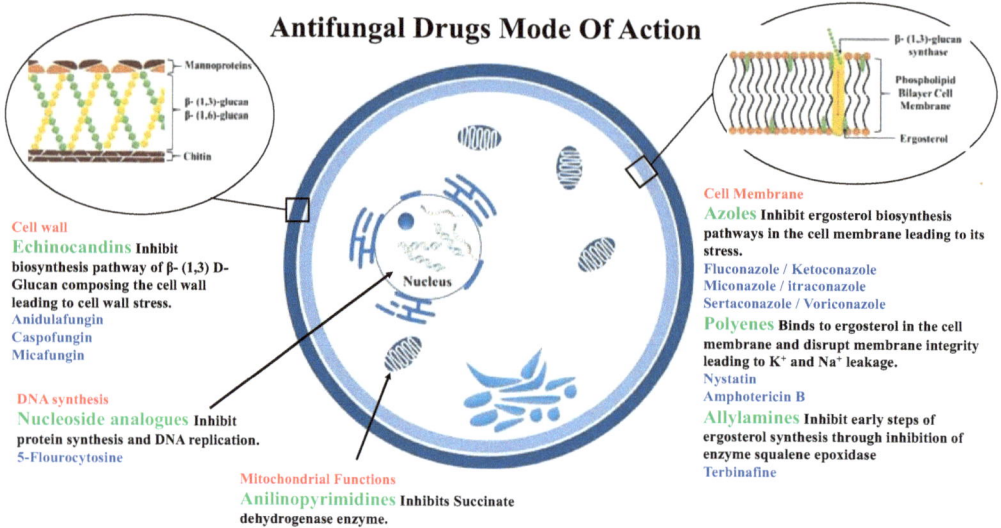

Fig. (1). Antifungal agents' mode of action.

Allylamines and Thiocarbamates

Naftifine and terbinafine are the most commonly used among this class, they exert their fungicidal action through inhibiting the squalene-epoxidase enzyme involved in the biosynthesis of ergosterol; the main cell wall component, which affects the cell integrity and disrupts the cell membrane. Griseofulvin was first isolated in 1939 as a metabolic product from the mold *Penicillium griseofulvum*, it acts by disrupting the spindle and cytoplasmic microtubule production, thereby inhibiting fungal mitosis [25]. Table (1) summarizes the antifungal classes with their corresponding mode of action.

Table 1. Antifungal classes with the mechanism of action.

Class	Members	Mode of Action	Ref.
Azoles	Fluconazole	Inhibition of ergosterol biosynthesis through inhibition of ERG11 gene; lanosterol 14α-demethylase.	[26 - 29]
	Itraconazole		
	Voriconazole		
	Posaconazole		
	Ravuconazole		
	Isavuconazole		
	Albaconazole		
	Miconazole		
	Ketoconazole		

(Table 1) cont.....

Class	Members	Mode of Action	Ref.
Polyenes	Amphotericin B	Cell membrane ergosterol (increased permeability and oxidative damage)	[30 - 32]
	Nystatin		
Echinocandins	Caspofungin	Interfere with cell wall biosynthesis, through inhibition of GSC1 gene product, β (1,3)-glucan synthase	[33, 34]
	Anidulafungin		
	Micafungin		
Nucleoside Analogues	5-fluorocytosine	DNA and RNA synthesis inhibition through misincorporation of 5-fluorouracil	[35, 36]
Allylamines	Terbinafine	Ergosterol biosynthesis inhibition through inhibition of ERG1 gene product squalene epoxidase)	[37, 38]
	Naftifine		

SUSCEPTIBILITY TESTING

Prompt initiation of appropriate antifungal agents is of utmost importance to achieve favorable outcomes in patients with invasive fungal infections. The selection of antifungal agents requires rapid identification of the infecting pathogen along with its susceptibility to that agent [39]. Susceptibility testing methods are required to be reproducible, reliable, clinically relevant and action-producing. Laboratory reference methods to define susceptibility to antifungal agents have been developed by two international institutions: Clinical Laboratory Standards Institute (CLSI) in the USA and European Committee on Antifungal Susceptibility testing (EUCAST). CLSI publishes the document M27A [40] "Reference method for broth dilution method for antifungal susceptibility testing of yeast; approved standards" and M38A [41] "Reference method for broth dilution method for antifungal susceptibility testing of filamentous fungi; approved standards".

EUCAST published [42] EUCAST definitive document E.DEF 7.3.1 "Method for the determination of broth dilution minimum inhibitory concentrations of antifungal agents for yeasts" and [43] " Method for the determination of broth dilution minimum inhibitory concentrations of antifungal agents for conidia forming molds " EUCAST definitive document E.DEF 9.3.1. Of note, both organizations have not established standards for dimorphic fungi until the time of writing this chapter.

The premise of antifungal susceptibility testing (AFST) is the concept of minimum inhibitory concentration (MIC); the minimum concentration that inhibits visible growth of the organism and clinical breakpoints (BP) which facilitate the categorization of fungal isolates into susceptible, susceptible dose-dependent and resistant. The definition of BP requires evaluation of several factors: CLSI reviews MIC distribution, MIC correlation with clinical outcomes and antifungal pharmacokinetics/ pharmacodynamics, on the other hand, EUCAST incorporates 5 variables in their review; the most common drug dosages used in the European Union, the determination of wild-type and the epidemiological cut-off for each species of the fungi in question, agent pharmacokinetics, pharmacodynamic target attainment (Monte Carlo simulations recognized), and MIC association with favorable outcomes [44]. Epidemiological cut-off value (ECV) designates if an isolate is equipped or devoid of intrinsic resistance and is defined as the upper limit of wild-type or the lower limit of non-wild-type MIC distribution [45]. The ECV does not imply that the isolate is categorized as susceptible or resistant and may not coincide with clinical BP. EUCAST has superseded CLSI in assigning BPs for molds including Aspergillus species (*A. fumigatus, A. niger, A nidulans, A. flavus and A. terreus*); however, both organizations introduced the concept of minimum effective concentration (MEC) to read echinocandins BP for molds which is based on the microscopic assessment of hyphae transition point from normal to aberrant forms [46].

The principal methods for MIC determination are the manually performed broth microdilution (BMD) and agar-based disc diffusion. There are several differences between the two organizations in their recommendation for BMD in AFST. While CLSI recommends round well shape, 0.2% glucose content, $0.5\text{-}2.5 \times 10^3$ inoculum size, azoles incubation time 48h, *Cryptococcus* incubation time 72h, visual method of reading, and amphotericin B endpoint inhibition of 100%, EUCAST recommends the following respectively; flat, 2%, $0.5\text{-}2.5 \times 10^5$, 24h, 48h, spectrophotometric, and 90% for the same parameters. Despite the different recommendations, there is reasonable concordance in the overall MIC determinations following the two standards and the corresponding BPs.

Commercial methods are available for clinical laboratories to determine antifungal susceptibility. Laboratories must perform the procedures strictly as instructed by the manufacturer and correlate with CLSI and EUCAST reference standards considering the essential agreement (no discrepancies in MICs > ± two-fold serial dilution and categorical agreement (if the clinical breakpoint is established). Commercial methods based on broth microdilution methods; SensititreYeastOne® [47] and SensiQuattro Candida EU® [48] employ colorimetric indicator, the color change can be detected visually or soft-ware facilitated signaling fungal growth, while Vitek 2® is a fully automated system employing miniature wells and computer-aided detection of growth, the system is accurate and reproducible with a strong correlation with reference methods [49]. Agar-based methods; Etest® and MIC Test Strip® use plastic or paper strips impregnated with a predefined gradient of the antifungal. When placed on an inoculated agar plates and incubated for an appropriate time, elliptical shape of inhibition appears due to antifungal diffusion. The results produced by the E-test methods demonstrate a moderate correlation with reference methods but are considered sensitive for discrimination of wild type *Candida species* from those carrying FKS mutations [50].

Non-conventional phenotypic assays are available which offer identification of a wide range of species, speed, and a high degree of reliability at a lower cost. An example of this technique is matrix-assisted laser desorption ionization time-o--flight mass spectrometry (MALDI-TOF MS) [51]; details and comparison of rapid diagnostics are presented in another chapter in this book. Lastly, *in vitro* susceptibility testing of fungi not only supports the clinical treatment decisions but also allows surveillance of resistance trends contributing to the elucidation of diseases epidemiology and the selection of empiric therapy.

FUNGAL RESISTANCE

A simple definition of fungal resistance is the lack of growth inhibition of fungi in the presence of the antifungal agent, or the requirement of an antifungal agent concentration too high to be safely feasible in patients. Resistance to antifungal agents can be; i) intrinsic or primary resistance which is manifested on the species level as an inherent resistance to certain drug or drug class, ii) extrinsic or secondary type is demonstrated by acquired resistance to a certain antifungal drug as a result of continuous exposure. Fungal species have managed to develop diversified mechanisms to combat antifungal agents comprising varying levels of resistance, the reversal of stability and fitness cost. Clinical resistance can be observed when the antifungal agent is administered at the highest possible dose and yet therapeutic failure ensues. Host immune status, site of infection, *in situ* drug availability or drug-drug interactions are factors that influence clinical response but irrelevant when categorizing the organism as resistant [52].

Resistance phenomenon in fungal cells is expressed through a diversity of mechanisms, over-expression of efflux pumps, alteration of target enzymes through genetic mutation in a way that impair drug binding ability, modification of key enzymes for biosynthetic pathways, drug inactivation through enzymatic degradation and finally; hindered entry of drugs molecules through cell wall consequent to altered permeability. There is a plethora of literature describing the findings of resistance mechanisms, in the following text we will highlight a variety of studies but the list is not meant to exhaustive.

Molecular and Genetic Basis for Fungal Resistance

Azole Antifungals

In the coming section, we will present a review of some literature that examined how fungal cells could potentially develop resistance to antifungal agents. Studies have utilized different approaches to detect several proposed mechanisms of resistance as evidence suggests that the resistance to azole antifungal can be attributed to several mechanisms.

Orozco and colleagues examined three fluconazole-resistant strains of *C. krusei* and one strain of susceptible *C. albicans*. Assays performed on cell extracts demonstrated that the fluconazole 50% inhibitory concentration was 24-48-fold higher in the resistant strains, insinuating that differences in enzyme affinity could be the culprit for the observed resistance. Analysis of fluconazole accumulation showed a decreased amount of fluconazole intracellularly probably implicating an active efflux mechanism and there was no significant difference in sterol content among the studied strains [53].

A clinical isolate of *C. albicans* collected from a patient relapsed after prolonged treatment, was found to have a difference in the cytochrome P450 enzyme pre and post-treatment through analysis of microsomal carbon monoxide spectra [54].

Van den Bossche and fellows studied a *C. glabrata* strain that became resistant to fluconazole after treatment for 9 days. The growth inhibitory concentration of not only fluconazole but ketoconazole and itraconazole significantly increased post-treatment indicating cross-resistance. The intracellular concentration was higher in the pre-treatment strain but could not solely explain the magnitude of observed resistance. However, there was a two-fold increase in the microsomal P-450 enzyme activity coincident with increased lanosterol synthesis. Of note, the amount of the enzyme and consequently lanosterol content decreased after serial sub-culturing in a drug-free medium [55] probably indicating the reversal of induced enzyme activity.

Boiron and others attempted to determine the penetration and intracellular concentration of ketoconazole using a radioactive labeled drug [^{3}H] KTZ and found that the intracellular concentration was 80-fold the extracellular concentration. The fungal cells have rapidly taken up 30% and 60% of the final concentration at 1 and 10 minutes respectively. The uptake of [^{3}H] KTZ was an active energy-required process (derived from glycolysis); dependent on the cellular viability, the temperature of the physiological environment and pH. Kinetic analysis of [^{3}H] KTZ uptake demonstrated that penetration of the drug was saturable suggesting carrier-mediated transport, while at higher concentration penetration was by simple diffusion. Interestingly, the study found no evidence for drug efflux probably because the energy level was inconsistent with the process [56].

In light of the above studies and others, it is evident that one of the major mechanisms of resistance to azole antifungals is the alteration of the target enzyme through several point mutations in the encoding gene ERG11/*cyp 51A/cyp51B* in resistant Candida and Aspergillus isolates leading to amino acid substitutions in the regions surrounding the heme-binding site of the enzyme [57, 58]. In addition to other mechanisms such as a constitutive overexpression of ERG11 found in resistant fungi, a gain-of-function mutations in the transcriptional activators; Upc2 in *C. albicans*, Sre1 in *C. neoformans* and SrbA in *A. fumigatus* was also observed. Interference with the function of other enzymes involved in the ergosterol biosynthesis pathway can confer antifungal resistance as well. Loss of function of Δ-5,6- desaturase enzyme (Erg 3) resulting from mutations in ERG3 culminates in depletion of ergosterol and accumulation of toxic alternative sterols leading to azole and polyenes resistance. Azole resistance originating from ERG3 mutations is closely related to key regulators of stress response; protein phosphate, calcineurin, protein kinase Pkc1 and molecular chaperone Hsp90. In a resistant clinical isolate of *C. albicans*, whole-genome sequencing demonstrated that a function nullifying 10-amino acid duplication in ERG5 gene coupled with amino acid substitutions in ERG11 gene product realized resistance to azoles and amphotericin B (polyene) owing to depletion of membrane ergosterol content [59].

Multidrug transporters and efflux mechanisms play a role in the acquired resistance through preventing the accumulation of lethal concentrations of antifungal drugs in the cytosol of fungal cells. The two major families of drug transporters are: ATP-binding cassette (ABC) superfamily that exploits energy generated from ATP hydrolysis; and major facilitator superfamily (MFS) dependent on proton gradient to efflux drugs. Members of the pleiotropic drug resistance family (PDR) of ABC transporters principally transport drugs and consequentially are implicated in the development of resistance. A couple of ABCs promiscuous proteins CDR1 and CDR2 [60] are overexpressed *via* mutations in the TAC1 transcriptional regulator leading to azole resistance in *C. albicans*. Similarly, mutations in CgPDR1 transcriptional regulator promote the expression of ABC transporters CgCDR1, CgCDR2 and CgSNQ2 in *C. glabrata*. In other fungi, ABC transporters have been reported to enhance resistance; up-regulation of CnAFR1 in *C. neoformans* [61] and AfuMDR4/atrF in *A. fumigatus* [62] imparts resistance to fluconazole and itraconazole respectively. Regarding the MFS, drug: H^+ antiporter families DHA1 and DHA2 (distinguished by the number of transmembrane helices) are linked to drug resistance [63]. Over-expression of CaMDR1 in *C. albicans* [64] and its homolog CdMDR1 in *C. dubliniensis* was found to be strongly associated with azole resistance [65]. All *C. albicans* isolates over-expressing CaMDR1 lodge a gain-of-function mutation of MRR1, the primary transcriptional factor, and the same applies to other species *C. dubliniensis* and *C, parapsilosis* [66]. Other genes encoding MFS transporters have been described in the literature. Fluconazole resistance 1(FLU1) gene has been shown to afford resistance to a mutant strain of *S. cerevisiae* [67], and modulate the transport of an intrinsic salivary antimicrobial peptide histatin 5 (Hst5) [68]. The two homolog proteins CgTpo 1-1 and 1-2 (regulated by the transcription factor CgPdr1) were overexpressed in *C. glabrata* in response to clotrimazole exposure and were illustrated to facilitate drug extrusion [69].

Fungal species are fraught with genomic plasticity in the face of diverse stressful stimuli. A common aneuploidy identified in *C. albicans* was the duplication of the left arm of chromosome 5 i(5L) which results in an augmented dosage of both ERG11 and TAG1 furnishing dual basis for resistance [70]. Another aneuploidy in *C. albicans* was described as multiple copies of chromosomes 3 and 6 in progeny cells with expanded ability to grow in the presence of fluconazole and progressive passaging of these strains yielded loss of chromosomal super numeracy with accompanying loss of decreased susceptibility [71]. Of note, the disomy of chromosome 1 carrying the ERG11 and AFR1 genes was observed in *C. neoformans* manifesting as an adaptive hetero-resistance to fluconazole [72].

Echinocandins

Resistance to echinocandins fundamentally arises from amino acid substitutions within highly conserved hot spot regions in *Candida species* (hot spot 1 and 2 encompass amino acids range Phe641-Pro649 and Asp1357-Leu1364, respectively). Substitutions in Fks subunits of glucan synthetase (Fksp the catalytic subunit and Rho1 the regulatory subunit) [73] manifest as different levels of resistance depending on the type of mutation and the level of expression of these genes. For example, in *C. glabrata*, FKS2 is regulated by calcineurin thus resistance can be reversed by the administration of an inhibitor (FK506). Mutations were observed in *C. tropicalis* and *A. fumigatus* as well. Intrinsic echinocandin resistance was observed in *C. parapslosis, C. orthopslosis, C. metapslosis and guilliermondii* that may be attributed to spontaneous proline-t--alanine substitution (P660A) [74]. One study showed that the production of melanin like pigments reduced the susceptibility of *C. neoformans and H. capsulatum* to caspofungin probably due to the binding of these antifungals by melanin [75]. It was reported that, in *A. fumigatus,* a mutation within the gene AfFKS1 encoding the putative catalytic subunit of glucan synthetase conferred a low-level resistance to caspofungin, another class of mutant laboratory strains exhibited resistance between 0.5-16 mcg/mL; therefore, the authors pointed out that neither target site mutations nor modified gene expression was responsible for observed resistance but probably due to the remodeling of cell wall structure [76]. In *A. fumigatus,* a single S678P substitution in Fks1p (equivalent to *C. albicans* Ser645 point mutation) was able to engender echinocandin cross-resistance [77], while the intrinsically resistant phenotype of *Fusarium graminearum* and *F. verticilloides* harboring amino acid substitutions in Fks1 hot spot 1(equivalent to *C. albicans* F641 point mutation) suggest that mutations in the conserved gene FKS hot spots are universal echinocandin resistance determinants.

Interestingly, an alternative to diminishing the drug affinity to a biological target, some mutations have decreased enzyme processivity [78]. It is noteworthy that multidrug efflux transporters do not impart a significant level of resistance; *C. albicans* and *S. cerevisiae* strains overexpressing drug transporters (CDR1, CDR2 and MDR1) did not exhibit elevated echinocandin MICs [79], and efflux pump hyper-expressing fluconazole-resistant *Candida species* had comparable resistance level to fluconazole-sensitive strains [80].

Polyenes

Fortuitously, resistance to polyenes remains uncommon despite decades of clinical utilization. This is probably attributed to the cost of mutations that confer resistance to polyenes in *C. albicans* which are associated with fitness trade-offs, in terms of increased vulnerability to oxidative stress, febrile temperature and neutrophil attacks besides the deleterious effects on morphogenesis and decreased ability for tissue penetration [81]. However, cases of a decrease in or lack of membrane ergosterol in *C. albicans* with maintained cellular viability, have been observed. Accumulation of sterol compounds replacing ergosterol has been attributed to alterations in the ERG3 gene [82]. In *C. albicans* biofilms, changing regulation of ERG1, ERG 25, SKN1 and KRE1 genes may lead to amphotericin B resistance [83]. Of note, a study observed that a mutation in ERG6 gene leads to loss of function and emerged decreased susceptibility to polyenes [84], additionally, the up-regulation of ERG6 expression contributes to resistance in *C. lusitaniae* [85]. Several mechanisms supposedly play a role in molds resistance to polyenes; altered membrane ergosterol content limiting target drug access, reduced oxidative damage secondary to increased catalase activity and accumulation of sterol with diminished intercalation affinity.

Nucleoside Analogues

Resistance to flucytosine (5-FC) was found in *C. albicans* and *C. lusitaniae* that harbor mutations in the FCY1 (encoding cytosine deaminase) and FCY2 (encoding cytosine permease) genes that mediate deamination and import of drugs, respectively or mutations in gene FUR1 (encoding uracil phosphoribosyltransferase) responsible for the conversion of 5-fluorouracil to 5-fluorouridine monophosphate. Notably, molecular resistance to 5-FC could signify cross-resistance to fluconazole [86]. Table **2** lists some examples of fungi resistance to different antifungal drugs.

Table 2. Examples of resistance mechanisms to different Antifungal drugs.

Organism	Drug	Mechanism	Ref.
Candida auris	Fluconazole	Mutation of Y132F or K143R in ERG11	[7]
Candida auris	Voriconazole	K143R mutation in ERG11	[7]
Candida auris	Micafungin	Mutation of S639F in FKS1.	[7]
Candida tropicalis	Fluconazole	Mutation Zinc Cluster Transcription Factor genes MRR1 (T255P, 647S), TAC1 (N164I, R47Q), and UPC2 (T241A, Q340H, T381S)	[87]
Candida tropicalis	Anidulafungin	Mutations in FKS1p	[88]
Candida glabrata	Echinocandin	Gene mutation of FKS1 and FKS2	[89]
Candida albicans	Azole Antifungals	Over- expression of the gene encoding the Cdr1 efflux pump	[90]
Candida albicans	Fluconazole	Mutation of Zinc Cluster Transcription Factor MRR2, TAC1, MRR1, and UPC2	[91]
Aspergillus spp.	Itraconazole	Cyp51 mutations	[92]
Aspergillus flavus	Voriconazole	Mutations in the cyp51C gene. Overexpression of efflux pumps	[93]
Candida glabrata	Fluconazole	Upregulated expression of ATP-binding cassette (ABC) transporter gene	[94]
Candida glabrata	Micafungin	13 amino acid substitutions in FKS1 and FKS2	[94]

Implications of Antifungal Resistance

The obvious consequence of increased fungal resistance to therapy is abysmal clinical outcomes for patients. Elevated MIC due to intrinsic or acquired resistance eventually leads to higher morbidity, mortality and health care costs. Studies have consistently shown that isolates with higher MICs were associated with treatment failure [95, 96]. In the setting of expanding immunologically vulnerable patient populations (HIV, transplant, cancer, immunocompromised…) who are using antifungal prophylaxis, another particularly worrisome consequence is the possibility of an outbreak of invasive fungal infections due to the selection of resistant strains. Two studies from Duke University Medical center reported an outbreak of invasive candidiasis in transplant patients caused by *C. glabrata* [97, 98].

FUTURE INSIGHTS INTO COMBATING FUNGAL RESISTANCE

The development of novel antifungal pharmacologic classes will extend the ambit of therapeutic choices that can counteract the resistance to other agents and provide clinical alternatives. Sordarin is a class of antifungals that blocks the function of Elongation Factor 2 (EF2) "an element in fungal RNA translation", thus inhibiting protein synthesis [99]. Sordarin derivatives display a variable spectrum of activity against fungal species; however, target specificity and simplicity of chemical synthesis accentuate the potential for future development. This new class comprises six tetracyclic diterpene glycosides (moriniafungins B to G) and soradaricin B. These compounds are isolated from marine-derived fungi. The new class showed activity against *C. albicans* [100]. Another class of novel antifungals comprises Melleolides which originate from the honey mushroom Armillaria mellea. This class showed antifungal activity against Aspergillus Spp. The mechanism of its action is through a delta 2, 4-double bond present in dihydroarmyillylorsellinate (DAO) or arnamial. However, the full mechanism of antifungal activity is not yet fully understood [101]. The third class of synthetic antifungals is a series of azasordarin analogs. This class is similar to the previously mentioned sordarin but with a broader spectrum of antifungal activity [102].

CONSENT FOR PUBLICATION

Not applicable.

CONFLICT OF INTEREST

The authors confirm that the contents of this chapter have no conflict of interest.

ACKNOWLEDGEMENTS

Declared none.

REFERENCES

[1]   Davies J, Davies D. Origins and evolution of antibiotic resistance. Microbiol Mol Biol Rev 2010; 74(3): 417-33.
        [http://dx.doi.org/10.1128/MMBR.00016-10] [PMID: 20805405]

[2]   Raymond B. Five rules for resistance management in the antibiotic apocalypse, a road map for integrated microbial management. Evol Appl 2019; 12(6): 1079-91.
        [http://dx.doi.org/10.1111/eva.12808] [PMID: 31297143]

[3]   Pfaller MA, Diekema DJ. Rare and emerging opportunistic fungal pathogens: concern for resistance beyond *Candida albicans* and *Aspergillus fumigatus*. J Clin Microbiol 2004; 42(10): 4419-31.
        [http://dx.doi.org/10.1128/JCM.42.10.4419-4431.2004] [PMID: 15472288]

[4]   Anaissie E, Bodey GP. Nosocomial fungal infections. Old problems and new challenges. Infect Dis Clin North Am 1989; 3(4): 867-82.

[PMID: 2687366]

[5]   Beck-Sagué C, Jarvis WR. Secular trends in the epidemiology of nosocomial fungal infections in the United States, 1980-1990. J Infect Dis 1993; 167(5): 1247-51.
[http://dx.doi.org/10.1093/infdis/167.5.1247] [PMID: 8486965]

[6]   Naglik JR, Moyes DL, Wächtler B, Hube B. *Candida albicans* interactions with epithelial cells and mucosal immunity. Microbes Infect 2011; 13(12-13): 963-76.
[http://dx.doi.org/10.1016/j.micinf.2011.06.009] [PMID: 21801848]

[7]   Ahmad S, Khan Z, Al-Sweih N, Alfouzan W, Joseph L. Candida auris in various hospitals across Kuwait and their susceptibility and molecular basis of resistance to antifungal drugs. Mycoses 2019.
[PMID: 31618799]

[8]   Pfaller MA, Diekema DJ. Epidemiology of invasive candidiasis: a persistent public health problem. Clin Microbiol Rev 2007; 20(1): 133-63.
[http://dx.doi.org/10.1128/CMR.00029-06] [PMID: 17223626]

[9]   Kidd SE, Hagen F, Tscharke RL, *et al.* A rare genotype of *Cryptococcus gattii* caused the cryptococcosis outbreak on Vancouver Island (British Columbia, Canada). Proc Natl Acad Sci USA 2004; 101(49): 17258-63.
[http://dx.doi.org/10.1073/pnas.0402981101] [PMID: 15572442]

[10]   Institute ClS. Wayne, PA: Reference Method for Broth Dilution Antifungal Susceptibility Testing of Yeasts 2017; p. 46.

[11]   EUCAST definitive document EDef 7.1: method for the determination of broth dilution MICs of antifungal agents for fermentative yeasts. Clin Microbiol Infect 2008; 14(4): 398-405.
[http://dx.doi.org/10.1111/j.1469-0691.2007.01935.x] [PMID: 18190574]

[12]   Fones HN, Fisher MC, Gurr SJ. Emerging fungal threats to plants and animals challenge agriculture and ecosystem resilience. Microbiol Spectr 2017; 5(2).
[PMID: 28361733]

[13]   Fisher MC, Gow NA, Gurr SJ. Tackling emerging fungal threats to animal health, food security and ecosystem resilience. Philos Trans R Soc Lond B Biol Sci 2016; 371(1709): 371.
[http://dx.doi.org/10.1098/rstb.2016.0332] [PMID: 28080997]

[14]   Podust LM, Poulos TL, Waterman MR. Crystal structure of cytochrome P450 14alpha -sterol demethylase (CYP51) from *Mycobacterium tuberculosis* in complex with azole inhibitors. Proc Natl Acad Sci USA 2001; 98(6): 3068-73.
[http://dx.doi.org/10.1073/pnas.061562898] [PMID: 11248033]

[15]   Kelly SL, Lamb DC, Baldwin BC, Corran AJ, Kelly DE. Characterization of *Saccharomyces cerevisiae* CYP61, sterol delta22-desaturase, and inhibition by azole antifungal agents. J Biol Chem 1997; 272(15): 9986-8.
[http://dx.doi.org/10.1074/jbc.272.15.9986] [PMID: 9092539]

[16]   Podust LM, Stojan J, Poulos TL, Waterman MR. Substrate recognition sites in 14alpha-sterol demethylase from comparative analysis of amino acid sequences and X-ray structure of *Mycobacterium tuberculosis* CYP51. J Inorg Biochem 2001; 87(4): 227-35.
[http://dx.doi.org/10.1016/S0162-0134(01)00388-9] [PMID: 11744060]

[17]   Zhang YQ, Gamarra S, Garcia-Effron G, Park S, Perlin DS, Rao R. Requirement for ergosterol in V-ATPase function underlies antifungal activity of azole drugs. PLoS Pathog 2010; 6(6): e1000939.
[http://dx.doi.org/10.1371/journal.ppat.1000939] [PMID: 20532216]

[18]   Odds FC, Cockayne A, Hayward J, Abbott AB. Effects of imidazole- and triazole-derivative antifungal compounds on the growth and morphological development of *Candida albicans* hyphae. J Gen Microbiol 1985; 131(10): 2581-9.
[PMID: 2999296]

[19]   Odds FC, Brown AJ, Gow NA. Antifungal agents: mechanisms of action. Trends Microbiol 2003;

11(6): 272-9.
[http://dx.doi.org/10.1016/S0966-842X(03)00117-3] [PMID: 12823944]

[20]   Douglas CM. Fungal beta(1,3)-D-glucan synthesis. Med Mycol 2001; 39 (Suppl. 1): 55-66.
       [http://dx.doi.org/10.1080/mmy.39.1.55.66] [PMID: 11800269]

[21]   Brajtburg J, Powderly WG, Kobayashi GS, Medoff G. Amphotericin B: current understanding of
       mechanisms of action. Antimicrob Agents Chemother 1990; 34(2): 183-8.
       [http://dx.doi.org/10.1128/AAC.34.2.183] [PMID: 2183713]

[22]   Kotler-Brajtburg J, Price HD, Medoff G, Schlessinger D, Kobayashi GS. Molecular basis for the
       selective toxicity of amphotericin B for yeast and filipin for animal cells. Antimicrob Agents
       Chemother 1974; 5(4): 377-82.
       [http://dx.doi.org/10.1128/AAC.5.4.377] [PMID: 15825391]

[23]   Dupont B. Overview of the lipid formulations of amphotericin B. J Antimicrob Chemother 2002; 49
       (Suppl. 1): 31-6.
       [http://dx.doi.org/10.1093/jac/49.suppl_1.31] [PMID: 11801578]

[24]   Pfaller MA, Messer SA, Boyken L, Huynh H, Hollis RJ, Diekema DJ. *In vitro* activities of 5-
       fluorocytosine against 8,803 clinical isolates of Candida spp.: global assessment of primary resistance
       using National Committee for Clinical Laboratory Standards susceptibility testing methods.
       Antimicrob Agents Chemother 2002; 46(11): 3518-21.
       [http://dx.doi.org/10.1128/AAC.46.11.3518-3521.2002] [PMID: 12384359]

[25]   Francois IE, Aerts AM, Cammue BP, Thevissen K. Currently used antimycotics: spectrum, mode of
       action and resistance occurrence. Curr Drug Targets 2005; 6(8): 895-907.
       [http://dx.doi.org/10.2174/138945005774912744] [PMID: 16375673]

[26]   Borgers M. Mechanism of action of antifungal drugs, with special reference to the imidazole
       derivatives. Rev Infect Dis 1980; 2(4): 520-34.
       [http://dx.doi.org/10.1093/clinids/2.4.520] [PMID: 7003674]

[27]   Kuchta T, Léka C, Farkas P, Bujdáková H, Belajová E, Russell NJ. Inhibition of sterol 4-
       demethylation in *Candida albicans* by 6-amino-2-n-pentylthiobenzothiazole, a novel mechanism of
       action for an antifungal agent. Antimicrob Agents Chemother 1995; 39(7): 1538-41.
       [http://dx.doi.org/10.1128/AAC.39.7.1538] [PMID: 7492100]

[28]   Smith EB, Henry JC. Ketoconazole: an orally effective antifungal agent. Mechanism of action,
       pharmacology, clinical efficacy and adverse effects. Pharmacotherapy 1984; 4(4): 199-204.
       [http://dx.doi.org/10.1002/j.1875-9114.1984.tb03356.x] [PMID: 6091064]

[29]   Yamaguchi H, Iwata K. Action mechanism of antifungal imidazole derivatives clotrimazole and
       miconazole: lipid specificity and binding sites. Nippon Saikingaku Zasshi 1975; 30(1): 261.
       [PMID: 765566]

[30]   Drouhet E, Hirth L, Lebeurier G. Mechanism of action of antifungal antibiotics. I. Action of
       amphotericin B on the respiratory metabolism of *Candida albicans*. Ann Inst Pasteur (Paris) 1960; 98:
       469-84.
       [PMID: 13818193]

[31]   Ghosh BK, Chatterjee AN. Leishmanicidal activity of nystatin, a polyene antifungal antibiotic. I. The
       probable mechanism of action of nystatin on *Leishmania donovani*. Antibiot Chemother (Northfield)
       1962; 12: 204-6.
       [PMID: 13898229]

[32]   Klimov AN, Litvinova VN. On the biochemical principles of the mechanism of action of the polyenic
       antifungal antibiotics. Antibiotiki 1968; 13(1): 88-94.

[33]   Denning DW. Echinocandins and pneumocandins--a new antifungal class with a novel mode of action.
       J Antimicrob Chemother 1997; 40(5): 611-4.
       [http://dx.doi.org/10.1093/jac/40.5.611] [PMID: 9421307]

[34] Fera MT, La Camera E, De Sarro A. New triazoles and echinocandins: mode of action, *in vitro* activity and mechanisms of resistance. Expert Rev Anti Infect Ther 2009; 7(8): 981-98.
[http://dx.doi.org/10.1586/eri.09.67] [PMID: 19803707]

[35] Drevets CC, Hummer LM. Therapeutic usefulness. 5-Fluorocytosine--a new anti-fungal agent. J Kans Med Soc 1975; 76(5): 103-7.
[PMID: 1168678]

[36] Pawlik B, Barylak J. Studies on deamination of 5-fluorocytosine in fungal cells. Mykosen 1979; 22(9): 328-35.
[http://dx.doi.org/10.1111/j.1439-0507.1979.tb01768.x] [PMID: 530295]

[37] Haraguchi H, Kataoka S, Okamoto S, Hanafi M, Shibata K. Antimicrobial triterpenes from Ilex integra and the mechanism of antifungal action. Phytother Res 1999; 13(2): 151-6.
[http://dx.doi.org/10.1002/(SICI)1099-1573(199903)13:2<151::AID-PTR391>3.0.CO;2-C] [PMID: 10190191]

[38] Danielli LJ, Pippi B, Duarte JA, *et al.* Antifungal mechanism of action of Schinus lentiscifolius Marchand essential oil and its synergistic effect *in vitro* with terbinafine and ciclopirox against dermatophytes. J Pharm Pharmacol 2018; 70(9): 1216-27.
[http://dx.doi.org/10.1111/jphp.12949] [PMID: 29956331]

[39] Patel GP, Simon D, Scheetz M, Crank CW, Lodise T, Patel N. The effect of time to antifungal therapy on mortality in Candidemia associated septic shock. Am J Ther 2009; 16(6): 508-11.
[http://dx.doi.org/10.1097/MJT.0b013e3181a1afb7] [PMID: 19531934]

[40] Clinical Laboratory Standards Institute. Reference Method for Broth Dilution Antifungal Susceptibility Testing of Yeasts. 4th Edition., Wayne, Clinical Laboratory Standards Institute 2017. CLSI document M27 A4.

[41] Reference Method for Broth Dilution Antifungal Susceptibility Testing of Filamentous Fundi. 3rd Edition., Wayne, Clinical Laboratory Standards Institute 2017. CLSI document M38 A3.

[42] Arendrup M C, Meletiadis J, Mouton J W, Lagrou K. Petr Hamal, J Guinea and the Subcommittee on Antifungal Susceptibility Testing (AFST) of the ESCMID European Committee for Antimicrobial Susceptibility Testing (EUCAST). Method for the determination of broth dilution minimum inhibitory concentrations of antifungal agents for yeasts EUCAST DEFINITIVE DOCUMENT EDEF 731 2017.

[43] Arendrup M C, Meletiadis J, Mouton J W, Lagrou K. Petr Hamal, J Guinea and the Subcommittee on Antifungal Susceptibility Testing (AFST) of the ESCMID European Committee for Antimicrobial Susceptibility Testing (EUCAST). Method for the determination of broth dilution minimum inhibitory concentrations of antifungal agents for conidia forming moulds EUCAST DEFINITIVE DOCUMENT EDEF 931 2017.

[44] Rodriguez-Tudela JL, Donnelly JP, Pfaller MA, *et al.* Statistical analyses of correlation between fluconazole MICs for Candida spp. assessed by standard methods set forth by the European Committee on Antimicrobial Susceptibility Testing (E.Dis. 7.1) and CLSI (M27-A2). J Clin Microbiol 2007; 45(1): 109-11.
[http://dx.doi.org/10.1128/JCM.01969-06] [PMID: 17093015]

[45] Arendrup MC, Cuenca-Estrella M, Lass-Flörl C, Hope WW. Breakpoints for antifungal agents: an update from EUCAST focussing on echinocandins against Candida spp. and triazoles against Aspergillus spp. Drug Resist Updat 2013; 16(6): 81-95.
[http://dx.doi.org/10.1016/j.drup.2014.01.001] [PMID: 24618110]

[46] Pfaller MA, Diekema DJ. Progress in antifungal susceptibility testing of candida spp. by use of clinical and laboratory standards institute broth microdilution methods, 2010 to 2012. J Clin Microbiol 2012; 50(9): 2846-56.
[http://dx.doi.org/10.1128/JCM.00937-12] [PMID: 22740712]

[47] Pfaller MA, Chaturvedi V, Diekema DJ, *et al.* Comparison of the Sensititre YeastOne colorimetric

antifungal panel with CLSI microdilution for antifungal susceptibility testing of the echinocandins against Candida spp., using new clinical breakpoints and epidemiological cutoff values. Diagn Microbiol Infect Dis 2012; 73(4): 365-8.
[http://dx.doi.org/10.1016/j.diagmicrobio.2012.05.008] [PMID: 22726528]

[48]   Koehling HL, Willinger B, Buer J, Rath P-M, Steinmann J. Comparative evaluation of a new commercial colorimetric microdilution assay (SensiQuattro Candida EU) with MIC test strip and EUCAST broth microdilution methods for susceptibility testing of invasive Candida isolates. J Clin Microbiol 2015; 53(1): 255-61.
[http://dx.doi.org/10.1128/JCM.02830-14] [PMID: 25392352]

[49]   Melhem MSC, Bertoletti A, Lucca HRL, Silva RBO, Meneghin FA, Szeszs MW. Use of the VITEK 2 system to identify and test the antifungal susceptibility of clinically relevant yeast species. Brazilian journal of microbiology : [publication of the Brazilian Society for Microbiology] 2014; 44(4): 1257-66.

[50]   Espinel-Ingroff A. Comparison of three commercial assays and a modified disk diffusion assay with two broth microdilution reference assays for testing zygomycetes, Aspergillus spp., Candida spp., and *Cryptococcus neoformans* with posaconazole and amphotericin B. J Clin Microbiol 2006; 44(10): 3616-22.
[http://dx.doi.org/10.1128/JCM.01187-06] [PMID: 16943356]

[51]   Clark AE, Kaleta EJ, Arora A, Wolk DM. Matrix-assisted laser desorption ionization-time of flight mass spectrometry: a fundamental shift in the routine practice of clinical microbiology. Clin Microbiol Rev 2013; 26(3): 547-603.
[http://dx.doi.org/10.1128/CMR.00072-12] [PMID: 23824373]

[52]   Alastruey-Izquierdo A, Melhem MSC, Bonfietti LX, Rodriguez-Tudela JL. Susceptibility test for fungi: clinical and laboratorial correlations in medical mycology. Revista do Instituto de Medicina Tropical de Sao Paulo 2015; 57(Suppl 19): 57-64.

[53]   Orozco AS, Higginbotham LM, Hitchcock CA, *et al.* Mechanism of fluconazole resistance in *Candida krusei*. Antimicrob Agents Chemother 1998; 42(10): 2645-9.
[http://dx.doi.org/10.1128/AAC.42.10.2645] [PMID: 9756770]

[54]   Smith KJ, Warnock DW, Kennedy CT, *et al.* Azole resistance in *Candida albicans*. J Med Vet Mycol 1986; 24(2): 133-44.
[http://dx.doi.org/10.1080/02681218680000201] [PMID: 3014106]

[55]   vanden Bossche H, Marichal P, Odds FC, Le Jeune L, Coene MC. Characterization of an azole-resistant *Candida glabrata* isolate. Antimicrob Agents Chemother 1992; 36(12): 2602-10.
[http://dx.doi.org/10.1128/AAC.36.12.2602] [PMID: 1482129]

[56]   Boiron P, Drouhet E, Dupont B, Improvisi L. Entry of ketoconazole into *Candida albicans*. Antimicrob Agents Chemother 1987; 31(2): 244-8.
[http://dx.doi.org/10.1128/AAC.31.2.244] [PMID: 3551831]

[57]   Marichal P, Koymans L, Willemsens S, *et al.* Contribution of mutations in the cytochrome P450 14alpha-demethylase (Erg11p, Cyp51p) to azole resistance in *Candida albicans*. Microbiology 1999; 145(Pt 10): 2701-13.
[http://dx.doi.org/10.1099/00221287-145-10-2701] [PMID: 10537192]

[58]   Balashov SV, Gardiner R, Park S, Perlin DS. Rapid, high-throughput, multiplex, real-time PCR for identification of mutations in the cyp51A gene of *Aspergillus fumigatus* that confer resistance to itraconazole. J Clin Microbiol 2005; 43(1): 214-22.
[http://dx.doi.org/10.1128/JCM.43.1.214-222.2005] [PMID: 15634974]

[59]   Martel CM, Parker JE, Bader O, *et al.* A clinical isolate of *Candida albicans* with mutations in ERG11 (encoding sterol 14alpha-demethylase) and ERG5 (encoding C22 desaturase) is cross resistant to azoles and amphotericin B. Antimicrob Agents Chemother 2010; 54(9): 3578-83.
[http://dx.doi.org/10.1128/AAC.00303-10] [PMID: 20547793]

[60] Prasad R, Banerjee A, Khandelwal NK, Dhamgaye S. The ABCs of *Candida albicans* Multidrug Transporter Cdr1. Eukaryot Cell 2015; 14(12): 1154-64.
[http://dx.doi.org/10.1128/EC.00137-15] [PMID: 26407965]

[61] Sanguinetti M, Posteraro B, La Sorda M, *et al.* Role of AFR1, an ABC transporter-encoding gene, in the *in vivo* response to fluconazole and virulence of *Cryptococcus neoformans*. Infect Immun 2006; 74(2): 1352-9.
[http://dx.doi.org/10.1128/IAI.74.2.1352-1359.2006] [PMID: 16428784]

[62] Nascimento AM, Goldman GH, Park S, *et al.* Multiple resistance mechanisms among *Aspergillus fumigatus* mutants with high-level resistance to itraconazole. Antimicrob Agents Chemother 2003; 47(5): 1719-26.
[http://dx.doi.org/10.1128/AAC.47.5.1719-1726.2003] [PMID: 12709346]

[63] Gaur M, Puri N, Manoharlal R, *et al.* MFS transportome of the human pathogenic yeast *Candida albicans*. BMC Genomics 2008; 9: 579.
[http://dx.doi.org/10.1186/1471-2164-9-579] [PMID: 19055746]

[64] Perea S, López-Ribot JL, Kirkpatrick WR, *et al.* Prevalence of molecular mechanisms of resistance to azole antifungal agents in *Candida albicans* strains displaying high-level fluconazole resistance isolated from human immunodeficiency virus-infected patients. Antimicrob Agents Chemother 2001; 45(10): 2676-84.
[http://dx.doi.org/10.1128/AAC.45.10.2676-2684.2001] [PMID: 11557454]

[65] Wirsching S, Moran GP, Sullivan DJ, Coleman DC, Morschhäuser J. MDR1-mediated drug resistance in *Candida dubliniensis*. Antimicrob Agents Chemother 2001; 45(12): 3416-21.
[http://dx.doi.org/10.1128/AAC.45.12.3416-3421.2001] [PMID: 11709317]

[66] Morschhäuser J, Barker KS, Liu TT, BlaB-Warmuth J, Homayouni R, Rogers PD. The transcription factor Mrr1p controls expression of the MDR1 efflux pump and mediates multidrug resistance in *Candida albicans*. PLoS Pathog 2007; 3(11): e164.
[http://dx.doi.org/10.1371/journal.ppat.0030164] [PMID: 17983269]

[67] Calabrese D, Bille J, Sanglard D. A novel multidrug efflux transporter gene of the major facilitator superfamily from *Candida albicans* (FLU1) conferring resistance to fluconazole. Microbiology 2000; 146(Pt 11): 2743-54.
[http://dx.doi.org/10.1099/00221287-146-11-2743] [PMID: 11065353]

[68] Bryant KA, Van Schooneveld TC, Thapa I, *et al.* KPC-4 Is encoded within a truncated Tn4401 in an IncL/M plasmid, pNE1280, isolated from *Enterobacter cloacae* and *Serratia marcescens*. Antimicrob Agents Chemother 2013; 57(1): 37-41.
[http://dx.doi.org/10.1128/AAC.01062-12] [PMID: 23070154]

[69] Pais P, Costa C, Pires C, Shimizu K, Chibana H, Teixeira MC. Membrane Proteome-Wide Response to the Antifungal Drug Clotrimazole in *Candida glabrata*: Role of the Transcription Factor CgPdr1 and the Drug:H+ Antiporters CgTpo1_1 and CgTpo1_2. Mol Cell Proteomics 2016; 15(1): 57-72.
[http://dx.doi.org/10.1074/mcp.M114.045344] [PMID: 26512119]

[70] Selmecki A, Gerami-Nejad M, Paulson C, Forche A, Berman J. An isochromosome confers drug resistance *in vivo* by amplification of two genes, ERG11 and TAC1. Mol Microbiol 2008; 68(3): 624-41.
[http://dx.doi.org/10.1111/j.1365-2958.2008.06176.x] [PMID: 18363649]

[71] Hirakawa MP, Chyou DE, Huang D, Slan AR, Bennett RJ. Parasex generates phenotypic diversity *de Novo* and impacts drug resistance and virulence in *Candida albicans*. Genetics 2017; 207(3): 1195-211.
[http://dx.doi.org/10.1534/genetics.117.300295] [PMID: 28912344]

[72] Sionov E, Lee H, Chang YC, Kwon-Chung KJ. *Cryptococcus neoformans* overcomes stress of azole drugs by formation of disomy in specific multiple chromosomes. PLoS Pathog 2010; 6(4): e1000848.
[http://dx.doi.org/10.1371/journal.ppat.1000848] [PMID: 20368972]

[73]   Kartsonis NA, Nielsen J, Douglas CM. Caspofungin: the first in a new class of antifungal agents. Drug resistance updates : reviews and commentaries in antimicrobial and anticancer chemotherapy 2003; 6(4): 197-218.
       [http://dx.doi.org/10.1016/S1368-7646(03)00064-5]

[74]   Garcia-Effron G, Katiyar SK, Park S, Edlind TD, Perlin DS. A naturally occurring proline-to-alanine amino acid change in Fks1p in *Candida parapsilosis*, *Candida orthopsilosis*, and *Candida metapsilosis* accounts for reduced echinocandin susceptibility. Antimicrob Agents Chemother 2008; 52(7): 2305-12.
       [http://dx.doi.org/10.1128/AAC.00262-08] [PMID: 18443110]

[75]   van Duin D, Casadevall A, Nosanchuk JD. Melanization of *Cryptococcus neoformans* and Histoplasma capsulatum reduces their susceptibilities to amphotericin B and caspofungin. Antimicrob Agents Chemother 2002; 46(11): 3394-400.
       [http://dx.doi.org/10.1128/AAC.46.11.3394-3400.2002] [PMID: 12384341]

[76]   Gardiner RE, Souteropoulos P, Park S, Perlin DS. Characterization of *Aspergillus fumigatus* mutants with reduced susceptibility to caspofungin. Med Mycol 2005; 43 (Suppl. 1): S299-305.
       [http://dx.doi.org/10.1080/13693780400029023] [PMID: 16110824]

[77]   Rocha EMF, Garcia-Effron G, Park S, Perlin DSA. A Ser678Pro substitution in Fks1p confers resistance to echinocandin drugs in *Aspergillus fumigatus*. Antimicrob Agents Chemother 2007; 51(11): 4174-6.
       [http://dx.doi.org/10.1128/AAC.00917-07] [PMID: 17724146]

[78]   Garcia-Effron G, Park S, Perlin DS. Correlating echinocandin MIC and kinetic inhibition of fks1 mutant glucan synthases for *Candida albicans*: implications for interpretive breakpoints. Antimicrob Agents Chemother 2009; 53(1): 112-22.
       [http://dx.doi.org/10.1128/AAC.01162-08] [PMID: 18955538]

[79]   Niimi K, Maki K, Ikeda F, *et al.* Overexpression of *Candida albicans* CDR1, CDR2, or MDR1 does not produce significant changes in echinocandin susceptibility. Antimicrob Agents Chemother 2006; 50(4): 1148-55.
       [http://dx.doi.org/10.1128/AAC.50.4.1148-1155.2006] [PMID: 16569823]

[80]   Bachmann SP, Patterson TF, López-Ribot JL. *In vitro* activity of caspofungin (MK-0991) against *Candida albicans* clinical isolates displaying different mechanisms of azole resistance. J Clin Microbiol 2002; 40(6): 2228-30.
       [http://dx.doi.org/10.1128/JCM.40.6.2228-2230.2002] [PMID: 12037093]

[81]   Vincent BM, Lancaster AK, Scherz-Shouval R, Whitesell L, Lindquist S. Fitness trade-offs restrict the evolution of resistance to amphotericin B. PLoS Biol 2013; 11(10): e1001692.
       [http://dx.doi.org/10.1371/journal.pbio.1001692] [PMID: 24204207]

[82]   Pemán J, Cantón E, Espinel-Ingroff A. Antifungal drug resistance mechanisms. Expert Rev Anti Infect Ther 2009; 7(4): 453-60.
       [http://dx.doi.org/10.1586/eri.09.18] [PMID: 19400764]

[83]   Khot PD, Suci PA, Miller RL, Nelson RD, Tyler BJ. A small subpopulation of blastospores in *Candida albicans* biofilms exhibit resistance to amphotericin B associated with differential regulation of ergosterol and beta-1,6-glucan pathway genes. Antimicrob Agents Chemother 2006; 50(11): 3708-16.
       [http://dx.doi.org/10.1128/AAC.00997-06] [PMID: 16966398]

[84]   Vandeputte P, Tronchin G, Bergès T, Hennequin C, Chabasse D, Bouchara JP. Reduced susceptibility to polyenes associated with a missense mutation in the ERG6 gene in a clinical isolate of *Candida glabrata* with pseudohyphal growth. Antimicrob Agents Chemother 2007; 51(3): 982-90.
       [http://dx.doi.org/10.1128/AAC.01510-06] [PMID: 17158937]

[85]   Young LY, Hull CM, Heitman J. Disruption of ergosterol biosynthesis confers resistance to amphotericin B in *Candida lusitaniae*. Antimicrob Agents Chemother 2003; 47(9): 2717-24.

[http://dx.doi.org/10.1128/AAC.47.9.2717-2724.2003] [PMID: 12936965]

[86] Papon N, Noël T, Florent M, *et al.* Molecular mechanism of flucytosine resistance in *Candida lusitaniae*: contribution of the FCY2, FCY1, and FUR1 genes to 5-fluorouracil and fluconazole cross-resistance. Antimicrob Agents Chemother 2007; 51(1): 369-71.
[http://dx.doi.org/10.1128/AAC.00824-06] [PMID: 17060521]

[87] Arastehfar A, Daneshnia F, Hafez A, *et al.* Antifungal susceptibility, genotyping, resistance mechanism, and clinical profile of *Candida tropicalis* blood isolates. Med Mycol 2019; myz124.
[http://dx.doi.org/10.1093/mmy/myz124] [PMID: 31828316]

[88] Chew KL, Octavia S, Lin RTP, Yan GZ, Teo JWP. Delay in effective therapy in anidulafungin-resistant *Candida tropicalis* fungaemia: Potential for rapid prediction of antifungal resistance with whole-genome-sequencing. J Glob Antimicrob Resist 2019; 16: 105-7.
[http://dx.doi.org/10.1016/j.jgar.2018.12.010] [PMID: 30583013]

[89] Fraser M, Borman AM, Thorn R, Lawrance LM. Resistance to echinocandin antifungal agents in the United Kingdom in clinical isolates of *Candida glabrata*: Fifteen years of interpretation and assessment. Med Mycol 2019.
[http://dx.doi.org/10.1093/mmy/myz053] [PMID: 31111912]

[90] Nishimoto AT, Sharma C, Rogers PD. Molecular and genetic basis of azole antifungal resistance in the opportunistic pathogenic fungus *Candida albicans*. J Antimicrob Chemother 2019.
[http://dx.doi.org/10.1093/jac/dkz400] [PMID: 31603213]

[91] Nishimoto AT, Zhang Q, Hazlett B, Morschhäuser J, Rogers PD. Contribution of clinically derived mutations in the gene encoding the zinc cluster transcription factor Mrr2 to fluconazole antifungal resistance and *CDR1* expression in *Candida albicans*. Antimicrob Agents Chemother 2019; 63(5): e00078-19.
[http://dx.doi.org/10.1128/AAC.00078-19] [PMID: 30833425]

[92] Rivero-Menendez O, Soto-Debran JC, Medina N, Lucio J, Mellado E, Alastruey-Izquierdo A. Molecular identification, antifungal susceptibility testing, and mechanisms of azole resistance in *Aspergillus* species received within a surveillance program on antifungal resistance in Spain. Antimicrob Agents Chemother 2019; 63(9): e00865-19.
[http://dx.doi.org/10.1128/AAC.00865-19] [PMID: 31285229]

[93] Rudramurthy SM, Paul RA, Chakrabarti A, Mouton JW, Meis JF. Invasive aspergillosis by *Aspergillus flavus*: epidemiology, diagnosis, antifungal resistance, and management. J Fungi (Basel) 2019; 5(3): E55.
[http://dx.doi.org/10.3390/jof5030055] [PMID: 31266196]

[94] Sakagami T, Kawano T, Yamashita K, *et al.* Antifungal susceptibility trend and analysis of resistance mechanism for Candida species isolated from bloodstream at a Japanese university hospital. J Infect Chemother 2019; 25(1): 34-40.
[http://dx.doi.org/10.1016/j.jiac.2018.10.007] [PMID: 30401513]

[95] Clancy CJ, Yu VL, Morris AJ, Snydman DR, Nguyen MH. Fluconazole MIC and the fluconazole dose/MIC ratio correlate with therapeutic response among patients with candidemia. Antimicrob Agents Chemother 2005; 49(8): 3171-7.
[http://dx.doi.org/10.1128/AAC.49.8.3171-3177.2005] [PMID: 16048920]

[96] Rex JH, Pfaller MA, Galgiani JN, *et al.* Subcommittee on Antifungal Susceptibility Testing of the National Committee for Clinical Laboratory Standards. Development of interpretive breakpoints for antifungal susceptibility testing: conceptual framework and analysis of *in vitro-in vivo* correlation data for fluconazole, itraconazole, and candida infections. Clin Infect Dis 1997; 24(2): 235-47.
[http://dx.doi.org/10.1093/clinids/24.2.235] [PMID: 9114154]

[97] Alexander BD, Schell WA, Miller JL, Long GD, Perfect JR. *Candida glabrata* fungemia in transplant patients receiving voriconazole after fluconazole. Transplantation 2005; 80(6): 868-71.
[http://dx.doi.org/10.1097/01.tp.0000173771.47698.7b] [PMID: 16210978]

[98]   Pfeiffer CD, Garcia-Effron G, Zaas AK, Perfect JR, Perlin DS, Alexander BD. Breakthrough invasive candidiasis in patients on micafungin. J Clin Microbiol 2010; 48(7): 2373-80.
[http://dx.doi.org/10.1128/JCM.02390-09] [PMID: 20421445]

[99]   Domínguez JM, Kelly VA, Kinsman OS, Marriott MS, Gómez de las Heras F, Martín JJ. Sordarins: A new class of antifungals with selective inhibition of the protein synthesis elongation cycle in yeasts. Antimicrob Agents Chemother 1998; 42(9): 2274-8.
[http://dx.doi.org/10.1128/AAC.42.9.2274] [PMID: 9736548]

[100]   Zhang MQ, Xu KX, Xue Y, *et al.* Sordarin diterpene glycosides with an unusual 1,3-dioxolan-4-one ring from the zoanthid-derived fungus *Curvularia hawaiiensis* TA26-15. J Nat Prod 2019; 82(9): 2477-82.
[http://dx.doi.org/10.1021/acs.jnatprod.9b00164] [PMID: 31478377]

[101]   Dörfer M, Heine D, König S, *et al.* Melleolides impact fungal translation *via* elongation factor 2. Org Biomol Chem 2019; 17(19): 4906-16.
[http://dx.doi.org/10.1039/C9OB00562E] [PMID: 31042251]

[102]   Wu Y, Dockendorff C. Synthesis of simplified azasordarin analogs as potential antifungal agents. J Org Chem 2019; 84(9): 5292-304.
[http://dx.doi.org/10.1021/acs.joc.9b00296] [PMID: 30919633]

CHAPTER 7

Evolving Rapid Diagnostics Tools

Diaa Alrahmany[1] and **Islam M. Ghazi[2,*]**

[1] *Inpatient Pharmacy, Sohar Hospital, Sultanate of Oman*

[2] *Philadelphia College of Pharmacy, University of the Sciences, Philadelphia, USA*

Abstract: The increasing threat of resistant bacterial phenotypes, leading to increased rates of treatment failure as well as prolonged hospitalization, necessitate early detection and more targeted therapy to improve clinical outcomes. Traditional microbiology laboratory diagnostic testing has been used for decades to identify the pathogens causing the infectious diseases and its susceptibility to antibiotics but these techniques are flawed particularly with long turnaround time. Rapid diagnostic platforms are able to identify the infective organisms as well as antibiotics susceptibility pattern within a significantly shorter period of time, which guides targeted antimicrobial treatment and limit the exposure to broad-spectrum antibiotics, the main trigger for bacterial resistance. Immuno-assay-based, nucleic acid probe-based, nucleic acid amplification-based and spectrometry-based techniques, in addition to the future development of whole genome sequencing and microfluidics are technological solutions that can be used by microbiology laboratories to minimize sample-to-answer time. This chapter aims to illustrate the rapid diagnostic testing platforms, discussing their scientific principle of operation, advantages and limitations. Also, the importance of effective incorporation of these techniques in patient care process.

Keywords: Antibiotics, Bacterial Resistance, Diagnostics Tools, Infectious Diseases, Pathogens, Techniques, Treatment.

INTRODUCTION

The microbiology laboratory plays a fundamental role in the process of rationalizing antibiotics use. The incorporation of point-of-care diagnostic testing (tests can be performed at the time and place of patient care), as well as rapid diagnostic tests (technology-based platforms able to identify the causative organism, determine susceptibility to tested antimicrobials and explore genetic

* **Corresponding author Islam M. Ghazi:** Philadelphia College of Pharmacy, University of the Sciences, Philadelphia, USA; Tel: +1 (215) 596-7121; Fax: +1 (215) 596-8585; E-mail: i.ghazi@usciences.edu

Islam M. Ghazi & Michael J. Cawley (Eds.)

resistance determinants), will definitely accelerate the availability of (hours instead of days) [1, 2] evidence-supported information, that guide the selection of definitive therapy and eventually minimize the exposure to broad-spectrum antibiotics, the principal culprit for acquired bacterial resistance. Advances in technology have facilitated the development of rapid diagnostic platforms utilizing diverse scientific principles including immunologic reactions, nucleic acid probe methods or molecular assays, to provide reliable and actionable information in much less time.

Historically, organism identification depended solely on the traditional microbiological methods; bacterial growth in specific culture media (*e.g.*, agar plates), followed by Gram-staining and visualization under a light microscope to identify bacterial shapes/staining patterns and conducting biochemical testing exploiting reactions specific to certain bacteria. The application of this methodology is limited by special growth media requirements of some pathogens in addition to long turnaround times (days to weeks) needed for growth and identification, and the need for extensive training and expertise for findings interpretation [3]. Antigens/antibodies detection tools were developed in mid of 20th century to replace conventional microbiological and histopathological techniques, they are based on the highly specific reaction between an antigen and its corresponding antibody in order to identify the presence of either one detected by a reactions indicator, *e.g.*, using fluorescein-tagged antibodies visible under light microscopy. However, the accuracy of these tests is limited by the cross-reactions between structurally similar molecules [4]. These techniques have significantly evolved after the introduction of monoclonal antibody-based immunochemical assays with improved affinity and specificity [5].

Molecular diagnostics are technologically-based platforms able to detect and analyze the biological markers and genomic components in order to aid diagnosis, anticipate prognosis and enable therapeutic monitoring. Molecular diagnostics are capable of rapidly distinguishing between viral and bacterial infections, specify the resistant determinants of the organism, and its susceptibility pattern with a high level of sensitivity/specificity, reproducible results, rapid turnaround time, maximum automation with affordable cost [6]. These systems are associated with the higher acquisition and operational costs when compared to conventional techniques, especially if not rationally managed, it may become an additional financial burden on the limited healthcare resources and shrivel the efficacy of antimicrobial stewardship (AMS) programs. In terms of true costs; reduction of antimicrobial treatment-related costs through using targeted instead of empiric treatment regimens, improved clinical outcomes, shortened length of hospitalization and halted microbial resistance, makes the incorporation of such platforms in healthcare systems cost-effective. Thus; it will be more realistic if we could direct part of the antimicrobials research and development budget toward the development and embedding of rapid diagnostic tests (RDTs) in the healthcare systems [7 - 9].

Laboratory stewardship programs (LSP) were developed in order to promote appropriate ordering, retrieval, interpretation and delivery of laboratory tests. LSPs aim to foster the collaboration between all the stakeholders including laboratory personnel and direct care providers (physicians, pharmacists and nurses). Education, protocols and effective communication are all tools to streamline the delivery of enhanced patient care maximize the benefits derived from RDTs [10, 11]. The following text provides a synopsis of the currently available RDTs, the impact of these techniques on improving the detection of infectious pathogens along with their limitations. In addition, a discussion on how to integrate the use of RDTs in the patient care process to achieve optimal outcomes in a cost-effective manner.

MICROSCOPY-BASED METHODS

The microscopical detection of pathogens through simple Gram-stain can confirm within minutes the presence of Gram-positive or Gram-negative isolates in a smear of sputum, urine or blood sample. Examining stained bacterial smear under a microscope remains the most economic technique for uncovering the underlying cause of infection. The lack of accuracy, the high dependability on personnel expertise, the incapability of visualizing certain pathogens, and the difficulty to distinguish between infections and colonization, collectively are the limitations to this technique [12].

Gram-Stain

A very small sample of a bacterial colony is gently stirred into the drop of saline on the slide to create a thin smear of bacterial suspension, before being heat-fixed to the slide. The smear is then flooded with crystal violet for one minute and washed by distilled water before flooded again by Gram's iodine for one minute then washed. The purple color turned smear is decolorized using 95% ethyl alcohol or acetone for 5-10 seconds until became almost clear. Then, the smear is gently flooded with safranin to counter-stain and let stand for 45 seconds, rinse again with distilled water, air dry, then examine using a light-microscope under oil-immersion. Gram-stain identifies the organism cell morphology (bacilli, cocci, rods) and cell arrangement (cluster, chains, ...) as well as its class (Gram-positive or Gram-negative) by detecting the organism ability to retain crystal violet stain (Gram-positive blue) or not (Gram-negative red) [13].

Acid-Fast and Modified Acid-Fast Stain

Acid-fast and modified acid-fast stains identify acid-fast Mycobacterium species with high specificity, although some moderately acid-fast organisms are difficult to be distinguished from Mycobacteria [14]. Using specific fluorescent nucleic acid probes and fluorescent stains like (acridine orange for bacteria and fungi), (auramine-rhodamine and auramine O for Mycobacteria), and (calcofluor white for fungi, especially dermatophytes) improve the visualization of micro-organisms using microscopical examination techniques [15 - 17].

Wet Mounts

In a wet mount, the specimen is suspended in a drop of distilled water, glycerol, saline or immersion oil, selected according to the natural habitat of the organism not to cause sample damage due to hyper/hypo-osmotic pressure, a phase-contrast or dark-field microscope should be used for clear observation of bacterial shape, arrangement and size [18, 19]. This procedure overcomes the probability of cell death or losing its natural shape and size due to heat-fixation and exposure to chemicals in Gram-stain.

Organism identification using microscopical examination guide other laboratory procedures to select appropriate isolation media, culture methods, susceptibility testing panel and aid the prescriber in selecting an empirical antibiotic therapy.

Microscopy-based techniques in low-resourced laboratories engaged in AMS programs (for example in primary healthcare facilities) can't adequately warrant delivery of robust guiding information to other AMS team members, although it can be helpful in identifying the targeted isolate for more evidence-based decisions, despite the resistance pattern of these isolates.

IMMUNOASSAYS

Manually-Performed Immunoassay-Based Techniques

A variety of RDTs available nowadays utilize mainly immunoassay platforms, from simple tests that can be performed in low-resource settings lacking advanced technology, equipment, and trained staff [20], to highly complicated, expensive technological equipment that needs trained personnel. Lateral flow, flow-through agglutination and dipstick tests are examples of simple point-of-care RDTs, the limitations and advantages of these RDT's are summarized in Table **1**.

Simple immunoassay platforms operation depends on flow of antigen (microbial particles) through nitrocellulose strips containing specific antibodies or aptamers that possess high binding affinity for microbial ultra-structures [21, 22]. The advantages of point-of-care devices are; rapid results (5-30 minutes), low price, simple, portable, qualitative/semi-quantitative RDT and long shelf life with no required special storage conditions. Due to aforementioned advantages its widely used in medical, environmental and agricultural fast samples analysis, in addition to low-resources settings, small ambulatory care units, remote regions and battlefields [23]. The parameters affecting the simple immunoassays are the selection of appropriate filter membranes, membrane pore size, capturing molecule, antibody binding capacity and the concentrations of immunoreagents [24, 25].

Table 1. Techniques, strengths and weaknesses of simple immunoassays.

Test	Lateral-flow [25]	Agglutination assays [26]	Flow-through [27]	Solid-phase assay [28] (dipstick)
Technique	Antigen ~ Antibody Technique called "sol particle immunoassay" (SPIA) Movement of a liquid sample along a strip of polymeric material, passing various zones where molecules have been attached that exert an interaction with the analyte.	Clumping of particles to form insoluble aggregates. These tests employ latex particles, gelatin beads, colloidal particles, or preserved mammalian blood cells to facilitate visualization of agglutination.	A flow of fluid analyte through a porous membrane into an absorbent pad. In which it is captured by analyte specific molecules and then visualized by the addition of analyte detection molecules.	solid, nonporous supports onto which analyte capture molecules are immobilized. Assay simply require the user to dip the test into a specimen and then wait for a color change indicating the test result.
Strengths	▪ Rapid (5-15 min) ▪ Designed to work bedside ▪ Works for multiple analytes (ex: urine, saliva, serum, *etc.*) ▪ Easy to use ▪ Works for non-medical specimen (soil, dust, vegetation,)	▪ Single-step ▪ Low cost per test ▪ Rapid results ▪ Semi-quantitative results in 2-10 folds specimen dilutions.	▪ Very rapid (3-5 min) ▪ Good sensitivity for antibody detection.	▪ One strip can test for multiple parameters

(Table 1) cont.....

Test	Lateral-flow [25]	Agglutination assays [26]	Flow-through [27]	Solid-phase assay [28] (dipstick)
Weaknesses	• Single use • Results are qualitative. • Semi-quantitative. • Less sensitive than an ELISA • Sample adequacy dependent. • Samples sometimes need to be mixed with a specific buffer.	• Low sensitivity • Some tests require training and a microscope to read results • Cross-reactions can cause sensitivity problems • Coagulate Pattern needs to be interpreted to get a result.	• Requires more training to perform • Less sensitive at antigen detection compared to lateral flow and other enzyme immuno-assays (EIA) • Requires attention.	• Requires several intermediate steps • Require some training. • completed ≥ 1hour. • Potentially expensive
Targets	• Antigens • Antibodies • Nucleic acid amplification tests.	• Antigens • Antibodies • Enzymes	• Antigens • Antibodies	• Antigens • Antibodies • Enzymes • Nucleic acid.
Examples	• Malaria RDTs. • Home pregnancy tests • Influenza A, influenza B	• HIV latex agglutination test • Leishmaniasis DAT	• *E. coli* detection	• HIV "comb" test

Based on the detection labels used in the assay, lateral flow assay can be distinguished into the lateral flow immunoassay (LFIA) and the nucleic acid lateral flow assay (NALFA).

Lateral Flow Immune-Assays (LFIA)

LFIA mechanism of action depends on the flow of a liquid or sample suspension by capillary force along a cardboard-supported strip of nitrocellulose [29], nylon [30], polyether-sulfone [31], polyethylene [32] or fused silica polymeric materials, the sample passes through the conjugate pad where specific immobilized nanoparticle antibodies complexes with the analyte. A typical LFIA platform consists of a surface layer (pore size 0.05 - 12 µm) to carry the sample from the sample application site *via* the conjugate pad along the strip encountering the detection zone up to the absorbent pad. Labels are made of easily visualized colored 15–800 nm nanoparticles made of colloidal gold, latex, selenium, carbon or liposomes. Labeling lines are allocated on the strip, at the test line, the recognition of the sample analyte by the reporter will result in the required response. Several test lines can be applied allowing simultaneous multianalyte detection or for semiquantitative results [29], Fig. (**1**) describes different components and the operation of LFIA platform.

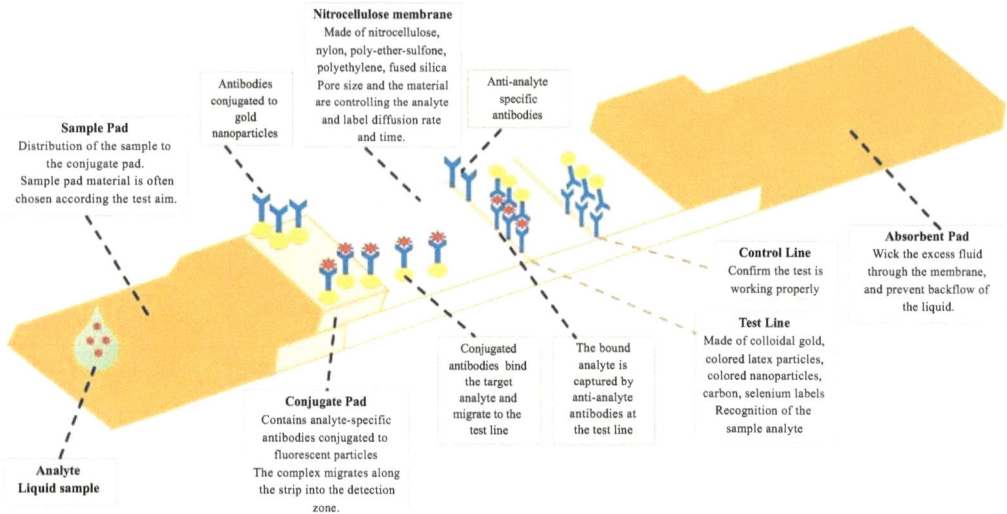

Fig. (1). Configuration and Operation of LFIA.

The sample application pad can be modified in order to allow sample pre-treatment (immersion, drying, components separation, …), this can be achieved through pH alteration, increase sample viscosity and decrease non-specific binding. While conjugate pads are typically composed of non-woven glass fibers into which the conjugate is added and easily released to interact with analyte, it is also modifiable by altering pH, adjustable wettability and viscosity in order to improve the binding specificity. The natural nitrocellulose diffusion membrane has a wide range of micropores that we can choose among them in order to modify the capillary flow rate and the capturing ability [33].

The 2 main formats of LFIA are sandwich and competitive formats, see Fig. (**2a** and **2b**).

Sandwich (Direct) Assay is applied mainly to large analytes with multiple antigenic determinants, the analyte sample migrates from the sample application site to conjugate pad, in which it is captured by a fluorescent-labeled aptamers resulting in the formation of labeled antibody conjugate/analyte complexes. The complexes migrate through the membrane by capillary flow up to the test line where it is again captured by another antibody. The analyte becomes sandwiched between the labeled and the primary antibodies forming a labeled antibody conjugate/analyte/primary-antibody complex. Color intensity visualized at the test line is directly proportional to the amount of analyte molecules.

Competitive Assay is mainly designed for small analytes with single antigen determinant which can't bind to more than one antibody at the same time. The analyte solution is applied to the sample pad leading to hydration of immobilized labeled conjugate which starts to flow with the flowing sample liquid. Test line contains pre-immobilized antigen (same analyte) which binds specifically to the labeled conjugate, when liquid sample reaches the test line, this pre-immobilized antigen will partially bind to the labeled conjugate - some sites of labeled antibody conjugate were vacant- whether target analyte in sample solution is absent or present. Antigen in the sample solution and the immobilized antigen at test line compete together to bind with the labeled conjugate. Absence of color at test line is an indication for the presence of analyte while the appearance of colored test lines and control lines indicates a negative result [34, 35].

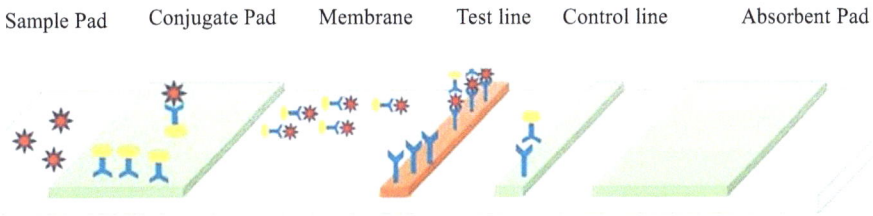

Sample Pad   Conjugate Pad   Membrane   Test line   Control line   Absorbent Pad

Fig. (2a). Sandwich (Direct) LFIA assay.

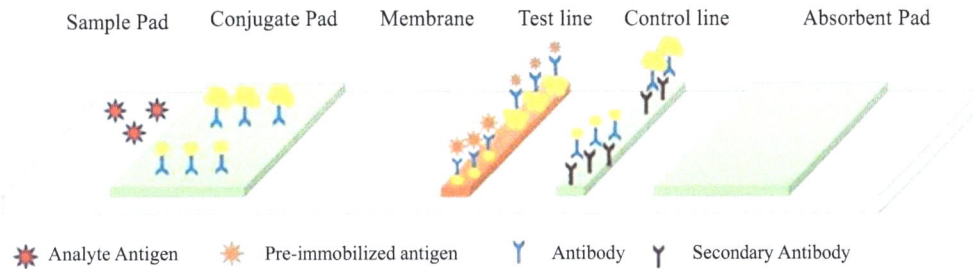

Sample Pad   Conjugate Pad   Membrane   Test line   Control line   Absorbent Pad

✳ Analyte Antigen   ✳ Pre-immobilized antigen   Y Antibody   Y Secondary Antibody

Fig. (2b). Competitive LFIA assay.

LFIA has spread widely in clinical diagnosis as a bed-side, low-tech, cost-effective diagnostic tool. Examples of the employment of LFIAs are found in veterinary, forensic, food safety, and environmental analysis, Examples of using LFIA in the diagnosis of infectious disease is summarized in Table **2**. In order to maximize LFIA cost effectiveness, the ability to detect more than one analyte at the same time is added, multiplexing LFIA (x-LFIA) can be achieved by embedding additional non-interfering reaction sites to the detection strip [36, 37].

Table 2. Overview of infections detected by LFIA.

Sample	Analyte	Technique	Organism	Sensitivity	Ref.
Serum and CSF	Cryptococcal capsular antigen (CrAg)	Latex-Cryptococcus antigen test using serotype-specific monoclonal antibodies	*Cryptococcus neoformans* and *Cryptococcus gattii.*	97.7%	[38]
Simulated clinical samples (mouse blood)	*Yersinia pestis* capsule like (F1) protein.	Paired monoclonal antibodies (MAbs) against *Yersinia pestis* capsule like fraction 1 (F1) protein.	*Yersinia pestis*	4 ng/ml of recombinant F1-protein	[39]
Urine sample	*S. pneumoniae* & *L. pneumophila* Urinary Antigen	BinaxNOW® lateral flow tests and the Binax® EIA test.	*Streptococcus pneumoniae* and *Legionella pneumophila*	Fast and sensitive	[40]
Serum	Antibodies to *Treponema pallidum* and hepatitis B antigen	Colloidal gold and oligonucleotide labelled antibody	*Treponema pallidum;* hepatitis B infection	5 µg L⁻¹ hepatitis B antigen	[41]
Serum	Antibody to Schistosoma Japonicum	Blue colloidal dye labelled egg antigen	Schistosomiasis	97% positives in acute form; 94% in chronic	[42]
Serum	Leptospira-serum-specific IgM	Colloidal dye labelled monoclonal antihuman IgM antibody	Leptospirosis	87% overall sensitivity	[43]
Respiratory sample	Influenza A, B and respiratory syncytial virus	Raman signature labelled antigen measures Raman scattering	Multianalyte detection of influenza A, influenza B and respiratory syncytial virus	n/a	[44]
Mosquito bloodmeal	Human or animal IgG in mosquito bloodmeal	Dye-labelled anti-IgG antibodies	IgG to detect different host sources of blood meal in insects	10 µg L⁻¹	[45]
Stool	*Helicobacter pylori* stool antigen (HpSA)	Two McAb pairs targeting *H. pylori*, DF2a/EE10b and IH10b/EE10b	*Helicobacter pylori*	$1.0 \times 10^{(4)}$ cfu/mL 100%	[46]
Serum	*Mycoplasma pneumoniae* specific IgM	anti-IgM-AF647 and anti-IgG-AF647	*Mycoplasma pneumoniae*	96.37%	[47]

Nucleic Acid Lateral Flow Immune-Assay (NALFIA)

NALFIA is mainly designed to explore pathogens in food and environmental samples, in which the analyte is an organism-specific double-stranded nucleic acid sequence (ds-amplicon), the ds-amplicon is amplified using PCR with two tagged primers, one strand is labelled with biotin and the other strand is labelled with fluorescein or digoxigenin, recognition of the analyte is done by binding to a tag-specific antibody sprayed at the test line. The biotin will bind to the avidin-labelled nanoparticles and the other tag will bind to the anti-tag-antibody, resulting in a colored signal, the color intensity depends mainly on analyte concentration [25, 48], Table **3** summarizes examples of testing infectious organisms by NALFIA

Table 3. Overview of infections detected by NALFIA.

Sample	Analyte	Technique	Organism	Sensitivity	Ref.
Food, shellfish	Invasion gene A (InvA)	Recombinase polymerase amplification (RPA) combined with lateral flow dipstick	Salmonella species	100 copies DNA per reaction (20 microL).	[49]
Blood & CSF	camp factor gene	Recombinase polymerase amplification with lateral flow strips	Group B streptococcus	100 genomic copies 100%	[50]
Synovial fluid	16s rDNA	PCR for amplification of 16s rDNA with a lateral flow immunoassay	Periprosthetic joint infection	97%	[51]
Cervical	HPV genotypes	Loop-mediated isothermal amplification with lateral flow dipstick tests.	human papilloma-virus HPV16 and HPV18	Very high sensitivity	[52]
Serum	Brucella-specific IgM antibodies	Colloidal labelled dye monoclonal antihuman IgM antibody	Brucellosis	93% positives	[53]
	Specific isothermally amplified RNA	Polystyrene dyed microsphere labelled	*Bacillus anthracis*	2 B. anthracis cells	[48]
Synovial Fluid	PCR amplified product of 23S ribosomal RNA	Colloidal gold labelled strands	Bacterial infections in arthroplasty	10 cells of *S. aureus*	[54]
Serum	4 dengue serotypes Isothermally amplified nucleic acid	Dye-entrapped liposome DNA probe	Viral infection	50–50,000 copies of RNA	[31]

(Table 3) cont.....

Sample	Analyte	Technique	Organism	Sensitivity	Ref.
Serum	Brucella-specific IgM antibodies	Isothermal amplification technique	Brucellosis	100%	[55]
Wound swabs and Respiratory sample	specific erm (41) gene	loop-mediated isothermal amplification coupled with lateral flow dipstick	*Mycobacterium abscessus* and *Mycobacterium massiliense*	100%	[56]

Flow-Through Assay FTA

It's one of the earliest devised RDT techniques, supplied as individual cassettes with extraction and wash reagents included. FTA is a rapid, simple, cheap, and user-friendly diagnostic test for bedside detection of antibodies/antigens of infectious organisms. A fluid sample of the analyte flows through a nitrocellulose porous immune-reactive membrane by capillary action into an absorbent membrane where it is captured by analyte-specific antibody, then the complex is bound to immobilized colloidal gold conjugate which can be visualized by the addition of signaling reagent [57], see Fig. (**3**).

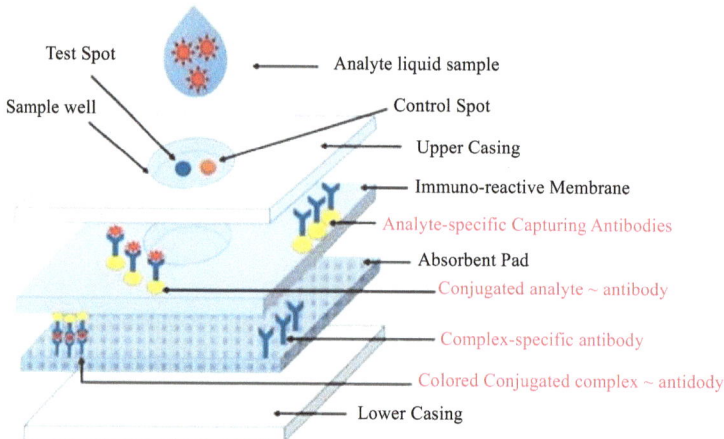

Fig. (3). Flow-through Assay.

Multiplex FTA is also applicable for diagnosis of up to 4 different target antigens/antibodies in the analyte sample by spotting multiple capture antibodies specific for different antigens at separated locations on the membrane [58, 59], it obtains results even faster than lateral flow tests (3-5 min), but requires an added wash and buffer steps as well as constant attention, which can limit its applicability.

Agglutination Test

The method principle is simply the observation of the binding between carrier particles and target analytes into visible clumps, seen either through a microscope or with the naked eye. However, if the binding of the particles is weak, this gives doubtful test results. See Fig. (**4**).

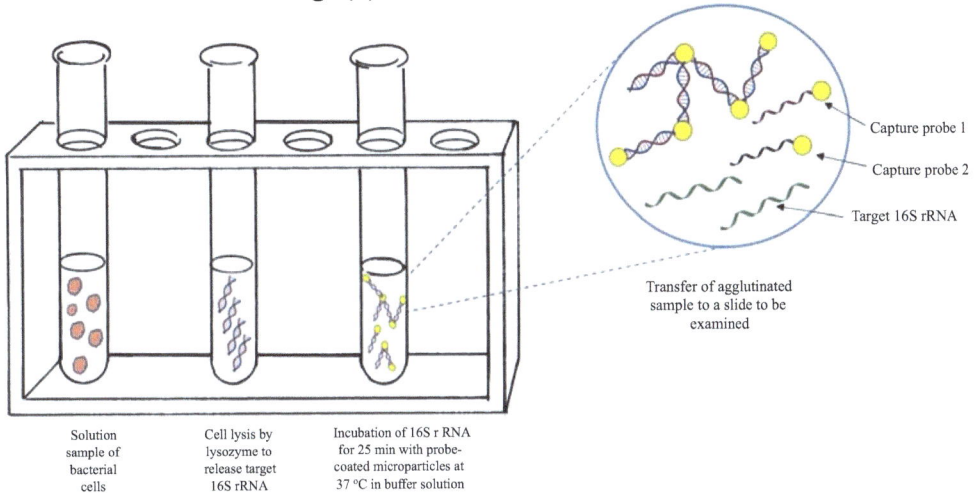

Fig. (4). Agglutination Test.

The agglutination carrier particles are added to the target analyte on a microscope slide or in a plate well, the mixture is agitated and allowed to settle for few minutes in order to allow visible agglutination. These tests employ latex particles, gelatin beads, colloidal particles, or preserved mammalian or avian blood cells to facilitate visualization of agglutination. Although it is an old technique, it is still showing high sensitivity towards some viral [60] and bacterial [61] strains. Agglutination tests are low-cost, rapid and semiquantitative in 2-10 folds specimen dilution, but it needs very precise interpretation for marginal results, as well as the lack of specificity due to interfering determinants.

Dipstick

Although it's not a typical LFIA, the LFA procedure is a rate determining step in its action. Original dipstick assays are based on the immunoblotting principle and don't rely on lateral fluid flow through a membrane. Dipstick is a solid, nonporous supported membrane onto which analyte capture molecules are immobilized. It works by placing the dipstick in a sample. The dipstick is then washed and incubated to prevent non-specific analyte binding. These additional steps can limit their usability in low-resource point of care. Most tests can be completed in one hour or less, and they allow individual patients to be tested for one or multiple parameters with a single assay. Nucleic acid dipstick assay (NADA) is a recent technique performed using dipstick platforms, it depends on visualization of thermally amplified nucleic acid using dipsticks [62]. Table **4**. gives some examples of using NADA in infections diagnosis.

Table 4. examples of nucleic acid dipstick assay NADA.

Sample	Analyte	Technique	Organism	Sensitivity	Time	Ref.
Rectal swab	Plasmid-mediated colistin resistance gene, mcr-1	PCR-dipstick technique	*Enterobacteriaceae*	100% sensitivity	< 2 hours	[63]
Live and heat inactivated cells	Salmonella RNA	DNA thermally amplified + dipstick	*S. enteritidis* *S. infantis.* *S. typhimurium*	$5 \times 10^{(5)} S.$ *typhimurium* cells	4-5 min	[64]
Rectal swab	Entamoeba RNA	DNA thermally amplified + dipstick	*Entamoeba histolytica* *Entamoeba dispar*	100% specificity	--	[65]
Clinical samples	Bovine ephemeral fever virus RNA	Recombinase polymerase amplification + dipstick	Bovine ephemeral fever virus (BEFV)	96.09%	25 min	[66]

Generally, simple immunoassay-based techniques provide a fast, low cost, simple, one-step procedure, applicable at the point of care to many types of fluid samples with minimal sample pre-treatment. Limitations related to its use are; results dependence on analyte volume and concentration, the avidity, reactivity, and cross-reactivity of the involved antigens and antibodies, and the unreliable outcomes with multi-analyte samples, which need further research and development of these assays and produce more microarray options to maximize accuracy and cost effectiveness [25]. Improved outcomes of immunoassays are related with recruitment of highly specific labels chemically linked to either enzymes, radioisotopes or fluorescent compounds in order to develop a measurable signal upon binding.

Automated Immunoassays

Enzyme-Linked Immunosorbent Assays (ELISA)

ELISA has been a commonly used technique since the early seventies of last century, the assay premise is the specific binding of enzyme-linked antibodies to detect the presence and quantity of a certain analyte in a liquid sample, chromogenic reporters are linked to the antibodies for the purpose of visualization and quantification of antigen-antibody complex using spectrophotometer, fluorometer or luminometer. The most commonly used enzyme labels are horseradish peroxidase (HRP), alkaline phosphatase (AP), β-galactosidase, acetylcholinesterase and catalase [67].

The analyte sample is immobilized into a polystyrene microtiter assay plate either by direct surface adsorption or by being indirectly captured by an immobilized antibody attached to the assay plate. The detection antibody-enzyme covalently-bonded complex is added to the analyte to make another complex with the antigen, washing using a detergent solution after each step is mandatory to remove non-specific antigens, then finally adding the enzymatic substrate to the complex produces a visualizable and measurable signal [68]. Monoclonal antibodies are used in direct ELISA, while polyclonal antibodies are more likely to be used in indirect ELISA. See Fig. (**5**).

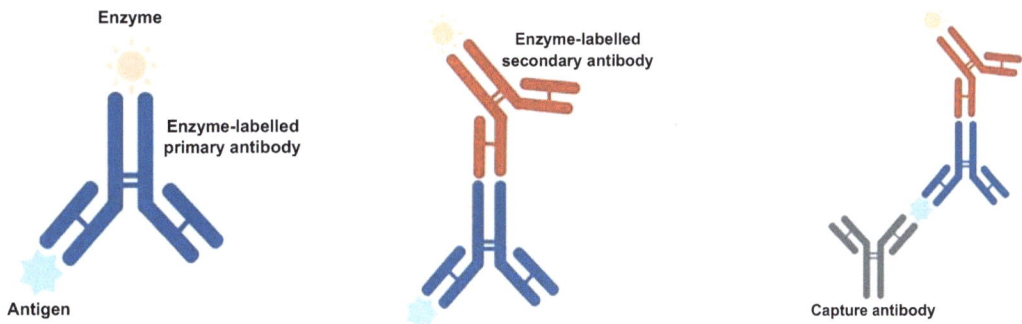

Fig. (5). Direct, indirect and sandwich ELISA.

In direct ELISA assays, the antigen is directly detected by a monoclonal enzyme-labelled antibody, fewer steps and reagents involved contributes to faster and more precise results [69], while indirect approach evolves immobilization of the antigen to the ELISA plate where its first captured by an antigen-specific unlabelled primary antibody, then another polyclonal enzyme-labelled secondary antibody is added to bound to the primary antibody, indirect ELISA offers increased sensitivity and cost-effectiveness [70].

As for sandwich ELISA, a pair of polyclonal matched antibodies, each is specific for different epitope of the antigen, are used for capture and detection of the antigen. The capture antibody is immobilized to ELISA well then, the labelled detection antibody is added. Any excess unbound enzyme-linked antibody is washed away after each step of the reaction, then substrate is added, and quantification of antigen in the specimen is possible by direct measurement of colour intensity resulting from substrate addition spectrophotometrically [68].

This approach is highly sensitive, which makes it suitable for low purity samples, as presence of antigen-specific capture antibody will roll-out other impurities. ELISA has been used successfully for precise identification and quantification of many viral infections, Zika virus [71], HIV antibodies [72], Hepatitis C antibodies [73], and Ebola virus [74], as well as some bacterial infections like *Mycobacterium tuberculosis* [75], *Escherichia coli* [76], and *Klebsiella pneumonia* [77].

Radioimmunoassay (RIA)

RIA is a highly sensitive and specific immunoassay technique; it allows the detection of as low as a few picograms of analyte using antibodies of high affinity to the analyte. It works through competitive binding interaction, where a radiolabeled antigen with gamma-radioactive isotopes of iodine (125-I), attached to tyrosine (the tracer), competes with unlabelled antigen (analyte) for fixed antibodies count, leading to the release of specified amount of labelled antigen. As the concentration of unlabeled antigen increases it will be able to displace the tracer from its binding site on the antibody, the ratio of labelled/unlabeled antigen is then measured to accurately quantify the analyte antigen using radioactivity measurement instrument, RIA required highly specialized fully-automated equipment as radioactive molecules are involved [78]. RIA have been used widely to identify hormones, peptides, viral infections (Mumps [79], Herpes simplex [80], Cytomegalovirus [81], Hepatitis B [82]), and bacterial infections; *Salmonella typhi* [83], *Pseudomonas aeruginosa* [84], and *E. coli* [85]).

Fluorescence Immunoassays (FIA)

Florescent immunoassay uses a fluorescent compound (fluorophore label) as a detection reagent. It is a competitive assay in which fluorophore-labelled antigen compete with the analyte to an available calculated number of antibodies, forming a stable antigen-antibody large complex and free rotating antigen in the sample solution. Exciting the fluorophore using polarized light will differentiate between both entities, as the fluorescence emitted by the stable complex will retain its original polarization, while fluorescence emitted by the unbound antigen will lose its polarization. The lost polarization degree represents the amount of unbound antigen which is proportional to the analyte amount in the specimen. Despite the high accuracy and specificity of this approach, it is of a limited use in infectious disease diagnosis and used mainly for hormonal and small sized biologicals assays. Newly developed FIA approaches are able to identify Dengue and Zika virus [86], Norwalk virus [87], Varicella zoster [88], and *E. coli* [89] infections.

Enzyme-Multiplied Immunoassay Technique (EMIT) and Microparticle enzyme immunoassay (MEIA) are other highly sensitive approaches belonging to automated immunoassays with no implication in diagnosis of infectious diseases, hopefully future researches and development will expand the utility of these techniques in this field.

Generally, automated immunoassays are the most well-established platforms in the laboratory, as they quickly and easily deliver highly precise results in assaying a wide variety of biological and chemical samples, like peptides, hormones, chemicals, drugs, cell markers and infectious diseases.

NUCLEIC ACID PROBE-BASED TECHNIQUES

Peptide Nucleic Acid (PNA) Fluorescence *In situ* Hybridization (FISH)

PNA-FISH is a molecular diagnostic tool for the rapid detection of pathogens from liquid media, approved by U.S. Food and Drug Administration (FDA) in 1986 for the detection of bacterial and fungal species [90]. It works through diffusion of synthetic fluorescent oligomers mimicking DNA or RNA (PNA probe) through cell wall to the organism-specific rRNA, binds to species-specific 16S rRNA directly. Visualization of this thermally-stable PNA-RNA fluorescent hybrids under fluorescent microscopy is possible. PNA probe length limit is 20 bases, with a modifiable structure in order to enhance the nucleic acid-binding properties [91 - 93], or to convey other desired properties to the molecule, like being able to detect analytes at very low concentrations [94].

PNA-FISH is widely used technique for understanding genetic mutations, it differs from most other techniques used for genetic studies in its ability to identify genetic determinants in non-actively dividing cells (no need for amplification) [95]. It is used for the detection and localization of blood-culture-negative endocarditis, respiratory infections, gastrointestinal diseases, mycobacterial infections, highly pathogenic microorganisms and other fastidious bacteria such as spirochetes with a turn-over time around 90 minutes [96]. Table **5** describes a panel of infectious diseases for which PNA-FISH diagnosis has proven its effectiveness.

Table 5. Overview of infections where PNA-FISH prove effectiveness.

Organism/s	Sample	Results	Platform	Time	Ref.
Pseudomonas aeruginosa *Staphylococcus aureus* *Candida albicans*	Burn wound infections	3 species were identifiable in tissue swabs, with minimal auto-fluorescence from any species.	AdvanDx	2.5 - 3 hours	[110]
Pseudomonas aeruginosa, Inquilinus limosus	Sputum samples	High predictive and experimental specificities and sensitivities	--	3-4 Hours	[111]
Escherichia coli, Klebsiella pneumoniae *Pseudomonas aeruginosa*	Blood cultures	PNA-FISH-AFC assay detect lower bacterial conc in shorter time compared to MALDI-TOF	BacTEC system	12 hours	[112]
Candida albicans *Candida glabrata* *Candida parapsilosis* *Candida tropicalis*	Blood cultures	concordance rate with the conventional methods was determined as 97.6%	AdvanDx	90 minutes	[104, 113]
enterococcal or streptococcal bacteremia	Blood cultures	Absence of guidance from an antibiotic stewardship program reduce the impact of PNA-FISH	--	30-90 minutes	[114]
Proteus species	Urine samples	98% sensitivity compared with CHROMagar	--	Approximately 2 hours	[115]
Lactobacillus species. *Gardnerella vaginalis*	Vaginal swabs	probes were able to differentiate Lactobacillus spp. And *Gardnerella vaginalis* from the other undefined bacterial species.	--	Approximately 2 hours	[116]
Staphylococcus aureus coagulase-negative staphylococcus	Blood cultures	Sensitivity for *S. aureus* and CoNS was 96.5% and 96.6%, respectively.	AdvanDx	Approximately 2 hours	[117]

PNA-FISH is performed by mixing of one drop of fixation solution with one drop of specimen on a PNA-FISH slide, this mixture is fixed in methanol followed by 80% ethanol for 10 minutes each, then allowed to air dry. A drop of the specific PNA probe is applied to the slide, then the slide is hybridized for 90 minutes at 55°C, followed by incubation in 55°C wash solution for 30 minutes. Once again, the slide is allowed to air dry before being mounted and examined using the microscope for the presence of multiple bright fluorescent (green, red, yellow) morphologically consistent microorganisms in multiple fields of view.

Quick FISH is a more developed, streamlined version of PNA-FISH to overcome multiple processes [97, 98], while preserving the sensitivity or signal detection quality [99]. Some techniques decreased the hybridization time from 1 hour in PNA-FISH to 150 seconds (Quick-FISH) through use of microwave to shorten the heating time [100]. (AdvanDx)ᵃ is PNA-FISH platform with an excellent specificity (95%–100%) towards Staphylococcus spp., Enterococcus spp [101], *Escherichia coli, Klebsiella pneumoniae, Pseudomonas aeruginosa* [102], and *Acinetobacter baumannii* [103], and Candida spp [104]. Of note, it requires the above mentioned sequence of procedures and reagents (fixation solution, methanol, ethanol, wash solution) in addition to a fluorescent microscopy [105]. Dana M Harris *et al.* reported that PNA-FISH (AdvanDx)ᵃ reduced the time needed for identification of bacteria and *candida species* originated from blood samples from 83.6 hours by conventional techniques to 11.2 hours with overall accuracy 98.8%, and in peritoneal fluid from 87.4 hours to 16.4 hours with overall accuracy 100% [105].

The (Verigeneᵃ) system nucleic acid-PCR amplification is another FDA approved PNA-FISH platform for Gram-positive and Gram-negative pathogens identification, where time-to-result is close to 2.5 hours. It is a microarray technique, where the organism DNA is sheared and then captured on a DNA microarray. Interaction of DNA with silver and gold nanoparticles allows the signal reader to interpret the results coming from the pathogen specific cartridge. (BC-GP) and (BC-GN) are the panel cartridges for Gram-positive and Gram-negative pathogens respectively, the BC-GP distinguishes coagulase-negative staphylococci CoNS from *S. aureus*, MRSA from MSSA, VRE from VSE, and several clinically significant streptococci to species level. Overall identification accuracy of panel targets, including mecA, vanA, and vanB resistance genes is reported to be more than 95% [106, 107]. While in a large multicentered study of 1847 blood cultures containing Gram-negative bacteria, the BC-GN had an overall sensitivity of 98% and specificity of 100% in organism identification from monomicrobial blood cultures, while both cartridges demonstrated low detection capabilities in case of polymicrobial infections ranging from 54% of cases with BC-GN to 70% with BC-GP [108]. Meanwhile, fungi detection probes beset of cross-reactivity of many fungal species *e.g.*: (*Candida orthopsilosisvs.Candida metapsilosis, Candida glabrata* or *Candida krusei*) [109].

NUCLEIC ACID AMPLIFICATION-BASED TECHNIQUES

Real-Time Polymerase Chain Reaction (RT-PCR)

PCR technique was developed in 1984 by Nobel prize winner Kary B. Mullis, it is based on amplifying small segments of DNA originating from tissues, organisms, or clinical samples, as a significant count of DNA copies is necessary for molecular and genetic analyses. To amplify a segment of DNA using PCR, the sample is heated and cooled in cycles by a programmed thermocycler (95°C), so the DNA strands separates into two pieces of single-stranded DNA, then the temperature is reduced to about 55 °C to let a heat-stable polymerase enzyme build two new strands of DNA (amplicon), using the original strands as templates and individual oligo-nucleotides bases (primers) – adenine, thymine, cytosine, and guanine. This process results in the duplication of the original DNA, which can be used to create two new copies within 5 minutes, and so on. The cycle of denaturing and synthesizing new DNA is repeated, and the number of copies doubles after each cycle until we have a measurable number of DNA copies within 25-30 minutes [118]. Amplified PCR can be visualized either by; staining of the amplified DNA product with a chemical dye such as ethidium bromide, or by pre-amplification labeling of the target PCR or free nucleotides with fluorescent dyes (fluorophores). See Fig. (**6**).

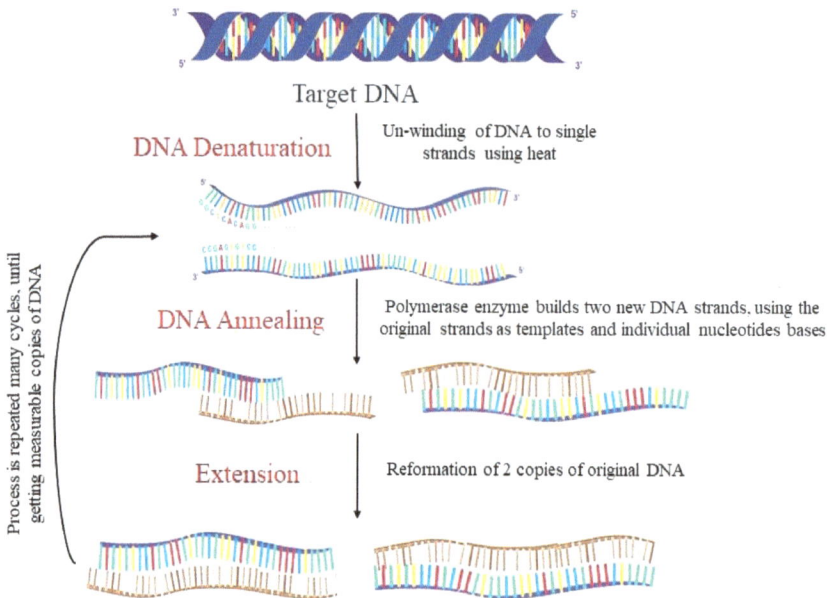

Fig. (6). Real-time PCR.

Most molecular biology protocols recommends performing PCR with a sample volume in the range of 5 μL to 100 μL. PCR technique used for detection of absence or presence of specific DNA is termed qualitative PCR, *e.g.* screening of patients on hemodialysis for detection of HCV infection using PCR [119]. While, quantitative real-time PCR (qRT-PCR) allows the detection and quantification of

DNA determinants, it works through reverse transcription PCR, in which the reverse transcriptase enzyme converts mRNA to single stranded complementary cDNA, the newly formed cDNA serves as the template for conventional PCR steps.

In real-time PCR, the amplicons are quantified after each cycle *via* fluorescent dyes that yield directly fluorescent signal proportional to the number of amplicons generated. Plotting fluorescence intensity against the amplification cycle number enables RT-PCR module to yield a robust quantification of amplicons over the whole period of PCR reaction. Table **6** gives examples of infections can be identified using PCR platforms.

Table 6. examples of infections detected by PCR technique.

Sample	Analyte	Technique	Organism	Specificity/Sensitivity	Ref.
Birds Secretions	Avian avula-virus 1 (AAvV-1) L-gene, using minor groove binding (MGB) probes	Real-time RT-PCR	Newcastle disease virus (NDV)	Enhanced sensitivity and specificity	[120]
Stool	*Schistosoma japonicum* DNA	Droplet digital (dd) PCR assays	*Schistosoma japonicum*	2.5 times higher than microscopy	[121]
Solid bovine manure	Bacterial DNA	Real-time quantitative PCR	*Escherichia coli* O157 & Salmonella species	Highly specific	[122]
Fermented dairy products	Bacterial DNA	Direct colony PCR using BOXA2R repetitive primers	*Lactococcus lactis*, *Leuconostoc mesenteroides*, *Streptococcus thermophilus*	Reproducible and rapid	[123]
Human serum and urine	ZIKV cDNA	Quantitative RT-PCR	Zika virus	(2.5 PFU/mL) in urine and in serum (250 PFU/mL)	[124]
Respiratory samples	*Mycobacterium tuberculosis* complex	Ethidium mono-azide EMA-PCR Method	*Mycobacterium tuberculosis*	Viable to dead cells 83% and 100%,	[125]
Blood	Herpesviruses DNA.	Multiplex PCR assay	Herpes viruses	--	[126]
Respiratory samples	RSV-A and RSV-B. DNA	Mismatch-tolerant Quantitative RT-PCR	Respiratory syncytial virus	Good specificity and sensitivity	[127]

(Table 6) cont.....

Sample	Analyte	Technique	Organism	Specificity/Sensitivity	Ref.
Gastric Biopsy	23S rRNA specific	Quantitative RT-PCR	*Helicobacter pylori*	PCR is more sensitive than microscopy.	[128]
Human serum samples	Plasmid-mediated colistin-resistant and CRE genes blaKPC, blaNDM, blaIMP, and blaOXA-48	Multiplex PCR	carbapenem-resistant *Enterobacteriaceae*	Good specificity and sensitivity	[129]

Real-Time Multiplex PCR (x-RT-PCR)

Multiplex real-time (x-RT-PCR) is used to produce qualitative or quantitative results, it can amplify more than one genetic sequence a time and detect the generated amplicons using a detector like gel electrophoresis. The cost-effectiveness is justified by increased throughput, reduced sample and reagents usage, x-RT-PCR usually involves multiple dyes in one well. The x-RT-PCR instrument must be capable of measuring those different dye signals in the same well with high accuracy. These measurements must remain specific for each dye, even when one dye signal is significantly higher than another.

SPECTROMETRY BASED TECHNIQUES

Matrix-Assisted Laser Desorption Ionization Time-of-Flight Mass Spectrometry (MALDI-TOF-MS)

MALDI-TOF-MS is a mass spectrometry based analytical technique suitable for peptides, lipids, saccharides, and other organic macromolecules, in which the sample particles are ionized, then their mass-to-charge ratio can be measured. The sample matrix is bombarded by a laser beam to convert the analyte molecules into gaseous state without causing fragmenting or decomposing of determinants.

The analyte is mixed with a sample-polarity-compatible, solid, energy-absorbent, organic compound matrix, the analyte/matrix solution ratio is optimized for MALDI-TOF spectra which fall into the range from (1000: 1) to (100,000: 1), then the mixture is spotted onto the metal target plate for analysis. After drying, the mixture of the sample and matrix co-crystallizes and forms a solid deposit of the sample embedded into the matrix. The choice of matrix depends on its polarity as highly polar analytes favor highly polar matrices, and nonpolar analytes are preferably combined with nonpolar matrices, the most commonly used matrixes are α-cyano-4-hydroxycinnamic acid, 2,5-dihydroxybenzoic acid, 3,5-dimethoxy-4-hydroxycinnamic acid, and 2,6-dihydroxyacetophenone.

The target plate is subsequently loaded into the MALDI-TOF instrument, the target is then irradiated by a laser pulse (ultraviolet or infra-red) to elevate its temperature and render it thermodynamically excited. The energetically activated matrix molecules dissociate from its surface and carry the analyte molecules into the gaseous phase as well. During this ablation process, the analyte molecules become ionized by protonation or deprotonation with the nearby matrix molecules.

The dispersed ions in the ionization chamber are of different mass/charge (m/z), they start their journey at the time of flight tube, ions of the same (m/z) ratio will reach the detector at the same time, with the lighter ones arrive earlier at the detector than the heavier ones, the m/z ratio of an ion is measured by determining the time required for it to travel the length of the flight tube. The ions are accelerated between series of ring electrodes with high voltage (reflectron) in order to homogenize the velocity of same (m/z) ions toward the detector, and a spectral representation of these ions is generated and analyzed by the MS analyzers, (quadrupole mass analyzers, ion trap analyzers, or time of flight (TOF) analyzers *etc.*) to generate a MS profile. The resulted MS can be compared with those of well-characterized organisms available in the reference library database to identify the isolate. The identified MS pattern of the ribosomal proteins, which represent about 60–70% of the dry weight of a microbial cell is used to identify a particular microorganism by matching it with MS profile of the ribosomal proteins archived database. Thus, the identity of organism can be established down to the genus, and in many cases to the species and strain level [130], as shown in Fig. (**7**).

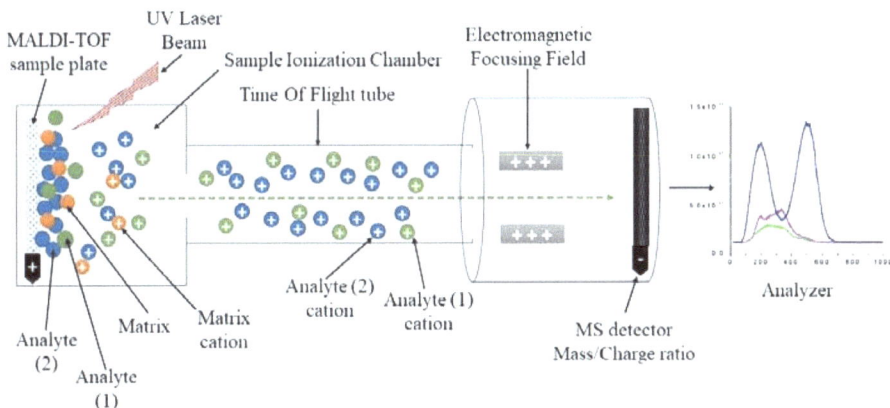

Fig. (7). MALDI-TOF operation.

MALDI-TOF is a suitable assay for thermo-labile proteins and enzymes that may undergo fragmentation upon exposure to extensive heating, also MALDI-TOF low dependence on reagents, buffers, detergents, and contaminants permits highly accurate identification, mass determination and fingerprinting of such molecules. Mass determination and complete sequencing of oligonucleotide fragments used as primers or probes in molecular techniques can be also performed accurately using MALDI-TOF to ensure complete synthesis of the right sequence (Table 7).

MALDI- Imaging Mass Spectrometry (MALDI-IMS)

This technique is introduced in the early 21st century, it provides detailed information through imaging of molecular composition and distribution of peptides directly from an intact thin tissue section that maintain the cells and its components integrity, up to a thousand lipid species can be detected, and the result provides both molecular–histological maps from the localization and identification of lipid biomolecules based on mass-to- charge ratio (m/z) [131].

MALDI-IMS incorporates 2 complementary modules; imaging and profiling. Imaging approach is performed to track the detailed distribution of certain analyte throughout the selected tissue section through mapping of the ionized molecules and correlation with histological features [132]. Profiling approach is more targeted as it allows the selective identification of individual analyte within the tissue section (*e.g.* distinguish malignant from normal cells) [133].

Although MALDI-TOF is a very rapid, fully automated, easy to use, cost effective with minimal requirement assay platform that can be applied for a wide range of analytes and sample types, there are still several limitations; like the inability to reliably detect some isolates such as *Shigella* species and *Streptococcus pneumoniae* [134], inability to determine the susceptibility pattern for the identified organism, and the need for human clinical samples processing before start the assay.

Table 7. Applications of MALDI-TOF MS in clinical diagnostic microbiology.

Sample	Technique	Organism	Sensitivity	Limitations	Ref.
Human clinical samples	MALDI Biotyper Selective Testing of Antibiotic Resistance-β-Lactamase	Carbapenemases-producing *Enterobacteriaceae*	Specificity and sensitivity of MBT STAR-BL were 100% and 98.69%	False-negative results for OXA-48 and OXA48+NDM-1 in K. pneumoniae.	[135]

(Table 7) cont.....

Sample	Technique	Organism	Sensitivity	Limitations	Ref.
Blood culture	MALDI-TOF MS analysis using Sepsi-Typer kit	Gram negative Gram positive Anaerobic bacteria	99% of the isolates were correctly identified by the Sepsi-Typer kit	MALDI-TOF use is limited with un-identified microorganisms	[136]
Blood culture	MALDI-TOF MS analysis	24 strains of eight Candida species.	Performance of identification reached 60%	The performance of the technique varied across Candida species	[137]
Human clinical samples	(MALDI-TOF) Vitek MS system	KPC-producing *Enterobacteriaceae*	95.5% detection of CRE	--	[138]
Human clinical samples	MALDI-TOF MS-Based Direct-on-Target Microdroplet Growth Assay	ESBL and AmpC β-Lactamases *Enterobacteriaceae*	ESBL, 94.44/100%; AmpC, 94.44/93.75% and ESBL+AmpC, 100/100%. Compared to PCR results	--	[139]
Human clinical samples	MALDI-TOF MS analysis (Bruker)	Non-tuberculous mycobacteria	MALDI-TOF MS classified significantly better than Geno-Type((R)).	--	[140]
Human clinical samples	MALDI-TOF MS analysis	Candida Species *C. auris*	MALDI-TOF MS gives more reliable results *vs* conventional Anti-fungal Susceptibility Testing	--	[141]

FUTURE RDTS IN DEVELOPMENT

Microfluidics (Lab-on-a-Chip)

Microfluidics are an emerging area of rapid diagnostic development. Using electrochemical sensors, these tests would include all detectors and reactants in a single portable chip. The whole microfluidic device has to be designed in advance and prepared using a cleanroom. Noteworthy, the considerably smaller volumes that can be introduced into the microfluidic device also necessitate that sufficient analyte should be present in such a small volume to be detectable [142]. Microfluidic devices can be designed for low-cost analysis of the minimum volume of samples, chemicals and reagents. It is elaborated to allow the user to generate multi-step uniform reactions requiring a low level of training and a lot of functionalities, thus it can be used in a wide range of research applications like molecular and cell biology research, genetics, fluid dynamics, micro-mixing, point of care diagnostics, lab on a chip, tissue engineering, organ on a chip, drug delivery device, fertility testing, and synthesis of chemicals or proteins. Yet; it is only a research tool and no diagnostic platform is designed based on microfluidics technique, but it remains a promising technological solution in microbiology diagnostics field due to low manufacturing and implementation costs compared to advanced platforms. The standardization, reagents and consumables costs, and automation applicability and reliability remain the barriers need to be overcame to develop an automated microfluidics-based platform [143].

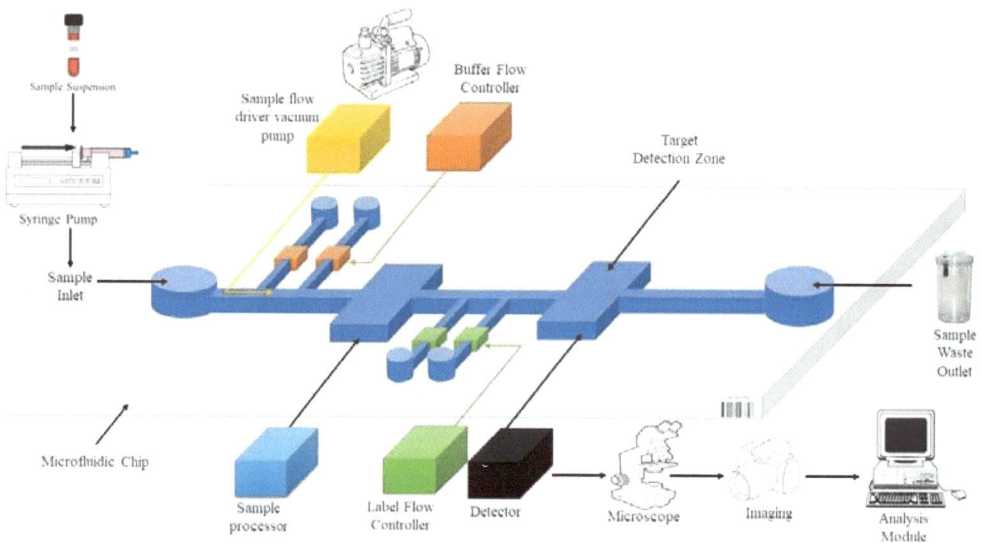

Fig. (8). Microfluidics technique.

A microfluidic chip is a set of micro-channels - ranging from submicron to few millimeters - molded into (glass, silicon or poly-dimethyl-siloxane). These micro-channels are connected together and to a macro-environment apparatus through inputs and outputs pierced through the chip. Liquid or gaseous samples are introduced and removed from the chip through tubing or syringe adapters with help of external active systems (valves, pressure controller, push-syringe, passive pressure or pump). Sample is directed, mixed, separated or manipulated to attain multiplexing, automation, and high-throughput systems. The pre-defined spots on the chip release specific probes that can bind selectively to certain target gene sequence, the gene-probe complex is analyzable by computer programs to identify the target determinants in the sample [144]. Fig. (**8**) demonstrates the operation of microfluidics technique.

Whole-Genome Sequencing (WGS)

WGS is a laboratory research tool designed to determine the order (sequence) of nucleotide bases building up the genome of an organism, in order to provide a precise DNA or RNA fingerprint. More advanced approaches are developed based on WGS can sequence both DNA and RNA faster and cheaper than the traditional approach, like (next-generation sequencing) and (massively parallel sequencing) [145].

The organism cells are treated chemically in order to release its DNA/RNA molecules, which are then purified and mechanically or enzymatically (molecular scissors) fragmented into specific length fragments, amplification of these fragmented copies is performed using PCR technique. The generated pool of genome fragments is called a genome library which is interpreted by a sequencer to build up a genome read. By means of specialized software, reconstruction of the whole genome is performed, which is then compared to already archived genome data bases for the purpose of identification.

Attempts are underway to deploy WGS in clinical practice to provide early prediction of inherited diseases [146, 147], unexplained chromosomal related diseases [148], identify the responsible genes for chronic comorbidities in high-risk patient groups [149], and recognition of genetic elements responsible for malignant cell mutations [150]. Regarding the implementation of WGS in infectious diseases, the actual transition from a mere research tool to practical diagnostic applications is still in development. The techniques is currently used in epidemiological studies and prediction of pandemic outbreaks [151 - 153], and identification of genetic determinants responsible for antimicrobial resistance in many species; for example, linezolid and vancomycin resistance in *Enterococcus faecium* [154], colonization controlling genes in MRSA [155], recurrence responsible genes for *Mycobacterium tuberculosis* [156], transmission and mixed-genotype adenoviruses infections genes in immunocompromised patients [157], and *Clostridium difficile* relapse responsible genes [158].

The integration of WGS into routine clinical laboratory workflow of organism and susceptibility pattern identification is facing the challenges of absence of standardized robust guidelines for sampling and sequencing per different isolates, lack of nucleotide sequence data for bacterial isolates, and how to interpret the available enormous sequencing data to serve clinical outcomes [159].

MILESTONES IN THE IMPLEMENTATION OF RAPID DIAGNOSTICS

Positioning and Priorities

RDTs have attracted global attention in the past two decades due to their significant role in predicting and diagnosing pandemic outbreaks and high-profile health emergencies, which led to the reassessment of positioning to be more inclined toward the development and adoption of RDTs in parallel to the development of antimicrobials and vaccines, and the incorporation of the novel diagnostics in the treatment protocols [160]. Detailed epidemiological and economical studies will direct the need, selection, and implementation of such platforms in a fashion to serve rapid, precise, cost-effective outcomes, and also how to rationalize and protocolize the requisition of RDT tests, either in governmental or private healthcare sectors.

Flexible-diagnostic-spectrum platforms that are able to detect polymicrobial infections (multiplex platforms), will be more favourable than single organism detectors, and in the same context updatable platforms will be more cost-effective compared to non-updatable. Tables **8** and **9** summarize advantages and disadvantages of many microbial detection methods in order to aid selection, use and positioning of each.

Nation-wide studies and decision models should be used for the assessment and tracking the convenience, compatibility, and the impact on patients of the incorporated RDT panels within healthcare systems. Comparisons with existing clinical practice, must be conducted on regular basis in order to supply researchers and manufacturers with further opportunities for development of the platforms to suit different organizations and conditions. Furthermore, adequate quality assurance policies should be applied to ensure that RDTs continue to generate precise and reliable results.

Table 8. Summarized comparison between microbial detection methods used in clinical microbiology.

Technique	Advantages	Limitations
Microscopy-based methods.	• Cheapest technique. • Highly accurate. • Suitable for mixed infections.	• Time consuming. • Need for expertise's professionals. • Needs sample processing. • Can't distinguish invasive organisms from colonizers. • Some organisms aren't stainable and visualizable.

(Table 8) cont.....

Technique	Advantages	Limitations
Culture on microbiological media	• Cheap • Highly accurate organism identification.	• Time consuming (48-72 hours). • Interpretation errors. • Liable to contamination.
Immunoassay based methods	• Faster than conventional. • Organisms and Toxins.	• Not as specific, sensitive, and rapid as nucleic-acid based methods.
Nucleic acid probe-based techniques PNA-FISH	• Rapid detection • Identification directly from slide smears. • Fast and ease-of-use of conventional staining methods combined with specificity of molecular methods.	• Multi-steps sample processing is required. • Test limited by the availability of specific antigens for detection • The need for fluorescent microscopy. • Cross-reactivity of the yeast PNA-FISH probes
Nucleic Acid Amplification-Based techniques A. RT-PCR B. Multiplex-PCR	• Culturing of the sample is not required. • Specific, sensitive, rapid, and accurate. • Closed-tube system reduces the risk of contamination. • Can detect many pathogens simultaneously.	• A highly precise thermal cycler is needed. • Trained laboratory personnel required for performing the test.
DNA sequencing MALDI-TOF MS	• 16S rDNA and 18S rDNA sequencing are the gold standards. • Can identify fastidious and uncultivable microorganisms. • Fast • Accurate • Less expensive than molecular and immunological-based detection methods • Trained laboratory personnel not required.	• Trained laboratory personnel and powerful interpretation software are required • High initial cost of the MALDI-TOF equipment • Not suitable for routine clinical use.
Microarrays	• Large scale screening system for simultaneous diagnosis and detection of many pathogens	• Expensive • • Trained laboratory personnel required.
Loop-mediated isothermal amplification (LAMP) assay	• Can generate large copies of DNA in less than an hour. • Easy to use. • No sophisticated equipment is required.	• Developed for only a small number of microorganisms as yet.

Infrastructure and Logistic Challenges

The includability of RDTs in healthcare systems is disserved by the inability of human resources and logistics to meet the operational demands. The abundance of consumable accessories supplies (plates, reagents, personal protection tools) is mandatory to guarantee consistent and efficient use of RDTs. National standardization of RDTs inclusion criteria in healthcare system on basis of epidemiological and economical studies will effectively minimize the supply chain failures. Lack of trained and knowledgeable personnel able to execute the diagnostic test and interpret results is a great barrier for implementation, staff development programs, training and qualifying practices will be the best way to overcome the obstacle of the inability of the human factor to keep pace with evolution of diagnostic tools [161].

The preparedness of the infrastructure to accommodate operational requirements such as the need for adjusted environmental factors of temperature and humidity, in addition to, the ability to provide essential services like refrigeration, waste disposals and reliable energy supply, could be a barricade that should be eliminated before starting the implementation of RDT in healthcare system. The accessibility of the majority of population to the centralized healthcare services with advanced laboratory facilities remains a challenge to RDTs, especially in low-resourced countries, the compulsory increased sample-to-result time will forfeit the most impactful feature of RTDs, the rapid results. Providing fast and hazards-free transportation of samples, parallel to interlinked computerized data bases will hasten as much as possible the results delivery either to the healthcare professionals or to the patients.

The integration of RTDs in healthcare system will be most effective when supported by a robust electronic medical record, data capture software, and epidemiological surveillance and transmission reports. The patient history of illness and clinical manifestations correlated with microbiological results will ensure proper delivery of antimicrobial therapies [162].

Cost-Effectiveness Challenges

Molecular diagnosis using amplification of pathogen genetic materials is found to be superior to conventional microscopy and culture-based methods, RDTs provided an influential decision-making support for prescribers to promptly initiate targeted antimicrobial treatment rather than using broad-spectrum empiric treatment. Although most of research work was directed towards the assessment of the RDT using outcomes and the comparison with conventional ways in respect to time, selectivity and accuracy which were the direct added values of using

RDT, the area of comprehensive cost-effectiveness is still in need for further investigation. The study of economic impacts of using RDT reflected by reducing antimicrobial treatment related costs, decreased length of hospitalization and treatment failures rates would correct the misconcept of considering RDT as an added expenditure burden on the healthcare budget due to its relatively high prices and operational complexity.

A decision analysis model designed for cost-savings attributed to the use of RT-PCR testing for diagnosis of enteroviral meningitis in children demonstrated a 17%–35% savings in total healthcare costs [163]. Also, Ramers *et al.* reported less ancillary tests (26% *vs* 72% ; P<.001), shorter durations of received antimicrobial treatment (median, 2.0 *vs* 3.5 days; P<.001) and more rapid hospital discharges (median, 42 *vs* 71.5 hours; P<.001) in aseptic meningitis patients with Enterovirus PCR results available before hospital discharge compared to patients diagnosed using conventional methods [164].

A 1000 USD cost molecular diagnostic test of blood samples of patients in septic shock, averted estimated incremental cost-effectiveness ratio (ICER) by < $20,000 per death, repoted by Shehadeh at al [165]. As per Ugandan national malaria treatment guidelines; RDT was most cost-effective with lowest ICER compared to microscopy in the high transmission setting, ICER was US$4.38 for RDT and US$12.98 for microscopy [17]. Patel *et al.* found that using MALDI-TOF assay decreased the total hospital costs per bloodstream infection by nearly $2,500 per patient [166].

LABORATORY STEWARDSHIP

The integration of the microbiological laboratory within AMS program is a garner of all the major components necessary for the success of such programs. The prevalence of target pathogens (resistant phenotypes), infectious diseases (bacteremias, respiratory tract, gastro-intestinal, *etc.*), related hospitalization costs, and health facility workload will guide the selection of RDTs that serve the AMS targets.

RDTs results reporting should be displayed in a fashion that serves the daily AMS activities and target actionable interventions, with post-implementation scheduled pilot studies to assess the outcomes, the impact on the healthcare process, and related expenditure. The impact of RDTs can be evaluated through the assessment of different parameters that reflects how useful is the RDTs, time to appropriate therapy, reduction in mortality, reduction in hospital length of stay, reduced treatment failures and days of therapy.

Table 9. Examples of marketed RDT platforms and Kits.

	Product	Technique	Sample	Target	Sens.	Autom.	Time
Mobidiag	**Amplidiag** *H. pylori*+ClariR	Multiplex PCR	Stool Gastric Biopsy	▪ *H. pylori* 23S rRNA gene ▪ Clarithromycin resistance	96% 93.2%	Yes	< 2 h.
	Amplidiag Stool Parasites	Multiplex PCR	Stool	▪ Cryptosporidium species. ▪ *Giardia lamblia* ▪ *Entamoeba histolytica* ▪ *Dientamoeba fragilis*	100% 100% 100% 87.5%	Yes	< 2 h.
	Amplidiag Bacterial GE	Multiplex PCR	DNA extracted from stool	▪ *Escherichia coli* ▪ Yersinia ▪ Campylobacter ▪ Shigella species ▪ Salmonella spp.	93.5-100% 100% 98.9% 98% 100%	Yes	< 2 h.
	Amplidiag CarbaR+VRE	Multiplex PCR	DNA extracted from stool Rectal swabs Pure culture	▪ KPC ▪ NDM ▪ VIM ▪ OXA-48, OXA-181 ▪ IMP ▪ Acinetobacter OXA ▪ VanA & VanB	96% 93% 100% 100% 100% 92% 100%	Yes	< 2 h.
	Amplidiag Viral GE	Multiplex PCR	stool	▪ Norovirus G ▪ Rotavirus A ▪ Sapovirus ▪ Adenovirus 40 and 41 ▪ Astrovirus 100%	100% 95.8% 100% 93.3%	Yes	<2.5 h.
	Novodiag Bacterial GE+	Micro-array qPCR	Stool	▪ *Escherichia coli* ▪ Yersinia ▪ Vibrio cholerae ▪ Shigella species ▪ Salmonella species ▪ *Clostridium difficile*	97.8-100% 100% n/a 100% 90% 100%	Yes	1 h
	Novodiag CarbaR+	Micro-array qPCR	Pure cultures	▪ ~100 Genetic markers	100%	Yes	1.5 h

(Table 9) cont.....

	Product	Technique	Sample	Target	Sens.	Autom.	Time
Curetis	Unyvero Hospitalized Pneumonia – HPN	Multiplex PCR	Sputum Tracheal aspirate Broncho-alveolar lavage.	■ 48 genetic markers ■ Gram-positive bacteria ■ Enterobacteriaceae ■ Non-fermenting bacteria ■ Fungal pathogens	92.3% 88.8% 88.8% 88.9-100% 94.4-100%	Yes	5-6 h
	Unyvero Urinary Tract Infection – UTI 103 organisms and resistance genes.	Multiplex PCR	Urine	■ Gram-positive bacteria ■ Enterobacteriaceae ■ Non-fermenting bacteria ■ Fungi ■ Anaerobic bacteria ■ Resistant genes	97-100% 80-100% 100% 100% 91%	Yes	5-6 h
	Unyvero Blood culture – BCU 103 DNA analytes from a single sample.	Multiplex PCR	Blood	■ Gram-positive bacteria ■ Gram-negative bacteria ■ Enterobacteriaceae ■ Non-fermenting bacteria ■ Mycobacteriaceae. ■ Anaerobic bacteria ■ Resistant genes	97.6-100% 100% 91-100% 86%-100% n/a 100% 91.4%	Yes	5-6 h
Nanosphere	Verigene BC-GP	Multiplex PCR	Blood	■ MSSA ■ S. epidermidis	95% 96%	Yes	150 min
	Verigene BC-GP	Multiplex PCR	Blood	■ Staphylococcus species ■ Streptococcus species ■ *Enterococcus faecalis* ■ Listeria species	96% 97% 67% 94% 100%	Yes	150 min
	Verigene gram-negative blood culture	Multiplex PCR	Blood	■ *Escherichia coli* ■ *Klebsiella pneumoniae* ■ *Pseudomonas aeruginosa* ■ *Klebsiella oxytoca* ■ *Serratia marcescens* ■ Acinetobacter species ■ Proteus species ■ Citrobacter species ■ Enterobacter species	93-100%	Yes	120 min

(Table 9) cont.....

	Product*	Technique	Sample	Target	Sens.	Autom.	Time
AdvanDx	*S. aureus*/CoNS PNA QuickFISH	PNA Quick-FISH	Blood	■ MSSA ■ CoNS	100%	No	20 min
	Enterococcus faecalis/OE PNA QuickFISH	PNA Quick-FISH	Blood	■ *Enterococcus faecalis*	100%	No	30 min
	GNR Traffic Light PNA QuickFISH	PNA Quick-FISH	Blood	■ *Escherichia coli* ■ *Pseudomonas aeruginosa* ■ *Klebsiella pneumoniae*	89.6-100%	No	30 min
	Yeast Traffic Light PNA Fish	PNA FISH	Blood	■ *Candida Species*	100%	No	90 min
Revogene	GenePOC* C. Diff test	Real-time PCR	Liquid or soft stool specimens	■ Toxin B gene of *C. Difficile*	96%	Yes	70 min
	GenePOC* (GBS) DS	Real-time PCR	Vaginal/rectal swab	■ Group B Streptococcus	96%	Yes	70 min
	GenePOC* Carba test	Real-time PCR	CRE colonies	■ blaKPC, blaNDM, blaVIM, blaOXA-48-,blaIMP gene sequences	n/a	Yes	70 min
Coris Bioconcept	Pylori-Strip	Dipstick	Stool	■ *H. pylori* antigen	92.3%	No	10 min
	RSV-Respi-Strip	Dipstick	Respiratory	■ Resp. Syncytial Virus	90%	No	15 min
	Adeno- Respi-Strip	Dipstick	Stool	■ Respiratory Adenovirus	~94%	No	15 min
	Influ-A&B-Uni-strip	Dipstick	Nasal swab	■ Influenza A & B Virus	100%	No	15 min
	O157 Coli-strips	Immunochromatography	Stool/urine	■ *Escherichia coli*	n/a	No	15 min
Quidel	Sofia* Influenza A+B FIA	LFIA	Nasal swab Nasopharyngeal	■ Influenza A & B Virus	n/a	No	15 min
	Sofia* Strep A+ FIA	LFIA	Throat swab	■ Group A streptococcus	n/a	No	5 min
	Sofia*S. pneumoniae	LFIA	Urine	■ *Streptococcus pneumoniae*	n/a	No	10 min
Bruker	MALDI Biotyper CA	MALDI-TOF MS	Pure colonies	■ Multiple bacterial and fungal pathogens	95%	Yes	15 min
Bio-Mérieux	VITEK MS	MALDI-TOF MS	Pure colonies	■ Multiple bacterial and fungal pathogens	95%	Yes	1 h

Laboratory stewardship program (LSP) should be incorporated in AMS activities in order to promote rational ordering, protocolized reporting, fast delivery and clear interpretation of RDTs results. Table **10** lists some examples of LSP interventions and its impact on healthcare process.

Table 10. Examples for the impact of LSP interventions on healthcare process.

Intervention	Impact	Ref.
Experiential learning lab embedded in a didactic course.	■ Increase application of acquired knowledge. ■ Build clinical reasoning skills. ■ Engage effectively in lab interventions.	[167]
Selective reporting of antimicrobial susceptibility reporting. (favor reporting of narrow-spectrum antimicrobials)	■ Improvement and standardization of antimicrobial susceptibility reporting reflect on antibiotic selection by AMS team.	[168]
Training of ID pharmacists about RDT's	■ Significantly influencing RDT familiarity.	[169]
Modify automated lab request to become more specific	■ 60% decrease in TSH testing without clinical indication.	[170]
Selective susceptibility reporting of Gram-negative susceptibility to ciprofloxacin	■ Reduce antimicrobial utilization and improve Gram-negative susceptibility to ciprofloxacin.	[171]
Automated electronic alert to stop inappropriate gastrointestinal pathogen panel GIPP ordering.	■ 30% reduction in total (GIPP) ordering	[172]
Optimizing the pre-analytical and analytic phases of blood culture management	■ Remarkable reduction in the time taken to detect most blood culture isolates	[173]

CLINICAL PEARLS

- The adoption of RDTs is an attractive option to provide fast and precise and microbiology results to rationalize antimicrobial treatment decisions, consequently ameliorating patient outcomes.
- Financial capacity, principally, the infrastructure and logistics availability direct the selection of suitable RDT platform for the organization considering direct cost, volume of patients and effective implementation.
- The implementation of RDTs may constitute a cost saving strategy when combined with active AMS practice, through decreased antibiotics consumption, de-escalation to more targeted treatment, improved clinical outcome, and reduced length of hospitalization and related costs.
- Microscopical examination remains the most cost-effective diagnostic tool with reliable results that suits low-resourced facilities and can reasonably guide appropriate empiric treatment. However, it does not obviate the need for more advanced automated diagnostic platforms like immunoassays, DNA-probes, PCR, MALDI-TOF-MS, that provides accurate identification of causative organism, and its susceptibility pattern that drive more definitive antimicrobial therapy, with microfluidics and WGS remains a glimpse into the horizon of diagnostic devices, that may provide more rapid, accurate and cost-effective outcomes.
- Application of laboratory stewardship is a vital component of switching to more

expensive RDTs to maximize the benefits of technology, justify the cost and enhance patient care outcomes.

CONSENT FOR PUBLICATION

Not applicable.

CONFLICT OF INTEREST

The author(s) confirm that this chapter content has no conflict of interest.

ACKNOWLEDGEMENTS

Declared none.

REFERENCES

[1]   Timbrook TT, Spivak ES, Hanson KE. Current and future opportunities for rapid diagnostics in antimicrobial stewardship. Med Clin North Am 2018; 102(5): 899-911.
        [http://dx.doi.org/10.1016/j.mcna.2018.05.004] [PMID: 30126579]

[2]   Bauer KA, Perez KK, Forrest GN, Goff DA. Review of rapid diagnostic tests used by antimicrobial stewardship programs. Clin Infect Dis 2014; 59 (Suppl. 3): S134-45.
        [http://dx.doi.org/10.1093/cid/ciu547] [PMID: 25261540]

[3]   Hamdy RF, Zaoutis TE, Seo SK. Antifungal stewardship considerations for adults and pediatrics. Virulence 2017; 8(6): 658-72.
        [http://dx.doi.org/10.1080/21505594.2016.1226721] [PMID: 27588344]

[4]   Caliendo AM, Gilbert DN, Ginocchio CC, *et al.* Better tests, better care: improved diagnostics for infectious diseases. Clin Infect Dis 2013; 57(suppl_3): S139-70.

[5]   Laurino JP, Shi Q, Ge J. Monoclonal antibodies, antigens and molecular diagnostics: a practical overview. Ann Clin Lab Sci 1999; 29(3): 158-66.
        [PMID: 10440578]

[6]   Acuna-Villaorduna C, Vassall A, Henostroza G, *et al.* Cost-effectiveness analysis of introduction of rapid, alternative methods to identify multidrug-resistant tuberculosis in middle-income countries. Clin Infect Dis 2008; 47(4): 487-95.
        [http://dx.doi.org/10.1086/590010] [PMID: 18636955]

[7]   Pliakos EE, Andreatos N, Shehadeh F, Ziakas PD, Mylonakis E. The cost-effectiveness of rapid diagnostic testing for the diagnosis of bloodstream infections with or without antimicrobial stewardship. Clin Microbiol Rev 2018; 31(3): e00095-17.
        [http://dx.doi.org/10.1128/CMR.00095-17] [PMID: 29848775]

[8]   Reuter CH, Palac HL, Kociolek LK, *et al.* Ideal and actual impact of rapid diagnostic testing and antibiotic stewardship on antibiotic prescribing and clinical outcomes in children with positive blood cultures. Pediatr Infect Dis J 2019; 38(2): 131-7.
        [http://dx.doi.org/10.1097/INF.0000000000002102] [PMID: 29750765]

[9]   Messacar K, Parker SK, Todd JK, Dominguez SR. Implementation of rapid molecular infectious disease diagnostics: the role of diagnostic and antimicrobial stewardship. J Clin Microbiol 2017; 55(3): 715-23.
        [http://dx.doi.org/10.1128/JCM.02264-16] [PMID: 28031432]

[10]   Baird G. The laboratory test utilization management toolbox. Biochem Med (Zagreb) 2014; 24(2):

223-34.
[http://dx.doi.org/10.11613/BM.2014.025] [PMID: 24969916]

[11] Meier FA, Badrick TC, Sikaris KA. What's to be done about laboratory quality? process indicators, laboratory stewardship, the outcomes problem, risk assessment, and economic value: responding to contemporary global challenges. Am J Clin Pathol 2018; 149(3): 186-96.
[http://dx.doi.org/10.1093/ajcp/aqx135] [PMID: 29471323]

[12] de Oliveira MR, de Castro Gomes A, Toscano CM. Cost effectiveness of OptiMal® rapid diagnostic test for malaria in remote areas of the Amazon Region, Brazil. Malar J 2010; 9: 277.
[http://dx.doi.org/10.1186/1475-2875-9-277] [PMID: 20937094]

[13] McClelland R. Gram's stain: the key to microbiology. MLO Med Lab Obs 2001; 33(4): 20-2.
[PMID: 11339101]

[14] Stone BL, Burman WJ, Hildred MV, Jarboe EA, Reves RR, Wilson ML. The diagnostic yield of acid-fast-bacillus smear-positive sputum specimens. J Clin Microbiol 1997; 35(4): 1030-1.
[http://dx.doi.org/10.1128/JCM.35.4.1030-1031.1997] [PMID: 9157126]

[15] Bissonnette L, Bergeron MG. Diagnosing infections--current and anticipated technologies for point-o--care diagnostics and home-based testing. Clin Microbiol Infect 2010; 16(8): 1044-53.
[http://dx.doi.org/10.1111/j.1469-0691.2010.03282.x] [PMID: 20670286]

[16] Chen IT, Aung T, Thant HN, Sudhinaraset M, Kahn JG. Cost-effectiveness analysis of malaria rapid diagnostic test incentive schemes for informal private healthcare providers in Myanmar. Malar J 2015; 14: 55.
[http://dx.doi.org/10.1186/s12936-015-0569-7] [PMID: 25653121]

[17] Batwala V, Magnussen P, Hansen KS, Nuwaha F. Cost-effectiveness of malaria microscopy and rapid diagnostic tests *versus* presumptive diagnosis: implications for malaria control in Uganda. Malar J 2011; 10: 372.
[http://dx.doi.org/10.1186/1475-2875-10-372] [PMID: 22182735]

[18] Mengist HM, Demeke G, Zewdie O, Belew A. Diagnostic performance of direct wet mount microscopy in detecting intestinal helminths among pregnant women attending ante-natal care (ANC) in East Wollega, Oromia, Ethiopia. BMC Res Notes 2018; 11(1): 276.
[http://dx.doi.org/10.1186/s13104-018-3380-z] [PMID: 29728136]

[19] Rivera-Sánchez R, Flores-Paz R, Arriaga-Alba M. Diagnostic effectiveness of wet mount examination *versus* nucleic acid hybridisation for the diagnosis of trichomoniasis. Aten Primaria 2010; 42(6): 347.
[PMID: 19892437]

[20] Costa MN, Veigas B, Jacob JM, *et al.* A low cost, safe, disposable, rapid and self-sustainable paper-based platform for diagnostic testing: lab-on-paper. Nanotechnology 2014; 25(9): 094006.
[http://dx.doi.org/10.1088/0957-4484/25/9/094006] [PMID: 24521980]

[21] Shamah SM, Healy JM, Cload ST. Complex target SELEX. Acc Chem Res 2008; 41(1): 130-8.
[http://dx.doi.org/10.1021/ar700142z] [PMID: 18193823]

[22] Dwarakanath S, Bruno JG, Shastry A, *et al.* Quantum dot-antibody and aptamer conjugates shift fluorescence upon binding bacteria. Biochem Biophys Res Commun 2004; 325(3): 739-43.
[http://dx.doi.org/10.1016/j.bbrc.2004.10.099] [PMID: 15541352]

[23] Koczula KM, Gallotta A. Lateral flow assays. Essays Biochem 2016; 60(1): 111-20.
[http://dx.doi.org/10.1042/EBC20150012] [PMID: 27365041]

[24] Abdel-Hamid I, Ivnitski D, Atanasov P, Wilkins E. Flow-through immunofiltration assay system for rapid detection of *E. coli* O157:H7. Biosens Bioelectron 1999; 14(3): 309-16.
[http://dx.doi.org/10.1016/S0956-5663(99)00004-4] [PMID: 10230031]

[25] Posthuma-Trumpie GA, Korf J, van Amerongen A. Lateral flow (immuno)assay: its strengths, weaknesses, opportunities and threats. A literature survey. Anal Bioanal Chem 2009; 393(2): 569-82.
[http://dx.doi.org/10.1007/s00216-008-2287-2] [PMID: 18696055]

[26] Wu TF, Chen YC, Wang WC, *et al.* A rapid and low-cost pathogen detection platform by using a molecular agglutination assay. ACS Cent Sci 2018; 4(11): 1485-94.
[http://dx.doi.org/10.1021/acscentsci.8b00447] [PMID: 30555900]

[27] Ramachandran S, Singhal M, McKenzie KG, *et al.* a rapid, multiplexed, high-throughput flow-through membrane immunoassay: a convenient alternative to ELISA. Diagnostics (Basel) 2013; 3(2): 244-60.
[http://dx.doi.org/10.3390/diagnostics3020244] [PMID: 26835678]

[28] Mambatta AK, Jayarajan J, Rashme VL, Harini S, Menon S, Kuppusamy J. Reliability of dipstick assay in predicting urinary tract infection. J Family Med Prim Care 2015; 4(2): 265-8.
[http://dx.doi.org/10.4103/2249-4863.154672] [PMID: 25949979]

[29] Zhang GP, Guo JQ, Wang XN, *et al.* Development and evaluation of an immunochromatographic strip for trichinellosis detection. Vet Parasitol 2006; 137(3-4): 286-93.
[http://dx.doi.org/10.1016/j.vetpar.2006.01.026] [PMID: 16487659]

[30] Buechler KF, Moi S, Noar B, *et al.* Simultaneous detection of seven drugs of abuse by the Triage panel for drugs of abuse. Clin Chem 1992; 38(9): 1678-84.
[http://dx.doi.org/10.1093/clinchem/38.9.1678] [PMID: 1525997]

[31] Edwards KA, Baeumner AJ. Optimization of DNA-tagged dye-encapsulating liposomes for lateral-flow assays based on sandwich hybridization. Anal Bioanal Chem 2006; 386(5): 1335-43.
[http://dx.doi.org/10.1007/s00216-006-0705-x] [PMID: 16943990]

[32] Fernández-Sánchez C, McNeil CJ, Rawson K, Nilsson O, Leung HY, Gnanapragasam V. One-step immunostrip test for the simultaneous detection of free and total prostate specific antigen in serum. J Immunol Methods 2005; 307(1-2): 1-12.
[http://dx.doi.org/10.1016/j.jim.2005.08.014] [PMID: 16277989]

[33] Kim DS, Kim YT, Hong SB, *et al.* Development of Lateral Flow Assay Based on Size-Controlled Gold Nanoparticles for Detection of Hepatitis B Surface Antigen. Sensors (Basel) 2016; 16(12): E2154.
[http://dx.doi.org/10.3390/s16122154] [PMID: 27999291]

[34] Liu C, Jia Q, Yang C, *et al.* Lateral flow immunochromatographic assay for sensitive pesticide detection by using Fe3O4 nanoparticle aggregates as color reagents. Anal Chem 2011; 83(17): 6778-84.
[http://dx.doi.org/10.1021/ac201462d] [PMID: 21793540]

[35] O'Farrell B. Lateral flow technology for field-based applications-basics and advanced developments. Top Companion Anim Med 2015; 30(4): 139-47.
[http://dx.doi.org/10.1053/j.tcam.2015.12.003] [PMID: 27154597]

[36] Taranova NA, Berlina AN, Zherdev AV, Dzantiev BB. 'Traffic light' immunochromatographic test based on multicolor quantum dots for the simultaneous detection of several antibiotics in milk. Biosens Bioelectron 2015; 63: 255-61.
[http://dx.doi.org/10.1016/j.bios.2014.07.049] [PMID: 25104435]

[37] Anfossi L, Di Nardo F, Cavalera S, Giovannoli C, Baggiani C. Multiplex lateral flow immunoassay: an overview of strategies towards high-throughput point-of-need testing. Biosensors (Basel) 2018; 9(1): E2.
[http://dx.doi.org/10.3390/bios9010002] [PMID: 30587769]

[38] Hansen J, Slechta ES, Gates-Hollingsworth MA, *et al.* Large-scale evaluation of the immuno-mycologics lateral flow and enzyme-linked immunoassays for detection of cryptococcal antigen in serum and cerebrospinal fluid. Clin Vaccine Immunol 2013; 20(1): 52-5.
[http://dx.doi.org/10.1128/CVI.00536-12] [PMID: 23114703]

[39] Hsu HL, Chuang CC, Liang CC, *et al.* Rapid and sensitive detection of *Yersinia pestis* by lateral-flow assay in simulated clinical samples. BMC Infect Dis 2018; 18(1): 402.
[http://dx.doi.org/10.1186/s12879-018-3315-2] [PMID: 30107826]

[40]   Jørgensen CS, Uldum SA, Sørensen JF, Skovsted IC, Otte S, Elverdal PL. Evaluation of a new lateral flow test for detection of *Streptococcus pneumoniae* and *Legionella pneumophila* urinary antigen. J Microbiol Methods 2015; 116: 33-6.
[http://dx.doi.org/10.1016/j.mimet.2015.06.014] [PMID: 26141796]

[41]   Oku Y, Kamiya K, Kamiya H, Shibahara Y, Ii T, Uesaka Y. Development of oligonucleotide lateral-flow immunoassay for multi-parameter detection. J Immunol Methods 2001; 258(1-2): 73-84.
[http://dx.doi.org/10.1016/S0022-1759(01)00470-7] [PMID: 11684125]

[42]   Zhu YC, Socheat D, Bounlu K, *et al.* Application of dipstick dye immunoassay (DDIA) kit for the diagnosis of *Schistosomiasis mekongi*. Acta Trop 2005; 96(2-3): 137-41.
[http://dx.doi.org/10.1016/j.actatropica.2005.07.008] [PMID: 16143289]

[43]   Gussenhoven GC, van der Hoorn MA, Goris MG, *et al.* LEPTO dipstick, a dipstick assay for detection of Leptospira-specific immunoglobulin M antibodies in human sera. J Clin Microbiol 1997; 35(1): 92-7.
[http://dx.doi.org/10.1128/JCM.35.1.92-97.1997] [PMID: 8968886]

[44]   Yguerabide J, Yguerabide EE. Light-scattering submicroscopic particles as highly fluorescent analogs and their use as tracer labels in clinical and biological applications. Anal Biochem 1998; 262(2): 137-56.
[http://dx.doi.org/10.1006/abio.1998.2759] [PMID: 9750128]

[45]   Snowden K, Hommel M. Antigen detection immunoassay using dipsticks and colloidal dyes. J Immunol Methods 1991; 140(1): 57-65.
[http://dx.doi.org/10.1016/0022-1759(91)90126-Z] [PMID: 2061614]

[46]   Lin Z, Cheng S, Yan Q, *et al.* Development of an immunochromatographic lateral flow device for rapid detection of *Helicobacter pylori* stool antigen. Clin Biochem 2015; 48(18): 1298-303.
[http://dx.doi.org/10.1016/j.clinbiochem.2015.08.004] [PMID: 26256542]

[47]   Ou L, Lv Q, Wu C, Hao H, Zheng Y, Jiang Y. Development of a lateral flow immunochromatographic assay for rapid detection of *Mycoplasma pneumoniae*-specific IgM in human serum specimens. J Microbiol Methods 2016; 124: 35-40.
[http://dx.doi.org/10.1016/j.mimet.2016.03.006] [PMID: 26979644]

[48]   Carter DJ, Cary RB. Lateral flow microarrays: a novel platform for rapid nucleic acid detection based on miniaturized lateral flow chromatography. Nucleic Acids Res 2007; 35(10): e74.
[http://dx.doi.org/10.1093/nar/gkm269] [PMID: 17478499]

[49]   Gao W, Huang H, Zhu P, *et al.* Recombinase polymerase amplification combined with lateral flow dipstick for equipment-free detection of Salmonella in shellfish. Bioprocess Biosyst Eng 2018; 41(5): 603-11.
[http://dx.doi.org/10.1007/s00449-018-1895-2] [PMID: 29349550]

[50]   Hu S, Zhong H, Huang W, *et al.* Rapid and visual detection of Group B streptococcus using recombinase polymerase amplification combined with lateral flow strips. Diagn Microbiol Infect Dis 2019; 93(1): 9-13.
[http://dx.doi.org/10.1016/j.diagmicrobio.2018.07.011] [PMID: 30122509]

[51]   Janz V, Schoon J, Morgenstern C, *et al.* Rapid detection of periprosthetic joint infection using a combination of 16s rDNA polymerase chain reaction and lateral flow immunoassay: A Pilot Study. Bone Joint Res 2018; 7(1): 12-9.
[http://dx.doi.org/10.1302/2046-3758.71.BJR-2017-0103.R2] [PMID: 29305426]

[52]   Kumvongpin R, Jearanaikoon P, Wilailuckana C, *et al.* Detection assay for HPV16 and HPV18 by loop-mediated isothermal amplification with lateral flow dipstick tests. Mol Med Rep 2017; 15(5): 3203-9.
[http://dx.doi.org/10.3892/mmr.2017.6370] [PMID: 28339040]

[53]   Clavijo E, Díaz R, Anguita A, García A, Pinedo A, Smits HL. Comparison of a dipstick assay for

detection of Brucella-specific immunoglobulin M antibodies with other tests for serodiagnosis of human brucellosis. Clin Diagn Lab Immunol 2003; 10(4): 612-5.
[http://dx.doi.org/10.1128/CDLI.10.4.612-615.2003] [PMID: 12853393]

[54]   Kalogianni DP, Goura S, Aletras AJ, *et al.* Dry reagent dipstick test combined with 23S rRNA PCR for molecular diagnosis of bacterial infection in arthroplasty. Anal Biochem 2007; 361(2): 169-75.
[http://dx.doi.org/10.1016/j.ab.2006.11.013] [PMID: 17196544]

[55]   Li S, Liu Y, Wang Y, Wang M, Liu C, Wang Y. Rapid detection of *Brucella* spp. and elimination of carryover using multiple cross displacement amplification coupled with nanoparticles-based lateral flow biosensor. Front Cell Infect Microbiol 2019; 9: 78.
[http://dx.doi.org/10.3389/fcimb.2019.00078] [PMID: 30984627]

[56]   Liu D, He W, Jiang M, *et al.* Development of a loop-mediated isothermal amplification coupled lateral flow dipstick targeting erm(41) for detection of *Mycobacterium abscessus* and *Mycobacterium massiliense*. AMB Express 2019; 9(1): 11.
[http://dx.doi.org/10.1186/s13568-019-0734-4] [PMID: 30673881]

[57]   Chennuru S, Pavuluri PR. Flow-through assay for detection of antibodies using protein-a colloidal gold conjugate as a probe. Methods Mol Biol 2015; 1318: 97-105.
[http://dx.doi.org/10.1007/978-1-4939-2742-5_10] [PMID: 26160568]

[58]   Li PQ, Yang ZF, Chen JX, *et al.* Simultaneous detection of different respiratory virus by a multiplex reverse transcription polymerase chain reaction combined with flow-through reverse dot blotting assay. Diagn Microbiol Infect Dis 2008; 62(1): 44-51.
[http://dx.doi.org/10.1016/j.diagmicrobio.2008.04.017] [PMID: 18639996]

[59]   Kolesnikova MD, Pak BJ. Simplified multiplex biomarker testing using flow-through microarray technology. MLO Med Lab Obs 2014; 46(9): 26-30.

[60]   Matsuura H, Akatsuka Y, Matsuno T, *et al.* Comparison of the tube test and column agglutination techniques for anti-A/-B antibody titration in healthy individuals. Vox Sang 2018; 113(8): 787-94.
[http://dx.doi.org/10.1111/vox.12713] [PMID: 30251432]

[61]   Felten A, Grandry B, Lagrange PH, Casin I. Evaluation of three techniques for detection of low-level methicillin-resistant *Staphylococcus aureus* (MRSA): a disk diffusion method with cefoxitin and moxalactam, the Vitek 2 system, and the MRSA-screen latex agglutination test. J Clin Microbiol 2002; 40(8): 2766-71.
[http://dx.doi.org/10.1128/JCM.40.8.2766-2771.2002] [PMID: 12149327]

[62]   Zhang S, Xue M, Zhang J, *et al.* A one-step dipstick assay for the on-site detection of nucleic acid. Clin Biochem 2013; 46(18): 1852-6.
[http://dx.doi.org/10.1016/j.clinbiochem.2013.10.013] [PMID: 24161476]

[63]   Shanmugakani RK, Akeda Y, Sugawara Y, *et al.* PCR-Dipstick-Oriented Surveillance and Characterization of *mcr-1-* and Carbapenemase-Carrying *Enterobacteriaceae* in a Thai Hospital. Front Microbiol 2019; 10: 149.
[http://dx.doi.org/10.3389/fmicb.2019.00149] [PMID: 30800104]

[64]   Çam D, Öktem HA. Development of rapid dipstick assay for food pathogens, Salmonella, by optimized parameters. J Food Sci Technol 2019; 56(1): 140-8.
[http://dx.doi.org/10.1007/s13197-018-3467-5] [PMID: 30728555]

[65]   Foo PC, Chan YY, Mohamed M, Wong WK, Nurul Najian AB, Lim BH. Development of a thermostabilised triplex LAMP assay with dry-reagent four target lateral flow dipstick for detection of *Entamoeba histolytica* and non-pathogenic Entamoeba spp. Anal Chim Acta 2017; 966: 71-80.
[http://dx.doi.org/10.1016/j.aca.2017.02.019] [PMID: 28372729]

[66]   Hou P, Zhao G, Wang H, He C, Huan Y, He H. Development of a recombinase polymerase amplification combined with lateral-flow dipstick assay for detection of bovine ephemeral fever virus. Mol Cell Probes 2018; 38: 31-7.
[http://dx.doi.org/10.1016/j.mcp.2017.12.003] [PMID: 29288049]

[67]   Engvall E, Perlmann P. Enzyme-linked immunosorbent assay (ELISA). Quantitative assay of immunoglobulin G. Immunochemistry 1971; 8(9): 871-4.
[http://dx.doi.org/10.1016/0019-2791(71)90454-X] [PMID: 5135623]

[68]   Sittampalam GS, Grossman A, Brimacombe K, Arkin M, Auld D, Austin CP, Eds. Assay Guidance Manual. Bethesda, MD: Eli Lilly & Company and the National Center for Advancing Translational Sciences 2004.

[69]   Singh G, Koerner T, Gelinas J-M, *et al.* Design and characterization of a direct ELISA for the detection and quantification of leucomalachite green. Food Addit Contam Part A Chem Anal Control Expo Risk Assess 2011; 28(6): 731-9.
[http://dx.doi.org/10.1080/19440049.2011.567360] [PMID: 21623496]

[70]   Lin AV. Indirect ELISA. Methods Mol Biol 2015; 1318: 51-9.
[http://dx.doi.org/10.1007/978-1-4939-2742-5_5] [PMID: 26160563]

[71]   Lustig Y, Koren R, Biber A, Zuckerman N, Mendelson E, Schwartz E. Screening and exclusion of Zika virus infection in travellers by an NS1-based ELISA and qRT-PCR. Clin Microbiol Infect 2020; S1198-743X(20)30141-5.
[http://dx.doi.org/10.1016/j.cmi.2020.02.037] [PMID: 32151598]

[72]   Rakovsky A, Gozlan Y, Bassal R, *et al.* Diagnosis of HIV-1 infection: Performance of Xpert Qual and Geenius supplemental assays in fourth generation ELISA-reactive samples. J Clin Virol 2018; 101: 7-10.
[http://dx.doi.org/10.1016/j.jcv.2018.01.007] [PMID: 29414189]

[73]   Major M, Law M. Detection of Antibodies to HCV E1E2 by Lectin-Capture ELISA. Methods Mol Biol 2019; 1911: 421-32.
[http://dx.doi.org/10.1007/978-1-4939-8976-8_28] [PMID: 30593642]

[74]   Cross RW, Ksiazek TG. ELISA Methods for the Detection of Ebolavirus Infection. Methods Mol Biol 2017; 1628: 363-72.
[http://dx.doi.org/10.1007/978-1-4939-7116-9_29] [PMID: 28573635]

[75]   Wang L, Tian XD, Yu Y, Chen W. Evaluation of the performance of two tuberculosis interferon gamma release assays (IGRA-ELISA and T-SPOT.TB) for diagnosing *Mycobacterium tuberculosis* infection. Data Brief 2018; 21: 2492-5.
[http://dx.doi.org/10.1016/j.dib.2018.08.112] [PMID: 30560159]

[76]   Zhao Y, Zeng D, Yan C, *et al.* Rapid and accurate detection of *Escherichia coli* O157:H7 in beef using microfluidic wax-printed paper-based ELISA. Analyst (Lond) 2020; 145(8): 3106-15.
[http://dx.doi.org/10.1039/D0AN00224K] [PMID: 32159201]

[77]   Trautmann M, Cross AS, Reich G, Held H, Podschun R, Marre R. Evaluation of a competitive ELISA method for the determination of Klebsiella O antigens. J Med Microbiol 1996; 44(1): 44-51.
[http://dx.doi.org/10.1099/00222615-44-1-44] [PMID: 8544211]

[78]   Goldsmith SJ. Radioimmunoassay: review of basic principles. Semin Nucl Med 1975; 5(2): 125-52.
[http://dx.doi.org/10.1016/S0001-2998(75)80028-6] [PMID: 164695]

[79]   Burkhardt F, Schilt U, Andres RY. Virologic diagnosis of mumps infection: a solid phase radioimmunoassay for the detection of mumps specific IgM antibodies (MACRIA). Schweiz Med Wochenschr 1982; 112(18): 638-43.
[PMID: 7079699]

[80]   Forghani B, Klassen T, Baringer JR. Radioimmunoassay of herpes simplex virus antibody: correlation with ganglionic infection. J Gen Virol 1977; 36(3): 371-5.
[http://dx.doi.org/10.1099/0022-1317-36-3-371] [PMID: 199689]

[81]   Griffiths PD. The presumptive diagnosis of primary cytomegalovirus infection in early pregnancy by means of a radioimmunoassay for specific-IgM antibodies. Br J Obstet Gynaecol 1981; 88(6): 582-7.
[http://dx.doi.org/10.1111/j.1471-0528.1981.tb01212.x] [PMID: 6264943]

[82]   Hsu CH, Liu JD, Wang CS, *et al.* Clinical application of detecting serum anti-HBc IgM in HBV infection by radioimmunoassay. Taiwan Yi Xue Hui Za Zhi 1984; 83(7): 675-81.
[PMID: 6594429]

[83]   Chau PY, Tsang RS, Lam SK, La Brooy JT, Rowley D. Antibody response to the lipopolysaccharide and protein antigens of Salmonella typhi during typhoid infection. II. Measurement of intestinal antibodies by radioimmunoassay. Clin Exp Immunol 1981; 46(3): 515-20.
[PMID: 7337978]

[84]   Kohler RB, Wheat LJ, White A. Rapid diagnosis of *Pseudomonas aeruginosa* urinary tract infections by radioimmunoassay. J Clin Microbiol 1979; 9(2): 253-8.
[PMID: 107191]

[85]   Shortliffe LM, Wehner N, Stamey TA. Use of a solid-phase radioimmunoassay and formalin-fixed whole bacterial antigen in the detection of antigen-specific immunoglobulin in prostatic fluid. J Clin Invest 1981; 67(3): 790-9.
[http://dx.doi.org/10.1172/JCI110096] [PMID: 7009649]

[86]   Zammarchi L, Colao MG, Mantella A, *et al.* Evaluation of a new rapid fluorescence immunoassay for the diagnosis of dengue and Zika virus infection. J Clin Virol 2019; 112: 34-9.
[http://dx.doi.org/10.1016/j.jcv.2019.01.011] [PMID: 30738366]

[87]   Kavanagh O, Estes MK, Reeck A, *et al.* Serological responses to experimental Norwalk virus infection measured using a quantitative duplex time-resolved fluorescence immunoassay. Clin Vaccine Immunol 2011; 18(7): 1187-90.
[http://dx.doi.org/10.1128/CVI.00039-11] [PMID: 21593238]

[88]   Chris Maple PA, Gray J, Brown K, Brown D. Performance characteristics of a quantitative, standardised varicella zoster IgG time resolved fluorescence immunoassay (VZV TRFIA) for measuring antibody following natural infection. J Virol Methods 2009; 157(1): 90-2.
[http://dx.doi.org/10.1016/j.jviromet.2008.12.007] [PMID: 19135089]

[89]   Bong JH, Kim J, Lee GY, *et al.* Fluorescence immunoassay of *E. coli* using anti-lipopolysaccharide antibodies isolated from human serum. Biosens Bioelectron 2019; 126: 518-28.
[http://dx.doi.org/10.1016/j.bios.2018.10.036] [PMID: 30476883]

[90]   Emmadi R, Boonyaratanakornkit JB, Selvarangan R, *et al.* Molecular methods and platforms for infectious diseases testing a review of FDA-approved and cleared assays. J Mol Diagn 2011; 13(6): 583-604.
[http://dx.doi.org/10.1016/j.jmoldx.2011.05.011] [PMID: 21871973]

[91]   Myers MC, Pokorski JK, Appella DH. Peptide nucleic acids with a flexible secondary amine in the backbone maintain oligonucleotide binding affinity. Org Lett 2004; 6(25): 4699-702.
[http://dx.doi.org/10.1021/ol0480980] [PMID: 15575664]

[92]   Jordan S, Schwemler C, Kosch W, *et al.* New hetero-oligomeric peptide nucleic acids with improved binding properties to complementary DNA. Bioorg Med Chem Lett 1997; 7(6): 687-90.
[http://dx.doi.org/10.1016/S0960-894X(97)00085-1]

[93]   Pokorski JK, Witschi MA, Purnell BL, Appella DH. (S,S)-trans-cyclopentane-constrained peptide nucleic acids. a general backbone modification that improves binding affinity and sequence specificity. J Am Chem Soc 2004; 126(46): 15067-73.
[http://dx.doi.org/10.1021/ja046280q] [PMID: 15548003]

[94]   Salimnia H, Fairfax MR, Lephart P, *et al.* An international, prospective, multicenter evaluation of the combination of AdvanDx Staphylococcus QuickFISH BC with mecA XpressFISH for detection of methicillin-resistant *Staphylococcus aureus* isolates from positive blood cultures. J Clin Microbiol 2014; 52(11): 3928-32.
[http://dx.doi.org/10.1128/JCM.01811-14] [PMID: 25165083]

[95]   Forrest GN. PNA FISH: present and future impact on patient management. Expert Rev Mol Diagn

2007; 7(3): 231-6.
[http://dx.doi.org/10.1586/14737159.7.3.231] [PMID: 17489730]

[96]   Prudent E, Raoult D. Fluorescence *in situ* hybridization, a complementary molecular tool for the clinical diagnosis of infectious diseases by intracellular and fastidious bacteria. FEMS Microbiol Rev 2019; 43(1): 88-107.
[http://dx.doi.org/10.1093/femsre/fuy040] [PMID: 30418568]

[97]   Koncelik DL, Hernandez J. The impact of implementation of rapid quickfish testing for detection of coagulase-negative staphylococci at a community-based hospital. Am J Clin Pathol 2016; 145(1): 69-74.
[http://dx.doi.org/10.1093/ajcp/aqv005] [PMID: 26657205]

[98]   Deck MK, Anderson ES, Buckner RJ, *et al.* Rapid detection of Enterococcus spp. direct from blood culture bottles using Enterococcus QuickFISH method: a multicenter investigation. Diagn Microbiol Infect Dis 2014; 78(4): 338-42.
[http://dx.doi.org/10.1016/j.diagmicrobio.2013.12.004] [PMID: 24439447]

[99]   Banerjee SK, Weston AP, Persons DL, Campbell DR. Quick-FISH: a rapid fluorescence *in situ* hybridization technique for molecular cytogenetic analysis. Biotechniques 1998; 24(5): 826-30.
[http://dx.doi.org/10.2144/98245dt03] [PMID: 9591133]

[100]   Cartwright IM, Genet MD, Kato TA. A simple and rapid fluorescence *in situ* hybridization microwave protocol for reliable dicentric chromosome analysis. J Radiat Res (Tokyo) 2013; 54(2): 344-8.
[http://dx.doi.org/10.1093/jrr/rrs090] [PMID: 23161278]

[101]   Laub RR, Knudsen JD. Clinical consequences of using PNA-FISH in *Staphylococcal bacteraemia*. Eur J Clin Microbiol Infect Dis 2014; 33(4): 599-601.
[http://dx.doi.org/10.1007/s10096-013-1990-x] [PMID: 24129501]

[102]   Parcell BJ, Orange GV. PNA-FISH assays for early targeted bacteraemia treatment. J Microbiol Methods 2013; 95(2): 253-5.
[http://dx.doi.org/10.1016/j.mimet.2013.09.004] [PMID: 24055387]

[103]   Peleg AY, Tilahun Y, Fiandaca MJ, *et al.* Utility of peptide nucleic acid fluorescence *in situ* hybridization for rapid detection of Acinetobacter spp. and *Pseudomonas aeruginosa*. J Clin Microbiol 2009; 47(3): 830-2.
[http://dx.doi.org/10.1128/JCM.01724-08] [PMID: 19116347]

[104]   Doğan Ö, İnkaya AC, Gülmez D, Uzun Ö, Akova M, Arıkan Akdağlı S. Evaluation of PNA-FISH method for direct identification of *Candida species* in blood culture samples and its potential impact on guidance of antifungal therapy. Mikrobiyol Bul 2016; 50(4): 580-9.
[PMID: 28124963]

[105]   Harris DM, Hata DJ. Rapid identification of bacteria and Candida using PNA-FISH from blood and peritoneal fluid cultures: a retrospective clinical study. Ann Clin Microbiol Antimicrob 2013; 12: 2.
[http://dx.doi.org/10.1186/1476-0711-12-2] [PMID: 23295014]

[106]   Bork JT, Leekha S, Heil EL, Zhao L, Badamas R, Johnson JK. Rapid testing using the Verigene Gram-negative blood culture nucleic acid test in combination with antimicrobial stewardship intervention against Gram-negative bacteremia. Antimicrob Agents Chemother 2015; 59(3): 1588-95.
[http://dx.doi.org/10.1128/AAC.04259-14] [PMID: 25547353]

[107]   Buchan BW, Ginocchio CC, Manii R, *et al.* Multiplex identification of gram-positive bacteria and resistance determinants directly from positive blood culture broths: evaluation of an automated microarray-based nucleic acid test. PLoS Med 2013; 10(7): e1001478.
[http://dx.doi.org/10.1371/journal.pmed.1001478] [PMID: 23843749]

[108]   Avdic E, Wang R, Li DX, *et al.* Sustained impact of a rapid microarray-based assay with antimicrobial stewardship interventions on optimizing therapy in patients with Gram-positive bacteraemia. J Antimicrob Chemother 2017; 72(11): 3191-8.
[http://dx.doi.org/10.1093/jac/dkx267] [PMID: 28961942]

[109] Hall L, Le Febre KM, Deml SM, Wohlfiel SL, Wengenack NL. Evaluation of the Yeast Traffic Light PNA FISH probes for identification of *Candidaspecies* from positive blood cultures. J Clin Microbiol 2012; 50(4): 1446-8.
[http://dx.doi.org/10.1128/JCM.06148-11] [PMID: 22238445]

[110] Weaver AJ, Brandenburg KS, Sanjar F, Wells AR, Peacock TJ, Leung KP. Clinical utility of pna-fish for burn wound diagnostics: a noninvasive, culture-independent technique for rapid identification of pathogenic organisms in burn wounds. J Burn Care Res 2019; 40(4): 464-70.
[http://dx.doi.org/10.1093/jbcr/irz047] [PMID: 30893424]

[111] Multiplex PNA-fish to detect cystic fibrosis polymicrobial communities. Biotechnol Bioeng 2017; 114(2): 244.
[http://dx.doi.org/10.1002/bit.26103] [PMID: 28005284]

[112] Huang XX, Urosevic N, Inglis TJJ. Accelerated bacterial detection in blood culture by enhanced acoustic flow cytometry (AFC) following peptide nucleic acid fluorescence *in situ* hybridization (PNA-FISH). PLoS One 2019; 14(2): e0201332.
[http://dx.doi.org/10.1371/journal.pone.0201332] [PMID: 30735489]

[113] Aydemir G, Koç AN, Atalay MA. Evaluation of peptide nucleic acid fluorescent in situ hybridization (PNA FISH) method in the identifi cation of *Candidaspecies* isolated from blood cultures. Mikrobiyol Bul 2016; 50(2): 293-9.
[http://dx.doi.org/10.5578/mb.22092] [PMID: 27175502]

[114] Cosgrove SE, Li DX, Tamma PD, *et al.* Use of PNA FISH for blood cultures growing Gram-positive cocci in chains without a concomitant antibiotic stewardship intervention does not improve time to appropriate antibiotic therapy. Diagn Microbiol Infect Dis 2016; 86(1): 86-92.
[http://dx.doi.org/10.1016/j.diagmicrobio.2016.06.016] [PMID: 27412814]

[115] Almeida C, Azevedo NF, Bento JC, *et al.* Rapid detection of urinary tract infections caused by Proteus spp. using PNA-FISH. Eur J Clin Microbiol Infect Dis 2013; 32(6): 781-6.
[http://dx.doi.org/10.1007/s10096-012-1808-2] [PMID: 23288291]

[116] Machado A, Cerca N. Multiplex Peptide Nucleic Acid Fluorescence *In Situ* Hybridization (PNA-FISH) for Diagnosis of Bacterial Vaginosis. Methods Mol Biol 2017; 1616: 209-19.
[http://dx.doi.org/10.1007/978-1-4939-7037-7_13] [PMID: 28600771]

[117] Hensley DM, Tapia R, Encina Y. An evaluation of the advandx *Staphylococcus aureus*/CNS PNA FISH assay. Clin Lab Sci 2009; 22(1): 30-3.
[PMID: 19354026]

[118] Garibyan L, Avashia N. Polymerase chain reaction. J Invest Dermatol 2013; 133(3): 1-4.
[http://dx.doi.org/10.1038/jid.2013.1] [PMID: 23399825]

[119] Khan N, Aswad S, Shidban H, *et al.* Improved detection of HCV Infection in hemodialysis patients using a new HCV RNA qualitative assay: experience of a transplant center. J Clin Virol 2004; 30(2): 175-82.
[http://dx.doi.org/10.1016/j.jcv.2003.10.004] [PMID: 15125874]

[120] Sutton DA, Allen DP, Fuller CM, *et al.* Development of an avian avulavirus 1 (AAvV-1) L-gene real-time RT-PCR assay using minor groove binding probes for application as a routine diagnostic tool. J Virol Methods 2019; 265: 9-14.
[http://dx.doi.org/10.1016/j.jviromet.2018.12.001] [PMID: 30579921]

[121] Cai P, Weerakoon KG, Mu Y, *et al.* Comparison of Kato Katz, antibody-based ELISA and droplet digital PCR diagnosis of *Schistosomiasis japonica*: Lessons learnt from a setting of low infection intensity. PLoS Negl Trop Dis 2019; 13(3): e0007228.
[http://dx.doi.org/10.1371/journal.pntd.0007228] [PMID: 30830925]

[122] Chen Z, Biswas S, Aminabadi P, Stackhouse JW, Jay-Russell MT, Pandey PK. Prevalence of *Escherichia coli* O157 and *Salmonella spp.* in solid bovine manure in California using real-time

quantitative PCR. Lett Appl Microbiol 2019; 69(1): 23-9.
[http://dx.doi.org/10.1111/lam.13156] [PMID: 30932223]

[123] Damnjanovic D, Harvey M, Bridge WJ. Application of colony BOXA2R-PCR for the differentiation and identification of lactic acid COCCI. Food Microbiol 2019; 82: 277-86.
[http://dx.doi.org/10.1016/j.fm.2019.02.011] [PMID: 31027784]

[124] Del Pilar Martinez Viedma M, Puri V, Oldfield LM, Shabman RS, Tan GS, Pickett BE. Optimization of qRT-PCR assay for zika virus detection in human serum and urine. Virus Res 2019; 263: 173-8.
[http://dx.doi.org/10.1016/j.virusres.2019.01.013] [PMID: 30742853]

[125] Fukuzawa S, Shiho H, Fujita T. Selective Detection of DNA from Viable *Mycobacterium tuberculosis* Complex Strains Using the EMA-PCR Method. Jpn J Infect Dis 2019; 72(1): 19-22.
[http://dx.doi.org/10.7883/yoken.JJID.2018.111] [PMID: 30270248]

[126] Ji YH, Zhu ZL, Yang LL, *et al.* Application of multiplex PCR assay to study early multiple herpesviruses infection during HSCT. Zhonghua Xue Ye Xue Za Zhi 2019; 40(2): 125-31.
[PMID: 30831627]

[127] Li Y, Wan Z, Hu Y, Zhou Y, Chen Q, Zhang C. A mismatch-tolerant RT-quantitative PCR: application to broad-spectrum detection of respiratory syncytial virus. Biotechniques 2019; 66(5): 225-30.
[http://dx.doi.org/10.2144/btn-2018-0184] [PMID: 31050303]

[128] Pokhrel N, Khanal B, Rai K, Subedi M, Bhattarai NR. Application of PCR and microscopy to detect *Helicobacter pylori* in Gastric biopsy specimen among acid peptic disorders at tertiary care centre in eastern Nepal. Can J Infect Dis Med Microbiol 2019; 2019: 3695307.
[http://dx.doi.org/10.1155/2019/3695307] [PMID: 30867850]

[129] Hatrongjit R, Kerdsin A, Akeda Y, Hamada S. Detection of plasmid-mediated colistin-resistant and carbapenem-resistant genes by multiplex PCR. MethodsX 2018; 5: 532-6.
[http://dx.doi.org/10.1016/j.mex.2018.05.016] [PMID: 30023315]

[130] Fagerquist CK, Garbus BR, Miller WG, *et al.* Rapid identification of protein biomarkers of *Escherichia coli* O157:H7 by matrix-assisted laser desorption ionization-time-of-flight-time-of-flight mass spectrometry and top-down proteomics. Anal Chem 2010; 82(7): 2717-25.
[http://dx.doi.org/10.1021/ac902455d] [PMID: 20232878]

[131] Andersson M, Groseclose MR, Deutch AY, Caprioli RM. Imaging mass spectrometry of proteins and peptides: 3D volume reconstruction. Nat Methods 2008; 5(1): 101-8.
[http://dx.doi.org/10.1038/nmeth1145] [PMID: 18165806]

[132] Stoeckli M, Chaurand P, Hallahan DE, Caprioli RM. Imaging mass spectrometry: a new technology for the analysis of protein expression in mammalian tissues. Nat Med 2001; 7(4): 493-6.
[http://dx.doi.org/10.1038/86573] [PMID: 11283679]

[133] Schwamborn K, Caprioli RM. MALDI imaging mass spectrometry--painting molecular pictures. Mol Oncol 2010; 4(6): 529-38.
[http://dx.doi.org/10.1016/j.molonc.2010.09.002] [PMID: 20965799]

[134] Ercibengoa M, Alonso M, Vicente D, Morales M, Garcia E, Marimón JM. Utility of MALDI-TOF MS as a new tool for *Streptococcus pneumoniae* serotyping. PLoS One 2019; 14(2): e0212022.
[http://dx.doi.org/10.1371/journal.pone.0212022] [PMID: 30753210]

[135] Akyar I, Kaya Ayas M, Karatuna O. Performance evaluation of MALDI-TOF MS MBT STAR-BL *versus* in-house carba np testing for the rapid detection of carbapenemase activity in *Escherichia coli* and *Klebsiella pneumoniae* strains. Microb Drug Resist 2019; 25(7): 985-90.
[http://dx.doi.org/10.1089/mdr.2018.0355] [PMID: 30939067]

[136] Azrad M, Keness Y, Nitzan O, *et al.* Cheap and rapid in-house method for direct identification of positive blood cultures by MALDI-TOF MS technology. BMC Infect Dis 2019; 19(1): 72.
[http://dx.doi.org/10.1186/s12879-019-3709-9] [PMID: 30658585]

[137] Bellanger AP, Gbaguidi-Haore H, Liapis E, Scherer E, Millon L. Rapid identification of Candida sp. by MALDI-TOF mass spectrometry subsequent to short-term incubation on a solid medium. APMIS 2019; 127(4): 217-21.
[http://dx.doi.org/10.1111/apm.12936] [PMID: 30803048]

[138] Centonze AR, Bragantini M, Lucchini E, Mazzariol A. Laboratory validation of a KPC-producing strain identification method based on the detection of a specific 11,109 Da peak *via* Maldi-Tof-Vitek MS in an endemic area. New Microbiol 2019; 42(2): 114-7.
[PMID: 31034082]

[139] Correa-Martínez CL, Idelevich EA, Sparbier K, Kostrzewa M, Becker K. Rapid detection of extended-spectrum β-Lactamases (ESBL) and AmpC β-Lactamases in *Enterobacterales*: development of a screening panel using the MALDI-TOF MS-based direct-on-target microdroplet growth assay. Front Microbiol 2019; 10: 13.
[http://dx.doi.org/10.3389/fmicb.2019.00013] [PMID: 30733710]

[140] Costa-Alcalde JJ, Barbeito-Castiñeiras G, González-Alba JM, Aguilera A, Galán JC, Pérez-De-Molino ML. Comparative evaluation of the identification of rapidly growing non-tuberculous mycobacteria by mass spectrometry (MALDI-TOF MS), GenoType Mycobacterium CM/AS assay and partial sequencing of the rpoβ gene with phylogenetic analysis as a reference method. Enferm Infecc Microbiol Clin 2019; 37(3): 160-6.
[http://dx.doi.org/10.1016/j.eimc.2018.04.012] [PMID: 29871765]

[141] Delavy M, Dos Santos AR, Heiman CM, Coste AT. Investigating antifungal susceptibility in *Candida* species with MALDI-TOF MS-based assays. Front Cell Infect Microbiol 2019; 9: 19.
[http://dx.doi.org/10.3389/fcimb.2019.00019] [PMID: 30792970]

[142] Situma C, Hashimoto M, Soper SA. Merging microfluidics with microarray-based bioassays. Biomol Eng 2006; 23(5): 213-31.
[http://dx.doi.org/10.1016/j.bioeng.2006.03.002] [PMID: 16905357]

[143] Whitesides GM. The origins and the future of microfluidics. Nature 2006; 442(7101): 368-73.
[http://dx.doi.org/10.1038/nature05058] [PMID: 16871203]

[144] Wissberg S, Ronen M, Oren Z, Gerber D, Kalisky B. Sensitive readout for microfluidic high-throughput applications using scanning squid microscopy. Sci Rep 2020; 10(1): 1573.
[http://dx.doi.org/10.1038/s41598-020-58307-w] [PMID: 32005843]

[145] Berg JS, Khoury MJ, Evans JP. Deploying whole genome sequencing in clinical practice and public health: meeting the challenge one bin at a time. Genet Med 2011; 13(6): 499-504.
[http://dx.doi.org/10.1097/GIM.0b013e318220aaba] [PMID: 21558861]

[146] Roach JC, Glusman G, Smit AF, *et al.* Analysis of genetic inheritance in a family quartet by whole-genome sequencing. Science 2010; 328(5978): 636-9.
[http://dx.doi.org/10.1126/science.1186802] [PMID: 20220176]

[147] Lupski JR, Reid JG, Gonzaga-Jauregui C, *et al.* Whole-genome sequencing in a patient with Charcot-Marie-Tooth neuropathy. N Engl J Med 2010; 362(13): 1181-91.
[http://dx.doi.org/10.1056/NEJMoa0908094] [PMID: 20220177]

[148] Vissers LE, de Ligt J, Gilissen C, *et al.* A de novo paradigm for mental retardation. Nat Genet 2010; 42(12): 1109-12.
[http://dx.doi.org/10.1038/ng.712] [PMID: 21076407]

[149] Ashley EA, Butte AJ, Wheeler MT, *et al.* Clinical assessment incorporating a personal genome. Lancet 2010; 375(9725): 1525-35.
[http://dx.doi.org/10.1016/S0140-6736(10)60452-7] [PMID: 20435227]

[150] Gerlinger M, Rowan AJ, Horswell S, *et al.* Intratumor heterogeneity and branched evolution revealed by multiregion sequencing. N Engl J Med 2012; 366(10): 883-92.
[http://dx.doi.org/10.1056/NEJMoa1113205] [PMID: 22397650]

[151] Arnold C. Outbreak breakthrough: using whole-genome sequencing to control hospital infection. Environ Health Perspect 2015; 123(11): A281-6.
[http://dx.doi.org/10.1289/ehp.123-A281] [PMID: 26523889]

[152] Roy S, Hartley J, Dunn H, Williams R, Williams CA, Breuer J. Whole-genome sequencing provides data for stratifying infection prevention and control management of nosocomial influenza a. Clin Infect Dis 2019; 69(10): 1649-56.
[http://dx.doi.org/10.1093/cid/ciz020] [PMID: 30993315]

[153] Popovich KJ, Snitkin ES. Whole genome sequencing-implications for infection prevention and outbreak investigations. Curr Infect Dis Rep 2017; 19(4): 15.
[http://dx.doi.org/10.1007/s11908-017-0570-0] [PMID: 28281083]

[154] Abbo L, Shukla BS, Giles A, *et al.* Linezolid and vancomycin-resistant *Enterococcus faecium* in solid organ transplant recipients: infection control and antimicrobial stewardship using whole genome sequencing. Clin Infect Dis 2019; 69(2): 259-65.
[http://dx.doi.org/10.1093/cid/ciy903] [PMID: 30339217]

[155] Bastos LR, Martins MCF, Albano RM, Marques EA, Leão RS. Whole genome sequencing of a ST2594 MRSA strain causing non-mucosal preoperative colonization and low-grade postoperative infection. Antonie van Leeuwenhoek 2019; 112(6): 961-4.
[http://dx.doi.org/10.1007/s10482-019-01229-z] [PMID: 30663019]

[156] Guerra-Assunção JA, Houben RM, Crampin AC, *et al.* Recurrence due to relapse or reinfection with *Mycobacterium tuberculosis*: a whole-genome sequencing approach in a large, population-based cohort with a high HIV infection prevalence and active follow-up. J Infect Dis 2015; 211(7): 1154-63.
[http://dx.doi.org/10.1093/infdis/jiu574] [PMID: 25336729]

[157] Houldcroft CJ, Roy S, Morfopoulou S, *et al.* Use of whole-genome sequencing of adenovirus in immunocompromised pediatric patients to identify nosocomial transmission and mixed-genotype infection. J Infect Dis 2018; 218(8): 1261-71.
[http://dx.doi.org/10.1093/infdis/jiy323] [PMID: 29917114]

[158] Zeng Z, Zhao H, Dorr MB, *et al.* Bezlotoxumab for prevention of *Clostridium difficile* infection recurrence: Distinguishing relapse from reinfection with whole genome sequencing. Anaerobe 2020; 61: 102137.
[http://dx.doi.org/10.1016/j.anaerobe.2019.102137] [PMID: 31846705]

[159] Croucher NJ, Harris SR, Grad YH, Hanage WP. Bacterial genomes in epidemiology--present and future. Philos Trans R Soc Lond B Biol Sci 2013; 368(1614): 20120202.
[http://dx.doi.org/10.1098/rstb.2012.0202] [PMID: 23382424]

[160] O'Neil J. Tackling drug-resistant infections globally: final report and recommendations.Resistance. ondon, United Kingdom 2016; pp. 1-84.

[161] Altaras R, Nuwa A, Agaba B, *et al.* How do patients and health workers interact around malaria rapid diagnostic testing, and how are the tests experienced by patients in practice? a qualitative study in Western Uganda. PLoS One 2016; 11(8): e0159525.
[http://dx.doi.org/10.1371/journal.pone.0159525] [PMID: 27494507]

[162] Palamountain KM, Baker J, Cowan EP, *et al.* Perspectives on introduction and implementation of new point-of-care diagnostic tests. J Infect Dis 2012; 205(Suppl 2): S181-90.
[http://dx.doi.org/10.1093/infdis/jis203]

[163] Marshall GS, Hauck MA, Buck G, Rabalais GP. Potential cost savings through rapid diagnosis of enteroviral meningitis. Pediatr Infect Dis J 1997; 16(11): 1086-7.
[http://dx.doi.org/10.1097/00006454-199711000-00015] [PMID: 9384344]

[164] Ramers C, Billman G, Hartin M, Ho S, Sawyer MH. Impact of a diagnostic cerebrospinal fluid enterovirus polymerase chain reaction test on patient management. JAMA 2000; 283(20): 2680-5.
[http://dx.doi.org/10.1001/jama.283.20.2680] [PMID: 10819951]

[165] Shehadeh F, Zacharioudakis IM, Zervou FN, Mylonakis E. Cost-effectiveness of rapid diagnostic assays that perform directly on blood samples for the diagnosis of septic shock. Diagn Microbiol Infect Dis 2019; 94(4): 378-84.
[http://dx.doi.org/10.1016/j.diagmicrobio.2019.02.018] [PMID: 30922592]

[166] Patel TS, Kaakeh R, Nagel JL, Newton DW, Stevenson JG. cost analysis of implementing matrix-assisted laser desorption ionization-time of flight mass spectrometry plus real-time antimicrobial stewardship intervention for bloodstream infections. J Clin Microbiol 2016; 55(1): 60-7.
[http://dx.doi.org/10.1128/JCM.01452-16] [PMID: 27795335]

[167] Benson JD, Provident I, Szucs KA. An experiential learning lab embedded in a didactic course: outcomes from a pediatric intervention course. Occup Ther Health Care 2013; 27(1): 46-57.
[http://dx.doi.org/10.3109/07380577.2012.756599] [PMID: 23855537]

[168] Graham M, Walker DA, Haremza E, Morris AJ. RCPAQAP audit of antimicrobial reporting in Australian and New Zealand laboratories: opportunities for laboratory contribution to antimicrobial stewardship. J Antimicrob Chemother 2019; 74(1): 251-5.
[PMID: 30295792]

[169] Foster RA, Kuper K, Lu ZK, Bookstaver PB, Bland CM, Mahoney MV. Pharmacists' familiarity with and institutional utilization of rapid diagnostic technologies for antimicrobial stewardship. Infect Control Hosp Epidemiol 2017; 38(7): 863-6.
[http://dx.doi.org/10.1017/ice.2017.67] [PMID: 28490386]

[170] Leis B, Frost A, Bryce R, Lyon AW, Coverett K. Altering standard admission order sets to promote clinical laboratory stewardship: a cohort quality improvement study. BMJ Qual Saf 2019; 28(10): 846-52.
[http://dx.doi.org/10.1136/bmjqs-2018-008995] [PMID: 31073090]

[171] Langford BJ, Seah J, Chan A, Downing M, Johnstone J, Matukas LM. Antimicrobial stewardship in the microbiology laboratory: impact of selective susceptibility reporting on ciprofloxacin utilization and susceptibility of gram-negative isolates to ciprofloxacin in a hospital setting. J Clin Microbiol 2016; 54(9): 2343-7.
[http://dx.doi.org/10.1128/JCM.00950-16] [PMID: 27385708]

[172] Marcelin JR, Brewer C, Beachy M, *et al.* Hardwiring diagnostic stewardship using electronic ordering restrictions for gastrointestinal pathogen testing. Infect Control Hosp Epidemiol 2019; 40(6): 668-73.
[http://dx.doi.org/10.1017/ice.2019.78] [PMID: 31012405]

[173] Weinbren MJ, Collins M, Heathcote R, *et al.* Optimization of the blood culture pathway: a template for improved sepsis management and diagnostic antimicrobial stewardship. J Hosp Infect 2018; 98(3): 232-5.
[http://dx.doi.org/10.1016/j.jhin.2017.12.023] [PMID: 29309813]

CHAPTER 8

Therapeutic Options for Difficult to Treat Bacteria and *Candida auris*

Viktorija O. Barr[1,2,*]**, Alyssa Christensen**[3]**, Morgan Anderson**[4] **and Addison Pang**[3]

[1] *Rosalind Franklin University, North Chicago, IL, USA*

[2] *T2Biosystems, Lexington, MA, USA*

[3] *Providence Health & Services, Portland, OR, USA*

[4] *Advocate Aurora Health, Downers Grove, IL, USA*

Abstract: The therapy of multidrug-resistant Gram-positive, Gram-negative, and *Candida auris* is challenging and has emerged as a major threat to human health. Commonly used drugs have become increasingly resistant, which has led to an absence of reliable options and use of current agents in combination. While this has led to the development of newer drugs, most of them are not available in the United States or are yet to be approved by the FDA. Described here is a comprehensive overview of antimicrobial resistance and recent developments in therapy for methicillin-resistant *Staphylococcus aureus*, vancomycin-resistant *Enterococcus spp*, extended-spectrum β-lactamases (ESBL's), carbapenemase-producing *Enterobacteriaceae* (CRE), multi-drug resistant *Pseudomonas aeruginosa* (PSA), multi-drug resistant *Acinetobacter* (ACB), and *Candida auris*.

Keywords: *AmpC*, Antimicrobial resistance, *Candida auris*, Carbapenemase-producing *Enterobacteriaceae* (CRE), *Enterococcus spp*, Extended-spectrum β-lactamases (ESBL's), Gram-negative, Gram-positive, Multidrug resistance, Multi-drug resistant *Acinetobacter*, *Pseudomonas aeruginosa*, *Staphylococcus aureus*.

INTRODUCTION

The objective of this chapter is to review the potential therapeutic options for the treatment of difficult to treat infections caused by some of the most common multidrug-resistant organisms identified in practice. Pathogens that will be discussed include *Staphylococcus aureus*, Enterococcus spp, extended-spectrum β-lactamases (ESBL's), carbapenemase-producing *Enterobacteriaceae* (CRE),

[*] **Corresponding author Viktorija O. Barr:** Rosalind Franklin University, North Chicago, IL, USA;
Tel: 847.578.8497; E-mail: viktorija.barr@rosalindfranklin.edu

Islam M. Ghazi & Michael J. Cawley (Eds.)

Pseudomonas aeruginosa (PSA), multi-drug resistant *Acinetobacter* (ACB), and *Candida auris*. This review mainly includes clinical studies, most of which are observational in design, and includes non-comparative studies only when these provide information relevant to specific populations. *In vitro* and animal studies are also included if considered necessary in the absence of clinical studies.

GRAM-POSITIVE ORGANISMS

Methicillin-Resistant *Staphylococcus aureus* (MRSA)

The US Centers for Disease Control and Prevention (CDC) and the European Antimicrobial Resistance Surveillance Network (EARS-Net) have shown that the prevalence of methicillin-resistant *Staphylococcus aureus* (MRSA) is decreasing in the USA and in some European countries [1]. Nevertheless, MRSA remains a serious concern in the inpatient setting due to its high rates of mortality and complications. This organism is implicated in a variety of infections, including those with skin and skin structure, pneumonia, and endovascular origins. Vancomycin is often positioned as the agent of choice for treatment of this organism, but an increase in vancomycin minimum inhibitory concentrations (MICs) and the development of heterogeneous vancomycin-intermediate *S. aureus* infections highlights the need for alternative therapeutic options.

Resistance Mechanisms

Methicillin resistance occurs after the acquisition of the *mecA* gene leading to the penicillin binding protein, PBP2a, that has a low affinity for β-lactams. Vancomycin, a glycopeptide antibiotic, is unaffected by this as it exerts its bactericidal effect by inhibiting the polymerization of peptidoglycans in the bacterial cell wall. MRSA isolates, with a decreased susceptibility to vancomycin, were identified in the late 1990s [2]. There are two distinct phenotypes associated with reduced vancomycin susceptibility in *Staphylococcus aureus*. Vancomycin-intermediate *Staphylococcus aureus* (VISA) does not have a clonal mechanism and involves an excess of cell wall material inhibiting the activity of the antibiotic. Heterogenous VISA (hVISA) refers to vancomycin-susceptible strains containing a subpopulation resistant to glycopeptides. The overall prevalence of VISA and hVISA is low, but outbreaks have been reported [3]. Both VISA and hVISA are an increasing public health problem and are associated with vancomycin treatment failure [4]. The second phenotype, vancomycin-resistant *S. aureus* (VRSA), carries transposon Tn1546, acquired from vancomycin-resistant *Enterococcus faecalis*. Tn1546 alters the cell wall structure and leads to modification of the target site of vancomycin. Rare isolates have been reported in the United States [5].

While resistance to linezolid and daptomycin remains low overall, point mutations leading to resistance have been described for linezolid, and horizontal transmission of *cfr*-mediated resistance to linezolid has been reported in clinical isolates [6]. Reports documenting the emergence of daptomycin resistance are often in the context of high-inoculum infections or after exposure to vancomycin. The most commonly implicated gene in this phenotype is *mprF,* but it is likely that there are many genes involved [3]. Additional drug resistance occurs through the creation of biofilm, a thick extracellular exopolysaccharide layer which protects bacteria. The formation of biofilm is a multifactorial event which is controlled by quorum sensing and proteins, such as the biofilm-associated protein (Bap), the accessory gene regulator (*Agr*), the intercellular adhesion protein (*Ica*), and the *S.aureus* surface protein (*SasC*). A summary of genes found to be involved in the development of resistance in *S. aureus,* to specific antimicrobials, is provided in Table **1**.

Table 1. *S. aureus* Resistance Genes.

Antibiotic	Gene(s) Involved	Resistance Strategy
Vancomycin (VRSA)	Tn1546/*vanA* gene cluster	Target replacement
Linezolid	*Cfr* 23S rRNA gene mutations	Target modification
Daptomycin	*MprF, dlt, vraRS, yycFG, pgsA, cls*	Changes in cell surface

Treatment Options

Vancomycin

Optimization of vancomycin dosing to achieve pharmacokinetic and pharma-codynamic targets can often lead to clinical success in MRSA infections. If the patient has not had a clinical or microbiologic response to vancomycin despite adequate debridement and removal of other foci of infection, an alternative to vancomycin is recommended regardless of MIC. For isolates with a vancomycin MIC's >2 µg/mL (*e.g.*, VISA or VRSA), an alternative to vancomycin should be used [7].

Daptomycin

Daptomycin is a bactericidal cyclic lipopeptide approved for the treatment of right-sided infective endocarditis (IE), complicated skin and skin structure infections (cSSSI), and *S. aureus* bacteremia. It is not appropriate for the treatment of pneumonia caused by MRSA due to the inactivation by lung surfactant. It has poor penetration into the cerebrospinal fluid and should only be used in central nervous system infections if no alternatives exist [8]. Although daptomycin dosing in MRSA infections is usually 6 mg/kg/day, clinical experts recommend higher dosing (8-10 mg/kg/day) when used for persistent MRSA bacteremia that has failed to respond to vancomycin [7].

Oxazolidinones

Linezolid, an oxazolidinone antimicrobial, only has bacteriostatic activity against *S. aureus* due to its mechanism of action. A notable advantage of this therapy option against MRSA is its high oral bioavailability (100%) that allows for the avoidance of intravenous access in long treatment courses. Linezolid is approved for the treatment of cSSSI and pneumonia suspected to be caused by Gram-positive bacteria. Linezolid achieves high levels in lung epithelial lining fluid and when compared with vancomycin, showed similar cure rates in patients with nosocomial pneumonia [9]. The 2016 hospital-acquired pneumonia/ventilator-associated pneumonia (HAP/VAP) guidelines positioned linezolid as an alternative first-line agent for MRSA, including in cases with secondary bacteremia [10]. The bacteriostatic activity of the drug against *S. aureus* limits its use in infective endocarditis, but retrospective studies and case reports suggest it may have a place as salvage therapy for persistent MRSA bacteremia [11 - 13]. The safety and efficacy of linezolid formulations given for longer than 28 days have not been evaluated in controlled clinical trials, therefore, patients receiving the drug for extended courses need close monitoring for its myelosuppressive effects.

Tedizolid is a newer oxazolidinone antimicrobial that was developed for the treatment of acute bacterial skin and skin structure infections (ABSSSI) caused by MRSA. Two Phase III trials proved tedizolid to be non-inferior to linezolid in the treatment of such infections, based on similar rates of clinical response [14, 15]. Tedizolid's several advantages over linezolid include once daily dosing, shorter duration of therapy, and increased tolerability. Tedizolid also maintains activity even in the presence of mutations on the *cfr* element conferring resistance to linezolid due to enhanced affinity for the target site. However, its cost may be prohibitive. Investigations are ongoing to determine its utility in other MRSA infections, including nosocomial pneumonia, diabetic foot, bone, and joint infections.

Lipoglycopeptides

Dalbavancin, oritavancin, and telavancin are lipoglycopeptides that exert their activity by interfering with cell wall biosynthesis. All three agents are approved to be used in acute bacterial skin and skin structure infections and have been shown to be non-inferior to IV vancomycin [16 - 18]. Telavancin also can be used for nosocomial pneumonia caused by *S. aureus* and a recent phase II trials' data showed similar cure rates in *S. aureus* bacteremia [19, 20]. Dalbavancin and oritavancin are unique in that they are given in short courses (two weekly infusions and a single infusion, respectively) but also maintain high, prolonged serum concentrations allowing for off-label use in complicated infections. Due to high cost, they are frequently reserved for outpatient use. Telavancin requires daily intravenous infusions for at least seven days, depending on the indication. Telavancin may possess superior bactericidal activity compared with vancomycin and linezolid in hVISA, but so far, data is limited to *In vitro* studies [21].

Ceftaroline

Ceftaroline is highly active against hVISA, VISA, and daptomycin-non-susceptible *S. aureus* due to its enhanced affinity for PBP2a. *In vitro* data has demonstrated the existence of a "seesaw effect", where β-lactam activity increases as vancomycin and daptomycin susceptibility decreases [22]. Reports of ceftaroline resistance (MICs between 4 and 8 µg/mL) have been published but are uncommon [23]. In addition to approved use for susceptible community-acquired bacterial pneumonia (CABP) and ABSSSI, ceftaroline is also used off-label for MRSA bacteremia salvage therapy. Like daptomycin, ceftaroline may be a promising alternative therapy in patients who fail vancomycin trials, have true vancomycin allergies or have certain infections with MRSA isolates with MIC's >1 µg/mL [24].

Delafloxacin

While approved for the treatment of ABSSSI, delafloxacin is also currently being evaluated in a phase III trial among patients with CABP. Delafloxacin is unique from other fluoroquinolones in that it exhibits balanced activity against DNA gyrase and topoisomerase IV. This may serve to limit resistance selection since double mutations are relatively rare genetic events. In a study, delafloxacin showed excellent *In vitro* activity and MIC values were not affected by the methicillin-resistant phenotype among levofloxacin-susceptible strains [25].

Omadacycline

Belonging to a subclass of tetracyclines, oral and intravenous formulations of omadacycline was approved by the FDA, in October 2018, for the treatment of CABP and ABSSSI [26, 27]. *In vitro* studies show that it displays broad-spectrum activity, including MRSA. In comparison with linezolid, omadacycline led to similar clinical response rates in acute skin and skin structure infections in one Phase III trial. The trial published in support of the agent in CABP had few

MRSA cases reported. More studies are needed to determine the optimal place of this agent in MRSA therapy.

Combination Therapy

Recent reports show a significant correlation between vancomycin MICs in the range of 1-2 µg/mL and higher daptomycin MICs [28]. Extensively resistant MRSA isolates may respond to daptomycin-based combination therapy with β-lactams due to the synergistic impact that they have on the surface charge of MRSA. Combination therapy with daptomycin and ceftaroline has been studied as salvage therapy in persistent MRSA bacteremia and led to the clearance of bacteremia in a median of 2 days [29]. Based on an *In vitro* analysis, ceftaroline may offer a potential dual benefit by its synergistic interaction with daptomycin, but also by sensitization of MRSA to the innate host defense peptide (HDP) catelicidin LL37. The addition of ceftaroline to daptomycin may even be beneficial in the treatment of daptomycin non-susceptible *S. aureus*. Other than ceftaroline, a case series of seven patients showed rapid clearance of MRSA after the addition of nafcillin to daptomycin therapy [30]. *In vitro* data suggests that other β-lactams may also provide a synergistic effect with daptomycin, but clinical evidence is lacking [31, 32].

Based on *In vitro* evidence, oritavancin and vancomycin may potentially be used in combination with β-lactams, especially in combination with ceftaroline, for the treatment of infections caused by multidrug-resistant *S. aureus* [33, 34].

Practical Applications

While vancomycin is often used first-line for MRSA infections, clinical or microbiologic failure can occur and daptomycin or linezolid should be considered as second-line options with selection based on susceptibility profile, type, and severity of the infection. Newer agents, such as tedizolid, omadacycline, delafloxacin, and the lipoglycopeptides, may be useful in skin and skin structure infections and pneumonia caused by MRSA, but evidence for use in severe infections, such as bacteremia, is limited. Ceftaroline can be used as salvage therapy for MRSA bacteremia and may be a valuable addition to daptomycin in cases of persistent bacteremia.

Vancomycin-resistant *Enterococcus spp.* (VRE)

Vancomycin-resistant *enterococcus* (VRE) is one of the most challenging causes of healthcare-associated infections and can be found as the source of a variety of infections, including urinary tract infections (UTI), bacteremia, IE, and meningitis. In general, enterococci are not regarded as highly virulent pathogens, but their increasing resistance profile adds to the complexity of selecting the most appropriate antibiotic regimen.

Resistance Mechanisms

Enterococcus spp. have intrinsic resistance to most of the β-lactam antibiotics, fluoroquinolones, clindamycin, trimethoprim/sulfamethoxazole (*in vivo*) and low concentrations of vancomycin or aminoglycosides. In the 1980s, some enterococcal strains were found to have acquired new resistance to high concentrations of vancomycin. Multiple types of VRE have been characterized on phenotypic bases, but the one most commonly associated with vancomycin resistance in *E. faecalis* and *E. faecium* is *VanA* [35]. Expression of this gene results in the synthesis of abnormal peptidoglycan precursors to which vancomycin binds with low affinity. This often results in a minimum inhibitory concentration to vancomycin ≥ 32 µg/mL.

Surveillance data shows that the prevalence of linezolid-resistant *enterococcus spp.* remains low. Isolates with resistance most frequently have mutations in the 23S rRNA genes [3]. Similar to in daptomycin-nonsusceptible *S. aureus*, it is likely that multiple genes are involved in non-susceptible VRE isolates. A summary of genes found to be involved in the development of resistance in *Enterococcus spp.* is provided in Table **2**.

Table 2. *Enterococcus spp.* Resistance Genes.

Antibiotic	Gene(s) Involved	Resistance Strategy
Vancomycin	*van* gene clusters	Target replacement
Linezolid	*Cfr*, 23S rRNA gene mutations	Target modification
Daptomycin	*LiaFSR, yycGF, gdpD, cls*	Changes in cell surface
β-lactams (Penicillin and Ampicillin)	PBP5	Target modification

Treatment Options

Ampicillin (+/- Gentamicin)

Ampicillin remains one of the most active anti-enterococcal β-lactams and resistance remains uncommon in *E. faecalis* isolates [3]. The most potent therapy for serious infections caused by strains of VRE, that remain susceptible, is a combination of intravenous ampicillin with gentamicin. It has been well documented that β-lactams are bactericidal *In vitro* for susceptible strains, however, monotherapy is considered to be inferior in serious infections, specifically in endocarditis [36]. Amoxicillin is able to achieve high concentrations in the urine (306-856 µg/mL), which suggests that urinary concentrations are well above the MICs of ampicillin-resistant VRE. A recent study evaluated the outcomes of aminopenicillin monotherapy for VRE-associated UTIs and found it to be effective regardless of susceptibility [37].

Daptomycin

Daptomycin has *In vitro* bactericidal activity against both *E. faecalis* and *E. faecium*, including VRE, which suggests that it may be a useful agent for more serious infections, such as VRE bacteremia [38]. Results are conflicting when daptomycin is compared to linezolid for VRE bacteremia, but further dose trials indicate that it is likely that daptomycin was under-dosed in those studies [39, 40]. Rather than the approved dose of 4-6 mg/kg/day, it is recommended that daptomycin be dosed at 8-12 mg/kg/day in the treatment of VRE infections, especially when the infection is invasive in nature [41].

Oxazolidinones

Linezolid is approved by the FDA for the treatment of VRE infections, including those with bacteremia. An open-label, non-randomized study demonstrated that treatment with linezolid led to a microbiologic eradication rate of 85% in vancomycin-resistant *E. faecalis* bacteremia [42]. As previously discussed, there is conflicting data when comparing the efficacy of linezolid *versus* daptomycin for the treatment of VRE-related bacteremia and both are considered as first-line therapies in the AHA Infective Endocarditis and IDSA Catheter-related Infection Guidelines [43]. There is currently no clinical data evaluating tedizolid use in serious enterococcal infections, but *In vitro* data suggest it maintains activity against *cfr*-mediated ribosomal mutations, present in linezolid-resistant isolates.

Lipoglycopeptides

Dalbavancin, oritavancin, and telavancin have demonstrated *In vitro* concentration-dependent bactericidal activity against enterococci isolates. The bactericidal activity of dalbavancin is restricted to specific genotypes of VRE, therefore, limiting its use in VRE infections. In a large susceptibility study, oritavancin had a potency 4- to 128-fold greater than active comparators, such as linezolid, daptomycin, and quinupristin/dalfopristin [44]. Further research with a focus on clinical outcomes is still needed.

Quinupristin-dalfopristin

The first antibiotic approved for the treatment of VRE infections was quinupristin-dalfopristin. It is bacteriostatic and historically has a broad spectrum of activity *In vitro* against Gram-positive organisms. When treating VRE infections, this antibiotic should only be used against *E. faecium* as it is not active against *E. faecalis*. One study found a clinical cure or improvement in 83% of patients treated with quinupristin/dalfopristin. Dose-related myalgias and arthralgias did occur in this study population and these adverse effects may be a limitation for use [45]. Due to these side effects, the drug has fallen out of favor and is rarely used unless there are no other viable options.

Fosfomycin

Fosfomycin is active against *Enterococcus spp.* and has approval from the FDA for the treatment of urinary tract infections (UTIs) caused by vancomycin-susceptible *E. faecalis*. Studies have reported variable susceptibility to VRE urine isolates, ranging from 0% to 100% and a published review of thirty-nine patients found that oral fosfomycin therapy resulted in a clinical cure rate of 82% in VRE UTIs [46, 47]. Fosfomycin provides a cost-effective alternative to more expensive VRE-active agents, such as daptomycin and linezolid, however, the utility is limited to UTIs. An intravenous formulation has been available in Asian and European countries for many years and a new drug application is currently under the FDA for approval, to treat complicated UTIs, including pyelonephritis.

Tigecycline

Tigecycline exhibits excellent bacteriostatic activity *In vitro* against both *E. faecalis* and *E. faecium*. It is approved by the FDA for the treatment of cSSSI, complicated intra abdominal infections (cIAI), and CABP. The use of tigecycline in bacteremia is controversial because of its high volume of distribution and a meta-analysis in 2010 that showed a 0.6% absolute increase in the risk of death with tigecycline, compared to other antibiotics [48].

Combination Therapy

The use of combination therapy for serious enterococcal infections is often recommended due to most monotherapy regimens being only bacteriostatic against the organism. As previously mentioned, using ampicillin with an aminoglycoside achieves bactericidal activity, however, the use of highly nephrotoxic agents, like aminoglycosides, can be difficult in patients with multiple comorbid conditions. Dual β-lactam therapy with ampicillin and ceftriaxone has shown to be successful in the treatment of enterococcal endocarditis, but mortality remains high, prompting the need for alternative options [49].

Combination regimens involving daptomycin and β-lactam antibiotics are supported by recent literature. *In vitro* data suggests that the presence of β-lactams increases the binding of daptomycin to daptomycin-nonsusceptible *E. faecium*. A few β-lactam agents have been specifically studied *In vitro* and ampicillin, ceftaroline, and ertapenem were shown to have synergistic activity when given in addition to daptomycin [50]. Limited clinical data exists, but a case report described a patient with ampicillin-resistant VRE *faecium* that responded to ampicillin and a high-dose of daptomycin [51].

Oritavancin also displays synergy with β-lactams in the treatment of VRE [33]. Linezolid, given with gentamicin, was successful in treating two serious VRE *faecium* infections, however, *In vitro* studies of the regimen have failed to show synergistic activity. While used infrequently due to better-tolerated alternatives, quinupristin-dalfopristin combined with minocycline or doxycycline has both *In vitro* data and case reports to support its use [52, 53].

Practical Applications

When susceptible, the combination of ampicillin and gentamicin should be considered initially in the treatment of VRE infections. When nephrotoxicity or severe β-lactam allergies preclude the use of this combination, daptomycin or linezolid should be considered with selection based on susceptibility profile, type, and severity of the infection. Alternative agents, such as quinupristin-dalfopristin, fosfomycin, tigecycline, and the lipoglycopeptides, can be considered, but the utility is affected by increased toxicities and pharmacodynamic limitations. Combination regimens are becoming more frequently utilized in persistent VRE bacteremias and should be considered in such cases where first-line regimens lead to clinical or microbiologic failure.

GRAM-NEGATIVE ORGANISMS

Enterobacteriaceae

Enterobacteriaceae are common pathogens that can cause infections in the community and healthcare settings. Treatment of infections due to multidrug-resistant (MDR) and extensively drug-resistant (XDR) *Enterobacteriaceae* is challenging. In recent years, it has been highlighted as a public health concern due to the fact that there are limited antimicrobials available and little evidence of their efficacy [54].

Resistance Mechanisms

Several schemes of classification have been proposed to characterize the vast number of β-lactamases identified. The Ambler class is a molecular classification scheme where enzymes are grouped based on protein homology [55]. Alternatively, the Bush–Jacoby functional classification system categorizes the β-lactamases into four main groups according to their substrate and inhibitory properties [56]. A list of β-lactamases in both classification systems is shown in Table **3**.

Table 3. ESBL Classification.

Ambler	Bush-Jacoby	Characteristics	Examples of Genes	Substrates
A	2a	Penicillinases inhibited by CA.	*PC1*	Penicillins
	2b	Broad-spectrum enzymes inhibited by CA.	*TEM-1, TEM-2, TEM-13, SHV-1,SHV-11*	Penicillins, cephalothin
	2be	Extended broad-spectrum enzymes inhibited by CA.	*TEM-3, TEM-10, TEM-26, SHV-2, SHV-3, Klebsiella oxytoca K1, CTXM, PER, VEB*	Penicillins, oxyimino-cephalosporins (cefotaxime, ceftazidime, ceftriaxone, cefepime), monobactams
	2br	Broad-spectrum enzymes with reduced binding to CA (inhibitor resistant TEMs).	*TEM-30, TEM-31, SHV-10, SHV-72*	Penicillins, resistant to CA, tazobactam and sulbactam
	2ber	Extended-spectrum enzymes with relative resistance to CA.	*TEM-50, TEM-158*	Penicillins, oxyimino-cephalosporins, monobactams, resistant to CA, tazobactam and sulbactam
	2c	Carbenicillin-hydrolyzing enzymes inhibited by CA.	*PSE-1, CARB-3*	Penicillins, carbenicillin
	2ce	Extended-spectrum carbenicillinase.	*RTG-4 (CARB-10)*	Carbenicillin, cefepime
	2e	Cephalosporinases inhibited by CA.	*CepA*	Cephalosporins
	2f	Carbapenem-hydrolyzing nonmetallo-β-lactamases.	*KPC, SME, GES, IMI-1*	All β-lactams, including carbapenems
B	3	Metallo-β-lactamases.	*IMP, VIM, IND*	All β-lactams, including carbapenems, with exception of monobactams
C	1	Cephalosporinases not inhibited by CA.	*ACT-1, FOX-1, MIR-1, CMY*	Narrow and extended-spectrum cephalosporins, including cephamycins

(Table 3) cont.....

Ambler	Bush-Jacoby	Characteristics	Examples of Genes	Substrates
D	2d	Cloxacillin-hydrolyzing enzymes with variable inhibition by CA.	*OXA-1, OXA-2, OXA-10*	Cloxacillin, oxacillin,
	2de		*OXA-11, OXA-15*	Cloxacillin, oxacillin, oxyimino cephalosporins, monobactams.
	2df		*OXA-23, OXA-51, OXA-58*	Cloxacillin, oxacillin, carbapenems
-	4	Penicillinases not inhibited by CA.	Penicillinases from *Burkholderia cepacia*	Penicillins

CA= clavulanic acid
Adapted from: Sarah S. Tang, Anucha Apisarnthanarak, Li Yang Hsu. Mechanisms of β-lactam antimicrobial resistance and epidemiology of major community and healthcare-associated multidrug-resistant bacteria. Advanced Drug Delivery Reviews; 78 (2014): 3-13.

Extended Spectrum β-lactamases (ESBL's) and AmpC's

ESBL's and *ampC's*, both are generally resistant to cephalosporins, but there are some notable differences between the two. ESBL's hydrolyze penicillins, cephalosporins, and aztreonam, but not cephamycins. They are also encoded by plasmid genes. The most frequently encountered ESBL's belong to the *CTX-M*, *SHV*, and *TEM* families [57]. *AmpC* β-lactamases hydrolyze many of the cephalosporins and, when hyper produced, may cause resistance to penicillins, aztreonam, cephamycins, and other cephalosporins with the exception of cefepime [54, 58, 59]. *AmpC* can be encoded by plasmid genes or be produced as a result of depression of chromosomal genes in some *Enterobacteriaceae* spp. [60]. *AmpC* expression varies among different *Enterobacteriaceae* spp. but is generally highest with *Enterobacter spp.*

For ESBL and *ampC* producing organisms, carbapenems have been the drugs of choice. However, due to the rising rates of carbapenem resistance, alternative therapies are needed and are outlined below.

Treatment Options

<u>Carbapenems</u>

Carbapenems have historically been the drug of choice for ESBL and *ampC* producing organisms [54, 59]. A meta-analysis that included 21 observational studies of bacteremic infections caused by ESBL producing organisms showed that mortality rates for patients who had received treatment with carbapenems were lower than those for patients treated with either an aminoglycoside, cephalosporin or fluoroquinolone [61].

The carbapenems that have been cited the most are the group one carbapenems, particularly imipenem and meropenem [61]. Some observational studies have compared ertapenem, the only group two carbapenem, to the other carbapenems. No differences in prognosis were identified, however, one study with a subgroup of septic shock patients, and primarily with urinary tract infection and hospital-acquired pneumonia (HAP), showed a slight increase in mortality in patients that were given ertapenem [62].

In regards to *Enterobacteriaceae* harboring the chromosomal *ampC* gene, a recent meta-analysis that included studies with limitations did not find that carbapenems were clearly superior to fluoroquinolones, cefepime, or β-lactam- β-lactamase inhibitors (BLBLI). In most studies reviewed, 20 to 35% of included isolates showed the derepressed *ampC* phenotype [63]. The data for plasmid-mediated *ampC* producers is limited.

Cephalosporins

ESBL and *ampC* producers are typically resistant to a majority of cephalosporins, but there are some notable differences. The organisms that produce *TEM* and *SHV* ESBL's are susceptible to cefotaxime, whereas *CTX-M* producers are more likely to be susceptible to ceftazidime and cefepime [54, 59]. ESBL's are unable to hydrolyze the cephamycins (cefoxitin and cefotetan), thus showing susceptibility to them. However, the use of these drugs against ESBL's has been discouraged due to reports of resistance

The clinical data to support the use of cephalosporins in ESBL infections has been found to be contradictory, but overall inclination has been to not use cephalosporins for ESBL infections, especially with higher MIC's of 2-8 mg/liter [64, 65].

AmpC producers are usually susceptible to cefepime unless other mechanisms of resistance exist. One retrospective study of *Enterobacter cloacae* bacteremia was conducted to evaluate the use of cefepime. In this multivariate analysis, a higher mortality was found for patients treated with cefepime than those treated with carbapenems when the isolates had cefepime MICs of 4 to 8 mg/liter [66]. Another study by Tamma and colleagues compared the mortality rates for hospitalized patients with blood, bronchoalveolar lavage, or intra-abdominal fluid cultures growing *ampC* producing *Enterobacter, Serratia*, or *Citrobacter spp.* with derepressed *ampC* and treated with cefepime (1 to 2 g every 8 h) or meropenem. In patients with hyper producing *ampC* organisms clinical outcomes were evaluated. After comparing the propensity score-matched pairs, there was no effect on mortality demonstrated between cefepime and meropenem (31% and 34%) [67].

BLBLI

ESBL's are inhibited by BLBLI, however, there have been concerns about their efficacy and there are a number of case reports regarding the use of piperacillin/tazobactam for ESBL infection with varying results. One study by Tamma and colleagues found that piperacillin-tazobactam was inferior to carbapenem therapy for the treatment of ESBL infections, particularly bacteremia's and concluded that early carbapenem therapy should be considered [68].

In regard to organisms with *ampC* genes, a meta-analysis of blood stream infections (BSI), caused by *Enterobacter, Citrobacter,* and *Serratia spp,* showed that treatment with piperacillin-tazobactam was not associated with increased mortality and could not state that they were inferior when compared to therapy with a carbapenems [63]. Additional literature is needed to truly asses the efficacy of these agents.

Cephalosporin-β Lactamase Combinations

Ceftazidime-avibactam (C/A) was approved by the FDA for the treatment of complicated urinary traction infections (cUTI), in combination with metronidazole for cIAI and VAP. Avibactam inhibits class A enzymes, including ESBL's and *Klebsiella pneumoniae* carbapenemases (*KPC*), as well as class C and some *OXA* β-lactamases, however, it is not against metallo- β -lactamases (*MBLs*) [69].

In the phase 3 trial looking at cUTI and cIAI, C/A was compared to the best available therapy, which was mainly a carbapenem. The primary endpoint was the clinical response of an ESBL infection at the test-of-cure visit, which was 7–10 days after the last infusion of study therapy. The overall proportion of patients with a clinical cure at the test-of-cure visit were similar with C/A (140 [91%; 95% CI 85·6–94·7]) and best available therapy [135 [91%; 85·9–95·0]). This study provided evidence of the efficacy of C/A as a potential alternative to carbapenems in patients with ESBL infections [70].

Ceftolozane-tazobactam (C/T) is a newer agent with enhanced antipseudomonal activity with a known β-lactamase inhibitor. The drug was approved by the FDA for the treatment of cUTI and cIAI (in combination with metronidazole). C/T has been shown to be active *In vitro* against ESBL producing organisms ranging from

41.8 to 98% [69]. One of the pivotal trials that included patients with cUTI and cIAI ESBL infections looked at C/T compared to levofloxacin and meropenem, respectively. Endpoints of the study were rates of clinical cure and microbiological eradication. In the cUTI patients, cure rates were higher with C/T (98.1% and 72.2%, respectively) than with levofloxacin (82.6% and 47.8%, respectively) and 82% of isolates were susceptible to C/T, whereas only 25% were susceptible to levofloxacin. In regards to the cIAI patients, C/T and meropenem outcomes were similar (clinical cure rates were 95.8% and 88.5%, respectively, and microbiological eradication was similar as well [71].

To date, there have been no studies for C/A and C/T providing clinical data on infections identified to be caused by *ampC* producing organisms.

Aminoglycosides

The use of aminoglycosides for serious infections, due to ESBL and *ampC* producing organisms, has been limited to combination therapy with β-lactam antibiotics, however, they have also shown to increase the risk of toxicity, particularly renal [72]. Amikacin has been the most extensively studied and tends to have superior Gram-negative coverage in comparison to other aminoglycosides for ESBL and organisms [73]. Plazomicin, a new aminoglycoside, shows promise against ESBL and *ampC* producing bacteria, however, more clinical data is needed [74, 75]. Empirical use of an aminoglycoside may be considered as a carbapenem sparing regimen, specifically in urosepsis cases.

Tigecycline

Tigecycline is a glycylcycline and is not affected by ESBL's or *ampC* β-lactamases. Its spectrum of activity covers the Gram-positive bacteria, *Enterobacteriaceae* (excluding *Proteus spp*), *A. baumannii*, and some anaerobes. It has a large volume of distribution and is not recommended to be used as the sole agent for a bacteremia. The drug was approved for the treatment of cSSSI, cIAI, and CABP. Since its approval, warnings of increased risk of mortality and clinical failure have been documented, and the reported clinical success is very limited [48, 76]. Although there is scant clinical experience with infections caused by ESBL and *ampC* producing organisms treated with tigecycline, they are expected to have similar results to non-ESBL organisms treated with tigecycline [77, 78]. Typically tigecycline is reserved as a last line agent or when other options are unavailable.

Fosfomycin

Fosfomycin remains active against most ESBL and *ampC*-producing *E. coli* and

K. pneumoniae organisms [79]. An oral formulation is available in the United States, which is used for the treatment of uncomplicated UTI, including ESBL producing organisms [80]. A retrospective cohort study was performed comparing fosfomycin and ertapenem. Ertapenem treated patients received longer outpatient antibiotic treatment (10 days *vs.* 6 days; *p* <0.001). The thirty day re-admission rates for fosfomycin and ertapenem were 14.6% *vs.* 13.5%. Fosfomycin was found to be non-inferior to ertapenem for treating outpatient ESBL UTIs and the authors speculated that it should be considered as appropriate step-down or carbapenem sparing therapy for these infections [81].

As previously stated, an intravenous formulation is available in Europe and is in development for the United States. In a systemic review evaluating fosfomycin and other antibiotics for sepsis, UTI, respiratory, bone, joint and CNS infections, there was no clinical nor microbiological difference between fosfomycin and other antibiotics observed [82]. There have been reports of emergence of resistance during monotherapy use of the drug and general studies have recommended fosfomycin to be used in combinations for severe infections caused by ESBL and *ampC* producing organisms [80, 83].

Carbapenamase Resistant *Enterobactereaciae* (CRE)

The CDC has labeled carbapenemases as a high-level health threat for multiple reasons. First, these organisms are often resistant to multiple classes of antimicrobials, limiting the potential treatment options. Infections caused by these organisms are associated with high mortality rates, up to 50% in some studies [84]. Additionally, many CRE possess carbapenemases that can be transmitted from one *Enterobacteriaceae* to another, potentially facilitating transmission of resistance. The reported incidence of CRE varies based on region. However, Greece (20–50%), India (4–24%), and the United States (4–11%) have the highest reported cases of incidence [85 - 87].

Carbapenemases are able to hydrolyze carbapenems and other β-lactams. Detection is a crucial infection control issue because it is often associated with extensive and sometimes complete antibiotic resistance. The carbapenem resistance is typically caused by the production of a carbapenemase and the ones that will be discussed are specifically caused by *KPC*, metallo β-lactamases (*MBLs*), particularly *NDM, IMP, VIM,* and *OXA* enzymes. There is minimal efficacy data to treat such infections with one agent, instead combination therapy is preferred. No such randomized control trial has been published, whereas multiple observational outcomes studies have been published and suggest that combination therapy may be beneficial in this patient population.

Treatment Options

Double Carbapenem Therapy

A study by Bulik and Nicolau was the first of its kind to mention the use of ertapenem and doripenem, specifically as dual carbapenem therapy for CRE infections. The thought behind the mechanism is similar to that of a β -lactam β -lactamase inhibitor combination. Ertapenem has increased affinity to *KPC*, which, in turn, prevents them from acting on the second carbapenem [88]. This *in-vitro* activity was studied and it was noted that this only works if the meropenem MIC is ≤ 128 mg/liter and does not apply to all strains of CREs [88, 89]. A retrospective observational study reported a clinical success rate of 70% and a crude mortality of 20% when treated with ertapenem and meropenem. However, in this study, roughly a third of patients also received an additional active antimicrobial agent [90].

Ceftazidime-Avibactam

As stated earlier, C/A inhibits ESBL's, *ampC*, *KPC*, and most of the *OXA*-48 enzymes, but not *MBLs* [91, 92]. Most literature available on C/A for the treatment of CRE infections is in retrospective study designs [93]. A study by Tumbarello and colleagues in which C/A was compared to a matched cohort with colistin in patients with CRE bacteremia showed that therapy with C/A was the sole independent predictor of survival [94]. Although more data is needed, C/A is gaining favorability for severe infections due to KPC and *OXA-48* producing *Enterobacteriaceae* infections.

Aminoglycosides

Aminoglycoside rates of susceptibility against CRE infections vary widely. Monotherapy use of aminoglycosides for CRE UTIs has been favorable when compared to polymyxin B [95], however, due to their pharmacokinetic profile, they should not be used as the sole agent for such infections since mortality has been associated to be as high as 80% [96]. Studies comparing outcomes for patients treated with and without aminoglycosides are limited and appropriate dosing based on patients' renal function and site of infection are imperative.

Plazomicin is a newly approved aminoglycoside and is active against CRE more so than the other aminoglycosides. In a phase 3 trial in patients with HAP, VAP or BSIs caused by CRE, plazomicin or colistin were given in combination with tigecycline or meropenem (investigators choice). Mortality rates at day 28 were 11.8% and 40%, respectively. Toxicity was less frequent with plazomicin, in particular renal toxicity [97].

Polymixins

Polymyxins (colistin and Polymixin B) are active against *Enterobacteriaceae*, except for *Proteus spp.*, *Serratia spp.*, *Morganella spp.* and *Providencia spp.* They have been considered the agents of last resort against CRE infections. There is more clinical information available on colistin however, cure rates and mortality seem to be similar between the two agents [98]. Overall, the polymixins have been used with carbapenems, tigecycline, aminoglycosides, and fosfomycin for combination therapy. A meta-analysis by Hirsch and colleagues reviewed articles on patients with KPC producing *Klebsiella pneumoniae* infections, treated with colistin and found that colistin in combination was more effective *vs.* monotherapy and concluded that polymyxin monotherapy was associated with higher mortality than that with colistin in combination with additional agents [99, 100]. In regards to the dosing of these agents, data has been controversial and discussion of optimal dosing schemes exceeds the scope of this text. Nephrotoxicity is commonly associated with these agents, which may drive a clinician to use alternate agents in patients. Overall, polymixins are sometimes the last agents available for CRE infections, and based on the literature, combination therapy may be more beneficial for this select patient population.

Tigecycline

Much like with ESBL infections, tigecycline has been used as a last resort treatment option for severe CRE as well as other MDR Gram-negative infections. A recent meta-analysis indicated that the efficacy of tigecycline is similar to that as other antimicrobials, however, in combination and high doses, it may be more effective than monotherapy and standard doses [101]. More data is needed to adequately compare the efficacy of tigecycline and CRE infections.

Eravacycline

Eravacycline is a new fluorocycline antibiotic active against many Gram-negative species and has been approved for use in intra-abdominal infections. *In-vitro* studies have shown susceptibility of ESBL's, *KPC, MBL* and *OXA*-48 enzymes. Eravacycline was tested against carbapenem and tigecycline resistant *Enterobacteriaceae*. It closely correlated with tigecycline, but a large amount of MIC's to eravacycline were 2-fold lower when compared to tigecycline MICs to CRE [102]. More clinical studies are required to assess its utility to CRE infections.

Fosfomyin

Fosfomycin IV has been used in combination for the treatment of CRE infections overseas. In a multicenter case series, mainly focusing on VAP and BSI, the twenty-eight day mortality rate was 37.5% and clinical success was identified in 54.2% of patients on day 14 of therapy [103]. However, resistance in three patients did occur while on therapy, which has been noted in other trials [104]. Administration with other active agents is likely necessary to reduce the mortality and risk of resistance [82].

Meropenem-Vaborbactam

Meropenem-vaborbactam is a known carbapenem with a new β-lactamase inhibitor combination with in-vitro activity against *KPC*-producing CRE and is inactive against CRE produced by *MBL*'s, specifically *NDM* (*VIM* and *IMI*) or *OXA*-48 enzymes [105]. Its efficacy in cUTI, as well as pyelonephritis, was proven in its phase 3 trial (TANGO I) and has shown clinical efficacy and decreased mortality against CRE infections (TANGO II) [106, 107]. More studies are needed to assess its toxicity, tolerability, and pharmacokinetic/pharmaco-dynamics profiles in comparison to other antimicrobials active against CRE infections.

Future Pipeline

A variety of new drugs are in the pipeline that display *in-vitro* CRE activity. They are currently being evaluated clinically. A high-level overview in regards to ESBL, *ampC* and CRE coverage is displayed in Table 4 below.

Table 4. New Agents with Activity Against CRE, ESBL, and ampC-producing Organisms.

Drug	Class	Spectrum Activity
Cefiderocol	Siderophore cephalosporin	ESBL, *KPC MBL* and *OXA*
Aztreonam-avibactam	BLBLI	ESBL, *ampC*, *KPC*, *MBL* and OXA
Ceftarolne fosamil-avibactam	BLBLI	ESBL, *KPC*, *ampC's* and variable *OXA*
Imipenem/cilistatin-relabactam	Carbapenem- β lactamase inhibitor	ESBL, *KPC*, *ampC's* and variable *OXA*
Meropenem-vaborbactam	Carbapenem- β lactamase inhibitor	Ambler class A and C β-lactamases

Adapted from: Tumbarello M *et al.* Curr Opin Infec Dis 2018;31:566-577.

Practical Application (ESBL, CRE)

When it comes to CRE infections, combination therapy may be warranted since it is associated with better outcomes for high-risk patients, particularly those in septic shock or with pneumonia, whereas ESBL and *ampC* infections might be treated with one agent.

Overall, therapy for ESBL, *ampC*, and CRE infections must be individualized according to the susceptibility profile, type, severity of infection, and the features of the patient. Newer agents show promising activity against ESBL, *ampC*, and CRE infections. Many will shortly be available for clinical use, however, studies will be required to truly asses their utility in treatment and patient care.

Multi-drug Resistant *Pseudomonas aeruginosa*

Approximately 21% of PSA isolates in the United States, in the year 2000, were resistant to 3 or more antibiotics and 1.0% were resistant to 6 antibiotics, including amikacin, ceftazidime, ciprofloxacin, gentamicin, imipenem, and piperacillin [108]. Risk factors for multi-drug resistant (MDR) PSA include intensive care unit (ICU) admission, use of invasive devices, treatment with broad-spectrum antibiotics, and immobility [109]. PSA is often associated with serious infections and is rarely considered a component of patients' normal microbial flora with the exception of cystic fibrosis and other chronic pulmonary diseases. Few antibiotics on the market have activity against PSA. Given the paucity of new antimicrobials targeting MDR-PSA, clinicians need to be equipped with multiple strategies to treat these infections.

Resistance Mechanism

PSA has been successful at evading eradication by antibiotics because of its intrinsic resistance to many antibiotic classes coupled with its ability to quickly acquire resistance *via* mutations. Much of PSA's intrinsic resistance is due to its cell wall impermeability, a combination of porin channel loss, and efficient efflux pumps. In particular, the *MexAB-OprM* efflux pump system removes β-lactams, fluoroquinolones, macrolides, sulfonamides, tetracyclines, and trimethoprim from the periplasmic space [108]. This efflux system is expressed in relatively constant amounts in all wild-type PSA strains but can also be hyper-expressed and result in increased resistance to fluoroquinolones and β-lactams, including meropenem [110]. PSA can also express a number of β-lactamases including an intrinsic *ampC* and acquired *TEM, OXA, Per-1, PSE-1, PSE-4* and rarely, *MBLs, IMP* and *VIM*. In addition to this, target-site mutations also contribute to antibiotic resistance. An example of this is topoisomerase II and IV mutations that confer resistance to fluoroquinolone antibiotics. MDR-PSA most likely occurs as a combination of up-regulated efflux pumps, porin loss (particularly *OprD*), and aminoglycoside-modifying enzymes, which can result from sequential and repeated antibiotic use. When combined, these mechanisms can confer resistance to nearly every drug class with the exception of polymyxin B [108]. Table **5** depicts the most common PSA resistance mechanisms.

Table 5. Select *Pseudomonas aeruginosa* Antibiotic Resistance Mechanisms.

Mechanism	Resistance
β-lactamases	
ampC	Nearly all β-lactams except carbapenems
TEM	Resistance to penicillins and cephalosporins
OXA	Resistant to all β-lactams except carbapenems
Per-1	Ceftazidime resistance and reduced susceptibility to piperacillin
PSE-1, PSE-4	
IMP, VIM	Nearly all β-lactams except aztreonam with resistance or reduced susceptibility to carbapenems
Porin Channel loss	
OprD	Resistance to imipenem and reduced susceptibility to meropenem
Efflux System	
MexAB-OprM	Piperacillin and ceftazidime
Target site mutations	
Topo II or IV (*gyrA* or *parC* mutation)	Fluoroquinolones
Combinations	
Upregulation of *MexAB-OprM* and loss of *OprD*	β-lactams, including carbapenems and fluoroquinolones
Upregulation of *MexEF-OprN*	Imipenem and fluoroquinolones. Reduced meropenem susceptibility

Resistance Prevention

Treatment Options

Unlike other organisms, the resistance mechanism expressed in clinical MDR-PSA is almost impossible to determine without extensive genetic testing. Because of this, treatment options are mainly guided by clinical susceptibility results. When treatment choices are limited by susceptibility results, clinicians often turn towards combination therapy even when one or both agents are resistant [111]. Other alternatives include extended infusion antibiotics, such as meropenem, or use of polymyxin antibiotics [112]. However, some of these agents should be used with caution. Colistin should only be utilized as salvage therapy because it is often associated with high failure rates, especially in the treatment of pneumonia [113]. Colistin and polymyxin B are usually used in combination with β-lactams when treatment options are limited and tend to be associated with high rates of adverse effects [114]. When these agents achieve clinical success, they are often associated with microbiologic failure and persistence of the organism at the site of infection [115]. Given the variability in resistance mechanisms and susceptibility results, this review focuses on new treatment strategies and recently developed antibiotics with activity against MDR-PSA.

Cephalosporin-β Lactamase Combinations

C/A and C/T both have potent *in-vitro* activity against PSA. In a large study across 75 US medical centers, Sader and colleagues demonstrated a 96.9% susceptibility rate of PSA isolates to C/A compared to 83.9% with ceftazidime alone [116]. More importantly, among MDR-PSA and extensively drug-resistant isolates, 81% and 73.7% were susceptible to C/A, respectively. C/T has also demonstrated high rates of susceptibility to MDR-PSA. An *in-vitro* study, by Buehrle and colleagues, revealed that 92% of meropenem-resistant PSA isolates were susceptible to C/T and C/A. Although both combinations are active against PSA, C/T tends to produce lower MICs against non-carbapenemase producing PSA strains [117].

Few studies have analyzed clinical outcomes in patients treated with C/T or C/A for MDR-PSA, however, the available data is promising. Munita and colleagues performed a multicenter, prospective study of C/T in patients with carbapenem-resistant PSA. They analyzed the outcomes of 35 patients who received C/T and observed a clinical success rate of 74% [118]. Several case series studies have documented successful clinical outcomes with the use of C/T [119, 120]. Unfortunately, clinical data with C/A for the treatment of MDR PSA is even sparser. One case series reported the outcomes of C/A used in patients with carbapenem-resistant organisms, however, only 2 patients with PSA were included making it hard to draw any meaningful conclusions [121]. Although data are limited, C/T appears to have more supporting evidence for use in MDR PSA and may be superior to C/A in patients with non-carbapenemase producing PSA.

Cefiderocol

Cefiderocol is a new siderophore cephalosporin antibiotic that takes advantage of iron uptake mechanisms in order to enter bacterial cells. This novel mechanism of cell entry allows for antibacterial activity even in the presence of porin channel loss or increased efflux pump expression. Cefiderocol is effective against many β-lactamases, including carbapenem-resistant organisms that express *VIM* or *IMP*-1 genes [122]. Cefiderocol was studied in a phase 2, multicenter, double-blind, non-inferior study for the treatment of cUTI compared to imipenem-cilastatin [123]. Results of this trial showed superiority of cefiderocol for the primary composite outcome, including microbiologic and clinical cure (73% *vs* 55%). Only a small percentage of PSA isolates were recovered from patients in this study, 7.1% in the cefiderocol group and 4.2% in the imipenem group. An *in-vitro* analysis of 100 imipenem-resistant PSA by Hsueh and colleagues, displayed a much higher *-in vitro* potency of cefiderocol when compared to C/T and C/A [124]. Although clinical data are lacking, one case report of cefiderocol compassionate use for a patient with MDR-PSA IE demonstrated positive clinical outcomes when used in combination with surgical intervention, colistin, and meropenem [125].

Imipenem-relebactam

Relebactam is a new diazabicyclooctane β-lactamase inhibitor that is structurally related to avibactam and has activity against a wide spectrum of β-lactamases. Imipenem-relebactam is an investigational new drug currently undergoing phase 3 trials for the treatment of bacterial HAP/VAP, cIAI, and cUTI compared with imipenem-cilastatin plus colistin among patients with carbapenem-resistant infections. Results from the SMART Global Surveillance Program found that out of 845 clinical PSA isolates, 94.3% were susceptible to imipemen-relebactam, whereas only 70.3% were susceptible to imipenem alone [126]. Another *in-vitro* study, by Lapuebla and colleagues, analyzed 490 clinical isolates in New York City and found that the addition of relebactam, increased susceptibility from 70% to 98%. In this study, imipenem-relebactam was effective against strains with a loss of *OprD* and those with increased *ampC* expression. While we are still waiting for FDA approval and clinical outcomes data for use in MDR-PSA, imipenem-relebactam appears to be a promising option for the treatment of carbapenem-resistant PSA [127].

Aztreonam/Avibactam

Aztreonam-avibactam is an investigational new drug currently being evaluated for the treatment of MDR Gram-negatives, including those harboring *MBLs*. An in-vitro study by Karlowski and colleagues, analyzed the activity of aztreonam-avibactam against 11,842 clinical PSA (452 harboring MBLs) isolates from 40 different countries [128]. They found that the addition of avibactam resulted in MICs that were 2-fold lower than aztreonam alone for PSA isolates. Avibactam offered no additional activity for isolates not containing *MBLs*, suggesting that aztreonam resistance in these organisms is driven by mechanisms other than β-lactamase enzymes. Similar to C/A, aztreonam-avibactam has activity against ESBL and *ampC* producing organisms [129]. It may be a treatment option for MDR PSA isolates that produce *MBLs*, ESBL, or *ampC* enzymes.

Plazomicin

Plazomicin is a next generation aminoglycoside with expanded coverage against MDR *Enterobacteriaceae*, including carbapenem-resistant strains and those harboring aminoglycoside-modifying enzymes, which are common among MDR-PSA. Plazomicin was recently studied alongside levofloxacin in a phase 2 randomized, double-blind trial of patients with cUTI, however, only two patients in this study had documented PSA infections [130]. Data regarding the efficacy of plazomicin against MDR-PSA isolates is insufficient. Similar to other aminoglycosides, plazomicin should not be used as a monotherapy for serious Gram-negative infections. However, there has been data to suggest that plazomicin achieves synergy with cefepime, piperacillin-tazobactam, imipenem, and doripenem for PSA isolates [131]. Until more data is available, it is difficult to determine if plazomicin is an effective treatment option for MDR-PSA, but it may play a role in combination therapy for difficult to treat infections.

Delafloxacin

Delafloxacin is a new fluoroquinolone antibiotic with broad Gram-positive and Gram-negative coverage. Although delafloxacin demonstrated *In vitro* activity against PSA, rates of susceptibility are similar to that of ciprofloxacin. Given that PSA can easily become resistant to all fluoroquinolones with *gyrZ* or *parC* mutations, delafloxacin appears to offer no additional benefits over existing fluoroquinolones on the market for the treatment of MDR-PSA infections [132].

Practical Applications

Many antibiotics, commonly used for the treatment of PSA, are vulnerable to mutational resistance mechanisms. When faced with an MDR-PSA isolate that is resistant to most antibiotics, including carbapenems, we recommend the following treatment strategies: If susceptible, C/T or C/A could be used as a first-line agent. If both are resistant, clinicians should closely examine susceptibility results to determine if combination therapy and/or extended infusion meropenem remains an option. If carbapenem MICs are excessively high and combination therapy is not an option, polymyxins may be used as salvage therapy in combination with other agents, preferably a β-lactam.

Fortunately, newer agents show promising activity against MDR-PSA and many are, or may soon be available for clinical use. Investigational agents, such as cefiderocol, imipenem-relabactam, and aztreonam-avibactam, have demonstrated promising *in-vitro* coverage of MDR-PSA, although clinical data is lacking. Aztreonam-avibactam may be a good option when resistance is due to β-lactamase enzymes. Plazomicin is an option for combination treatment of MDR-PSA when susceptible. Delafloxacin may play a role in combination therapy for MDR-PSA but is unlikely to add any additional benefits over other fluoroquinolone antibiotics. Unfortunately, meropenem-vaborbactam is not an effective treatment option for MDR-PSA. Once available, these new agents will be a welcomed addition to the armamentarium of antibiotics used for MDR-PSA infections.

Multi-drug Resistant *Acinteobacter baumanii*

Acinetobacter baumanii has a unique ability to remain on environmental surfaces, making it a concerning healthcare-associated infection (HAI) often associated with localized outbreaks [133]. In 2014, nearly half of those strains isolated from patients with HAI were carbapenem-non-susceptible and the frequency appears to be increasing [134]. In 1999, 6.3% of ACB isolates were non-susceptible to imipenem compared to 11.4% in 2001 [135]. *A. baumanii* shares many similarities with PSA, including its propensity to accumulate resistance mechanisms resulting in multi-drug resistant strains that are difficult to treat. While attributable mortality has been debated due to the severe underlying comorbidities of these patients, there is certainly an associated increase in mortality that accompanies infections with *A. baumanii* [136].

Resistance Mechanisms

Multi-drug resistant *A. baumanii* (MDR-ACB) has both intrinsic and acquired resistance mechanisms. Similar to PSA, *A. baumanii* has a chromosomally located *ampC* β-lactamase. All strains also carry class D β-lactamase *OXA*-51 gene variants, but most strains express low levels of carbapenemase activity [137]. ACB can quickly become MDR resulting in carbapenem-resistant *Acinetobacter baumanii* (CRAB) *via* the acquisition of enzymes, decreased outer membrane permeability, or a combination of the two [138]. A variety of ESBL enzymes have been isolated for *A. baumanii*, including class A (*PER*, *GES*, and *VEB*), class B (*IMP*, *VIM*, and *SIM*), and class D (*OXA*).

The most common carbapenemase produced by ACB are *MBLs* like *IMP*, *VIM*, or *SIM*, or high level carbapenem hydrolyzing oxacillinase enzymes (*OXA*-23, *OXA*-27, and *OXA*-49) [137]. Porin loss or modification can also result in carbapenem resistance [139]. Specifically, the *CarO* protein is involved in the entry of carbapenem into ACB cells and loss of this porin can result in resistance to imipenem and meropenem [140]. In addition to this, ACB also carries an *OprD*-like porin similar to PSA, the loss of which may play a role in carbapenem resistance [141]. Other less common mechanisms that may play a role in ACB drug resistance include penicillin-binding protein (PBP) modification and efflux systems like the *AdeABC* efflux. For example, tigecycline resistance may be due to the up-regulation of the *AdeABC* efflux pump, whereas colistin resistance is likely due to alterations in Lipopolysaccharide (LPS) or loss of LPS production [142].

Treatment Options

Treatment options for MDR-ACB remain limited and depend upon individual susceptibility patterns. Lack of randomized controlled trials makes it difficult to prefer one treatment strategy over another. Potential treatment options include minocycline, ampicillin-sulbactam (sometimes given as a continuous infusion), colistin, and tigecycline (for non-bacteremic infections) [143, 144]. Ampicillin-sulbactam is often considered the drug of choice when susceptible and has demonstrated efficacy in the treatment of MDR-ACB. Combination therapy has also been used successfully for the treatment of MDR-ACB. Several *in vivo* studies have demonstrated synergy with the combination of imipenem and aminoglycosides, colistin, tobramycin, or rifampicin for CRAB [145]. Although *in vivo* data is limited, trimethoprim-sulfamethoxazole has demonstrated *In vitro* efficacy against CRAB when used in combination with colistin [146]. Combination therapy with carbapenems has repeatedly demonstrated superior mortality rates compared to alternative combinations, such as tigecycline and colistin [147]. Tigecycline combinations should only be used as a last resort due to the high mortality and lower microbial eradication rates that have been observed [148]. Cephalosporin, carbapenem, and aztreonam β-lactamase combinations have no reliable activity against MDR-ACB.

Unfortunately, strains with no apparent susceptible antibiotic options have been identified and proven difficult to treat. One option may be combination therapy, even when all agents are resistant. A study by Lenhard and colleagues demonstrated *In vitro* efficacy of triple antimicrobial therapy with polymyxin B, meropenem, and ampicillin/sulbactam and may be an option when no other alternatives are available [149]. Fortunately, newer agents on the market have shown promising results in the treatment of MDR-ACB and will be the focus of the following section.

Cefiderocol

An *In vitro* study by Hsueh and colleagues compared the activity of C/T, C/A, and cefiderocol against 100 CRAB isolates, out of which 42% were colistin-resistant [124]. In this analysis, cefiderocol had the lowest MIC90 values and interestingly, the authors noted that carbapenemase activity did not appear to be a significant source of resistance to cefiderocol.

Eravacycline

A study by Livermore and colleagues analyzed the *In vitro* activity of eravacycline compared to tigecycline for CRAB isolates [102]. They demonstrated a small increase in antibacterial activity of eravacycline. Another *In vitro* study by Seifert and colleagues compared activity of eravacycline, *amikacin, colistin, doxycycline, imipenem, levofloxacin, meropenem, minocycline, sulbactam, tigecycline and tobramycin for carbapenem-nonsusceptible A.baumanii* with acquired *OXA* or up-regulated *OXA*-51 enzymes [150]. They also showed greater activity of eravacycline than tigecycline, minocycline, levofloxacin, amikacin, tobramycin, and colistin. The demonstrated higher potency, higher serum levels, and a lower rate of adverse effects of eravacycline offer many advantages in the treatment MDR-ACB.

Plazomicin

Plazomicin has shown synergistic activity *In vitro* when used in combination with a carbapenem for the treatment of *A. baumannii* infections, including those caused by carbapenem-resistant isolates [151]. Similar to the treatment of MDR PSA, plazomicin may play a role in combination therapy when susceptible.

Practical Application

Treatment recommendations of MDR-ACB or CRAB are closely aligned with those recommended for MDR-PSA. The volume and complexity of resistance mechanisms in these organisms require careful evaluation of susceptibility and MIC results. Bactericidal agents, such as ampicillin-sulbactam or carbapenems should be used as first-line agents. Minocycline may be considered in strains resistant to β-lactams. Tigecycline and colistin should be reserved for salvage therapy and only used in combination therapy with other agents. Lastly, combination therapy should be utilized when front line agents are resistant or demonstrate elevated MIC results. Combinations, including β-lactams are preferred over those containing tigecycline and colistin.

Based on extremely limited data, eravacycline may be preferred over treatment with tigecycline and colistin due to its improved pharmacokinetic and adverse effect profile, combined with superior *In vitro* activity. When susceptible, plazomicin may be a valid component of combination therapy for MDR-ACB. Cefiderocol shows promising *In vitro* activity against carbapenemase-producing ACB strains and may become a front-line agent in the future.

Candida auris

Over the past decade, *Candida auris* has surfaced as a new multidrug-resistant yeast that has impacted many parts of the world and has been associated with high mortality [152]. An international, collaborative study with the Center for Disease Control and Prevention found that in 54 patients, 93% of *C. auris* isolates were resistant to fluconazole, 35% to amphotericin B, and 7% to echinocandins. Even more worrisome, 41% of isolates were resistant to two antifungal classes, 4% of isolates were resistant to 3 antifungal classes, and 59% of patients died [153]. A more recent review of 28 cases in a US multisite health system observed more favorable clinical outcomes with 14% of isolates resistant to fluconazole and a 17% mortality rate [154]. *C. auris* was first described in 2009, but the earliest isolate was discovered in 1996 [155]. Historical incidence may be higher than what has been described in the literature, as there is a concern with the difficulty in identifying *C. auris* due to its close phylogenic resemblance with other *candida species* and the lack of yeast available in the databases of commercially available biochemical identifications systems. In fact, Kathuria and colleagues discovered that among 102 isolates initially determined to be either *C. haemulonii* or *C. famata* by a VITEK identification system, 88.2% were actually *C. auris* [156]. *C. auris* has primarily been identified in blood, wound, and ear infections, but isolates have also been found in respiratory and urine cultures. Currently, *C. auris* is a relatively uncommon pathogen, but given its propensity for resistance, difficulty with identification and poor associated outcomes, it is important for clinicians to understand current and emerging treatment strategies.

Resistance Mechanisms

C. auris has been found to overcome antifungals through several intrinsic mechanisms. Many of which are similar to those possessed by other *Candida* species. Two mechanisms that have been discovered consistently in resistant *C. auris* isolates are alterations to lanosterol 14-α-demethylase and upregulation of efflux pumps [157]. Mutations to *ERG*11, specifically substitutions at *Y132F* and *K143R*, have led to phenotypic modification at the azole-binding site of lanosterol 14-α-demethylase that decreases affinity to azole antifungals [152]. The efflux pumps responsible for the removal of antifungals from *C. auris* are known as ATP-bind cassette (ABC) transporters. The two most prominent ABC transporters utilized by *C. auris* are *CDR1* and *MDR1*, which have been found to be more abundant in *C. auris* than other *Candida* species [158]. Other mechanisms that may also attribute to resistance include biofilm formation and mutations to fungal genes responsible for ergosterol production (*ERG*2, 3, 5 and 6) and regulation of host and medication-induced stress (HSP90 and HOG1) [159]. Unique to echinocandin resistant isolates, resistance has been caused by mutations to *FKS*1 (substitution at S639F) and *FKS*2 genes, which encode for the production of β-1,3-D-glucan synthase [157].

Treatment Options

Currently, the three antifungal classes utilized for invasive candidiasis are azoles, polyenes, and echinocandins. Among the azoles, fluconazole resistance rates (86-93%) have been almost universal for *C. auris* isolates, whereas voriconazole resistance has been variable (15-54%). Broader spectrum azoles have shown to have relatively low resistance rates: itraconazole (2-3%), posaconazole (0-2%), and isavuconazole (2-3%). The primarily utilized polyene antifungal is amphotericin B, which has shown to have resistance rates similar to voriconazole (8-43% and 15-54%, respectively) [160, 161]. Moreover, while resistance rates have slightly risen over the years, echinocandins have shown to have the lowest resistance rates and experts have recommended that this class should be used as first-line against *C. auris:* micafungin (1-4%), caspofungin (3-7%), anidulafungin (1-4%) [162]. New literature has found promising efficacy with combination therapy with two of the three main antifungal classes, as well as the addition of sulfamethoxazole to azole regimens [163].

Ibrexafungerp

Ibrexafungerp is a triterpene glucan synthase inhibitor. It is available in both in an oral and intravenous formulation. It has a broad spectrum of activities against *Candida* species, including *C. auris*. In an *In vitro* study by Berkow and colleagues, 100 *C. auris* isolates were examined and discovered that 100% had an ibrexafungerp MIC of ≤ 2 µg/ml. In addition, among the isolates that were shown to be resistant to one or more echinocandins, the ibrexafungerp MIC ranged between 0.5-1.0 µg/ml [164]. While the breakpoints for ibrexafungerp have not been established yet, these data are promising given that the achievable serum concentration is above 2 µg/mL. Currently, ibrexafungerp is not FDA approved, but has shown promising results in a phase 2, double-blind, randomized control trial (DOVE) and recruitment for a phase 3 randomized control trial began at the end of 2018 (CARES) [165].

Rezafungin

Rezafungin is a novel echinocandin and differs from others in its class because of choline moiety at the C5 ornithine position, which results in a longer half-life (T½ = 80 hrs). This pharmacokinetic advantage allows for less frequent dosing (*i.e.* once-weekly) and an improved safety profile. *In vitro* and *in vivo* studies have demonstrated potent efficacy of rezafungin against both *Candida* and *Aspergillus* species, including strains resistant to other echinocandins [166]. In an *in vivo* study by Hager and colleagues, inspected the effectiveness of rezafungin against *C. auris* in immunocompromised mice. This study revealed that mice treated with rezafungin had less *C. auris* CFU/g of tissue on day 10 of treatment compared to those treated with micafungin ($p = 0.0128$) or amphotericin B ($p < 0.0001$) [167]. Like ibrexafungerp, rezafungin is currently not FDA approved. However, after positive efficacy and safety results from the phase 2 STRIVE trial, recruitment began at the beginning of 2019 for a phase 3 randomized control trial (ReSTORE).

VT-1598

VT-1598 is tetrazole that inhibits CYP51A (lanosterol 14-α-demethylase), similar to the mechanism of action of triazole antifungals. VT-1598 differs from triazoles in that it has a greater selectivity for fungal CYP51A, compared to mammalian CYP51A. This selectivity is also seen among other CYP450 enzymes, which suggest less potential for drug-drug interactions [168]. In an *In vitro* and *in vivo* study by Wiederhold and colleagues, the authors found that *C. auris* isolates were more susceptible to VT-1598 than fluconazole and had similar susceptibility to caspofungin. It was found that VT-1598 increased survival and decreased fungal burden as well [169]. VT-1598 is still in the early stages of drug approval, but literature shows that it may be an advantageous and effective agent against *C. auris*.

APX001/APX001A

APX001 is the first in a new drug class that targets the fungal enzyme Gwt1. Inhibition of Gwt1 halts the inositol acylation step during the production of glycosylphosphatidylinositol-anchored proteins of the cell wall, which leads to the degradation of cell wall integrity [168]. APX001 is a phosphate pro-drug that is quickly converted to APX001A by systemic phosphatases. *In vitro* studies have revealed that APX001A has activity against *Candida, Cryptococcus, Aspergillus, Scedosporium, Fusarium, and Mucorales* species. In terms of *C. auris*, Hager and colleagues compared the *In vitro* efficacy of APX001A with 9 other antifungals, including azoles, amphoteric B, echinocandins, and flucytosine. The investigators found that APX001A had the lowest MIC with a range of 0.002-0.063 µg/ml. In the same study, the *in vivo* efficacy of APX001A was compared to anidulafungin. APX001A was found to have a greater rate of survival ($p = 0.034$). Also, a decrease in fungal burden was similar for the two antifungals for kidney and lungs, but APX001A was superior to anidulafungin for fungal burden reduction in the brain [170]. Similar to VT-1598, APX001 is early in drug development, but studies have revealed that its broad-spectrum activity could be a potent option for *C. auris* in the future.

Practical Application

C. auris has emerged as a new multidrug-resistant yeast that has been associated with poor outcomes around the world. Among currently available antifungals, echinocandins have displayed the lowest rates of resistance and should be considered first-line for *C. auris* infections. However, for patients who cannot take an echinocandin or if an echinocandin is not available, broader spectrum azoles (itraconazole, posaconazole, and isavuconazole) or a combination of antifungal classes can be utilized as second-line therapy. Moreover, many promising antifungals are in the pipeline with novel mechanisms of action or pharmacokinetic properties. Ibrexafungerp, rezafungin, VT-1598, and APX001 have all shown to be effective against *C. auris* and may be beneficial options in the future.

CONSENT FOR PUBLICATION

Not applicable.

CONFLICT OF INTEREST

The authors confirm that the contents of this chapter have no conflict of interest.

ACKNOWLEDGEMENTS

Declared none.

REFERENCES

[1]   US Centers for Disease Control and Prevention. 2012. http://www.cdc.gov/abcs/reports-findings/survreports/mrsa12.pdf

[2]   Hiramatsu K, Hanaki H, Ino T, Yabuta K, Oguri T, Tenover FC. Methicillin-resistant *Staphylococcus aureus* clinical strain with reduced vancomycin susceptibility. J Antimicrob Chemother 1997; 40(1): 135-6.
        [http://dx.doi.org/10.1093/jac/40.1.135] [PMID: 9249217]

[3]   Munita JM, Bayer AS, Arias CA. Evolving resistance among Gram-positive pathogens. Clin Infect Dis 2015; 61 (Suppl. 2): S48-57.
        [http://dx.doi.org/10.1093/cid/civ523] [PMID: 26316558]

[4]   Zhang S, Sun X, Chang W, Dai Y, Ma X. Systematic review and meta-analysis of the epidemiology of vancomycin-intermediate and heterogeneous vancomycin-intermediate *Staphylococcus aureus* isolates. PLoS One 2015; 10(8): e0136082.
        [http://dx.doi.org/10.1371/journal.pone.0136082] [PMID: 26287490]

[5]   Sievert DM, Rudrik JT, Patel JB, McDonald LC, Wilkins MJ, Hageman JC. Vancomycin-resistant *Staphylococcus aureus* in the United States, 2002-2006. Clin Infect Dis 2008; 46(5): 668-74.
        [http://dx.doi.org/10.1086/527392] [PMID: 18257700]

[6]   Stryjewski ME, Corey GR. Methicillin-resistant *Staphylococcus aureus*: an evolving pathogen. Clin Infect Dis 2014; 58 (Suppl. 1): S10-9.
        [http://dx.doi.org/10.1093/cid/cit613] [PMID: 24343827]

[7]   Liu C, Bayer A, Cosgrove SE, *et al.* Clinical practice guidelines by the infectious diseases society of america for the treatment of methicillin-resistant *Staphylococcus aureus* infections in adults and children: executive summary. Clin Infect Dis 2011; 52(3): 285-92.
        [http://dx.doi.org/10.1093/cid/cir034] [PMID: 21217178]

[8]   Riser MS, Bland CM, Rudisill CN, Bookstaver PB. Cerebrospinal fluid penetration of high-dose daptomycin in suspected *Staphylococcus aureus* meningitis. Ann Pharmacother 2010; 44(11): 1832-5. [http://dx.doi.org/10.1345/aph.1P307] [PMID: 20959502]

[9]   Wunderink RG, Cammarata SK, Oliphant TH, Kollef MH. Continuation of a randomized, double-blind, multicenter study of linezolid *versus* vancomycin in the treatment of patients with nosocomial pneumonia. Clin Ther 2003; 25(3): 980-92. [http://dx.doi.org/10.1016/S0149-2918(03)80118-2] [PMID: 12852712]

[10]   Kalil AC, Metersky ML, Klompas M, *et al.* Management of adults with hospital-acquired and ventilator-associated pneumonia: 2016 clinical practice guidelines by the infectious diseases society of america and the american thoracic society. Clin Infect Dis 2016; 63(5): e61-e111. [http://dx.doi.org/10.1093/cid/ciw353] [PMID: 27418577]

[11]   Jang HC, Kim SH, Kim KH, *et al.* Salvage treatment for persistent methicillin-resistant *Staphylococcus aureus* bacteremia: efficacy of linezolid with or without carbapenem. Clin Infect Dis 2009; 49(3): 395-401. [http://dx.doi.org/10.1086/600295] [PMID: 19569970]

[12]   Park HJ, Kim SH, Kim MJ, *et al.* Efficacy of linezolid-based salvage therapy compared with glycopeptide-based therapy in patients with persistent methicillin-resistant *Staphylococcus aureus* bacteremia. J Infect 2012; 65(6): 505-12. [http://dx.doi.org/10.1016/j.jinf.2012.08.007] [PMID: 22902942]

[13]   Pistella E, Campanile F, Bongiorno D, *et al.* Successful treatment of disseminated cerebritis complicating methicillin-resistant *Staphylococcus aureus* Endocarditis unresponsive to vancomycin therapy with linezolid. Scand J Infect Dis 2004; 36(3): 222-5. [http://dx.doi.org/10.1080/00365540410019345] [PMID: 15119370]

[14]   Prokocimer P, De Anda C, Fang E, Mehra P, Das A. Tedizolid phosphate *vs* linezolid for treatment of acute bacterial skin and skin structure infections: the ESTABLISH-1 randomized trial. JAMA 2013; 309(6): 559-69. [http://dx.doi.org/10.1001/jama.2013.241] [PMID: 23403680]

[15]   Moran GJ, Fang E, Corey GR, Das AF, De Anda C, Prokocimer P. Tedizolid for 6 days *versus* linezolid for 10 days for acute bacterial skin and skin-structure infections (ESTABLISH-2): a randomised, double-blind, phase 3, non-inferiority trial. Lancet Infect Dis 2014; 14(8): 696-705. [http://dx.doi.org/10.1016/S1473-3099(14)70737-6] [PMID: 24909499]

[16]   Boucher HW, Wilcox M, Talbot GH, Puttagunta S, Das AF, Dunne MW. Once-weekly dalbavancin *versus* daily conventional therapy for skin infection. N Engl J Med 2014; 370(23): 2169-79. [http://dx.doi.org/10.1056/NEJMoa1310480] [PMID: 24897082]

[17]   Corey GR, Good S, Jiang H, *et al.* Single-dose oritavancin *versus* 7-10 days of vancomycin in the treatment of gram-positive acute bacterial skin and skin structure infections: the SOLO II noninferiority study. Clin Infect Dis 2015; 60(2): 254-62. [http://dx.doi.org/10.1093/cid/ciu778] [PMID: 25294250]

[18]   Stryjewski ME, Graham DR, Wilson SE, *et al.* Telavancin *versus* vancomycin for the treatment of complicated skin and skin-structure infections caused by gram-positive organisms. Clin Infect Dis 2008; 46(11): 1683-93. [http://dx.doi.org/10.1086/587896] [PMID: 18444791]

[19]   Wilson SE, Graham DR, Wang W, Bruss JB, Castaneda-Ruiz B. Telavancin in the Treatment of Concurrent *Staphylococcus aureus* Bacteremia: A Retrospective Analysis of ATLAS and ATTAIN Studies. Infect Dis Ther 2017; 6(3): 413-22. [http://dx.doi.org/10.1007/s40121-017-0162-1] [PMID: 28695347]

[20]   Rubinstein E, Lalani T, Corey GR, *et al.* Telavancin *versus* vancomycin for hospital-acquired pneumonia due to gram-positive pathogens. Clin Infect Dis 2011; 52(1): 31-40. [http://dx.doi.org/10.1093/cid/ciq031] [PMID: 21148517]

[21]   Leonard SN, Szeto YG, Zolotarev M, Grigoryan IV. Comparative *In vitro* activity of telavancin, vancomycin and linezolid against heterogeneously vancomycin-intermediate *Staphylococcus aureus* (hVISA). Int J Antimicrob Agents 2011; 37(6): 558-61.
[http://dx.doi.org/10.1016/j.ijantimicag.2011.02.007] [PMID: 21497067]

[22]   Barber KE, Ireland CE, Bukavyn N, Rybak MJ. Observation of "seesaw effect" with vancomycin, teicoplanin, daptomycin and ceftaroline in 150 unique MRSA strains. Infect Dis Ther 2014; 3(1): 35-43.
[http://dx.doi.org/10.1007/s40121-014-0023-0] [PMID: 25134810]

[23]   Alm RA, McLaughlin RE, Kos VN, Sader HS, Iaconis JP, Lahiri SD. Analysis of *Staphylococcus aureus* clinical isolates with reduced susceptibility to ceftaroline: an epidemiological and structural perspective. J Antimicrob Chemother 2014; 69(8): 2065-75.
[http://dx.doi.org/10.1093/jac/dku114] [PMID: 24777906]

[24]   Arshad S, Huang V, Hartman P, Perri MB, Moreno D, Zervos MJ. Ceftaroline fosamil monotherapy for methicillin-resistant *Staphylococcus aureus* bacteremia: a comparative clinical outcomes study. Int J Infect Dis 2017; 57: 27-31.
[http://dx.doi.org/10.1016/j.ijid.2017.01.019] [PMID: 28131729]

[25]   McCurdy S, Lawrence L, Quintas M, *et al.* In vitro activity of delafloxacin and microbiological response against fluoroquinolone-susceptible and nonsusceptible *Staphylococcus aureus* isolates from two phase 3 studies of acute bacterial skin and skin structure infections. Antimicrob Agents Chemother 2017; 61(9): e00772-17.
[http://dx.doi.org/10.1128/AAC.00772-17] [PMID: 28630189]

[26]   Stets R, Popescu M, Gonong JR, *et al.* Omadacycline for community-acquired bacterial pneumonia. N Engl J Med 2019; 380(6): 517-27.
[http://dx.doi.org/10.1056/NEJMoa1800201] [PMID: 30726692]

[27]   O'Riordan W, Green S, Overcash JS, *et al.* Omadacycline for acute bacterial skin and skin-structure infections. N Engl J Med 2019; 380(6): 528-38.
[http://dx.doi.org/10.1056/NEJMoa1800170] [PMID: 30726689]

[28]   Moise PA, North D, Steenbergen JN, Sakoulas G. Susceptibility relationship between vancomycin and daptomycin in *Staphylococcus aureus*: facts and assumptions. Lancet Infect Dis 2009; 9(10): 617-24.
[http://dx.doi.org/10.1016/S1473-3099(09)70200-2] [PMID: 19778764]

[29]   Sakoulas G, Moise PA, Casapao AM, *et al.* Antimicrobial salvage therapy for persistent *staphylococcal bacteremia* using daptomycin plus ceftaroline. Clin Ther 2014; 36(10): 1317-33.
[http://dx.doi.org/10.1016/j.clinthera.2014.05.061] [PMID: 25017183]

[30]   Dhand A, Sakoulas G. Reduced vancomycin susceptibility among clinical *Staphylococcus aureus* isolates ('the MIC Creep'): implications for therapy. F1000 Med Rep 2012; 4: 4.
[http://dx.doi.org/10.3410/M4-4] [PMID: 22312414]

[31]   Dhand A, Bayer AS, Pogliano J, *et al.* Use of antistaphylococcal β-lactams to increase daptomycin activity in eradicating persistent bacteremia due to methicillin-resistant *Staphylococcus aureus*: role of enhanced daptomycin binding. Clin Infect Dis 2011; 53(2): 158-63.
[http://dx.doi.org/10.1093/cid/cir340] [PMID: 21690622]

[32]   Leonard SN, Rolek KM. Evaluation of the combination of daptomycin and nafcillin against vancomycin-intermediate *Staphylococcus aureus*. J Antimicrob Chemother 2013; 68(3): 644-7.
[http://dx.doi.org/10.1093/jac/dks453] [PMID: 23152482]

[33]   Smith JR, Yim J, Raut A, Rybak MJ. Oritavancin Combinations with β-Lactams against Multidrug-Resistant *Staphylococcus aureus* and Vancomycin-Resistant Enterococci. Antimicrob Agents Chemother 2016; 60(4): 2352-8.
[http://dx.doi.org/10.1128/AAC.03006-15] [PMID: 26833159]

[34]   Werth BJ, Vidaillac C, Murray KP, *et al.* Novel combinations of vancomycin plus ceftaroline or

oxacillin against methicillin-resistant vancomycin-intermediate *Staphylococcus aureus* (VISA) and heterogeneous VISA. Antimicrob Agents Chemother 2013; 57(5): 2376-9.
[http://dx.doi.org/10.1128/AAC.02354-12] [PMID: 23422917]

[35]   Arias CA, Murray BE. The rise of the Enterococcus: beyond vancomycin resistance. Nat Rev Microbiol 2012; 10(4): 266-78.
[http://dx.doi.org/10.1038/nrmicro2761] [PMID: 22421879]

[36]   Murray BE. Vancomycin-resistant enterococcal infections. N Engl J Med 2000; 342(10): 710-21.
[http://dx.doi.org/10.1056/NEJM200003093421007] [PMID: 10706902]

[37]   Cole KA, Kenney RM, Perri MB, *et al.* Outcomes of aminopenicillin therapy for vancomycin-resistant enterococcal urinary tract infections. Antimicrob Agents Chemother 2015; 59(12): 7362-6.
[http://dx.doi.org/10.1128/AAC.01817-15] [PMID: 26369973]

[38]   Steenbergen JN, Alder J, Thorne GM, Tally FP. Daptomycin: a lipopeptide antibiotic for the treatment of serious Gram-positive infections. J Antimicrob Chemother 2005; 55(3): 283-8.
[http://dx.doi.org/10.1093/jac/dkh546] [PMID: 15705644]

[39]   Balli EP, Venetis CA, Miyakis S. Systematic review and meta-analysis of linezolid *versus* daptomycin for treatment of vancomycin-resistant enterococcal bacteremia. Antimicrob Agents Chemother 2014; 58(2): 734-9.
[http://dx.doi.org/10.1128/AAC.01289-13] [PMID: 24247127]

[40]   Britt NS, Potter EM, Patel N, Steed ME. Comparison of the effectiveness and safety of linezolid and daptomycin in vancomycin-resistant enterococcal bloodstream infection: a national cohort study of veterans affairs patients. Clin Infect Dis 2015; 61(6): 871-8.
[http://dx.doi.org/10.1093/cid/civ444] [PMID: 26063715]

[41]   Britt NS, Potter EM, Patel N, Steed ME. Comparative Effectiveness and Safety of Standard-, Medium- and High-Dose Daptomycin Strategies for the Treatment of Vancomycin-Resistant Enterococcal Bacteremia Among Veterans Affairs Patients. Clin Infect Dis 2017; 64(5): 605-13.
[PMID: 28011602]

[42]   Birmingham MC, Rayner CR, Meagher AK, Flavin SM, Batts DH, Schentag JJ. Linezolid for the treatment of multidrug-resistant, gram-positive infections: experience from a compassionate-use program. Clin Infect Dis 2003; 36(2): 159-68.
[http://dx.doi.org/10.1086/345744] [PMID: 12522747]

[43]   Mermel LA, Allon M, Bouza E, *et al.* Clinical practice guidelines for the diagnosis and management of intravascular catheter-related infection: 2009 Update by the Infectious Diseases Society of America. Clin Infect Dis 2009; 49(1): 1-45.
[http://dx.doi.org/10.1086/599376] [PMID: 19489710]

[44]   Mendes RE, Woosley LN, Farrell DJ, Sader HS, Jones RN. Oritavancin activity against vancomycin-susceptible and vancomycin-resistant Enterococci with molecularly characterized glycopeptide resistance genes recovered from bacteremic patients, 2009-2010. Antimicrob Agents Chemother 2012; 56(3): 1639-42.
[http://dx.doi.org/10.1128/AAC.06067-11] [PMID: 22183169]

[45]   Winston DJ, Emmanouilides C, Kroeber A, *et al.* Quinupristin/Dalfopristin therapy for infections due to vancomycin-resistant *Enterococcus faecium.* Clin Infect Dis 2000; 30(5): 790-7.
[http://dx.doi.org/10.1086/313766] [PMID: 10817685]

[46]   Fuchs PC, Barry AL, Brown SD. Fosfomycin tromethamine susceptibility of outpatient urine isolates of *Escherichia coli* and *Enterococcus faecalis* from ten North American medical centres by three methods. J Antimicrob Chemother 1999; 43(1): 137-40.
[http://dx.doi.org/10.1093/jac/43.1.137] [PMID: 10381112]

[47]   Krause R, Mittermayer H, Feierl G, *et al.* Austrian Carbapenem Susceptibility Surveillance Group. *In vitro* activity of newer broad spectrum β-lactam antibiotics against *Enterobacteriaceae* and non-fermenters: a report from Austrian intensive care units. Wien Klin Wochenschr 1999; 111(14): 549-54.

[PMID: 10467641]

[48]   Yahav D, Lador A, Paul M, Leibovici L. Efficacy and safety of tigecycline: a systematic review and meta-analysis. J Antimicrob Chemother 2011; 66(9): 1963-71.
[http://dx.doi.org/10.1093/jac/dkr242] [PMID: 21685488]

[49]   Baddour LM, Wilson WR, Bayer AS, *et al.* American heart association committee on rheumatic fever, endocarditis, and kawasaki disease of the council on cardiovascular disease in the young, council on clinical cardiology, council on cardiovascular surgery and anesthesia, and stroke council. Infective endocarditis in adults: diagnosis, antimicrobial therapy, and management of complications: a scientific statement for healthcare professionals from the american heart association. Circulation 2015; 132(15): 1435-86.
[http://dx.doi.org/10.1161/CIR.0000000000000296] [PMID: 26373316]

[50]   Smith JR, Barber KE, Raut A, Aboutaleb M, Sakoulas G, Rybak MJ. β-Lactam combinations with daptomycin provide synergy against vancomycin-resistant *Enterococcus faecalis* and *Enterococcus faecium.* J Antimicrob Chemother 2015; 70(6): 1738-43.
[http://dx.doi.org/10.1093/jac/dkv007] [PMID: 25645208]

[51]   Sakoulas G, Bayer AS, Pogliano J, *et al.* Ampicillin enhances daptomycin- and cationic host defense peptide-mediated killing of ampicillin- and vancomycin-resistant *Enterococcus faecium.* Antimicrob Agents Chemother 2012; 56(2): 838-44.
[http://dx.doi.org/10.1128/AAC.05551-11] [PMID: 22123698]

[52]   Aeschlimann JR, Zervos MJ, Rybak MJ. Treatment of vancomycin-resistant *Enterococcus faecium* with RP 59500 (quinupristin-dalfopristin) administered by intermittent or continuous infusion, alone or in combination with doxycycline, in an *in vitro* pharmacodynamic infection model with simulated endocardial vegetations. Antimicrob Agents Chemother 1998; 42(10): 2710-7.
[http://dx.doi.org/10.1128/AAC.42.10.2710] [PMID: 9756782]

[53]   Raad I, Hachem R, Hanna H, *et al.* Treatment of vancomycin-resistant enterococcal infections in the immunocompromised host: quinupristin-dalfopristin in combination with minocycline. Antimicrob Agents Chemother 2001; 45(11): 3202-4.
[http://dx.doi.org/10.1128/AAC.45.11.3202-3204.2001] [PMID: 11600379]

[54]   Pitout JD, Laupland KB. Extended-spectrum β-lactamase-producing *Enterobacteriaceae*: an emerging public-health concern. Lancet Infect Dis 2008; 8(3): 159-66.
[http://dx.doi.org/10.1016/S1473-3099(08)70041-0] [PMID: 18291338]

[55]   Hall BG, Barlow M. Revised Ambler classification of β-lactamases. J Antimicrob Chemother 2005; 55(6): 1050-1.
[http://dx.doi.org/10.1093/jac/dki130] [PMID: 15872044]

[56]   Bush K, Jacoby GA. Updated functional classification of β-lactamases. Antimicrob Agents Chemother 2010; 54(3): 969-76.
[http://dx.doi.org/10.1128/AAC.01009-09] [PMID: 19995920]

[57]   Bradford PA. Extended-spectrum β-lactamases in the 21st century: characterization, epidemiology, and detection of this important resistance threat. Clin Microbiol Rev 2001; 14(4): 933-51. [table of contents.].
[http://dx.doi.org/10.1128/CMR.14.4.933-951.2001] [PMID: 11585791]

[58]   Jacoby GA. AmpC β-lactamases. Clin Microbiol Rev 2009; 22(1): 161-82. [Table of Contents.].
[http://dx.doi.org/10.1128/CMR.00036-08] [PMID: 19136439]

[59]   Paterson DL, Bonomo RA. Extended-spectrum β-lactamases: a clinical update. Clin Microbiol Rev 2005; 18(4): 657-86.
[http://dx.doi.org/10.1128/CMR.18.4.657-686.2005] [PMID: 16223952]

[60]   Jones RN. Important and emerging β-lactamase-mediated resistances in hospital-based pathogens: the Amp C enzymes. Diagn Microbiol Infect Dis 1998; 31(3): 461-6.
[http://dx.doi.org/10.1016/S0732-8893(98)00029-7] [PMID: 9635237]

[61]   Vardakas KZ, Tansarli GS, Rafailidis PI, Falagas ME. Carbapenems *versus* alternative antibiotics for the treatment of bacteraemia due to *Enterobacteriaceae* producing extended-spectrum β-lactamases: a systematic review and meta-analysis. J Antimicrob Chemother 2012; 67(12): 2793-803.
[http://dx.doi.org/10.1093/jac/dks301] [PMID: 22915465]

[62]   Gutiérrez-Gutiérrez B, Bonomo RA, Carmeli Y, *et al.* Ertapenem for the treatment of bloodstream infections due to ESBL-producing *Enterobacteriaceae*: a multinational pre-registered cohort study. J Antimicrob Chemother 2016; 71(6): 1672-80.
[http://dx.doi.org/10.1093/jac/dkv502] [PMID: 26907184]

[63]   Harris PN, Wei JY, Shen AW, *et al.* Carbapenems *versus* alternative antibiotics for the treatment of bloodstream infections caused by Enterobacter, Citrobacter or Serratia species: a systematic review with meta-analysis. J Antimicrob Chemother 2016; 71(2): 296-306.
[http://dx.doi.org/10.1093/jac/dkv346] [PMID: 26542304]

[64]   Chopra T, Marchaim D, Veltman J, *et al.* Impact of cefepime therapy on mortality among patients with bloodstream infections caused by extended-spectrum-β-lactamase-producing *Klebsiella pneumoniae* and *Escherichia coli.* Antimicrob Agents Chemother 2012; 56(7): 3936-42.
[http://dx.doi.org/10.1128/AAC.05419-11] [PMID: 22547616]

[65]   Lee NY, Lee CC, Huang WH, Tsui KC, Hsueh PR, Ko WC. Cefepime therapy for monomicrobial bacteremia caused by cefepime-susceptible extended-spectrum β-lactamase-producing *Enterobacteriaceae*: MIC matters. Clin Infect Dis 2013; 56(4): 488-95.
[http://dx.doi.org/10.1093/cid/cis916] [PMID: 23090931]

[66]   Lee NY, Lee CC, Li CW, *et al.* Cefepime therapy for monomicrobial enterobacter cloacae bacteremia: unfavorable outcomes in patients infected by cefepime-susceptible dose-dependent isolates. Antimicrob Agents Chemother 2015; 59(12): 7558-63.
[http://dx.doi.org/10.1128/AAC.01477-15] [PMID: 26416853]

[67]   Tamma PD, Girdwood SC, Gopaul R, *et al.* The use of cefepime for treating AmpC β-lactamas-producing *Enterobacteriaceae.* Clin Infect Dis 2013; 57(6): 781-8.
[http://dx.doi.org/10.1093/cid/cit395] [PMID: 23759352]

[68]   Tamma PD, Han JH, Rock C, *et al.* Carbapenem therapy is associated with improved survival compared with piperacillin-tazobactam for patients with extended-spectrum β-lactamase bacteremia. Clin Infect Dis 2015; 60(9): 1319-25.
[http://dx.doi.org/10.1093/cid/civ003] [PMID: 25586681]

[69]   van Duin D, Bonomo RA. Ceftazidime/avibactam and ceftolozane/tazobactam: second-generation β-Lactam/β-lactamase inhibitor combinations. Clin Infect Dis 2016; 63(2): 234-41.
[http://dx.doi.org/10.1093/cid/ciw243] [PMID: 27098166]

[70]   Carmeli Y, Armstrong J, Laud PJ, *et al.* Ceftazidime-avibactam or best available therapy in patients with ceftazidime-resistant *Enterobacteriaceae* and *Pseudomonas aeruginosa* complicated urinary tract infections or complicated intra-abdominal infections (REPRISE): a randomised, pathogen-directed, phase 3 study. Lancet Infect Dis 2016; 16(6): 661-73.
[http://dx.doi.org/10.1016/S1473-3099(16)30004-4] [PMID: 27107460]

[71]   Popejoy MW, Paterson DL, Cloutier D, *et al.* Efficacy of ceftolozane/tazobactam against urinary tract and intra-abdominal infections caused by ESBL-producing *Escherichia coli* and *Klebsiella pneumoniae*: a pooled analysis of Phase 3 clinical trials. J Antimicrob Chemother 2017; 72(1): 268-72.
[http://dx.doi.org/10.1093/jac/dkw374] [PMID: 27707990]

[72]   Paul M, Lador A, Grozinsky-Glasberg S, Leibovici L. Beta lactam antibiotic monotherapy *versus* beta lactam-aminoglycoside antibiotic combination therapy for sepsis. Cochrane Database Syst Rev 2014; (1): CD003344.
[http://dx.doi.org/10.1002/14651858.CD003344.pub3] [PMID: 24395715]

[73]   Jean SS, Coombs G, Ling T, *et al.* Epidemiology and antimicrobial susceptibility profiles of pathogens causing urinary tract infections in the Asia-Pacific region: Results from the Study for Monitoring

Antimicrobial Resistance Trends (SMART), 2010-2013. Int J Antimicrob Agents 2016; 47(4): 328-34.
[http://dx.doi.org/10.1016/j.ijantimicag.2016.01.008] [PMID: 27005459]

[74]   Haidar G, Alkroud A, Cheng S, *et al.* Association between the Presence of Aminoglycoside-Modifying Enzymes and *In vitro* Activity of Gentamicin, Tobramycin, Amikacin, and Plazomicin against *Klebsiella pneumoniae* Carbapenemase- and Extended-Spectrum-β-Lactamase-Producing Enterobacter Species. Antimicrob Agents Chemother 2016; 60(9): 5208-14.
[http://dx.doi.org/10.1128/AAC.00869-16] [PMID: 27297487]

[75]   López-Diaz MD, Culebras E, Rodríguez-Avial I, *et al.* Plazomicin Activity against 346 Extended-Spectrum-β-Lactamase/AmpC-Producing *Escherichia coli* Urinary Isolates in Relation to Aminoglycoside-Modifying Enzymes. Antimicrob Agents Chemother 2017; 61(2): e02454-16.
[http://dx.doi.org/10.1128/AAC.02454-16] [PMID: 27919895]

[76]   Tasina E, Haidich AB, Kokkali S, Arvanitidou M. Efficacy and safety of tigecycline for the treatment of infectious diseases: a meta-analysis. Lancet Infect Dis 2011; 11(11): 834-44.
[http://dx.doi.org/10.1016/S1473-3099(11)70177-3] [PMID: 21784708]

[77]   Vasilev K, Reshedko G, Orasan R, *et al.* 309 Study Group. A Phase 3, open-label, non-comparative study of tigecycline in the treatment of patients with selected serious infections due to resistant Gram-negative organisms including Enterobacter species, *Acinetobacter baumannii* and *Klebsiella pneumoniae.* J Antimicrob Chemother 2008; 62 (Suppl. 1): i29-40.
[http://dx.doi.org/10.1093/jac/dkn249] [PMID: 18684704]

[78]   Poulakou G, Kontopidou FV, Paramythiotou E, *et al.* Tigecycline in the treatment of infections from multi-drug resistant gram-negative pathogens. J Infect 2009; 58(4): 273-84.
[http://dx.doi.org/10.1016/j.jinf.2009.02.009] [PMID: 19344841]

[79]   Vardakas KZ, Legakis NJ, Triarides N, Falagas ME. Susceptibility of contemporary isolates to fosfomycin: a systematic review of the literature. Int J Antimicrob Agents 2016; 47(4): 269-85.
[http://dx.doi.org/10.1016/j.ijantimicag.2016.02.001] [PMID: 27013000]

[80]   Falagas ME, Kastoris AC, Kapaskelis AM, Karageorgopoulos DE. Fosfomycin for the treatment of multidrug-resistant, including extended-spectrum β-lactamase producing, *Enterobacteriaceae* infections: a systematic review. Lancet Infect Dis 2010; 10(1): 43-50.
[http://dx.doi.org/10.1016/S1473-3099(09)70325-1] [PMID: 20129148]

[81]   Veve MP, Wagner JL, Kenney RM, Grunwald JL, Davis SL. Comparison of fosfomycin to ertapenem for outpatient or step-down therapy of extended-spectrum β-lactamase urinary tract infections. Int J Antimicrob Agents 2016; 48(1): 56-60.
[http://dx.doi.org/10.1016/j.ijantimicag.2016.04.014] [PMID: 27234673]

[82]   Grabein B, Graninger W, Rodríguez Baño J, Dinh A, Liesenfeld DB. Intravenous fosfomycin-back to the future. Systematic review and meta-analysis of the clinical literature. Clin Microbiol Infect 2017; 23(6): 363-72.
[http://dx.doi.org/10.1016/j.cmi.2016.12.005] [PMID: 27956267]

[83]   Karageorgopoulos DE, Wang R, Yu XH, Falagas ME. Fosfomycin: evaluation of the published evidence on the emergence of antimicrobial resistance in Gram-negative pathogens. J Antimicrob Chemother 2012; 67(2): 255-68.
[http://dx.doi.org/10.1093/jac/dkr466] [PMID: 22096042]

[84]   Patel G, Huprikar S, Factor SH, Jenkins SG, Calfee DP. Outcomes of carbapenem-resistant *Klebsiella pneumoniae* infection and the impact of antimicrobial and adjunctive therapies. Infect Control Hosp Epidemiol 2008; 29(12): 1099-106.
[http://dx.doi.org/10.1086/592412] [PMID: 18973455]

[85]   Vatopoulos A. High rates of metallo-β-lactamase-producing *Klebsiella pneumoniae* in Greece--a review of the current evidence. Euro Surveill 2008; 13(4): 8023.
[PMID: 18445397]

[86]   Kumarasamy KK, Toleman MA, Walsh TR, *et al.* Emergence of a new antibiotic resistance

mechanism in India, Pakistan, and the UK: a molecular, biological, and epidemiological study. Lancet Infect Dis 2010; 10(9): 597-602.
[http://dx.doi.org/10.1016/S1473-3099(10)70143-2] [PMID: 20705517]

[87]   Hidron AI, Edwards JR, Patel J, *et al.* NHSN annual update: antimicrobial-resistant pathogens associated with healthcare-associated infections: annual summary of data reported to the National Healthcare Safety Network at the Centers for Disease Control and Prevention, 2006-2007. Infect Control Hosp Epidemiol 2008; 29(11): 996-1011.
[http://dx.doi.org/10.1086/591861] [PMID: 18947320]

[88]   Bulik CC, Nicolau DP. Double-carbapenem therapy for carbapenemase-producing *Klebsiella pneumoniae*. Antimicrob Agents Chemother 2011; 55(6): 3002-4.
[http://dx.doi.org/10.1128/AAC.01420-10] [PMID: 21422205]

[89]   Oliva A, D'Abramo A, D'Agostino C, *et al.* Synergistic activity and effectiveness of a double-carbapenem regimen in pandrug-resistant *Klebsiella pneumoniae* bloodstream infections. J Antimicrob Chemother 2014; 69(6): 1718-20.
[http://dx.doi.org/10.1093/jac/dku027] [PMID: 24521856]

[90]   Karaiskos I, Antoniadou A, Giamarellou H. Combination therapy for extensively-drug resistant gram-negative bacteria. Expert Rev Anti Infect Ther 2017; 15(12): 1123-40.
[http://dx.doi.org/10.1080/14787210.2017.1410434] [PMID: 29172792]

[91]   Shirley M. Ceftazidime-avibactam: a review in the treatment of serious gram-negative bacterial infections. Drugs 2018; 78(6): 675-92.
[http://dx.doi.org/10.1007/s40265-018-0902-x] [PMID: 29671219]

[92]   MacVane SH, Crandon JL, Nichols WW, Nicolau DP. *In vivo* efficacy of humanized exposures of Ceftazidime-Avibactam in comparison with Ceftazidime against contemporary *Enterobacteriaceae* isolates. Antimicrob Agents Chemother 2014; 58(11): 6913-9.
[http://dx.doi.org/10.1128/AAC.03267-14] [PMID: 25223999]

[93]   Shields RK, Potoski BA, Haidar G, *et al.* Clinical outcomes, drug toxicity, and emergence of ceftazidime-avibactam resistance among patients treated for carbapenem-resistant *Enterobacteriaceae* infections. Clin Infect Dis 2016; 63(12): 1615-8.
[http://dx.doi.org/10.1093/cid/ciw636] [PMID: 27624958]

[94]   Tumbarello M, Trecarichi EM, Corona A, *et al.* Efficacy of Ceftazidime-Avibactam Salvage Therapy in Patients With Infections Caused by *Klebsiella pneumoniae* Carbapenemase-producing *K. pneumoniae*. Clin Infect Dis 2019; 68(3): 355-64.
[http://dx.doi.org/10.1093/cid/ciy492] [PMID: 29893802]

[95]   Satlin MJ, Kubin CJ, Blumenthal JS, *et al.* Comparative effectiveness of aminoglycosides, polymyxin B, and tigecycline for clearance of carbapenem-resistant *Klebsiella pneumoniae* from urine. Antimicrob Agents Chemother 2011; 55(12): 5893-9.
[http://dx.doi.org/10.1128/AAC.00387-11] [PMID: 21968368]

[96]   Tzouvelekis LS, Markogiannakis A, Piperaki E, Souli M, Daikos GL. Treating infections caused by carbapenemase-producing *Enterobacteriaceae*. Clin Microbiol Infect 2014; 20(9): 862-72.
[http://dx.doi.org/10.1111/1469-0691.12697] [PMID: 24890393]

[97]   Connolly LJA, O'Keeffe B, Serio A, *et al.* 2017.

[98]   Vardakas KZ, Falagas ME. Colistin *versus* polymyxin B for the treatment of patients with multidrug-resistant Gram-negative infections: a systematic review and meta-analysis. Int J Antimicrob Agents 2017; 49(2): 233-8.
[http://dx.doi.org/10.1016/j.ijantimicag.2016.07.023] [PMID: 27686609]

[99]   Hirsch EB, Tam VH. Detection and treatment options for *Klebsiella pneumoniae* carbapenemases (KPCs): an emerging cause of multidrug-resistant infection. J Antimicrob Chemother 2010; 65(6): 1119-25.
[http://dx.doi.org/10.1093/jac/dkq108] [PMID: 20378670]

[100] Zusman O, Altunin S, Koppel F, Dishon Benattar Y, Gedik H, Paul M. Polymyxin monotherapy or in combination against carbapenem-resistant bacteria: systematic review and meta-analysis. J Antimicrob Chemother 2017; 72(1): 29-39.
[http://dx.doi.org/10.1093/jac/dkw377] [PMID: 27624572]

[101] Ni W, Han Y, Liu J, *et al.* Tigecycline Treatment for Carbapenem-Resistant *Enterobacteriaceae* Infections: A Systematic Review and Meta-Analysis. Medicine (Baltimore) 2016; 95(11): e3126.
[http://dx.doi.org/10.1097/MD.0000000000003126] [PMID: 26986165]

[102] Livermore DM, Mushtaq S, Warner M, Woodford N. *In vitro* Activity of Eravacycline against Carbapenem-Resistant *Enterobacteriaceae* and *Acinetobacter baumannii*. Antimicrob Agents Chemother 2016; 60(6): 3840-4.
[http://dx.doi.org/10.1128/AAC.00436-16] [PMID: 27044556]

[103] Pontikis K, Karaiskos I, Bastani S, *et al.* Outcomes of critically ill intensive care unit patients treated with fosfomycin for infections due to pandrug-resistant and extensively drug-resistant carbapenemase-producing Gram-negative bacteria. Int J Antimicrob Agents 2014; 43(1): 52-9.
[http://dx.doi.org/10.1016/j.ijantimicag.2013.09.010] [PMID: 24183799]

[104] Karageorgopoulos DE, Miriagou V, Tzouvelekis LS, Spyridopoulou K, Daikos GL. Emergence of resistance to fosfomycin used as adjunct therapy in KPC *Klebsiella pneumoniae* bacteraemia: report of three cases. J Antimicrob Chemother 2012; 67(11): 2777-9.
[http://dx.doi.org/10.1093/jac/dks270] [PMID: 22782489]

[105] Castanheira M, Huband MD, Mendes RE, Flamm RK. Meropenem-vaborbactam tested against contemporary gram-negative isolates collected worldwide during 2014, including carbapenem-resistant, kpc-producing, multidrug-resistant, and extensively drug-resistant *Enterobacteriaceae*. Antimicrob Agents Chemother 2017; 61(9): e00567-17.
[http://dx.doi.org/10.1128/AAC.00567-17] [PMID: 28652234]

[106] Kaye KS, Bhowmick T, Metallidis S, *et al.* Effect of meropenem-vaborbactam *vs* piperacillin-tazobactam on clinical cure or improvement and microbial eradication in complicated urinary tract infection: the tango i randomized clinical trial. JAMA 2018; 319(8): 788-99.
[http://dx.doi.org/10.1001/jama.2018.0438] [PMID: 29486041]

[107] Wunderink RG, Giamarellos-Bourboulis EJ, Rahav G, *et al.* Effect and Safety of Meropenem-Vaborbactam *versus* Best-Available Therapy in Patients with Carbapenem-Resistant *Enterobacteriaceae* Infections: The TANGO II Randomized Clinical Trial. Infect Dis Ther 2018; 7(4): 439-55.
[http://dx.doi.org/10.1007/s40121-018-0214-1] [PMID: 30270406]

[108] Livermore DM. Multiple mechanisms of antimicrobial resistance in *Pseudomonas aeruginosa*: our worst nightmare? Clin Infect Dis 2002; 34(5): 634-40.
[http://dx.doi.org/10.1086/338782] [PMID: 11823954]

[109] Aloush V, Navon-Venezia S, Seigman-Igra Y, Cabili S, Carmeli Y. Multidrug-resistant *Pseudomonas aeruginosa*: risk factors and clinical impact. Antimicrob Agents Chemother 2006; 50(1): 43-8.
[http://dx.doi.org/10.1128/AAC.50.1.43-48.2006] [PMID: 16377665]

[110] Li XZ, Zhang L, Poole K. Interplay between the MexA-MexB-OprM multidrug efflux system and the outer membrane barrier in the multiple antibiotic resistance of *Pseudomonas aeruginosa*. J Antimicrob Chemother 2000; 45(4): 433-6.
[http://dx.doi.org/10.1093/jac/45.4.433] [PMID: 10747818]

[111] Dubois V, Arpin C, Melon M, *et al.* Nosocomial outbreak due to a multiresistant strain of *Pseudomonas aeruginosa* P12: efficacy of cefepime-amikacin therapy and analysis of β-lactam resistance. J Clin Microbiol 2001; 39(6): 2072-8.
[http://dx.doi.org/10.1128/JCM.39.6.2072-2078.2001] [PMID: 11376037]

[112] Domenig C, Traunmüller F, Kozek S, *et al.* Continuous β-lactam antibiotic therapy in a double-lung transplanted patient with a multidrug-resistant *Pseudomonas aeruginosa* infection. Transplantation

2001; 71(6): 744-5.
[http://dx.doi.org/10.1097/00007890-200103270-00009] [PMID: 11330535]

[113] Levin AS, Barone AA, Pénço J, *et al.* Intravenous colistin as therapy for nosocomial infections caused by multidrug-resistant *Pseudomonas aeruginosa* and *Acinetobacter baumannii*. Clin Infect Dis 1999; 28(5): 1008-11.
[http://dx.doi.org/10.1086/514732] [PMID: 10452626]

[114] Ouderkirk JP, Nord JA, Turett GS, Kislak JW. Polymyxin B nephrotoxicity and efficacy against nosocomial infections caused by multiresistant gram-negative bacteria. Antimicrob Agents Chemother 2003; 47(8): 2659-62.
[http://dx.doi.org/10.1128/AAC.47.8.2659-2662.2003] [PMID: 12878536]

[115] Linden PK, Kusne S, Coley K, Fontes P, Kramer DJ, Paterson D. Use of parenteral colistin for the treatment of serious infection due to antimicrobial-resistant *Pseudomonas aeruginosa*. Clin Infect Dis 2003; 37(11): e154-60.
[http://dx.doi.org/10.1086/379611] [PMID: 14614688]

[116] Sader HS, Castanheira M, Mendes RE, Flamm RK, Farrell DJ, Jones RN. Ceftazidime-avibactam activity against multidrug-resistant *Pseudomonas aeruginosa* isolated in U.S. medical centers in 2012 and 2013. Antimicrob Agents Chemother 2015; 59(6): 3656-9.
[http://dx.doi.org/10.1128/AAC.05024-14] [PMID: 25845861]

[117] Alatoom A, Elsayed H, Lawlor K, *et al.* Comparison of antimicrobial activity between ceftolozane-tazobactam and ceftazidime-avibactam against multidrug-resistant isolates of *Escherichia coli*, *Klebsiella pneumoniae*, and *Pseudomonas aeruginosa*. Int J Infect Dis 2017; 62: 39-43.
[http://dx.doi.org/10.1016/j.ijid.2017.06.007] [PMID: 28610832]

[118] Munita JM, Aitken SL, Miller WR, *et al.* Multicenter evaluation of ceftolozane/tazobactam for serious infections caused by carbapenem-resistant *Pseudomonas aeruginosa*. Clin Infect Dis 2017; 65(1): 158-61.
[http://dx.doi.org/10.1093/cid/cix014] [PMID: 28329350]

[119] Haidar G, Philips NJ, Shields RK, *et al.* Ceftolozane-tazobactam for the treatment of multidrug-resistant *Pseudomonas aeruginosa* infections: clinical effectiveness and evolution of resistance. Clin Infect Dis 2017; 65(1): 110-20.
[http://dx.doi.org/10.1093/cid/cix182] [PMID: 29017262]

[120] Castón JJ, De la Torre Á, Ruiz-Camps I, Sorlí ML, Torres V, Torre-Cisneros J. Salvage therapy with ceftolozane-tazobactam for multidrug-resistant *Pseudomonas aeruginosa* infections. Antimicrob Agents Chemother 2017; 61(3): e02136-16.
[http://dx.doi.org/10.1128/AAC.02136-16] [PMID: 27956431]

[121] Temkin E, Torre-Cisneros J, Beovic B, *et al.* Ceftazidime-avibactam as salvage therapy for infections caused by carbapenem-resistant organisms. Antimicrob Agents Chemother 2017; 61(2): e01964-16.
[http://dx.doi.org/10.1128/AAC.01964-16] [PMID: 27895014]

[122] Ito A, Sato T, Ota M, *et al. In vitro* antibacterial properties of cefiderocol, a novel siderophore cephalosporin, against gram-negative bacteria. Antimicrob Agents Chemother 2017; 62(1): e01454-17.
[http://dx.doi.org/10.1128/AAC.01454-17] [PMID: 29061741]

[123] Portsmouth S, van Veenhuyzen D, Echols R, *et al.* Cefiderocol *versus* imipenem-cilastatin for the treatment of complicated urinary tract infections caused by Gram-negative uropathogens: a phase 2, randomised, double-blind, non-inferiority trial. Lancet Infect Dis 2018; 18(12): 1319-28.
[http://dx.doi.org/10.1016/S1473-3099(18)30554-1] [PMID: 30509675]

[124] Hsueh SC, Lee YJ, Huang YT, Liao CH, Tsuji M, Hsueh PR. *In vitro* activities of cefiderocol, ceftolozane/tazobactam, ceftazidime/avibactam and other comparative drugs against imipenem-resistant *Pseudomonas aeruginosa* and *Acinetobacter baumannii*, and *Stenotrophomonas maltophilia*, all associated with bloodstream infections in Taiwan. J Antimicrob Chemother 2019; 74(2): 380-6.
[http://dx.doi.org/10.1093/jac/dky425] [PMID: 30357343]

[125] Edgeworth JD, Merante D, Patel S, *et al.* Compassionate use of cefiderocol as adjunctive treatment of native aortic valve endocarditis due to XDR-*Pseudomonas aeruginosa*. Clin Infect Dis 2019; 68(11): 1932-4.

[126] Lob SH, Hackel MA, Kazmierczak KM, *et al. In vitro* Activity of Imipenem-Relebactam against Gram-Negative ESKAPE Pathogens Isolated by Clinical Laboratories in the United States in 2015 (Results from the SMART Global Surveillance Program). Antimicrob Agents Chemother 2017; 61(6): e02209-16.
[http://dx.doi.org/10.1128/AAC.02209-16] [PMID: 28320716]

[127] Lapuebla A, Abdallah M, Olafisoye O, *et al.* Activity of imipenem with relebactam against gram-negative pathogens from New York City. Antimicrob Agents Chemother 2015; 59(8): 5029-31.
[http://dx.doi.org/10.1128/AAC.00830-15] [PMID: 26014931]

[128] Karlowsky JA, Kazmierczak KM, de Jonge BLM, Hackel MA, Sahm DF, Bradford PA. *In vitro* Activity of Aztreonam-Avibactam against *Enterobacteriaceae* and *Pseudomonas aeruginosa* Isolated by Clinical Laboratories in 40 Countries from 2012 to 2015. Antimicrob Agents Chemother 2017; 61(9): e00472-17.
[http://dx.doi.org/10.1128/AAC.00472-17] [PMID: 28630192]

[129] Crandon JL, Nicolau DP. Human simulated studies of aztreonam and aztreonam-avibactam to evaluate activity against challenging gram-negative organisms, including metallo-β-lactamase producers. Antimicrob Agents Chemother 2013; 57(7): 3299-306.
[http://dx.doi.org/10.1128/AAC.01989-12] [PMID: 23650162]

[130] Connolly LE, Riddle V, Cebrik D, Armstrong ES, Miller LGA. A Multicenter, Randomized, Double-Blind, Phase 2 Study of the Efficacy and Safety of Plazomicin Compared with Levofloxacin in the Treatment of Complicated Urinary Tract Infection and Acute Pyelonephritis. Antimicrob Agents Chemother 2018; 62(4): e01989-17.
[http://dx.doi.org/10.1128/AAC.01989-17] [PMID: 29378708]

[131] Thwaites M, Hall D, Stoneburner A, *et al.* Activity of plazomicin in combination with other antibiotics against multidrug-resistant *Enterobacteriaceae*. Diagn Microbiol Infect Dis 2018; 92(4): 338-45.
[http://dx.doi.org/10.1016/j.diagmicrobio.2018.07.006] [PMID: 30097297]

[132] Mogle BT, Steele JM, Thomas SJ, Bohan KH, Kufel WD. Clinical review of delafloxacin: a novel anionic fluoroquinolone. J Antimicrob Chemother 2018; 73(6): 1439-51.
[http://dx.doi.org/10.1093/jac/dkx543] [PMID: 29425340]

[133] Molter G, Seifert H, Mandraka F, *et al.* Outbreak of carbapenem-resistant *Acinetobacter baumannii* in the intensive care unit: a multi-level strategic management approach. J Hosp Infect 2016; 92(2): 194-8.
[http://dx.doi.org/10.1016/j.jhin.2015.11.007] [PMID: 26778130]

[134] https://gis.cdc.gov/grasp/PSA/MapView.html

[135] Livermore DM. The threat from the pink corner. Ann Med 2003; 35(4): 226-34.
[http://dx.doi.org/10.1080/07853890310001609] [PMID: 12846264]

[136] Falagas ME, Kopterides P, Siempos II. Attributable mortality of *Acinetobacter baumannii* infection among critically ill patients. Clin Infect Dis 2006; 43: 388-9.

[137] Poirel L, Nordmann P. Carbapenem resistance in *Acinetobacter baumannii*: mechanisms and epidemiology. Clin Microbiol Infect 2006; 12(9): 826-36.
[http://dx.doi.org/10.1111/j.1469-0691.2006.01456.x] [PMID: 16882287]

[138] Bou G, Cerveró G, Domínguez MA, Quereda C, Martínez-Beltrán J. Characterization of a nosocomial outbreak caused by a multiresistant *Acinetobacter baumannii* strain with a carbapenem-hydrolyzing enzyme: high-level carbapenem resistance in *A. baumannii* is not due solely to the presence of β-lactamases. J Clin Microbiol 2000; 38(9): 3299-305.
[http://dx.doi.org/10.1128/JCM.38.9.3299-3305.2000] [PMID: 10970374]

[139] Costa SF, Woodcock J, Gill M, *et al.* Outer-membrane proteins pattern and detection of β-lactamases

in clinical isolates of imipenem-resistant *Acinetobacter baumannii* from Brazil. Int J Antimicrob Agents 2000; 13(3): 175-82.
[http://dx.doi.org/10.1016/S0924-8579(99)00123-5] [PMID: 10724021]

[140] Mussi MA, Limansky AS, Viale AM. Acquisition of resistance to carbapenems in multidrug-resistant clinical strains of *Acinetobacter baumannii*: natural insertional inactivation of a gene encoding a member of a novel family of β-barrel outer membrane proteins. Antimicrob Agents Chemother 2005; 49(4): 1432-40.
[http://dx.doi.org/10.1128/AAC.49.4.1432-1440.2005] [PMID: 15793123]

[141] Dupont M, Pagès JM, Lafitte D, Siroy A, Bollet C. Identification of an OprD homologue in *Acinetobacter baumannii*. J Proteome Res 2005; 4(6): 2386-90.
[http://dx.doi.org/10.1021/pr050143q] [PMID: 16335991]

[142] Potron A, Poirel L, Nordmann P. Emerging broad-spectrum resistance in *Pseudomonas aeruginosa* and *Acinetobacter baumannii*: Mechanisms and epidemiology. Int J Antimicrob Agents 2015; 45(6): 568-85.
[http://dx.doi.org/10.1016/j.ijantimicag.2015.03.001] [PMID: 25857949]

[143] Levin AS. Multiresistant Acinetobacter infections: a role for sulbactam combinations in overcoming an emerging worldwide problem. Clin Microbiol Infect 2002; 8(3): 144-53.
[http://dx.doi.org/10.1046/j.1469-0691.2002.00415.x] [PMID: 12010169]

[144] Michalopoulos A, Kasiakou SK, Rosmarakis ES, Falagas ME. Cure of multidrug-resistant *Acinetobacter baumannii* bacteraemia with continuous intravenous infusion of colistin. Scand J Infect Dis 2005; 37(2): 142-5.
[http://dx.doi.org/10.1080/00365540410020776-1] [PMID: 15764204]

[145] Montero A, Ariza J, Corbella X, *et al.* Antibiotic combinations for serious infections caused by carbapenem-resistant *Acinetobacter baumannii* in a mouse pneumonia model. J Antimicrob Chemother 2004; 54(6): 1085-91.
[http://dx.doi.org/10.1093/jac/dkh485] [PMID: 15546972]

[146] Nepka M, Perivolioti E, Kraniotaki E, Politi L, Tsakris A, Pournaras S. *In vitro* Bactericidal Activity of Trimethoprim-Sulfamethoxazole Alone and in Combination with Colistin against Carbapenem-Resistant *Acinetobacter baumannii* Clinical Isolates. Antimicrob Agents Chemother 2016; 60(11): 6903-6.
[http://dx.doi.org/10.1128/AAC.01082-16] [PMID: 27550356]

[147] Cheng A, Chuang YC, Sun HY, *et al.* Excess Mortality Associated With Colistin-Tigecycline Compared With Colistin-Carbapenem Combination Therapy for Extensively Drug-Resistant *Acinetobacter baumannii* Bacteremia: A Multicenter Prospective Observational Study. Crit Care Med 2015; 43(6): 1194-204.
[http://dx.doi.org/10.1097/CCM.0000000000000933] [PMID: 25793437]

[148] Ni W, Han Y, Zhao J, *et al.* Tigecycline treatment experience against multidrug-resistant *Acinetobacter baumannii* infections: a systematic review and meta-analysis. Int J Antimicrob Agents 2016; 47(2): 107-16.
[http://dx.doi.org/10.1016/j.ijantimicag.2015.11.011] [PMID: 26742726]

[149] Lenhard JR, Thamlikitkul V, Silveira FP, *et al.* Polymyxin-resistant, carbapenem-resistant *Acinetobacter baumannii* is eradicated by a triple combination of agents that lack individual activity. J Antimicrob Chemother 2017; 72(5): 1415-20.
[http://dx.doi.org/10.1093/jac/dkx002] [PMID: 28333347]

[150] Seifert H, Stefanik D, Sutcliffe JA, Higgins PG. *In-vitro* activity of the novel fluorocycline eravacycline against carbapenem non-susceptible *Acinetobacter baumannii*. Int J Antimicrob Agents 2018; 51(1): 62-4.
[http://dx.doi.org/10.1016/j.ijantimicag.2017.06.022] [PMID: 28705668]

[151] García-Salguero C, Rodríguez-Avial I, Picazo JJ, Culebras E. Can Plazomicin Alone or in

Combination Be a Therapeutic Option against Carbapenem-Resistant *Acinetobacter baumannii*? Antimicrob Agents Chemother 2015; 59(10): 5959-66.
[http://dx.doi.org/10.1128/AAC.00873-15] [PMID: 26169398]

[152] Arikan-Akdagli S, Ghannoum M, Meis JF. Antifungal Resistance: Specific Focus on Multidrug Resistance in *Candida auris* and Secondary Azole Resistance in *Aspergillus fumigatus*. J Fungi (Basel) 2018; 4(4): E129.
[http://dx.doi.org/10.3390/jof4040129] [PMID: 30563053]

[153] Lockhart SR, Etienne KA, Vallabhaneni S, *et al.* Simultaneous Emergence of Multidrug-Resistant *Candida auris* on 3 Continents Confirmed by Whole-Genome Sequencing and Epidemiological Analyses. Clin Infect Dis 2017; 64(2): 134-40.
[http://dx.doi.org/10.1093/cid/ciw691] [PMID: 27988485]

[154] Arensman K, Miller JL, Chiang A, *et al.* Clinical outcomes of patients treated for *Candida auris* infections in a multisite health system, Illinois, USA. Emerg Infect Dis 2020; 26(5): 876-80.
[http://dx.doi.org/10.3201/eid2605.191588] [PMID: 32310077]

[155] Kwon YJ, Shin JH, Byun SA, *et al. Candida auris* Clinical Isolates from South Korea: Identification, Antifungal Susceptibility, and Genotyping. J Clin Microbiol 2019; 57(4): e01624-18.
[http://dx.doi.org/10.1128/JCM.01624-18] [PMID: 30728190]

[156] Kathuria S, Singh PK, Sharma C, *et al.* Multidrug-Resistant *Candida auris* Misidentified as Candida haemulonii: Characterization by Matrix-Assisted Laser Desorption Ionization-Time of Flight Mass Spectrometry and DNA Sequencing and Its Antifungal Susceptibility Profile Variability by Vitek 2, CLSI Broth Microdilution, and Etest Method. J Clin Microbiol 2015; 53(6): 1823-30.
[http://dx.doi.org/10.1128/JCM.00367-15] [PMID: 25809970]

[157] Cortegiani A, Misseri G, Fasciana T, Giammanco A, Giarratano A, Chowdhary A. Epidemiology, clinical characteristics, resistance, and treatment of infections by *Candida auris*. J Intensive Care 2018; 6: 69.
[http://dx.doi.org/10.1186/s40560-018-0342-4] [PMID: 30397481]

[158] Rybak JM, Doorley LA, Nishimoto AT, Barker KS, Palmer GE, Rogers PD. Abrogation of triazole resistance upon deletion of CDR1 in a clinical isolate of *Candida auris*. Antimicrob Agents Chemother 2019; 63(4): e00057-19.
[http://dx.doi.org/10.1128/AAC.00057-19] [PMID: 30718246]

[159] Arendrup MC, Patterson TF. 2017.

[160] Osei Sekyere J. *Candida auris*: A systematic review and meta-analysis of current updates on an emerging multidrug-resistant pathogen. MicrobiologyOpen 2018; 7(4): e00578.
[http://dx.doi.org/10.1002/mbo3.578] [PMID: 29345117]

[161] Chowdhary A, Prakash A, Sharma C, *et al.* A multicentre study of antifungal susceptibility patterns among 350 *Candida auris* isolates (2009-17) in India: role of the ERG11 and FKS1 genes in azole and echinocandin resistance. J Antimicrob Chemother 2018; 73(4): 891-9.
[http://dx.doi.org/10.1093/jac/dkx480] [PMID: 29325167]

[162] Chowdhary A, Sharma C, Meis JF. *Candida auris*: A rapidly emerging cause of hospital-acquired multidrug-resistant fungal infections globally. PLoS Pathog 2017; 13(5): e1006290.
[http://dx.doi.org/10.1371/journal.ppat.1006290] [PMID: 28542486]

[163] Eldesouky HE, Li X, Abutaleb NS, Mohammad H, Seleem MN. Synergistic interactions of sulfamethoxazole and azole antifungal drugs against emerging multidrug-resistant *Candida auris*. Int J Antimicrob Agents 2018; 52(6): 754-61.
[http://dx.doi.org/10.1016/j.ijantimicag.2018.08.016] [PMID: 30145250]

[164] Berkow EL, Angulo D, Lockhart SR. *In vitro* Activity of a novel glucan synthase inhibitor, scy-078, against clinical isolates of *Candida auris*. Antimicrob Agents Chemother 2017; 61(7): e00435-17.
[http://dx.doi.org/10.1128/AAC.00435-17] [PMID: 28483955]

[165] Angulo D, Tufa M, Azie N. A phase 2b, dose-selection study evaluating the efficacy and safety of oral ibrexafungerp *vs* fluconazole in vulvovaginal candidiasis (DOVE). Amer J Obs and Gyn 2019.
[http://dx.doi.org/10.1016/j.ajog.2019.10.088]

[166] Sofjan AK, Mitchell A, Shah DN, *et al.* Rezafungin (CD101), a next-generation echinocandin: A systematic literature review and assessment of possible place in therapy. J Glob Antimicrob Resist 2018; 14: 58-64.
[http://dx.doi.org/10.1016/j.jgar.2018.02.013] [PMID: 29486356]

[167] Hager CL, Larkin EL, Long LA, Ghannoum MA. Evaluation of the efficacy of rezafungin, a novel echinocandin, in the treatment of disseminated *Candida auris* infection using an immunocompromised mouse model. J Antimicrob Chemother 2018; 73(8): 2085-8.
[http://dx.doi.org/10.1093/jac/dky153] [PMID: 29897469]

[168] Wiederhold NP. Antifungal resistance: current trends and future strategies to combat. Infect Drug Resist 2017; 10: 249-59.
[http://dx.doi.org/10.2147/IDR.S124918] [PMID: 28919789]

[169] Wiederhold NP, Lockhart SR, Najvar LK, *et al.* The Fungal Cyp51-Specific Inhibitor VT-1598 Demonstrates *In vitro* and *In Vivo* Activity against *Candida auris*. Antimicrob Agents Chemother 2019; 63(3): e02233-18.
[http://dx.doi.org/10.1128/AAC.02233-18] [PMID: 30530603]

[170] Hager CL, Larkin EL, Long L, Zohra Abidi F, Shaw KJ, Ghannoum MA. *In vitro* and *In Vivo* Evaluation of the Antifungal Activity of APX001A/APX001 against *Candida auris*. Antimicrob Agents Chemother 2018; 62(3): e02319-17.
[http://dx.doi.org/10.1128/AAC.02319-17] [PMID: 29311065]

CHAPTER 9

Antimicrobial Therapeutic Drug Monitoring

Rim W. Rafeh[1], Kamilia Abdelraouf[2], Nisrine Haddad[3], Nesrine Rizk[4] and Ahmed F. El-Yazbi[1,5], *

[1] *Department of Pharmacology and Toxicology, Faculty of Medicine and Medical Center, the American University of Beirut, Beirut, Lebanon*

[2] *Center of Anti-infective Research and Development, Hartford Hospital, Hartford, Connecticut, USA*

[3] *Department of Pharmacy, the American University of Beirut Medical Center, Beirut, Lebanon*

[4] *Division of Infectious Diseases, Department of Internal Medicine and Medical Center, the American University of Beirut, Lebanon*

[5] *Department of Pharmacology and Toxicology, Faculty of Pharmacy, Alexandria University, Egypt*

Abstract: Therapeutic Drug Monitoring (TDM) is the art of measuring the levels of a therapeutic agent in body fluids, most commonly plasma, and interpreting the results in order to adjust dosing such that therapeutic benefit is maximized and toxic effects are prevented. With respect to antibiotics, TDM was traditionally viewed as a method to curtail the side effects of agents with narrow therapeutic indices. However, with improved understanding of pharmacokinetic differences in various patient populations, TDM is evolving to a method by which to ensure adequate benefit in patients whose pharmacokinetic status is in question. Moreover, the ever-increasing surge in antimicrobial-resistant organisms is calling for this practice once more, this time to ensure that drug concentrations are maintained sufficiently large in order to combat infections with such organisms. This book chapter details the use of TDM in different patient populations and for different antimicrobials, with emphasis on how reference PK/PD parameters and drug levels are determined.

Keywords: Aminoglycosides, Antimicrobial Agents, Beta Lactams, Critically Ill Patients, Fluoroquinolones, Glycopeptides, Linezolid, Minimum Inhibitory Concentration, Pharmacodynamics, Pharmacokinetics, PK/PD index, Therapeutic Drug Monitoring, Vancomycin.

INTRODUCTION

Therapeutic drug monitoring (TDM) is the practice of measuring the levels of a

* **Corresponding Author Ahmed F. El-Yazbi:** Department of Pharmacology and Toxicology, Faculty of Medicine and Medical Center, the American University of Beirut, Beirut, Lebanon; Tel: +961 1350 000; EXT: 4779; E-mail: ae88@aub.edu.lb

Islam M. Ghazi & Michael J. Cawley (Eds.)

substance in whole blood, serum, or plasma, and interpreting the results in order to inform clinical decisions regarding dose adjustments and prescribing procedures. The rationale for TDM stems from the fact that certain drugs, although highly effective, have a narrow therapeutic index or exhibit significant interpatient pharmacokinetic variability, such that the dose calculated based on established pharmacokinetic parameters may greatly exceed or fall short of the actual dose required to land within the therapeutic window of the drug. Thus, TDM is used in this context as a mode of individualizing drug therapy in a pharmacokinetically diverse population, by assessing whether the administered dose of the drug is sufficient to attain an effective level while remaining below toxic levels [1].

TDM: RATIONALE AND DRUG CHARACTERISTICS

The success of any antimicrobial treatment depends on the selection of adequate antibiotics, and their administration at the appropriate dosage using the most effective route for an appropriate duration [2]. Drug dosage can usually be adjusted by monitoring clinical parameters that are indicative of the drug's therapeutic benefit or failure. In the case of antimicrobials, clinical parameters that reflect antimicrobial therapeutic effect include signs and symptoms (*e.g.* a decrease in fever, tachycardia, or confusion), laboratory values (*e.g.* a decrease in leukocyte count), and radiologic findings (*e.g.* a decrease in the size of an abscess or consolidation). Thus, TDM is usually carried out in order to prevent adverse outcomes of treatment, rather than ensure therapeutic success. For example, TDM of vancomycin was advocated after the drug was associated with nephrotoxicity, infusion-related toxicity, and ototoxicity [3, 4]. Moreover, the benefits of TDM in aminoglycosides have been demonstrated since 1979, when Bootman *et al.* reported that burn patients with gram-negative sepsis who were treated with gentamicin had a lower mortality rate if their gentamicin doses were individualized by TDM [5].

However, the incidence of side effects is not the only pre-requisite to recommend TDM of a certain antimicrobial. Drugs must possess a number of criteria in order to be suitable for TDM, including having a narrow target range, significant pharmacokinetic variability, a correlation between plasma concentration and clinical effects (both toxic and therapeutic), an established target concentration range, and the availability of a cost-effective drug assay [6].

The goal of any drug therapy is to achieve an adequate therapeutic response while minimizing toxicity. In the case of antimicrobials, mounting challenges related to the emergence of antimicrobial resistance render the need for therapy optimization to minimize resistance crucial [7, 8]. As will be discussed below in more detail, TDM could be utilized to achieve these purposes.

MECHANISTIC BASIS OF TDM

Appropriate dosing decisions are driven by the principles of pharmacokinetics (PK) and pharmacodynamics (PD), and PK/PD studies are usually performed to identify the dosage at which to administer a novel drug in clinical trials [9]. The use of PK/PD studies to individualize therapy involving marketed antimicrobials has garnered minimal support, mainly due to insufficient clinical evidence and the potential of increased cost and personnel requirement [10]; yet the information provided by these studies forms the basis for the models and procedures employed in antimicrobial TDM. Selection of the parameters measured in routine TDM including peak and/or trough serum concentrations, together with the timing of such measurements, is based on information supplied by these basic PK/PD studies.

From a PD perspective, antibiotics are classified into three categories based on the index that best correlates with their antimicrobial effect: concentration-dependent killing, time-dependent killing, or a combination of both. Time-dependent antibiotics, like beta-lactams, require the amount of antibiotic in the bloodstream to be maintained above a low cutoff point, usually the minimal inhibitory concentration (MIC), for a sufficient amount of time. Increasing the concentration of antibiotic beyond this cutoff point serves no additional benefit. In contrast, concentration-dependent antibiotics such as aminoglycosides increase in efficacy as their bloodstream concentration increases. A number of drugs exhibit a combination of both concentration-dependent and time-dependent characteristics [11, 12]. As such, each of these groups will require a different set of parameters in order to adequately describe the relationship between antibiotic exposure and bacterial response [13]. The commonly used indices are the maximal plasma concentration (C_{max}) of the antibacterial/MIC, area under the plasma concentration vs. time curve (AUC)/MIC, and time where plasma concentration is above MIC (T>MIC). It is noteworthy that all PK parameters measured pertain to the free (plasma protein-unbound) fraction of the antibacterial.

The PK/PD index most representative of *in vivo* efficacy, and thus most useful for the purpose of TDM, will differ among antimicrobial classes due to the previously described variations on their PD parameters. For instance, beta-lactams, which exhibit time-dependent killing, are best described by the duration that the unbound antibiotic concentration exceeds the MIC ($fT_{>MIC}$). In contrast, aminoglycosides, which demonstrate concentration-dependent killing, are better represented by the ratio of the maximal unbound drug concentration to the MIC

$((fC_{max})/MIC)$. On the other hand, drugs that follow a combination of time- and concentration-dependent killing are best described by the ratio of the area under the unbound drug concentration-time curve to the MIC ($fAUC/MIC$). The decision to use one of these parameters will determine the optimal timing for serum sampling and the reference values for drug concentration. In this section, we will provide an outline of the series of experiments used to determine the type and magnitude of PK/PD parameter that is best-suited to describe the efficacy of a given antimicrobial.

In vitro Infection Models

PK/PD investigation commences *in vitro*, where time- *vs.* concentration-dependent killing properties are assessed using time-kill experiments. Several studies utilized PK/PD modelling of time-kill data to draw conclusions about optimal antimicrobial plasma concentrations and doses necessary to provide antibacterial synergistic effects, especially against resistant organisms [14 - 16]. *In vitro* investigation also includes establishing infection models that can aid the decision-making process in terms of dosing levels and schedules. Several systems are available for the *in vitro* estimation of PK/PD parameters. Those commonly used include the one-compartment and hollow fiber infection models [17]. Both systems function by dynamically varying the antimicrobial concentration in contact with a specific infectious agent, while determining the effect of antimicrobial exposure on the microbe. The most effective maximal concentration or exposure time is determined, and parameters such as fC_{max}/MIC, $fT>MIC$, or $fAUC/MIC$ can be estimated from this data, as will be described below. One-compartment systems involve the incubation of the antimicrobial with the desired organism in a single compartment, with a series of dilutions to simulate the decline in serum antimicrobial concentration. On the other hand, the hollow-fiber infection model involves the separation of sites of infection, which occurs by inoculating the organism in the hollow-fiber cartridge, and the antimicrobial dilution in a separate reservoir. However, both systems are not without limitations. *In vitro* systems in general fall short of replicating the anatomical barriers and physiological microenvironment that might limit the exposure of the infectious organism to the antimicrobial. In addition, both systems suffer limitations that are inherent to their design. Specifically, the one-compartment systems suffer from an over-estimation of the effect of the antimicrobial due to a concurrent dilution of the organism that happens simultaneously. This effect is not always accounted for appropriately by mathematical correction [17]. Apart from the expense, hollow-fiber infection models might suffer from inaccurate assessment of emergence of resistant strains should the antibiotic-degrading enzymes get concentrated in the hollow-fiber cartridges.

In vivo Infection Models

During the pre-clinical phase of development of investigational antibacterial agents, the use of animal infection models can provide valuable predictions of clinical outcomes as well as effective dosing regimens for clinical trials. Unlike *in vitro* models of infection, animal models can reasonably replicate the anatomical and physiological conditions of the *in vivo* infection, which is essential for forecasting clinical efficacy in patients. The most widely utilized *in vivo* models are the murine thigh infection model, as a model of soft tissue infections, and the murine lung infection model, which mimics pneumonia. Neutropenia is usually induced in mice *via* cyclophosphamide injections to facilitate the establishment of infection and minimize the contribution of the immune function to the outcome. Using these *in vivo* models, a series of studies are conducted to characterize drug PK/PD profile.

Dose-Fractionation Studies

The purpose of these experiments is to determine the PK/PD index (fCmax/MIC, fAUC/MIC and fT>MIC) that correlates most closely with efficacy of the antimicrobial agent [18, 19]. One or more total daily dose(s) of the compound are usually evaluated against several bacterial strains. Each of the total daily doses is fractionated into multiple regimens with various dosing frequencies. For example, one quarter, one half or the entire dose is administered 4 times, 2 times or once over a 24-hour period for a total of 3 different regimens per each total daily dose. Treatment is usually continued for 24 hours, albeit some drugs with long half-lives in the murine infection models may be compared following 36- and 72-hour dosing to allow for sufficient discrimination in fT>MIC between regimens. After the treatment period, the bacterial burdens are compared across the different dosing regimens to determine if an increase in fCmax/MIC (single-daily dose) or fT>MIC (fractionated, more frequent administration) are related to improvement in bacterial kill. If neither of these alterations in exposure results in a significantly different degree of killing, then fAUC /MIC would be considered the index best predictive of outcome, as this index remains constant at the same total daily dose irrespective of the dosing frequency.

Dose-Ranging Studies

In addition to the identification of the PK/PD index for the antibacterial activity, additional experiments aim to assess the magnitude of the index that is required to derive efficacy [20, 21]. As such, dose-ranging studies are conducted to evaluate the *in vivo* bactericidal activity of various escalating exposures of the antibacterial agent against a wide selection of bacterial isolates with variable MICs. For the pharmacodynamic analysis of the test compound, efficacy is calculated as the change in bacterial density ($\log_{10}$ CFU) obtained at the end of the study period, usually 24-hours, compared with the initial bacterial burdens. The plot of $\log_{10}$ CFU *versus* the PK/PD index that best predicts bacterial killing of the compound (fC_{max}/MIC, $fAUC$/MIC or $fT>$MIC), calculated for each of the doses examined, is constructed for each isolate. The bioactive, free-drug exposures are determined using values obtained from protein binding and pharmacokinetic studies. A sigmoid inhibitory efficacy (E_{max}) model is fitted to the data based on the four parameter Hill equation and is used to predict the magnitude of index required to produce various efficacy endpoints *i.e.* bacteriostasis, 1- and 2-log kill. The predicted exposure targets are used to guide the selection of the doses of the test compounds for Phase II and/or III clinical trials.

Efficacy of Human-Simulated Exposures

Evaluating the efficacy of antimicrobial agents at murine doses that provide systemic exposures simulating those clinically achievable in humans can provide complementary information to traditional PK/PD assessments, as well as support the establishment of antimicrobial susceptibility breakpoints [22, 23]. The antimicrobial doses administered to mice are selected to resemble the mean or median exposure achieved in humans on the basis of the index that correlates with the efficacy of the agent, for example $fT_{>MIC}$ for ß-lactams. Since the half-lives of renally-eliminated drugs are generally shorter in mice compared to humans, renal insufficiency is often induced in mice to assist with humanizing the regimens. These types of modifications should take drug exposure at infection site into consideration. For example, drug concentration in lung epithelial lining fluid may substantially differ from that in plasma and thus *in vivo* studies utilizing murine pneumonia models should aim to simulate actual exposure in patients [24]. Additionally, if a difference in drug protein binding exists between mice and humans, the use of free drug concentrations becomes extremely important for proper exposure simulation in these investigations.

Limitations of *In vivo* Assessments and Outcome Translation

While animal infection models play an important role in assisting with clinical dose selection, there are several limitations to the *in vivo* PK/PD models. Variabilities in the PK exposures, the severity of infection and the degree of immune suppression in animals can result in inconsistency in PK/PD target values across different studies. Different targets can also be obtained from different bacterial isolates. Furthermore, a point of controversy is the specific efficacy endpoint, *i.e.* bacteriostasis, 1-log or 2-log bacterial killing, that should be used to define the magnitude of PK/PD index required for efficacy and subsequently clinical dose prediction. While it is generally accepted that bacteriostasis in infection models is sufficient to predict clinical efficacy for less invasive infection such as cystitis, there is lack of consensus regarding the target for deep-seeded infections such as pyelonephritis and pneumonia.

Certain pharmacokinetic concerns should also be considered such as potential differences in the extent and rate of penetration of drugs into infection sites between murine and human tissue (*e.g.* for oritavancin and tedizolid) [24, 25], which highlights the importance of assessing drug concentrations at infection site. While the *in vivo* models that utilize human-simulated exposures of antibacterial agents can improve the translational application of outcomes from pre-clinical studies into clinical practice, the simulated exposures in these models are typically built around the mean or median drug PK profiles obtained from patients or oftentimes healthy volunteers in Phase I clinical trials. Thus, they do not usually take into account the wide inter-subject variability in exposures between patients as well as special patient populations. The aforementioned considerations can impact the effective translation of outcomes from preclinical models to clinic.

Models of Population Kinetics

Population pharmacokinetic models are built with experimental values obtained from the analysis of serum concentration-time courses from individual subjects. Datasets accumulated from a large number of individuals are then pooled and subjected to several types of modelling calculations, that include different numbers of compartments, types of elimination, and inter- and intra-subject variabilities [13]. For most antibiotics, the information generated from these and PK/PD studies is enough to reliably calculate optimal antibiotic dosages for a large number of patients. However, there remain classes of antibiotics and patient groups where TDM is necessary. For instance, observations of early trials with large dose once daily regimens of aminoglycosides revealed that they were accompanied with a lack of standardization, as evidenced by the wide range of dosages administered and peak concentrations observed. This might have been because aminoglycosides exhibit large interpatient pharmacokinetic variability but is nevertheless quite concerning given the small therapeutic index that characterizes this class of antimicrobials [26]. Moreover, the lack of prospective validation of simulation population kinetics data poses an additional challenge against the clinical utility of these recommendations. For instance, comparing several simulation studies on a dosing recommendation of 1200 mg/day for ciprofloxacin for resistant Gram-negative infections showed significant heterogeneity in patient population, dosing algorithms, and dosing adjustment for renal impairment, thus limiting the clinical translation of these recommendations [27 - 31]. Thus, TDM of these antimicrobials is necessary to achieve therapeutic benefit and circumvent negative consequences.

ANTIMICROBIAL TDM IN SPECIAL PATIENT POPULATION: CLINICAL NECESSITY *VS.* INVESTIGATIONAL LUXURY

A major limitation of the population pharmacokinetic models on which dosing decisions are made is the study sample from which the results are derived. Most studies obtain data from healthy, young volunteers representing a stark contrast to the extremes of pathophysiology and age that characterize a large number of patients [32]. Particularly problematic is the fact that the pathophysiology of disease and age of patients may bring about different rates of drug absorption, metabolism, distribution, and elimination, creating a pharmacokinetic profile for the antibiotic that is distinct from that used to inform dosing decisions, as treatment guidelines do not usually include guidance for effective dosing in special patient populations. In clinical practice, dosing strategies for these patients are extrapolated from those available on the product information package for each medication, accounting for the changes in pharmacokinetics that each disease state may convey [33]. However, this strategy has proven to be far from satisfactory, as a multinational study that measured the serum levels of beta lactams in critically-ill patients noted that minimal therapeutic PK/PD targets were not attained in a large fraction of patients, whom in turn were less likely to have a positive clinical outcome [34]. Thus, after years of adopting a 'one dose fits all' therapeutic strategy, it is time to explore other options, especially since the attitude within healthcare is shifting towards individualized therapy. In this section, we will provide an outline of the available data regarding the value of antimicrobial drug monitoring in specific patient populations.

Critically Ill Patients

The term critical illness is a broad umbrella under which are classified a range of pathologies resulting in life-threatening, multisystem disorders [35]. In terms of pharmacokinetics, critically ill patients usually have a diverse array of changes depending on the pathology at hand. Systemic inflammatory response syndrome (SIRS) is a condition that frequently afflicts intensive care unit (ICU) patients and is characterized by a systemic inflammatory reaction leading to mass fluid extravasation from the intravascular compartment to the interstitial space, essentially concentrating administered drugs in this 'third space' [36]. In an attempt to correct for the hypotension that results from this extreme capillary leakage, large amounts of fluids are administered that may also distribute into the interstitial space, further increasing its volume. The consequences of these changes are magnified for hydrophilic antibiotics like aminoglycosides, beta lactams, glycopeptides, and linezolid, that normally remain in the aqueous environment of the intravascular compartment and have a relatively smaller volume of distribution [37 - 42]. In fact, studies have shown that it is common to observe up to two-fold increases in these antibiotics' volume of distribution, drastically increasing the dose required for them to be of therapeutic benefit. In contrast, the volumes of distribution of lipophilic antibiotics like fluoroquinolones and macrolides are relatively unaffected by such fluid movements by virtue of their initially large volumes of distribution [43].

Another condition that is highly common among ICU patients is hypoalbuminemia, where the level of albumin in the bloodstream decreases to a concentration less than 25 g/L [44]. Serum albumin normally binds a fraction of administered drugs, essentially trapping them in a form that leaves them incapable of performing their therapeutic functions. A decrease in albumin level renders more of the drug available not only to distribute to tissues and exert its therapeutic (or toxic) effect, but also to be metabolized and eliminated. There is controversy as to what the increase in amount of albumin-free drug in the serum means in terms of dosing adjustments. It is well established that the effective drug serum concentration is that of the unbound drug, as it is the portion through which the therapeutic effect is mediated. This implies that patients with hypoalbuminemia may require lower doses of antibiotics to achieve the same therapeutic outcome as those with normal levels of albumin and may even experience toxicity with unadjusted dosages [45, 46]. However, some authors argue that by freeing the drug from its intravascular albumin bind, hypoalbuminemia increases its volume of distribution, which is likely to *decrease* the drug plasma concentration at a faster rate than usual, risking potential under-dosing, especially for time-dependent antibiotics like the beta lactams [44, 47] This effect is further enhanced by the fact that the kidneys and liver can only clear albumin-free drugs from the body, and thus hypoalbuminemia shortens the half-life of antimicrobials by making them more available for clearance. This is especially exaggerated in patients with sepsis who may develop augmented renal clearance of drugs due to a hyperdynamic state that results in increased renal blood flow [48].

As previously mentioned, the greatest impact of these pharmacokinetic changes is on time-dependent antimicrobials. This is because the augmented clearance and increased volume of distribution resulting from lower albumin levels evoke a steep decrease in antimicrobial levels, in turn diminishing the time the antimicrobial concentration is above the MIC. For example, ceftriaxone, a third-generation cephalosporin, has failed to attain the PK/PD targets of therapy when dosed conventionally in burn patients with hypoalbuminemia [49]. The serum levels of flucloxacillin, an isoxazolyl penicillin, were reported to fall to 1mg/L only four hours after the bolus dose of 2g has been administered to patients with hypoalbuminemia, when its MIC for methicillin-susceptible *Staphylococcus aureus* (MSSA) is 2mg/L, double that concentration [50]. The carbapenem ertapenem showed a similar trend with two studies reporting its failure to achieve its optimal PK/PD target in a large number of patients with hypoalbuminemia [51] [52] The volume of distribution and clearance of cephalothin, a first-generation cephalosporin, however, were not affected by hypoalbuminemia in a study done on burn patients, possibly due to the fact that the study was carried out during the initial phase of burn injury which is characterized by hypovolemia and cardiac dysfunction that are likely to offset the changes caused by hypoalbuminemia [53]. This serves as a reminder that critically ill patients often suffer from multiple pathologies that each cast a massive fingerprint on antimicrobial pharmacokinetic parameters and therapeutic effect, accentuating the ever-increasing need to employ TDM to inform dosing decisions for individual patients that are unique in their changing pharmacokinetic profile.

However, changes in pharmacokinetic parameters due to hypoalbuminemia do only not affect the outcome of time-dependent antimicrobials. Glycopeptides, whose optimal PK/PD parameter is fAUC/MIC, exhibit fluctuating serum concentrations in patients with hypoalbuminemia, but unlike beta lactams, there is no reliable trend towards a decrease in PK/PD values to subtherapeutic levels, though their volume of distribution and clearance increase [49, 54] A study finding that serum variations in teicoplanin levels range between 8% and 42% in patients with hypoalbuminemia, rendering conventional dosing strategies akin to random dose selection [54]. More studies are needed to characterize the consequences of these pharmacokinetic changes on glycopeptide dosing strategies as it remains clear that these fluctuations do occur and are clinically relevant. Authors have thus advocated for the use of glycopeptide TDM as essential to guide dosing decisions in populations with such variable pharmacokinetics [47, 55].

The effect of hypoalbuminemia on concentration-dependent antibiotics is multifaceted. On one hand, by increasing their volume of distribution, hypoalbuminemia decreases their C_{max}. The PK/PD index by which the therapeutic efficacy of many of these antibiotics, including the aminoglycosides, is gauged is C_{max}/MIC, and thus hypoalbuminemia essentially decreases the therapeutic efficacy of conventional antibiotic dosing [56, 57]. On the other hand, the paucity of albumin allows a greater fraction of the drug to exist in its free form in the plasma, thus increasing the concentration of free antibiotic in the intravascular compartment. Since the free proportion of antibiotic is responsible for the therapeutic action, the latter effect appears to increase therapeutic efficacy, creating a situation that is at odds with what would be predicted based on volume of distribution and PK/PD parameters alone. One would conclude that hypoalbuminemia might not impose different dosing strategies for concentration-dependent antibiotics due to its opposing effects on pharmacokinetic parameters. In reality, the outcomes are dependent on the specific antibiotic at hand. For example, daptomycin, a lipopeptide antibiotic with normal protein binding levels of 90-93%, is expected to achieve greater therapeutic benefit in patients with hypoalbuminemia because a small decrease in albumin levels would free a large proportion of therapeutically active drug [58]. The opposing effect on volume of distribution is expected to be limited, since the lipophilicity of daptomycin already contributes to enhanced distribution [51, 58 - 62]. Thus, it is expected that daptomycin will require a downgrade in dosing regimen in order for it not to exceed the threshold of toxicity. Surprisingly, it is the exact opposite that happens. A study evaluating daptomycin dosing strategies in burn patients with hypoalbuminemia concluded that these patients required a dose of 10-20 mg/kg of body weight/day of daptomycin treatment in order to achieve the same therapeutic benefit that a dose of 6 mg/kg of body weight/day would confer in healthy patients [58]. The authors hypothesized that this may be due to augmented daptomycin clearance that is also a result of hypoalbuminemia. Equally surprising is the fact that amikacin, an aminoglycoside antibiotic whose efficacy is expected to decrease due to the drastic increase in volume of distribution and clearance hydrophilic antibiotics undergo in patients with hypoalbuminemia, actually exhibits greater toxicity and higher serum concentrations in these patients [63]. Given the unpredictability of pharmacokinetic changes in this context, therapeutic drug monitoring will be necessary to deliver antibiotic therapy that is efficacious and safe.

Drug clearance is one of the four pillars of pharmacokinetics, and one that is especially important to consider in critically ill patients whose renal function is frequently affected by various pathologies. In fact, it is standard practice to reduce antibiotic dosing in the presence of renal dysfunction, acute kidney injury, or renal replacement therapy in order to avoid toxicity from reduced renal clearance. On the other hand, conditions leading to increased renal elimination are not equally well-studied. Augmented renal clearance is a condition characterized by an increase in glomerular filtration driven by pathophysiological responses to infection, fluid resuscitation, or use of vasopressors [33, 64]. This leads to increased drug delivery to the kidney which in turn augments drug elimination, effectively decreasing the concentration of drug in the plasma and risking therapeutic failure. A study done on 54 adult ICU patients with moderate kidney function treated with imipenem concluded that critically-ill patients had consistently lower serum concentrations of the drug than healthy volunteers receiving the same dose, with mean concentrations below the MICs of several ICU pathogens, rendering the treatment futile and risking the emergence of antibiotic-resistant organisms [65]. In fact, it is estimated that 82% of patients with augmented renal clearance that will not achieve therapeutic antibiotic concentrations with standard antibiotic doses [66].

Considering the derangements in individual pharmacokinetic parameters that characterize critically ill patients, it is difficult to make dosing decisions tailored to these pharmacokinetic changes, prompting the need for TDM to achieve therapeutic efficacy and avoid toxicity. Critical illness leads to significant changes in pharmacokinetics within the same patient, necessitating the need to regularly monitor serum concentrations of antimicrobial agents and adjust dosing strategies accordingly [32]. In addition, the exhaustive list of medications these patients receive further complicates dosing and creates problems of toxicity and drug-drug interactions, emphasizing the need for an objective measure that accurately portrays whether therapeutic benefit is being achieved before the occurrence of adverse events due to ineffectively treated disease or toxic drug dose.

However, there is a main fundamental limitation to using plasma TDM as this objective measure. Many critically ill patients have end-organ dysfunction that may impair drug distribution and clearance, creating a situation where the antimicrobial may reach toxic concentrations in one compartment while remaining at subtherapeutic levels where it is required to act [33, 48]. This is due to an impairment in microvascular function that hinders drug delivery to peripheral tissues while maintaining an elevated plasma drug concentration, of which only a small portion will reach the intended site of action, thus masking the therapeutic ineffectiveness that characterizes this state [67]. This has been reported for cefpirome, fosfomycin, piperacillin, and levofloxacin, and at least for these antibiotics, the conventional PK/PD indices do not hold true by virtue of their plasma concentrations being false indicators of therapeutic efficacy [68 - 71]. In this case, using plasma concentrations as a vehicle for TDM may be futile, and perhaps better replaced by tissue sampling, which in itself is invasive and problematic.

Obese and Overweight Patients

Pharmacokinetic diversity is not confined to critically ill patients. This is especially important in the wake of the obesity epidemic of today, as obese patients exhibit antibiotic pharmacokinetic parameters that differ significantly from the non-obese [72, 73]. Obese patients have been shown to have delayed gastric emptying, which may lead to a lower maximum serum drug concentration (C_{max}) or reduced absorption of certain antibiotics [74, 75]. In terms of distribution, obese patients tend to have a larger volume of distribution; for a given dose of antibiotic, an individual with obesity will have a lower serum concentration of drug than his/her healthy counterpart [73]. Although obesity is associated with augmented renal clearance, this is countered by a higher incidence of renal dysfunction over time, resulting in an antibiotic exposure that is difficult to predict [73]. The impact of this on antimicrobial therapy has been demonstrated by a study that concluded that obese patients require lower weight-based doses of vancomycin to achieve target concentrations compared to their non-obese counterparts, emphasizing the fact that dosing guidelines that apply to healthy individuals are not optimal for use in obese patients, regardless of whether the dose is adjusted for weight [76].

TDM USING ALTERNATIVE BIOLOGICAL MATRICES

TDM is usually thought of as a drug optimization method based on plasma sampling. However, this mode of sampling relies on the fact that the level of drug at the site of action can be predicted based on plasma concentration. This is not always true, for example, in critically ill patients, and is particularly problematic since the critically ill are the main population in which TDM is necessary. In addition, plasma sampling may be impossible, impractical, or unethical in some patient populations, including elderly, pediatric, and anemic patients, and those with fragile veins [77]. Initially utilized because of its convenience, relative noninvasiveness, and for lack of other optimized sampling methods, the limitations of plasma sampling were previously foregone in favor of the benefit that it confers. However, efforts to identify alternative, less invasive biological matrices for TDM are underway, and saliva and interstitial fluid have emerged as potential candidates due to the demonstrated ability to reliably quantify drug concentrations in these matrices [78].

Saliva is routinely used as a matrix to measure xenobiotic concentrations for forensic and toxicological purposes. Drug penetration into saliva generally occurs by simple diffusion, the final concentration of drug largely determined by its acid dissociation constant (pK_a), partition coefficient, molar mass and the salivary pH. Drugs that are unionized at salivary pH are more likely to be distributed to the saliva. Relatively low in protein, saliva provides a convenient method by which to sample the pharmacologically active concentration of a drug at a given time, which is reflective of free drug levels in the plasma in many cases. This has prompted several clinical studies to adopt salivary analysis of drugs in routine protocols of pharmacokinetic and pharmacodynamic assessment of drug development. In case of TDM, salivary analysis could possibly propel the practice from something that is performed by a skilled professional on high risk inpatients to a drug optimization method that can be done by the patient at home. This will become particularly important to avoid the emergence of antibiotic-resistant organisms. However, this comes with challenges, as extrapolating data obtained from salivary sampling to plasma drug concentrations can be problematic. For one, there may be a need to account for the preferential distribution of some compounds to the saliva due to a pH difference between saliva and plasma [79]. If the pK_a of a basic drug is greater than 6 or that of an acidic drug is less than 8, then it is likely that these drugs will be ionized at salivary pH, inhibiting their distribution to saliva and creating disparities between drug concentration in plasma and that in saliva. This is further complicated by the fact that salivary pH fluctuates with variations in flow rate, rendering time of sampling with respect to meals crucial to providing samples that are suitable for comparison to predetermined drug ranges. Changes in salivary flow rate may also accompany multiple clinical conditions including chronic obstructive pulmonary disease and xerostomia, and may be a result of the administration of a long list of drugs frequented by a large portion of patients, including diuretics, beta blockers, and antihistamines, limiting the use of this technique in these patient populations. Moreover, salivary pH is characterized by extreme intra- and inter-individual variation, with documented pH ranges from 5.8 to 8.4 [80]. In fact, a study assessing the ratio of salivary to unbound plasma fluoroquinolone concentration (S/Pu) reported a range of ciprofloxacin, norfloxacin, lomefloxacin, ofloxacin, and sparfloxacin S/Pu ratios from 0.014 to 1.497, much larger than the theoretically calculated pH-based range of 1.0 to 1.3 [81].

Correlations between salivary and plasma drug levels may also be complicated by the protein-binding pattern the drug adopts. As previously mentioned, plasma proteins do not pass to the saliva, limiting the salivary drug composition to the non-protein bound, pharmacologically active drug component. While this might be beneficial by removing the analytical steps required to isolate the free drug fraction, it creates a novel problem in which drugs with dose-dependent protein-binding patterns may be underrepresented in the saliva when administered at high concentrations, while appearing falsely high in patients administered low drug doses. Nevertheless, saliva sampling holds promise as a surrogate for plasma-based TDM, at least for drugs that are low in molecular weight, unionized at salivary pH, and exhibit low protein binding. For example, plasma levels of ofloxacin, a quinolone antibiotic, have been shown to closely correlate with its salivary levels in patients with chronic respiratory infections, holding promise for use in these patients who require a plethora of antibiotics and in whom monitoring for drug resistance is so necessary [82]. Once plasma-independent, saliva-optimized target drug ranges are developed for drugs in which correlations with plasma concentrations cannot be made with much confidence, salivary TDM may be used in patients where plasma sampling is not feasible or practical and may even be used as an assay that facilitates outpatient TDM. Efforts are currently focused on optimizing salivary antimicrobial detection assays, the use of salivary drug monitoring for the purpose of studying drug pharmacokinetics, and the evaluation of plasma-to-saliva drug ratios for a multitude of antimicrobials including antibacterial, antiviral, and antifungal agents [83]. How soon these efforts will translate to a large-scale evolution in TDM is unclear.

Interstitial fluid is a matrix that is lower in protein content than plasma, much like saliva. However, while saliva is a convenient matrix for TDM, antimicrobial action in saliva is only necessary when the infection is of the oral cavity. Interstitial fluid, on the other hand, bathes tissues that are frequently targeted by antimicrobial action, and may provide a local update on drug penetration at different sites in patients with altered pharmacokinetic profiles [84]. However, interstitial fluid is difficult to sample by conventional methods due to its limited availability in the skin and the invasive nature of obtaining it. Therefore, the development of microneedle technologies that can be applied as a pain-free patch on the skin and contain integrated biosensors capable of analyzing minute volumes of fluid propelled interstitial fluid TDM into something that is not only clinically and commercially feasible but also to a possible replacement of plasma-based TDM. Moreover, by bypassing the requirement of professional personnel for plasma collection, interstitial fluid sampling using microneedle technologies is a possible technique by which TDM can be performed in outpatient settings [77].

Unlike saliva, drug penetration from the plasma to the interstitial fluid is less understood and more difficult to predict. There is a general consensus that antibiotics exhibit different degrees of penetration into adipose tissue and muscle, and that drug protein binding profiles heavily impact their interstitial fluid distribution. A comprehensive review of the available data on antimicrobial distribution concluded that protein binding was the only factor that affected distribution into interstitial fluid [84]. The observed disparities between muscle and adipose tissue distribution could not be predicted based on differences in solubility or molecular weight. However, pathological tissue alterations were not accounted for, since the data used for regression was obtained from healthy volunteers. Despite this, studies describing the status of interstitial distribution in healthy and diseased tissues might exist for individual antibiotics. For example, early studies using *in* vivo microdialysis sampling showed parallels between plasma concentration of piperacillin and its free tissue distribution patterns [85], in pneumonia patients [86]. Studies on daptomycin shown that its distribution to skin was not affected by the disease state in patients with confirmed diabetic foot infection [87].

Interestingly, reduced drug levels are observed in interstitial fluid compared to plasma even in non-critically ill patients, which is at odds with the assumption that plasma drug levels are representative of distributed drug concentrations. For instance, studies on piperacillin, a penicillin antibiotic, have shown that the concentration of this drug in interstitial fluid is reduced compared to plasma in moderately-ill patients and is more extensively reduced in critically-ill patients, further validating the claim that plasma drug levels are not suitable for TDM in the critically-ill. This was also observed for a variety of other antimicrobials including cefpirome, cefazolin, and meropenem. Although interstitial fluid exposure values may differ from those of plasma for the penicillins, cephalosporins, and carbapenems, the elimination rate is similar, making these drugs suitable candidates for TDM using interstitial fluid. Of note, inconsistent distribution ratios between adipose tissue and muscle were reported among different studies conducted on imipenem, emphasizing the importance of standardizing calibration and analysis techniques before employing this method of TDM in clinical settings. Nevertheless, interstitial fluid TDM using microneedle technologies presents a less invasive technique which may justify using TDM for antimicrobials with a large therapeutic window to which organisms are developing resistance.

As for drugs that are normally plasma monitored in the clinical setting, like vancomycin, studies have shown that vancomycin distributes well to tissues in patients with peripheral infections but exhibits reduced penetration into interstitial fluid in diabetic patients [88 - 90]. This imposes the important limitation of using skin interstitial fluid to monitor vancomycin levels to avoid toxicity, as dangerously high plasma vancomycin levels may be underscored by moderate interstitial fluid microneedle assay results in diabetic patients. Thus, using interstitial fluid for TDM may be futile, and quite dangerous, in some situations. No studies to date have assessed the feasibility of interstitial fluid TDM for aminoglycosides. This innovative technique is anticipated to meet the newly encountered need to monitor for resistance, while the conventional plasma sampling method may be better suited for conventional TDM carried out on toxic drugs with low therapeutic indices.

TDM OF ANTIMICROBIALS TO AVOID EMERGENCE OF RESISTANCE

While typically TDM targets for antimicrobials are recommended to ensure positive therapeutic outcomes, and reduce potential side effects, sometimes the target recommendations are set to prevent the emergence of bacterial resistance. Exposure to low antibiotic levels are associated with selection of resistant bacterial strains, and thus setting targets for minimum levels of systemic antibiotic exposure could help reduce the likelihood of this selection process. Alongside TDM targets for vancomycin appropriate for methicillin-resistant *S. aureus* infections, the Infectious Disease society of America set an additional target, above which the vancomycin serum concentration should be maintained, to avoid the emergence of Vancomycin-intermediately susceptible *S. aureus* [91]. Similarly, retrospective TDM-based studies demonstrated that arbitrary dosing and dosing adjustment of fluoroquinolones based on renal function provided little impact on drug accumulation while leading to serum profiles below the pharmacodynamics break points for resistant organisms, and hence a recommendation of a TDM-guided dosage adjustment to attain a target of $C_{max}/MIC > 10$ or $AUC/MIC > 125$ was made [92, 93].

COMMON AND RECENT TDM RECOMMENDATIONS FOR SPECIFIC ANTIBIOTICS AND ANTIBIOTIC CLASSES

Therapeutic drug monitoring is considered standard practice for aminoglycosides (*e.g.* gentamicin, tobramycin, and amikacin) and glycopeptides (*e.g.* vancomycin and teicoplanin). Initially introduced as a method to minimize the nephrotoxicity associated with these classes of antibiotics, TDM is now also used to maximize efficacy by ensuring that the dose administered achieves the target concentration [94]. The target concentration of antibiotic in the bloodstream is defined by studying the PK/PD index that is best associated with efficacy of the antimicrobial class at hand, and then determining the minimal PK/PD value that ensures a high probability of successful treatment. To attain a specific PK/PD level, adequate exposure to the drug should be ensured, and this depends on the dose administered and the pharmacokinetic parameters of the drug, which may exhibit marked interpatient variability. For this purpose, studies are designed to determine the ideal serum sampling parameters for optimal forecasting of the relevant PK/PD index using models of population pharmacokinetics.

Vancomycin

Vancomycin is a glycopeptide antibiotic that was developed as an alternative to penicillin to treat penicillinase-producing bacteria. Due to the availability of semi-synthetic penicillins (*e.g.* methicillin, oxacillin, nafcillin) that confer similar therapeutic benefit without the side effects of nephrotoxicity and ototoxicity, the use of vancomycin was initially uncalled-for. However, the emergence of methicillin-resistant *Staphylococcus aureus* (MRSA) strains has plunged vancomycin back into the frontline of antimicrobial therapy, accompanied by TDM to curtail its side effects. Despite significant clinical controversy regarding the establishment of a causal relationship between high serum concentrations of vancomycin and nephro- or ototoxicity [95 - 99], the general consensus remains that TDM of vancomycin improves clinical outcomes, is associated with less incidence of toxicities, and reduces the emergence of resistance [93].

Vancomycin is generally considered to follow time-dependent killing kinetics. The ideal PK/PD parameter that most correlates with vancomycin's therapeutic benefit has been debatable in research. For instance, *in vivo* experiments on a rabbit model of *S aureus* aortic valve endocarditis and clinical studies of *S aureus* septicemia and endocarditis yielded a time-dependent action for glycolipids that is best represented by trough plasma concentration of protein free vancomycin greater than MIC [100 - 102]. On the other hand, a study of MRSA lower respiratory tract infection patients showed that clinical improvement and bacterial eradication was correlated with the 24-hour AUC/MIC value [103]. The use of this parameter is supported by evidence from several *in vitro*, animal models, and human studies [12, 104 - 108]. However, it is difficult to obtain multiple plasma samples in the clinical setting in order to construct an individualized vancomycin concentration-time curve, necessitating the need to determine the timepoint at which drug measurement best correlates with AUC. Since vancomycin's bactericidal effect is time-dependent and its concentration-time curve exhibits a multiexponential decline, it is not useful to measure peak vancomycin concentration as a surrogate for AUC. Trough serum concentration, obtained just prior to the administration of the next dose of vancomycin, has proven to be the most optimal method to ensure that the levels of vancomycin are efficacious and non-toxic. Trough serum concentration measurements should be taken at pharmacokinetic steady state, assumed to be achieved before the fourth dose in a 12-hour dosing schedule [93]. Vancomycin clearance is mainly dependent on renal function, and thus patients with renal impairment will demonstrate an extended half-life, causing the steady state not to be achieved at the same time interval. As such, a trough concentration at this time may underestimate steady-state antibiotic exposure [109]. This should be taken into consideration when making any dose adjustment.

Trough serum vancomycin concentration levels are usually determined using commercial immunoassays, though studies have reported challenges with inter-assay variability and lack of standardization among different methods available [110]. Dose adjustment is done based on the assay results and the target serum levels. A higher continuous infusion target is required to ensure the achievement of the same AUC compared to intermittent dosing, thus the target concentrations commonly used are 15–20 mg/L and 20–25 mg/L for intermittent and continuous dosing, respectively [91]. Although methodologies do exist for vancomycin dose adjustment based on calculation of individual patient pharmacokinetic parameters and AUC/MIC, they are not widely adopted in clinical practice [111]. Dose adjustment is best done by PK forecasting coupled with TDM [91]. However, these practices have been recently challenged, especially that for more resistant organisms with MIC > 2 mg/L, the AUC/MIC target of 400 mg.hr/L would not be achievable without using doses that produce serious renal toxicity, with calculations based on serum trough levels. A large-scale simulation study (5000 patients] showed that 60% of patients could achieve therapeutic AUC values with trough concentrations below 15 mg/L, assuming a vancomycin MIC value of ≤1 mg/L [112]. This has caused the American Society for Health Systems Pharmacists to advocate for a new TDM strategy for vancomycin [113]. The new strategy called for an improved AUC estimation based on two serum levels, ideally from the same dosing interval at steady state, one representing a post-distribution peak obtained 1–2 hours after the end of the infusion, and the other a trough level. Early levels, after the first dose, could be obtained in patient groups with challenging pharmacokinetic profiles, including obese, elderly, or critically-ill patients. Afterwards, repeat trough levels obtained weekly should be sufficient to ascertain that the AUC is within target ranges. More frequent trough levels are recommended for hemodynamically unstable patients or patients at high risk for nephrotoxicity. Additional two-level calculations might be necessary if follow-up trough levels reveal AUC values that are out of range.

The value of antimicrobials lies in their ability to eradicate, or assist the immune system in eradicating, infecting microbes. The emergence of vancomycin-intermediate susceptible *S. aureus* (VISA) and vancomycin-resistant *S. aureus* (VRSA) in recent years has prompted caretakers to evaluate the utility of this antibiotic, fearing that continued use of vancomycin will increase the prevalence of resistant organisms. However, recent studies have uncovered an important correlation linking serum levels of less than 10mg/dL of vancomycin to the emergence of VISA or VRSA, introducing a novel way by which to use TDM in order to monitor resistance to antimicrobials in addition to efficacy and toxicity [114, 115]. Based on the data acquired from these studies, it is now recommended that serum vancomycin concentration be maintained at 10-15 mg/L in adult patients [116] with mild-moderate skin and soft tissue infections or for *S. aureus* and MIC <1 mcg/mL. On the other hand, for patients with more severe and deep-seated infections such as endocarditis, osteomyelitis, meningitis, hospital-acquired or ventilator-associated pneumonia, prosthetic infections, bacteremia, and necrotizing fasciitis, a trough level of 15-20 mg/L is recommended [91, 117]. The following cases are an example of how vancomycin TDM is carried out in hospital settings given the information presented above.

Aminoglycosides

Aminoglycosides are an inexpensive class of antimicrobials with efficacy against Gram-negative bacteria, making them an ideal choice for severe infections of nosocomial origin or in critically ill patients. Because aminoglycosides are concentration-dependent antibiotics, treatment optimization involves the maintenance of bloodstream antibiotic concentrations at the highest possible level in order to achieve the best microbiological outcome, without evoking the time-dependent consequences of ototoxicity and nephrotoxicity. For these reasons, caregivers have adopted the approach of administering a large dose of aminoglycosides once daily, as opposed to smaller doses over a 24-hour period, thus maximizing the peak concentration of antibiotic while minimizing the time that the antibiotic is in the bloodstream. Studies investigating this approach concluded that these once-daily regimens are therapeutically effective, minimize toxicity, and prevent the emergence of aminoglycoside-resistant pathogens when the ratio of peak concentration to MIC is at least 10:1 [9, 118]. Note that the once-daily dosing strategy is not recommended when aminoglycosides are used synergistically in enterococcal endocarditis. This approach is also less studied in patients who are younger than 13 years of age, pregnant, have cystic fibrosis, renal impairment (eCrCl<20 mL/min), burns affecting > 20% of body surface area [BSA), ascites, or febrile neutropenia [119].

Vancomycin Case 1

NM is a 72 y.o. septic male patient (weight=120 kg, estimated creatinine clearance (eCrCl) >80 mL/min) who was started on Vancomycin 1 g intravenously (IV) q8h (every 8 hours) for MRSA bacteremia. A trough level was drawn one hour before the next expected dose and turned out to be 25.7 mg/L.

The following kinetics parameters are calculated for this patient:
True vancomycin trough = 26.81 mg/L
Vancomycin volume of distribution (Vd) = 84 L
Vancomycin elimination rate constant (Ke) = 0.0423 h^{-1}
Vancomycin half-life = 16.39 h

The adjusted dosing regimen of vancomycin of 1g IV infused over 1 hour q12h (every 12 hours) would yield a predicted vancomycin trough of 18.39 mg/L, which is within the desired target range of 15-20 mg/L.

This change in dosing regimen is recommended for this patient, as well as a trough level to be drawn 30 minutes before the 4th dose of the new dosing regimen. An important factor would be to emphasize the need to not hold the upcoming dose of vancomycin until the trough level is out but rather adjust the drug regimen starting from the next scheduled dose if need be.
Adapted for educational purposes from a real-life clinical case.

Vancomycin Case 2

KL is an 86 y.o. female patient (weight=47 kg) on intermittent hemodialysis who was started on Vancomycin empirically for MRSA coverage. The desired target trough range is 15-20 mg/L. The patient's last dose was 500 mg administered after her dialysis session.

As part of vancomycin TDM, the recommendation would be to draw a pre-dialysis random level on the morning of next scheduled dialysis. Then, the patient may be re-dosed after hemodialysis depending on the level obtained. Note that high-flux hemodialysis may decrease vancomycin levels by approximately 40%.

Vancomycin level obtained on the morning of next dialysis was 17 mg/L. The recommendation would be to give the patient a dose of 5-7.5 mg/kg (~250 mg) once after dialysis to maintain the level at target. A random level should be requested prior to next dialysis session.

Adapted for educational purposes from a real-life clinical case.

Aminoglycoside TDM is done utilizing the Hartford or Urban & Craig Nomogram methods, whereby the initial dose is calculated based on the patient's body weight and then monitored by drawing blood 8-12 hours after the beginning of infusion. The drug serum concentration is measured and then plotted on a standardized concentration-time graph called a nomogram, and the dosage is adjusted according to where this level lies on the graph [118]. The Hartford Nomogram has been shown to be effective in reducing the incidence of nephrotoxicity from 3-5% to 1.2% in a study on more than 2000 patients treated with aminoglycosides, while maintaining a similar clinical response. However, the predictability of aminoglycoside PK is very poor in several patient classes including critically-ill and burn patients [120], decreasing the likelihood of achieving the target maximal concentration. As such, estimation of C_{max} and AUC is preferred in patients with conditions leading to alterations in volume of distribution. This can be achieved by TDM with two samples, one drawn at 1 hour and the other at 6–22 hours post administration [121, 122]. Peak concentrations and AUC can then be estimated using linear regression or Bayesian approaches with more accurate forecasting of future dosing requirements. Similar to vancomycin, commercially available immunoassays are the most frequently used method for aminoglycoside TDM. They have relatively lower cost and are validated for routine clinical use [123]. For patients who do not qualify for once-daily dosing, a peak and trough is recommended to be drawn before and after the fourth dose in adult patients, and before and after the third dose in pediatric patients. The following cases are an example of how aminoglycoside TDM is carried out in hospital settings given the information presented above.

Aminoglycosides Case 1

KT is a 30-year old male (Weight 75 kg, eCrCl >100 mL/min) who was started on gentamicin 460 mg IV q24h (every 24 hours) for osteomyelitis.

The patient is an adult and does not have any conditions that may lead to a variable volume of distribution. He thus qualifies for the once-daily dose of aminoglycosides. One level should be drawn 8-12 hours after the dose.

The patient's 8-hour level turned out to be 10.5. When plotting it on the Hartford nomogram, the level falls within the 48-h interval. The most appropriate step would be to extend the interval to 48h, making the dosing regimen 460 mg IV q48h (every 48 hours). Another random level is recommended at 8-12 hours after the change in dosing regimen. *Adapted for educational purposes from a real-life clinical case.*

Aminoglycosides Case 2

HF is a 7-year old female (Weight 27kg, Height 110 cm) with choroid plexus carcinoma s/p autologous stem cell transplant. She was started on amikacin for suspected gram-negative bacteremia. Her serum creatinine was 0.3 mg/dL.

The dose the patient was started on was 230 mg IV q8h. You are asked to recommend a monitoring plan for the patient.

Since this is a pediatric patient, the once-daily dosing regimen is less favored as it is less studied in this patient population. In this specific case, the conventional more frequent dosing is recommended. Rather than carrying out one-level testing, it becomes important to ask for a trough and peak level respectively before and after the third dose of this dosing regimen. The trough level should be drawn 30 minutes prior to the dose while the peak is drawn 30 minutes after the half hour infusion of amikacin.

For this specific patient, the trough level was 1.7 and the peak 12.8. The target peak is 25-30 while the target trough is <5. Since both the peak and the trough are low, it is imperative to increase the total daily dose while keeping the same interval (which is the minimal accepted dosing interval for this drug). Though no clear guidelines are available for exact dosing increment, it may be reasonable to increase the individual dose by 10 % in this specific case. The recommended new dosing regimen for this patient is 250 mg IV q8h. A more accurate way of dose increase, though less practical at the bedside, can be obtained by calculating specific kinetic parameters for this patient.
Adapted for educational purposes from a real-life clinical case.

Beta Lactams

Beta lactam antibiotics are a group of bactericidal agents that have formed the cornerstone of antimicrobial therapy since the discovery of their parent compound, penicillin, in 1928. United by their structural beta lactam ring, this family of antimicrobials has expanded to meet the needs of an ever-evolving group of beta-lactam-resistant bacteria. Thousands of new members have been developed with time, but the rate of antibiotic-resistant bacteria has steadily kept up, with ceftobiprole, a 5th generation cephalosporin, starting to show signs of resistance [124].

This group of antibiotics exhibits time-dependent killing properties, and hence its optimal PK/PD index is the percentage of dosing interval during which the unbound serum antibiotic concentration remains above the MIC for a given organism ($\%f\,T_{>\,\text{MIC}}$). In keeping with the increase in MIC of beta lactams for most bacteria, the optimal PK/PD value has increased from the traditional target range of 40-60% of the dosing interval to 100%. Thus, a family of drugs with a therapeutic index that was traditionally viewed as large is being re-evaluated due to the increase in dose that is considered therapeutic. To further complicate the issue, higher beta lactam concentrations have proven difficult to attain particularly in critically-ill patients [125].

The narrowing of their therapeutic window brought about a problem not previously experienced with the beta lactams, with doses that are considered therapeutic increasingly approaching toxic concentrations, bringing about the need to re-evaluate and optimize dosing strategies. Without a currently well-defined toxic threshold, TDM could help avert drug-related toxicities particularly in patients susceptible to neurological toxicities. Various methods to accomplish this have been suggested, including dosing nomograms and creatinine-clearance adjusted dosing strategies, both of which have proven to be unsuccessful thus far [32]. This is accompanied by a change in attitude towards TDM from a method that curtails toxicity to one that optimizes therapy, with the purpose of TDM in this case being to correct for under-dosing. In fact, as of 2015, 30 hospitals worldwide have been documented to perform beta lactam TDM on a routine basis, the majority of cases being on critically ill patients. However, there is a lack of standardization in the way TDM is carried out in these hospitals, as each hospital has developed its own strategy. Generally, steady state trough serum samples are collected (after 3-4 doses) and analyzed using liquid chromatography methods. Dose adjustment can be performed using dosing nomograms or Bayesian-driven PK models, neither of which has been standardized or validated [93].

Linezolid

Linezolid is an oxazolidinone class antibiotic, which blocks the initiation of bacterial protein synthesis [126]. It exhibits mainly time-dependent activity against Gram-positive pathogens with limited concentration dependence. The AUC/MIC is the PK/PD index best correlated with Linezolid's efficacy [127]. Linezolid demonstrates a favorable pharmacokinetic profile where it is rapidly and completely absorbed with 100% oral bioavailability, consistent plasma protein binding that is concentration independent, homogenous distribution to well-perfused tissues and linear elimination over the therapeutic dosing range [126]. An excellent pulmonary, cerebrospinal fluid, and skin and soft tissue distribution profile led to linezolid being considered as an agent of choice for multi-drug resistant Gram-positive infections of these tissues.

Although, owing to the high consistency of linezolid's PK profile, dosage adjustment in renal and hepatic dysfunction were considered unnecessary [128], studies have shown that linezolid accumulation in renal insufficiency patients was likely, and resulted in toxicities such as pancytopenia, thrombocytopenia and liver dysfunction [129 - 131]. Moreover, studies have observed a wide variability of systemic linezolid exposure among patients receiving fixed dose regiments [132] and that these PK variations occurred more frequently in critically ill patients with burn injuries [133] leading to sub-therapeutic exposure. On the other hand, attempts to use higher doses in critically-ill patients to ensure attainment of PK/PD targets were associated with hematological toxicities [134]. As such, while routine TDM of linezolid is not currently supported by current clinical data, it might be warranted at least in certain patient categories with critical illness or multi-drug resistant organisms. Steady state trough serum levels on the third day of therapy correlate well with linezolid AUC and can be used for estimation of AUC/MIC [132]. High performance liquid chromatography (HPLC) methods on patient plasma [135] or oral fluids [136] are available and validated for the purpose of linezolid TDM.

Fluoroquinolones

A large body of evidence showed that 80% of therapeutic failure in patients treated with quinolones was due to the development of microbial resistance resulting from under-treatment [137]. This issue becomes particularly problematic in critically ill patients where fluoroquinolone PK becomes less predictable [138]. On the other hand, quinolone accumulation to levels requiring dose reduction was reported in non-critically-ill patients [139]. Moreover, factors like renal replacement therapy could further contribute to the observed PK variability of fluoroquinolones [140]. As such, a select group of patients including critically-ill patients with infections caused by organisms with a high MIC could benefit from TDM. Steady state serum measurements of peak (30 minutes after bolus infusion) and trough serum concentrations are required for the estimation of AUC and AUC/MIC, which is the index used for fluoroquinolones [92]. HPLC methods are available for estimation of ciprofloxacin concentration in serum [125].

CONCLUDING REMARKS

As personalized medicine is making its way into clinical reality, TDM is emerging as a method to maximize individual patient benefit from a set of routinely used drugs. A body of evidence has shown that the application of this technique that is currently reserved to curtail toxicity for the most part, may maximize antimicrobial therapeutic potential and minimize the constant threat of drug resistance. Multiple innovative approaches including saliva and non-invasive interstitial fluid sampling are being developed, which may help maximize the benefit of TDM and propel it into the frontiers of routine medical care.

ABBREVIATIONS

PK	Pharmaco kinetics
PD	Pharmacodynamics
MIC	Minimal inhibitory concentration
C_{max}	Maximal plasma concentration
AUC	Area under the plasma concentration *versus* time curve
$FT>_{MIC}$	The duration of time that the concentration of unbound antibiotic exceeds MIC
FC_{max}/MIC	The ratio of maximal unbound drug concentration to MIC
FAUC/MIC	The ratio of the area under the unbound drug concentration-time curve to the MIC
CFU	Colony forming units
pK_a	Negative log of the acid dissociation constant
IV	Intravenous
V_d	Volume of distribution
K_e	Elimination rate constant
$_eC_rCL$	Estimated creatinine clearance

CONSENT FOR PUBLICATION

Not applicable.

CONFLICT OF INTEREST

The authors confirm that the contents of this chapter have no conflict of interest.

ACKNOWLEDGEMENTS

Declared none.

REFERENCES

[1]   Touw DJ, Neef C, Thomson AH, Vinks AA. Cost-effectiveness of therapeutic drug monitoring committee of the international association for therapeutic drug monitoring and clinical toxicology. Cost-effectiveness of therapeutic drug monitoring: a systematic review. Ther Drug Monit 2005; 27(1): 10-7.
[http://dx.doi.org/10.1097/00007691-200502000-00004] [PMID: 15665740]

[2]   Nicolau DP, Dimopoulos G, Welte T, Luyt C-E. Can we improve clinical outcomes in patients with pneumonia treated with antibiotics in the intensive care unit? Expert Rev Respir Med 2016; 10(8): 907-18.
[http://dx.doi.org/10.1080/17476348.2016.1190277] [PMID: 27181707]

[3]   Moellering RC Jr. Vancomycin: a 50-year reassessment. Clin Infect Dis 2006; 42 (Suppl. 1): S3-4.
[http://dx.doi.org/10.1086/491708] [PMID: 16323117]

[4]   Levine DP. Vancomycin: a history. Clin Infect Dis 2006; 42 (Suppl. 1): S5-S12.
[http://dx.doi.org/10.1086/491709] [PMID: 16323120]

[5]   Bootman JL, Wertheimer AI, Zaske D, Rowland C. Individualizing gentamicin dosage regimens in burn patients with gram-negative septicemia: a cost--benefit analysis. J Pharm Sci 1979; 68(3): 267-72.
[http://dx.doi.org/10.1002/jps.2600680304] [PMID: 106108]

[6]   Ghiculesco R. Abnormal laboratory results: Therapeutic drug monitoring: which drugs, why, when and how to do it. Aust Prescr 2008; 31(2): 42-4.
[http://dx.doi.org/10.18773/austprescr.2008.025]

[7]   Craig WA. The hidden impact of antibacterial resistance in respiratory tract infection Reevaluating current antibiotic therapy Respir Med 2001. Suppl A:S12-19;.

[8]   Joint commission on hospital accreditation. APPROVED: New Antimicrobial Stewardship Standard Jt Comm Perspect Jt Comm Accreditation Healthc Organ. 36(7): 3-4.

[9]   Motos A, Kidd JM, Nicolau DP. Optimizing Antibiotic Administration for Pneumonia. Clin Chest Med 2018; 39(4): 837-52.
[http://dx.doi.org/10.1016/j.ccm.2018.08.006] [PMID: 30390753]

[10]   Kalil AC, Metersky ML, Klompas M, *et al.* Management of adults with hospital-acquired and ventilator-associated pneumonia: Clinical Practice Guidelines by the Infectious Diseases Society of America and the American Thoracic Society. Clin Infect Dis 2016; 63(5): e61-e111.
[http://dx.doi.org/10.1093/cid/ciw353] [PMID: 27418577]

[11]   Craig WA. Pharmacokinetic/pharmacodynamic parameters: rationale for antibacterial dosing of mice and men. Clin Infect Dis Off Publ Infect Dis Soc Am 1998 ; 26(1): 1- 10. quiz 11–2..

[12]   Drusano GL. Antimicrobial pharmacodynamics: critical interactions of 'bug and drug'. Nat Rev Microbiol 2004; 2(4): 289-300.
[http://dx.doi.org/10.1038/nrmicro862] [PMID: 15031728]

[13]   de Velde F, Mouton JW, de Winter BCM, van Gelder T, Koch BCP. Clinical applications of population pharmacokinetic models of antibiotics: Challenges and perspectives. Pharmacol Res 2018; 134: 280-8.
[http://dx.doi.org/10.1016/j.phrs.2018.07.005] [PMID: 30033398]

[14]   Zhou Y-F, Tao M-T, Feng Y, *et al.* Increased activity of colistin in combination with amikacin against *Escherichia coli* co-producing NDM-5 and MCR-1. J Antimicrob Chemother 2017; 72(6): 30-1723.

[15] Mohamed AF, Kristoffersson AN, Karvanen M, Nielsen EI, Cars O, Friberg LE. Dynamic interaction of colistin and meropenem on a WT and a resistant strain of *Pseudomonas aeruginosa* as quantified in a PK/PD model. J Antimicrob Chemother 2016; 71(5): 1279-90.
[http://dx.doi.org/10.1093/jac/dkv488] [PMID: 26850719]

[16] Rao GG, Ly NS, Diep J, *et al.* Combinatorial pharmacodynamics of polymyxin B and tigecycline against heteroresistant *Acinetobacter baumannii.* Int J Antimicrob Agents 2016; 48(3): 331-6.
[http://dx.doi.org/10.1016/j.ijantimicag.2016.06.006] [PMID: 27449542]

[17] Drusano GL. Pre-clinical *in vitro* infection models. Curr Opin Pharmacol 2017; 36: 100-6.
[http://dx.doi.org/10.1016/j.coph.2017.09.011] [PMID: 29035729]

[18] Louie A, Kaw P, Liu W, Jumbe N, Miller MH, Drusano GL. Pharmacodynamics of daptomycin in a murine thigh model of *Staphylococcus aureus* infection. Antimicrob Agents Chemother 2001; 45(3): 845-51.
[http://dx.doi.org/10.1128/AAC.45.3.845-851.2001] [PMID: 11181370]

[19] Gumbo T, Angulo-Barturen I, Ferrer-Bazaga S. Pharmacokinetic-pharmacodynamic and dose-response relationships of antituberculosis drugs: recommendations and standards for industry and academia. J Infect Dis 2015; 211 (Suppl. 3): S96-S106.
[http://dx.doi.org/10.1093/infdis/jiu610] [PMID: 26009618]

[20] Andes D, Craig WA. *In vivo* pharmacodynamic activity of the glycopeptide dalbavancin. Antimicrob Agents Chemother 2007; 51(5): 1633-42.
[http://dx.doi.org/10.1128/AAC.01264-06] [PMID: 17307987]

[21] Mavridou E, Melchers RJB, van Mil ACHAM, Mangin E, Motyl MR, Mouton JW. Pharmacodynamics of imipenem in combination with β-lactamase inhibitor MK7655 in a murine thigh model. Antimicrob Agents Chemother 2015; 59(2): 790-5.
[http://dx.doi.org/10.1128/AAC.03706-14] [PMID: 25403667]

[22] Abdelraouf K, Kim A, Krause KM, Nicolau DP. *In Vivo* efficacy of plazomicin alone or in combination with meropenem or tigecycline against enterobacteriaceae isolates exhibiting various resistance mechanisms in an immunocompetent murine septicemia model. Antimicrob Agents Chemother 2018; 62(8): e01074-18.
[http://dx.doi.org/10.1128/AAC.01074-18] [PMID: 29866866]

[23] Monogue ML, Tsuji M, Yamano Y, Echols R, Nicolau DP. Efficacy of humanized exposures of cefiderocol (S-649266) against a diverse population of gram-negative bacteria in a murine thigh infection model. Antimicrob Agents Chemother 2017; 61(11): e01022-17.
[http://dx.doi.org/10.1128/AAC.01022-17] [PMID: 28848004]

[24] Kidd JM, Abdelraouf K, Nicolau DP. Comparative efficacy of human-simulated epithelial lining fluid exposures of tedizolid, linezolid and vancomycin in neutropenic and immunocompetent murine models of *Staphylococcal pneumonia.* J Antimicrob Chemother 2019; 74(4): 970-7.
[http://dx.doi.org/10.1093/jac/dky513] [PMID: 30561650]

[25] Ambrose PG, Drusano GL, Craig WA. *In vivo* activity of oritavancin in animal infection models and rationale for a new dosing regimen in humans. Clin Infect Dis 2012; 54 (Suppl. 3): S220-8.
[http://dx.doi.org/10.1093/cid/cis001] [PMID: 22431852]

[26] Gilbert DN. Once-daily aminoglycoside therapy. Antimicrob Agents Chemother 1991; 35(3): 399-405.
[http://dx.doi.org/10.1128/AAC.35.3.399] [PMID: 2039189]

[27] Forrest A, Nix DE, Ballow CH, Goss TF, Birmingham MC, Schentag JJ. Pharmacodynamics of intravenous ciprofloxacin in seriously ill patients. Antimicrob Agents Chemother 1993; 37(5): 1073-81.
[http://dx.doi.org/10.1128/AAC.37.5.1073] [PMID: 8517694]

[28] van Zanten ARH, Polderman KH, van Geijlswijk IM, van der Meer GYG, Schouten MA, Girbes ARJ. Ciprofloxacin pharmacokinetics in critically ill patients: a prospective cohort study. J Crit Care 2008;

23(3): 422-30.
[http://dx.doi.org/10.1016/j.jcrc.2007.11.011] [PMID: 18725050]

[29]   Zelenitsky S, Ariano R, Harding G, Forrest A. Evaluating ciprofloxacin dosing for *Pseudomonas aeruginosa* infection by using clinical outcome-based Monte Carlo simulations. Antimicrob Agents Chemother 2005; 49(10): 4009-14.
[http://dx.doi.org/10.1128/AAC.49.10.4009-4014.2005] [PMID: 16189073]

[30]   Khachman D, Conil J-M, Georges B, *et al.* Optimizing ciprofloxacin dosing in intensive care unit patients through the use of population pharmacokinetic-pharmacodynamic analysis and Monte Carlo simulations. J Antimicrob Chemother 2011; 66(8): 1798-809.
[http://dx.doi.org/10.1093/jac/dkr220] [PMID: 21653603]

[31]   Haeseker M, Stolk L, Nieman F, *et al.* The ciprofloxacin target AUC : MIC ratio is not reached in hospitalized patients with the recommended dosing regimens. Br J Clin Pharmacol 2013; 75(1): 180-5.
[http://dx.doi.org/10.1111/j.1365-2125.2012.04337.x] [PMID: 22616681]

[32]   Huttner A, Harbarth S, Hope WW, Lipman J, Roberts JA. Therapeutic drug monitoring of the β-lactam antibiotics: what is the evidence and which patients should we be using it for? J Antimicrob Chemother 2015; 70(12): 3178-83.
[http://dx.doi.org/10.1093/jac/dkv201] [PMID: 26188037]

[33]   Roberts JA, Abdul-Aziz MH, Lipman J, *et al.* International society of anti-infective pharmacology and the pharmacokinetics and pharmacodynamics study group of the european society of clinical microbiology and infectious diseases. Individualised antibiotic dosing for patients who are critically ill: challenges and potential solutions. Lancet Infect Dis 2014; 14(6): 498-509.
[http://dx.doi.org/10.1016/S1473-3099(14)70036-2] [PMID: 24768475]

[34]   Roberts JA, Paul SK, Akova M, *et al.* DALI Study. DALI: defining antibiotic levels in intensive care unit patients: are current β-lactam antibiotic doses sufficient for critically ill patients? Clin Infect Dis 2014; 58(8): 1072-83.
[http://dx.doi.org/10.1093/cid/ciu027] [PMID: 24429437]

[35]   Robertson LC, Al-Haddad M. Recognizing the critically ill patient. Anaesth Intensive Care Med 2013; 14(1): 11-4.
[http://dx.doi.org/10.1016/j.mpaic.2012.11.010]

[36]   van der Poll T. Immunotherapy of sepsis. Lancet Infect Dis 2001; 1(3): 165-74.
[http://dx.doi.org/10.1016/S1473-3099(01)00093-7] [PMID: 11871493]

[37]   Gonçalves-Pereira J, Póvoa P. Antibiotics in critically ill patients: a systematic review of the pharmacokinetics of β-lactams. Crit Care 2011; 15(5): R206.
[http://dx.doi.org/10.1186/cc10441] [PMID: 21914174]

[38]   Conil JM, Georges B, Breden A, *et al.* Increased amikacin dosage requirements in burn patients receiving a once-daily regimen. Int J Antimicrob Agents 2006; 28(3): 226-30.
[http://dx.doi.org/10.1016/j.ijantimicag.2006.04.015] [PMID: 16908121]

[39]   Marik PE. Aminoglycoside volume of distribution and illness severity in critically ill septic patients. Anaesth Intensive Care 1993; 21(2): 172-3.
[http://dx.doi.org/10.1177/0310057X9302100206] [PMID: 8517507]

[40]   Sime FB, Roberts MS, Peake SL, Lipman J, Roberts JA. Does beta-lactam pharmacokinetic variability in critically ill patients justify therapeutic drug monitoring? a systematic review. Ann Intensive Care 2012; 2(1): 35.
[http://dx.doi.org/10.1186/2110-5820-2-35] [PMID: 22839761]

[41]   Roberts JA, Taccone FS, Udy AA, Vincent J-L, Jacobs F, Lipman J. Vancomycin dosing in critically ill patients: robust methods for improved continuous-infusion regimens. Antimicrob Agents Chemother 2011; 55(6): 2704-9.
[http://dx.doi.org/10.1128/AAC.01708-10] [PMID: 21402850]

[42] Buerger C, Plock N, Dehghanyar P, Joukhadar C, Kloft C. Pharmacokinetics of unbound linezolid in plasma and tissue interstitium of critically ill patients after multiple dosing using microdialysis. Antimicrob Agents Chemother 2006; 50(7): 2455-63.
[http://dx.doi.org/10.1128/AAC.01468-05] [PMID: 16801426]

[43] Gous A, Lipman J, Scribante J, *et al.* Fluid shifts have no influence on ciprofloxacin pharmacokinetics in intensive care patients with intra-abdominal sepsis. Int J Antimicrob Agents 2005; 26(1): 50-5.
[http://dx.doi.org/10.1016/j.ijantimicag.2005.04.005] [PMID: 15955670]

[44] Ulldemolins M, Roberts JA, Rello J, Paterson DL, Lipman J. The effects of hypoalbuminaemia on optimizing antibacterial dosing in critically ill patients. Clin Pharmacokinet 2011; 50(2): 99-110.
[http://dx.doi.org/10.2165/11539220-000000000-00000] [PMID: 21142293]

[45] Gurevich KG. Effect of blood protein concentrations on drug-dosing regimes: practical guidance. Theor Biol Med Model 2013; 10: 20.
[http://dx.doi.org/10.1186/1742-4682-10-20] [PMID: 23506635]

[46] Vanstraelen K, Wauters J, Vercammen I, *et al.* Impact of hypoalbuminemia on voriconazole pharmacokinetics in critically ill adult patients. Antimicrob Agents Chemother 2014; 58(11): 6782-9.
[http://dx.doi.org/10.1128/AAC.03641-14] [PMID: 25182655]

[47] Theuretzbacher U. Pharmacokinetic and pharmacodynamic issues for antimicrobial therapy in patients with cancer. Clin Infect Dis 2012; 54(12): 1785-92.
[http://dx.doi.org/10.1093/cid/cis210] [PMID: 22437238]

[48] Ulldemolins M, Roberts JA, Lipman J, Rello J. Antibiotic dosing in multiple organ dysfunction syndrome. Chest 2011; 139(5): 1210-20.
[http://dx.doi.org/10.1378/chest.10-2371] [PMID: 21540219]

[49] Mimoz O, Rolland D, Adoun M, *et al.* Steady-state trough serum and epithelial lining fluid concentrations of teicoplanin 12 mg/kg per day in patients with ventilator-associated pneumonia. Intensive Care Med 2006; 32(5): 775-9.
[http://dx.doi.org/10.1007/s00134-006-0136-3] [PMID: 16550370]

[50] Ulldemolins M, Roberts JA, Wallis SC, Rello J, Lipman J. Flucloxacillin dosing in critically ill patients with hypoalbuminaemia: special emphasis on unbound pharmacokinetics. J Antimicrob Chemother 2010; 65(8): 1771-8.
[http://dx.doi.org/10.1093/jac/dkq184] [PMID: 20530507]

[51] Burkhardt O, Kumar V, Katterwe D, *et al.* Ertapenem in critically ill patients with early-onset ventilator-associated pneumonia: pharmacokinetics with special consideration of free-drug concentration. J Antimicrob Chemother 2007; 59(2): 277-84.
[http://dx.doi.org/10.1093/jac/dkl485] [PMID: 17185298]

[52] Boselli E, Breilh D, Saux M-C, Gordien J-B, Allaouchiche B. Pharmacokinetics and lung concentrations of ertapenem in patients with ventilator-associated pneumonia. Intensive Care Med 2006; 32(12): 2059-62.
[http://dx.doi.org/10.1007/s00134-006-0401-5] [PMID: 17039351]

[53] Bonate PL. Pathophysiology and pharmacokinetics following burn injury. Clin Pharmacokinet 1990; 18(2): 118-30.
[http://dx.doi.org/10.2165/00003088-199018020-00003] [PMID: 2180612]

[54] Soy D, López E, Ribas J. Teicoplanin population pharmacokinetic analysis in hospitalized patients. Ther Drug Monit 2006; 28(6): 737-43.
[http://dx.doi.org/10.1097/01.ftd.0000249942.14145.ff] [PMID: 17164688]

[55] MacGowan AP. Pharmacodynamics, pharmacokinetics, and therapeutic drug monitoring of glycopeptides. Ther Drug Monit 1998; 20(5): 473-7.
[http://dx.doi.org/10.1097/00007691-199810000-00005] [PMID: 9780121]

[56] Etzel JV, Nafziger AN, Bertino JS Jr. Variation in the pharmacokinetics of gentamicin and tobramycin

in patients with pleural effusions and hypoalbuminemia. Antimicrob Agents Chemother 1992; 36(3): 679-81.
[http://dx.doi.org/10.1128/AAC.36.3.679] [PMID: 1622185]

[57] Ronchera-Oms CL, Tormo C, Ordovás JP, Abad J, Jiménez NV. Expanded gentamicin volume of distribution in critically ill adult patients receiving total parenteral nutrition. J Clin Pharm Ther 1995; 20(5): 253-8.
[http://dx.doi.org/10.1111/j.1365-2710.1995.tb00659.x] [PMID: 8576291]

[58] Mohr JF III, Ostrosky-Zeichner L, Wainright DJ, Parks DH, Hollenbeck TC, Ericsson CD. Pharmacokinetic evaluation of single-dose intravenous daptomycin in patients with thermal burn injury. Antimicrob Agents Chemother 2008; 52(5): 1891-3.
[http://dx.doi.org/10.1128/AAC.01321-07] [PMID: 18299410]

[59] Stoeckel K, McNamara PJ, Brandt R, Plozza-Nottebrock H, Ziegler WH. Effects of concentration-dependent plasma protein binding on ceftriaxone kinetics. Clin Pharmacol Ther 1981; 29(5): 650-7.
[http://dx.doi.org/10.1038/clpt.1981.90] [PMID: 7053242]

[60] Joynt GM, Lipman J, Gomersall CD, Young RJ, Wong EL, Gin T. The pharmacokinetics of once-daily dosing of ceftriaxone in critically ill patients. J Antimicrob Chemother 2001; 47(4): 421-9.
[http://dx.doi.org/10.1093/jac/47.4.421] [PMID: 11266414]

[61] Pletz MWR, Rau M, Bulitta J, et al. Ertapenem pharmacokinetics and impact on intestinal microflora, in comparison to those of ceftriaxone, after multiple dosing in male and female volunteers. Antimicrob Agents Chemother 2004; 48(10): 3765-72.
[http://dx.doi.org/10.1128/AAC.48.10.3765-3772.2004] [PMID: 15388432]

[62] Landersdorfer CB, Kirkpatrick CMJ, Kinzig-Schippers M, et al. Population pharmacokinetics at two dose levels and pharmacodynamic profiling of flucloxacillin. Antimicrob Agents Chemother 2007; 51(9): 3290-7.
[http://dx.doi.org/10.1128/AAC.01410-06] [PMID: 17576847]

[63] Gamba G, Contreras AM, Cortés J, et al. Hypoalbuminemia as a risk factor for amikacin nephrotoxicity. Rev Invest Clin 1990; 42(3): 204-9.
[PMID: 2270367]

[64] Di Giantomasso D, May CN, Bellomo R. Vital organ blood flow during hyperdynamic sepsis. Chest 2003; 124(3): 1053-9.
[http://dx.doi.org/10.1378/chest.124.3.1053] [PMID: 12970037]

[65] Huttner A, Von Dach E, Renzoni A, et al. Augmented renal clearance, low β-lactam concentrations and clinical outcomes in the critically ill: an observational prospective cohort study. Int J Antimicrob Agents 2015; 45(4): 385-92.
[http://dx.doi.org/10.1016/j.ijantimicag.2014.12.017] [PMID: 25656151]

[66] Udy AA, Varghese JM, Altukroni M, et al. Subtherapeutic initial β-lactam concentrations in select critically ill patients: association between augmented renal clearance and low trough drug concentrations. Chest 2012; 142(1): 30-9.
[http://dx.doi.org/10.1378/chest.11-1671] [PMID: 22194591]

[67] Joukhadar C, Frossard M, Mayer BX, et al. Impaired target site penetration of beta-lactams may account for therapeutic failure in patients with septic shock. Crit Care Med 2001; 29(2): 385-91.
[http://dx.doi.org/10.1097/00003246-200102000-00030] [PMID: 11246321]

[68] Zeitlinger MA, Dehghanyar P, Mayer BX, et al. Relevance of soft-tissue penetration by levofloxacin for target site bacterial killing in patients with sepsis. Antimicrob Agents Chemother 2003; 47(11): 3548-53.
[http://dx.doi.org/10.1128/AAC.47.11.3548-3553.2003] [PMID: 14576116]

[69] Roberts JA, Roberts MS, Robertson TA, Dalley AJ, Lipman J. Piperacillin penetration into tissue of critically ill patients with sepsis--bolus *versus* continuous administration? Crit Care Med 2009; 37(3): 926-33.

[http://dx.doi.org/10.1097/CCM.0b013e3181968e44] [PMID: 19237898]

[70] Joukhadar C, Klein N, Dittrich P, *et al.* Target site penetration of fosfomycin in critically ill patients. J Antimicrob Chemother 2003; 51(5): 1247-52.
[http://dx.doi.org/10.1093/jac/dkg187] [PMID: 12668580]

[71] Joukhadar C, Klein N, Mayer BX, *et al.* Plasma and tissue pharmacokinetics of cefpirome in patients with sepsis. Crit Care Med 2002; 30(7): 1478-82.
[http://dx.doi.org/10.1097/00003246-200207000-00013] [PMID: 12130965]

[72] Pai MP, Bearden DT. Antimicrobial dosing considerations in obese adult patients. Pharmacotherapy 2007; 27(8): 1081-91.
[http://dx.doi.org/10.1592/phco.27.8.1081] [PMID: 17655508]

[73] Janson B, Thursky K. Dosing of antibiotics in obesity. Curr Opin Infect Dis 2012; 25(6): 634-49.
[http://dx.doi.org/10.1097/QCO.0b013e328359a4c1] [PMID: 23041773]

[74] Maddox A, Horowitz M, Wishart J, Collins P. Gastric and oesophageal emptying in obesity. Scand J Gastroenterol 1989; 24(5): 593-8.
[http://dx.doi.org/10.3109/00365528909093095] [PMID: 2762759]

[75] Jackson SJ, Leahy FE, McGowan AA, Bluck LJC, Coward WA, Jebb SA. Delayed gastric emptying in the obese: an assessment using the non-invasive (13)C-octanoic acid breath test. Diabetes Obes Metab 2004; 6(4): 264-70.
[http://dx.doi.org/10.1111/j.1462-8902.2004.0344.x] [PMID: 15171750]

[76] Lin H, Yeh DD, Levine AR. Daily vancomycin dose requirements as a continuous infusion in obese *versus* non-obese SICU patients. Crit Care 2016; 20(1): 205.
[http://dx.doi.org/10.1186/s13054-016-1363-9] [PMID: 27363312]

[77] Kiang TKL, Ranamukhaarachchi SA, Ensom MHH. Revolutionizing therapeutic drug monitoring with the use of interstitial fluid and microneedles technology. Pharmaceutics 2017; 9(4): E43.
[http://dx.doi.org/10.3390/pharmaceutics9040043] [PMID: 29019915]

[78] Raju KSR, Taneja I, Singh SP, Wahajuddin . Utility of noninvasive biomatrices in pharmacokinetic studies. Biomed Chromatogr 2013; 27(10): 1354-66.
[http://dx.doi.org/10.1002/bmc.2996] [PMID: 23939915]

[79] Drobitch RK, Svensson CK. Therapeutic drug monitoring in saliva. An update. Clin Pharmacokinet 1992; 23(5): 365-79.
[http://dx.doi.org/10.2165/00003088-199223050-00003] [PMID: 1478004]

[80] Gorodischer R, Koren G. Salivary excretion of drugs in children: theoretical and practical issues in therapeutic drug monitoring. Dev Pharmacol Ther 1992; 19(4): 161-77.
[http://dx.doi.org/10.1159/000457481] [PMID: 1343619]

[81] Li Q, Naora K, Hirano H, Okunishi H, Iwamoto K. Comparative study on salivary distribution of fluoroquinolones in rats. Biol Pharm Bull 2002; 25(8): 1084-9.
[http://dx.doi.org/10.1248/bpb.25.1084] [PMID: 12186414]

[82] Koizumi F, Ohnishi A, Takemura H, Okubo S, Kagami T, Tanaka T. Effective monitoring of concentrations of ofloxacin in saliva of patients with chronic respiratory tract infections. Antimicrob Agents Chemother 1994; 38(5): 1140-3.
[http://dx.doi.org/10.1128/AAC.38.5.1140] [PMID: 8067752]

[83] Mullangi R, Agrawal S, Srinivas NR. Measurement of xenobiotics in saliva: is saliva an attractive alternative matrix? Case studies and analytical perspectives. Biomed Chromatogr 2009; 23(1): 3-25.
[http://dx.doi.org/10.1002/bmc.1103] [PMID: 18816455]

[84] Kiang TKL, Häfeli UO, Ensom MHH. A comprehensive review on the pharmacokinetics of antibiotics in interstitial fluid spaces in humans: implications on dosing and clinical pharmacokinetic monitoring. Clin Pharmacokinet 2014; 53(8): 695-730.
[http://dx.doi.org/10.1007/s40262-014-0152-3] [PMID: 24972859]

[85] Dalla Costa T, Nolting A, Kovar A, Derendorf H. Determination of free interstitial concentrations of piperacillin-tazobactam combinations by microdialysis. J Antimicrob Chemother 1998; 42(6): 769-78.
[http://dx.doi.org/10.1093/jac/42.6.769] [PMID: 10052901]

[86] Tomaselli F, Dittrich P, Maier A, *et al.* Penetration of piperacillin and tazobactam into pneumonic human lung tissue measured by *in vivo* microdialysis. Br J Clin Pharmacol 2003; 55(6): 620-4.
[http://dx.doi.org/10.1046/j.1365-2125.2003.01797.x] [PMID: 12814459]

[87] Traunmüller F, Schintler MV, Metzler J, *et al.* Soft tissue and bone penetration abilities of daptomycin in diabetic patients with bacterial foot infections. J Antimicrob Chemother 2010; 65(6): 1252-7.
[http://dx.doi.org/10.1093/jac/dkq109] [PMID: 20375031]

[88] Housman ST, Bhalodi AA, Shepard A, Nugent J, Nicolau DP. Vancomycin tissue pharmacokinetics in patients with lower-limb infections *via In Vivo* Microdialysis. J Am Podiatr Med Assoc 2015; 105(5): 381-8.
[http://dx.doi.org/10.7547/14-033] [PMID: 26429605]

[89] Hamada Y, Kuti JL, Nicolau DP. Vancomycin serum concentrations do not adequately predict tissue exposure in diabetic patients with mild to moderate limb infections. J Antimicrob Chemother 2015; 70(7): 2064-7.
[http://dx.doi.org/10.1093/jac/dkv074] [PMID: 25802284]

[90] Skhirtladze K, Hutschala D, Fleck T, *et al.* Impaired target site penetration of vancomycin in diabetic patients following cardiac surgery. Antimicrob Agents Chemother 2006; 50(4): 1372-5.
[http://dx.doi.org/10.1128/AAC.50.4.1372-1375.2006] [PMID: 16569854]

[91] Rybak MJ, Lomaestro BM, Rotschafer JC, *et al.* Vancomycin therapeutic guidelines: a summary of consensus recommendations from the infectious diseases Society of America, the American Society of Health-System Pharmacists, and the Society of Infectious Diseases Pharmacists. Clin Infect Dis 2009; 49(3): 325-7.
[http://dx.doi.org/10.1086/600877] [PMID: 19569969]

[92] Pea F, Poz D, Viale P, Pavan F, Furlanut M. Which reliable pharmacodynamic breakpoint should be advised for ciprofloxacin monotherapy in the hospital setting? A TDM-based retrospective perspective. J Antimicrob Chemother 2006; 58(2): 380-6.
[http://dx.doi.org/10.1093/jac/dkl226] [PMID: 16735422]

[93] Wong G, Sime FB, Lipman J, Roberts JA. How do we use therapeutic drug monitoring to improve outcomes from severe infections in critically ill patients? BMC Infect Dis 2014; 14: 288.
[http://dx.doi.org/10.1186/1471-2334-14-288] [PMID: 25430961]

[94] Roberts JA, Norris R, Paterson DL, Martin JH. Therapeutic drug monitoring of antimicrobials. Br J Clin Pharmacol 2012; 73(1): 27-36.
[http://dx.doi.org/10.1111/j.1365-2125.2011.04080.x] [PMID: 21831196]

[95] Minejima E, Choi J, Beringer P, Lou M, Tse E, Wong-Beringer A. Applying new diagnostic criteria for acute kidney injury to facilitate early identification of nephrotoxicity in vancomycin-treated patients. Antimicrob Agents Chemother 2011; 55(7): 3278-83.
[http://dx.doi.org/10.1128/AAC.00173-11] [PMID: 21576448]

[96] Prabaker KK, Tran TP-H, Pratummas T, Goetz MB, Graber CJ. Elevated vancomycin trough is not associated with nephrotoxicity among inpatient veterans. J Hosp Med 2012; 7(2): 91-7.
[http://dx.doi.org/10.1002/jhm.946] [PMID: 22086511]

[97] Jeffres MN, Isakow W, Doherty JA, Micek ST, Kollef MH. A retrospective analysis of possible renal toxicity associated with vancomycin in patients with health care-associated methicillin-resistant *Staphylococcus aureus* pneumonia. Clin Ther 2007; 29(6): 1107-15.
[http://dx.doi.org/10.1016/j.clinthera.2007.06.014] [PMID: 17692725]

[98] Bosso JA, Nappi J, Rudisill C, *et al.* Relationship between vancomycin trough concentrations and nephrotoxicity: a prospective multicenter trial. Antimicrob Agents Chemother 2011; 55(12): 5475-9.

[http://dx.doi.org/10.1128/AAC.00168-11] [PMID: 21947388]

[99]   Forouzesh A, Moise PA, Sakoulas G. Vancomycin ototoxicity: a reevaluation in an era of increasing doses. Antimicrob Agents Chemother 2009; 53(2): 483-6.
[http://dx.doi.org/10.1128/AAC.01088-08] [PMID: 19001107]

[100]   Chambers HF, Kennedy S. Effects of dosage, peak and trough concentrations in serum, protein binding, and bactericidal rate on efficacy of teicoplanin in a rabbit model of endocarditis. Antimicrob Agents Chemother 1990; 34(4): 510-4.
[http://dx.doi.org/10.1128/AAC.34.4.510] [PMID: 2140496]

[101]   Harding I, MacGowan AP, White LO, Darley ES, Reed V. Teicoplanin therapy for *Staphylococcus aureus* septicaemia: relationship between pre-dose serum concentrations and outcome. J Antimicrob Chemother 2000; 45(6): 835-41.
[http://dx.doi.org/10.1093/jac/45.6.835] [PMID: 10837438]

[102]   Wilson AP, Grüneberg RN, Neu H. A critical review of the dosage of teicoplanin in Europe and the USA. Int J Antimicrob Agents 1994; 4 (Suppl. 1): 1-30.
[http://dx.doi.org/10.1016/0924-8579(94)90049-3] [PMID: 18611626]

[103]   Moise-Broder PA, Forrest A, Birmingham MC, Schentag JJ. Pharmacodynamics of vancomycin and other antimicrobials in patients with *Staphylococcus aureus* lower respiratory tract infections. Clin Pharmacokinet 2004; 43(13): 925-42.
[http://dx.doi.org/10.2165/00003088-200443130-00005] [PMID: 15509186]

[104]   Löwdin E, Odenholt I, Cars O. *In vitro* studies of pharmacodynamic properties of vancomycin against *Staphylococcus aureus* and *Staphylococcus epidermidis*. Antimicrob Agents Chemother 1998; 42(10): 2739-44.
[http://dx.doi.org/10.1128/AAC.42.10.2739] [PMID: 9756787]

[105]   Ackerman BH, Vannier AM, Eudy EB. Analysis of vancomycin time-kill studies with Staphylococcus species by using a curve stripping program to describe the relationship between concentration and pharmacodynamic response. Antimicrob Agents Chemother 1992; 36(8): 1766-9.
[http://dx.doi.org/10.1128/AAC.36.8.1766] [PMID: 1416862]

[106]   Rybak MJ. Pharmacodynamics: relation to antimicrobial resistance. Am J Med 2006; 119(6) (Suppl. 1): S37-44.
[http://dx.doi.org/10.1016/j.amjmed.2006.04.001] [PMID: 16735150]

[107]   Craig WA. Basic pharmacodynamics of antibacterials with clinical applications to the use of beta-lactams, glycopeptides, and linezolid. Infect Dis Clin North Am 2003; 17(3): 479-501.
[http://dx.doi.org/10.1016/S0891-5520(03)00065-5] [PMID: 14711073]

[108]   Rybak MJ. The pharmacokinetic and pharmacodynamic properties of vancomycin. Clin Infect Dis 2006; 42 (Suppl. 1): S35-9.
[http://dx.doi.org/10.1086/491712] [PMID: 16323118]

[109]   Takahashi Y, Takesue Y, Takubo S, *et al.* Preferable timing of therapeutic drug monitoring in patients with impaired renal function treated with once-daily administration of vancomycin. J Infect Chemother 2013; 19(4): 709-16.
[http://dx.doi.org/10.1007/s10156-013-0551-7] [PMID: 23345049]

[110]   Wilson JF, Davis AC, Tobin CM. Evaluation of commercial assays for vancomycin and aminoglycosides in serum: a comparison of accuracy and precision based on external quality assessment. J Antimicrob Chemother 2003; 52(1): 78-82.
[http://dx.doi.org/10.1093/jac/dkg296] [PMID: 12805260]

[111]   Shahrami B, Najmeddin F, Mousavi S, *et al.* Achievement of vancomycin therapeutic goals in critically ill patients: early individualization may be beneficial. Crit Care Res Pract 2016; 2016: 1245815.
[http://dx.doi.org/10.1155/2016/1245815] [PMID: 27073695]

[112] Neely MN, Youn G, Jones B, *et al.* Are vancomycin trough concentrations adequate for optimal dosing? Antimicrob Agents Chemother 2014; 58(1): 309-16.
[http://dx.doi.org/10.1128/AAC.01653-13] [PMID: 24165176]

[113] Heil EL, Claeys KC, Mynatt RP, *et al.* Making the change to area under the curve-based vancomycin dosing. Am J Health Syst Pharm 2018; 75(24): 1986-95.
[http://dx.doi.org/10.2146/ajhp180034] [PMID: 30333114]

[114] Sakoulas G, Gold HS, Cohen RA, Venkataraman L, Moellering RC, Eliopoulos GM. Effects of prolonged vancomycin administration on methicillin-resistant *Staphylococcus aureus* (MRSA) in a patient with recurrent bacteraemia. J Antimicrob Chemother 2006; 57(4): 699-704.
[http://dx.doi.org/10.1093/jac/dkl030] [PMID: 16464892]

[115] Howden BP, Ward PB, Charles PGP, *et al.* Treatment outcomes for serious infections caused by methicillin-resistant *Staphylococcus aureus* with reduced vancomycin susceptibility. Clin Infect Dis 2004; 38(4): 521-8.
[http://dx.doi.org/10.1086/381202] [PMID: 14765345]

[116] Ye Z-K, Chen Y-L, Chen K, *et al.* Guideline steering group, the guideline development group and the guideline secretary group. Therapeutic drug monitoring of vancomycin: a guideline of the division of therapeutic drug monitoring, chinese pharmacological society. J Antimicrob Chemother 2016; 71(11): 3020-5.
[http://dx.doi.org/10.1093/jac/dkw254] [PMID: 27494905]

[117] Wieczorkiewicz SM, Sincak CA. American Society of Health-System Pharmacists. The pharmacist's guide to antimicrobial therapy and stewardship. Bethesda, MD: ASHP Publications 2016.

[118] Nicolau DP, Freeman CD, Belliveau PP, Nightingale CH, Ross JW, Quintiliani R. Experience with a once-daily aminoglycoside program administered to 2,184 adult patients. Antimicrob Agents Chemother 1995; 39(3): 650-5.
[http://dx.doi.org/10.1128/AAC.39.3.650] [PMID: 7793867]

[119] Banerjee S, Narayanan M, Gould K. Monitoring aminoglycoside level. BMJ 2012; 345: e6354.
[http://dx.doi.org/10.1136/bmj.e6354]

[120] Conil J-M, Georges B, Ruiz S, *et al.* Tobramycin disposition in ICU patients receiving a once daily regimen: population approach and dosage simulations. Br J Clin Pharmacol 2011; 71(1): 61-71.
[http://dx.doi.org/10.1111/j.1365-2125.2010.03793.x] [PMID: 21143502]

[121] Botha FJ, van der Bijl P, Seifart HI, Parkin DP. Fluctuation of the volume of distribution of amikacin and its effect on once-daily dosage and clearance in a seriously ill patient. Intensive Care Med 1996; 22(5): 443-6.
[http://dx.doi.org/10.1007/BF01712162] [PMID: 8796397]

[122] Begg EJ, Barclay ML, Duffull SB. A suggested approach to once-daily aminoglycoside dosing. Br J Clin Pharmacol 1995; 39(6): 605-9.
[http://dx.doi.org/10.1111/j.1365-2125.1995.tb05719.x] [PMID: 7654477]

[123] Dasgupta A. Advances in antibiotic measurement. Adv Clin Chem 2012; 56: 75-104.
[http://dx.doi.org/10.1016/B978-0-12-394317-0.00013-3] [PMID: 22397029]

[124] Thakuria B, Lahon K. The beta lactam antibiotics as an empirical therapy in a developing country: an update on their current status and recommendations to counter the resistance against them. J Clin Diagn Res 2013; 7(6): 1207-14.
[http://dx.doi.org/10.7860/JCDR/2013/5239.3052] [PMID: 23905143]

[125] van Geijlswijk IM, van Zanten ARH, van der Meer YG. Reliable new high-performance liquid chromatographic method for the determination of ciprofloxacin in human serum. Ther Drug Monit 2006; 28(2): 278-81.
[http://dx.doi.org/10.1097/01.ftd.0000189823.43236.90] [PMID: 16628145]

[126] Roger C, Roberts JA, Muller L. Clinical pharmacokinetics and pharmacodynamics of oxazolidinones.

Clin Pharmacokinet 2018; 57(5): 559-75.
[http://dx.doi.org/10.1007/s40262-017-0601-x] [PMID: 29063519]

[127] Andes D, van Ogtrop ML, Peng J, Craig WA. *In vivo* pharmacodynamics of a new oxazolidinone (linezolid). Antimicrob Agents Chemother 2002; 46(11): 3484-9.
[http://dx.doi.org/10.1128/AAC.46.11.3484-3489.2002] [PMID: 12384354]

[128] Stalker DJ, Jungbluth GL. Clinical pharmacokinetics of linezolid, a novel oxazolidinone antibacterial. Clin Pharmacokinet 2003; 42(13): 1129-40.
[http://dx.doi.org/10.2165/00003088-200342130-00004] [PMID: 14531724]

[129] Tsuji Y, Hiraki Y, Mizoguchi A, *et al.* Pharmacokinetics of repeated dosing of linezolid in a hemodialysis patient with chronic renal failure. J Infect Chemother 2008; 14(2): 156-60.
[http://dx.doi.org/10.1007/s10156-008-0587-2] [PMID: 18622681]

[130] Tsuji Y, Hiraki Y, Matsumoto K, *et al.* Thrombocytopenia and anemia caused by a persistent high linezolid concentration in patients with renal dysfunction. J Infect Chemother 2011; 17(1): 70-5.
[http://dx.doi.org/10.1007/s10156-010-0080-6] [PMID: 20582446]

[131] Nukui Y, Hatakeyama S, Okamoto K, *et al.* High plasma linezolid concentration and impaired renal function affect development of linezolid-induced thrombocytopenia. J Antimicrob Chemother 2013; 68(9): 2128-33.
[http://dx.doi.org/10.1093/jac/dkt133] [PMID: 23625638]

[132] Pea F, Furlanut M, Cojutti P, *et al.* Therapeutic drug monitoring of linezolid: a retrospective monocentric analysis. Antimicrob Agents Chemother 2010; 54(11): 4605-10.
[http://dx.doi.org/10.1128/AAC.00177-10] [PMID: 20733043]

[133] Lovering AM, Le Floch R, Hovsepian L, *et al.* Pharmacokinetic evaluation of linezolid in patients with major thermal injuries. J Antimicrob Chemother 2009; 63(3): 553-9.
[http://dx.doi.org/10.1093/jac/dkn541] [PMID: 19153078]

[134] Lopez-Garcia B, Luque S, Roberts JA, Grau S. Pharmacokinetics and preliminary safety of high dose linezolid for the treatment of Gram-positive bacterial infections. J Infect 2015; 71(5): 604-7.
[http://dx.doi.org/10.1016/j.jinf.2015.06.007] [PMID: 26099449]

[135] Polillo M, Tascini C, Lastella M, *et al.* A rapid high-performance liquid chromatography method to measure linezolid and daptomycin concentrations in human plasma. Ther Drug Monit 2010; 32(2): 200-5.
[http://dx.doi.org/10.1097/FTD.0b013e3181d3f5cb] [PMID: 20216115]

[136] Bolhuis MS, van Altena R, van Hateren K, *et al.* Clinical validation of the analysis of linezolid and clarithromycin in oral fluid of patients with multidrug-resistant tuberculosis. Antimicrob Agents Chemother 2013; 57(8): 3676-80.
[http://dx.doi.org/10.1128/AAC.00558-13] [PMID: 23689722]

[137] Fish DN, Piscitelli SC, Danziger LH. Development of resistance during antimicrobial therapy: a review of antibiotic classes and patient characteristics in 173 studies. Pharmacotherapy 1995; 15(3): 279-91.
[PMID: 7667163]

[138] Kontou P, Chatzika K, Pitsiou G, *et al.* Pharmacokinetics of ciprofloxacin and its penetration into bronchial secretions of mechanically ventilated patients with chronic obstructive pulmonary disease. Antimicrob Agents Chemother 2011; 55(9): 4149-53.
[http://dx.doi.org/10.1128/AAC.00566-10] [PMID: 21670178]

[139] Gasser TC, Ebert SC, Graversen PH, Madsen PO. Ciprofloxacin pharmacokinetics in patients with normal and impaired renal function. Antimicrob Agents Chemother 1987; 31(5): 709-12.
[http://dx.doi.org/10.1128/AAC.31.5.709] [PMID: 3300537]

[140] Fish DN, Bainbridge JL, Peloquin CA. Variable disposition of ciprofloxacin in critically ill patients undergoing continuous arteriovenous hemodiafiltration. Pharmacotherapy 1995; 15(2): 236-45.

CHAPTER 10

Worldwide Antimicrobial Pipeline and Development

Enas A. Almohammadi, Lamia S. Alzahrani, Hadeel N. Alshaikh and **Abrar K. Thabit**[*]

Pharmacy Practice Department, Faculty of Pharmacy, King Abdulaziz University, Jeddah, Saudi Arabia

Abstract: Antimicrobials are a cornerstone of the medical armamentarium due to the increased prevalence of infectious diseases, particularly those caused by drug-resistant pathogens. As organisms that infect humans become smarter through the development of different resistance mechanisms to some of the currently available antimicrobials, the development of new agents with novel mechanisms of action becomes imperative. Many antimicrobials, including antibacterials, antifungals, and antiparasitics, have recently been approved for clinical use or are currently at some stage in the pipeline. This chapter provides a brief description of these antimicrobials with regards to their mechanisms of action, spectra of activity, indications, and pharmaceutical formulations and describes whether they were recently approved or are currently under development or in clinical trials. The wise use of these antimicrobials is essential to maintain their effectiveness for more tenacious infections.

Keywords: Antibacterial, Antibiotic, Antifungal, Antimicrobial, Antiparasitic, Antiprotozoal, β-lactamase, Development, Novel, Pipeline, Resistance, Trials.

INTRODUCTION

As the global battle against antimicrobial resistance continues with the evolution of new resistance mechanisms, antimicrobial therapy has become more challenging over time. Therefore, the development of new weapons (*i.e.,* antimicrobials) with novel mechanisms of actions that are effective against pathogens exhibiting resistance to currently available antimicrobials has become a necessity. The call for the development of new antimicrobials to combat resistance has been made by several health organizations worldwide (such as the World Health Organization, the Infectious Diseases Society of America, and the Wellcome Trust Foundation of the UK) and leaders of several countries.

---

[*] **Corresponding author Abrar K. Thabit:** Pharmacy Practice Department, Faculty of Pharmacy, King Abdulaziz University, Jeddah, Saudi Arabia; Tel: +966-503692243; E-mail: akthabit@kau.edu.sa

Islam M. Ghazi & Michael J. Cawley (Eds.)

This chapter provides a summary of new antimicrobials, whether they were recently approved by the U.S. Food and Drug Administration (FDA; from January 2014 to date for antibacterials, from January 2011 to date for antifungals and antiparasitics, or are still in the pipeline. The summary includes information about the mechanisms of action, spectra of activity, indications, and pharmaceutical formulations and describes whether the agent was recently approved or is currently in development or in a clinical trial. The chapter is divided into three major sections, depending on the target organism: antibacterials, antifungals, and antiparasitics (collectively including antiprotozoals). Due to a large number of antibacterial agents listed, this section was further divided into two subsections: antibacterials that were recently approved and antibacterials that are still under development (*i.e.*, in the pipeline).

ANTIBACTERIAL AGENTS

Approved Antibacterial Agents

Bezlotoxumab

It is a human monoclonal antibody that was approved by the U.S. FDA at the end of 2016 to prevent the recurrence of *Clostridioides difficile* infection (CDI) in adults receiving antibacterial drug treatment for CDI who are at high risk for CDI recurrence [1, 2]. A single molecule of bezlotoxumab neutralizes toxin B by binding to it and thus preventing the toxin from binding to host cells [3]. The most common adverse reactions are nausea, pyrexia, and headache [1]. A study of 2655 participants conducted to measure the safety and efficacy of bezlotoxumab and found that bezlotoxumab was more effective in reducing the rate of CDI recurrence compared with a placebo and had a safety profile similar to that of the placebo [4]. Bezlotoxumab is available as a solution for intravenous (IV) administration.

Cefiderocol

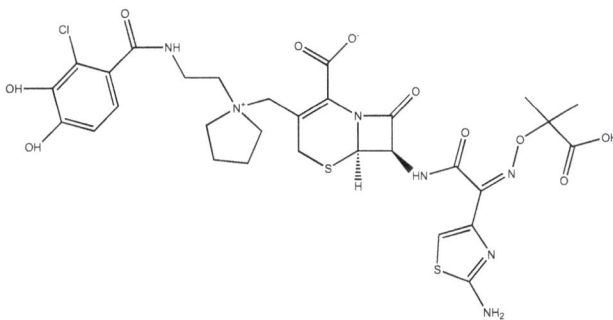

It is a siderophore bactericidal cephalosporin antibiotic that binds to ferric iron and is transported into bacterial cells through the outer membrane, in addition to having a β-lactam effect of inhibiting cell wall synthesis. Cefiderocol covers Gram-negative bacteria including *Escherichia coli, Enterobacter cloacae, Klebsiella pneumoniae, Proteus mirabilis,* and *Pseudomonas aeruginosa. In vitro,* cefiderocol has shown broad-spectrum activity against extended-spectrum β-lactamase (ESBL)-producing organisms, CRE, carbapenem-resistant *P. aeruginosa, Stenotrophomonas maltophilia,* and *Acinetobacter baumannii.* Cefiderocol was approved for complicated urinary tract infections (cUTIs), including pyelonephritis [5]. The most common adverse effects are infusion site reactions, candidiasis, and elevations in liver tests [5]. A phase III clinical trial for the treatment of nosocomial pneumonia caused by Gram-negative bacteria and the treatment of serious infections caused by carbapenem-resistant, Gram-negative bacteria, showed an increase in all-cause mortality in patients treated with cefiderocol as compared to the best available therapy [6, 7]. Cefiderocol was approved by the U.S. FDA in 2019 and is available as a lyophilized powder for IV injection.

Ceftazidime/Avibactam

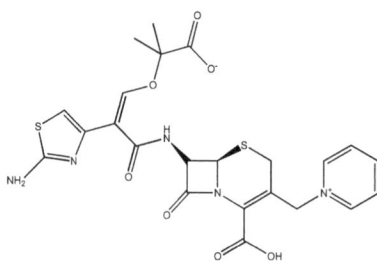
Ceftazidime

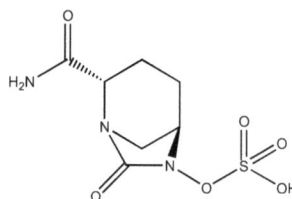
Avibactam

It is a combination of a cephalosporin and a synthetic non-β-lactam, β-lactamase inhibitor that was approved in 2015 [8]. As a β-lactam, ceftazidime kills by inhibiting bacterial cell wall synthesis, whereas avibactam inactivates some β-lactamases (ESBLs, *AmpC* β-lactamase, *K. pneumoniae* carbapenemase [KPC], and OXA-48) to protect ceftazidime from degradation [9]. However, avibactam does not protect against degradation by New Delhi metallo-β-lactamase-1 (NDM-1). Ceftazidime/avibactam was approved for the treatment of the following infections caused by Gram-negative bacteria such as Enterobacteriaceae, *P. aeruginosa,* and *Haemophilus influenza*: complicated intra-abdominal infections (cIAI), used in combination with metronidazole; cUTIs, including pyelonephritis; and hospital-acquired bacterial pneumonia and ventilator-associated bacterial pneumonia (HABP/VABP) [10 - 12]. A pharmacokinetic/pharmacodynamic study in cystic fibrosis patients showed the potential utility of ceftazidime/avibactam for the treatment of acute pulmonary exacerbations in this patient population [10]. Common adverse reactions include gastrointestinal upset and rash [13]. Ceftazidime/avibactam is available as a powder for IV infusion.

Ceftobiprole

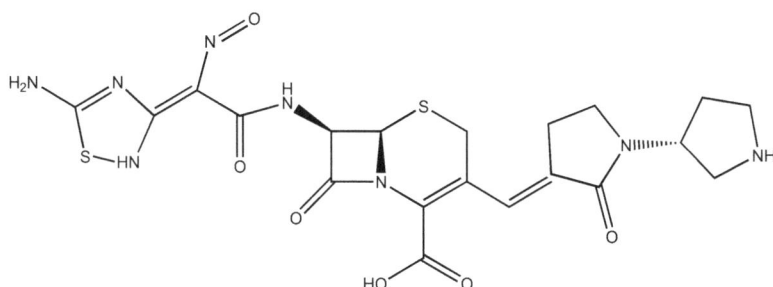

It is a β-lactam that inhibits cell wall synthesis *via* binding to penicillin-binding proteins. It has good activity against many Gram-positive and Gram-negative aerobes, including MRSA, *Enterococcus faecalis*, Enterobacteriaceae, and *P. aeruginosa* [14, 15]. It is being studied for the treatment of HABP and complicated skin and skin structure infection (cSSSI) [14]. It is currently available in Europe as an IV formulation.

Ceftolozane/Tazobactam

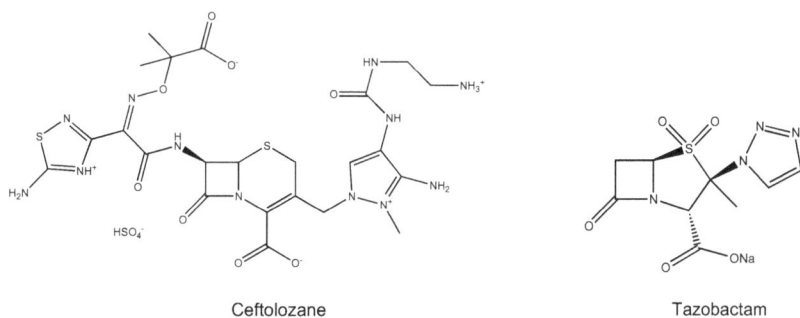

Ceftolozane   Tazobactam

Ceftolozane is a cephalosporin bactericidal antibiotic that inhibits cell wall synthesis, while tazobactam is an irreversible β-lactamase inhibitor (mainly ESBL). Ceftolozane/tazobactam mainly covers Gram-negative bacteria including Enterobacteriaceae and *P. aeruginosa* (including multidrug-resistant [MDR] isolates) [16]. Among Gram-positive bacteria, ceftolozane/tazobactam have activity against *Streptococcus anginosus, S. constellatus* and *S. salivarius*. The anaerobic *Bacteroides fragilis* is also susceptible to the drug. Approved indications include cIAI and cUTI, including pyelonephritis [16]. The most common adverse effects are hypersensitivity reactions, pyrexia, hyperglycemia, renal impairment, venous thrombosis, and hypokalemia. Its efficacy decreases in patients with moderate renal impairment (creatinine clearance = 30-50 mL/min) [16]. Recently, Ceftolozane/ tazobactam completed phase III for ventilator-associated nosocomial pneumonia, but FDA approval remains pending for this indication [17]. The drug is available as a powder for IV infusion.

Dalbavancin

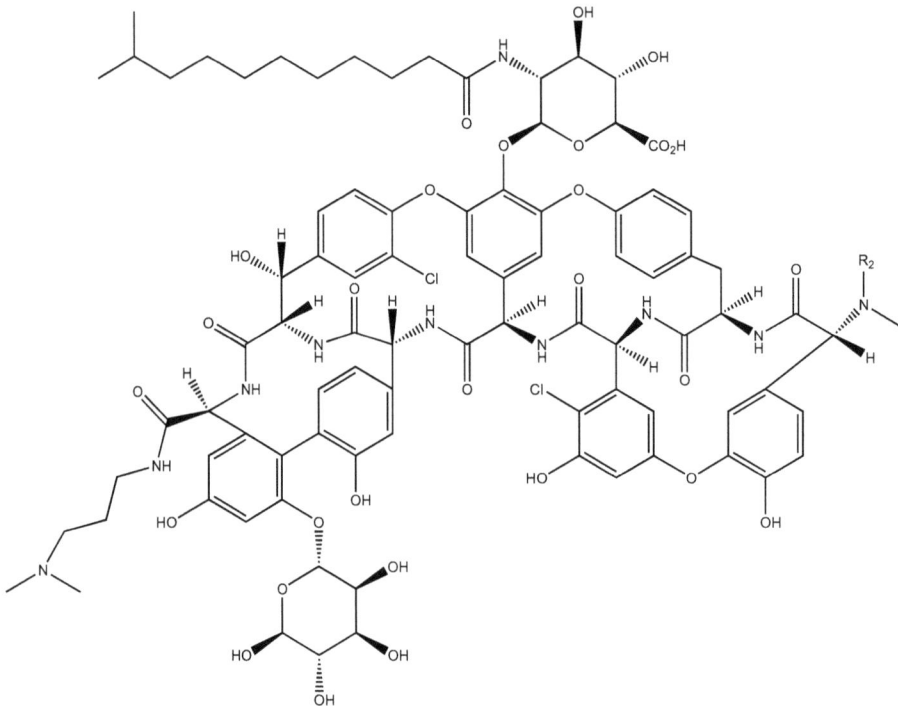

It is a semisynthetic lipoglycopeptide bactericidal antibiotic that binds to the D-alanyl-D-alanine terminus leading to inhibition of cell wall synthesis. Dalbavancin covers Gram-positive bacteria such as *Staphylococcus aureus* (including methicillin-resistant *Staphylococcus aureus*; MRSA), *Streptococcus pyogenes, Streptococcus agalactiae, Streptococcus dysgalactiae, Streptococcus anginosus*, and *E. faecalis* (vancomycin-susceptible only) [18]. Dalbavancin was approved for acute bacterial skin and skin structure infections (ABSSSI) as single or two-dose (separated by one week) regimens given as 30-minute IV infusion. The most common adverse effects are hypersensitivity reactions, infusion-related reactions, hepatotoxicity, international normalized ratio (INR) elevation, hypoglycemia, and bronchospasm [18]. Phase II clinical trial in osteomyelitis has just completed [19]. Dalbavancin is available as a powder for IV infusion.

Delafloxacin

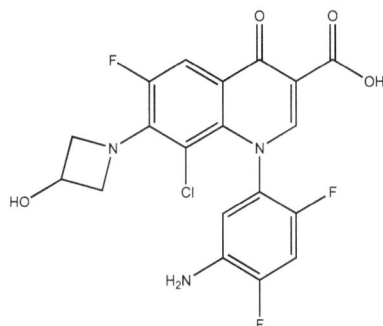

It is a fluoroquinolone antibacterial that was approved by the U.S. FDA in 2017 for the treatment of ABSSSIs caused by Gram-positive organisms such as *Staphylococcus aureus* (including methicillin-resistant [MRSA; first anti-MRSA fluoroquinolone] and methicillin susceptible [MSSA] isolates), *Staphylococcus haemolyticus*, *Streptococcus anginosus*, *S. pyogenes*, and *E. faecalis*. It also has activity against Gram-negative organisms including Enterobacteriaceae and *P. aeruginosa*. Delafloxacin inhibits the activity of bacterial DNA topoisomerase IV and DNA gyrase (topoisomerase II) [20 - 22]. Delafloxacin was also approved for community-acquired bacterial pneumonia (CABP) caused by these pathogens and by *Streptococcus pneumoniae* and atypical pathogens [20 - 22]. A study to evaluate the pharmacokinetics and pharmacodynamics of delafloxacin showed remarkable low minimum inhibitory concentrations (MIC) against Gram-positive organisms and anaerobes, and similar to those of ciprofloxacin against Gram-negative bacteria [23]. Delafloxacin has the advantage of being active against most fluoroquinolone-resistant strains, except *Enterococci*. Its potency is further increased in the acidic environment [24]. Interestingly, delafloxacin is active on *Staphylococci* growing intracellularly or in biofilms [20, 21]. The most common adverse reactions include gastrointestinal upset, liver transaminase elevations, and headache. Serious adverse reactions are similar to other fluoroquinolones and include tendonitis, tendon rupture, peripheral neuropathy, central nervous system effects, and exacerbation of myasthenia gravis, Delafloxacin available as an oral and powder for IV infusion [22].

Eravacycline

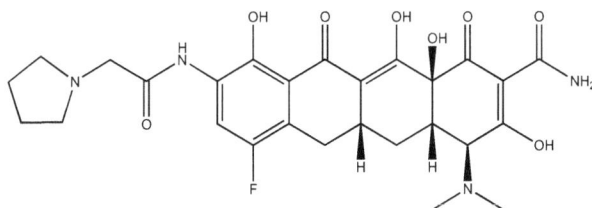

It is a fluorocycline (a derivative of tetracycline) bacteriostatic antibiotic that inhibits protein synthesis. Eravacycline covers both Gram-positive, Gram-negative, and anaerobic bacteria including *A. baumannii*, but not *P. aeruginosa* [25 - 27]. Eravacycline was approved in 2018 for cIAIs and the most common adverse effects reported in the trial were anemia, nausea, pyrexia, and phlebitis [28]. Phase III clinical trial in complicated urinary tract infections cUTI has just completed, but FDA approval was not obtained because of the higher rate of failure in the eravacycline arm, particularly among patients who were early switched from the IV formulation of eravacycline to oral tablets [29]. Eravacycline is currently available as a powder for IV injection.

Finafloxacin

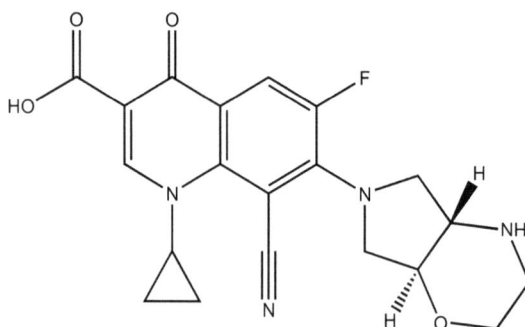

It is a fluoroquinolone antibiotic that inhibits topoisomerase IV and DNA gyrase leading to inhibition of DNA synthesis. Finafloxacin mainly covers *S. aureus and P. aeruginosa*. Finafloxacin was approved for acute otitis externa (AOE) as an otic suspension only. The most common adverse effects are ear pruritus, ear pain, cerumen impaction and hypoacusis [30]. Recently, finafloxacin completed phase II for cUTI [31]. Finafloxacin is available as a sterile suspension ear drops.

Imipenem/Cilastatin/Relebactam

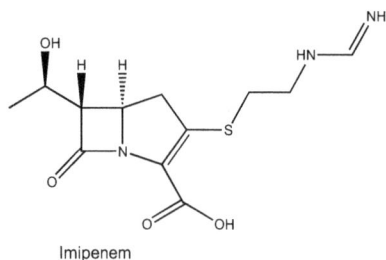

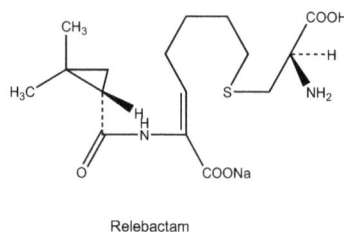

Imipenem

Relebactam

Relebactam is a novel class A and C β-lactamase inhibitor. Imipenem is a broad-spectrum carbapenem bactericidal antibiotic co-formulated with cilastatin which is a dehydropeptidase inhibitor (that protects imipenem from degradation by dehydropeptidase enzyme in the kidneys). Imipenem/cilastatin/relebactam has broad-spectrum activity against β-lactamase-producing Gram-negative bacteria, including CRE [32]. The drug has received U.S. FDA approval in 2019 for cIAIs and cUTIs [33] and the Phase III trial is also completed for HABP/VABP [34]. The drug is available as an IV formulation.

Lascufloxacin

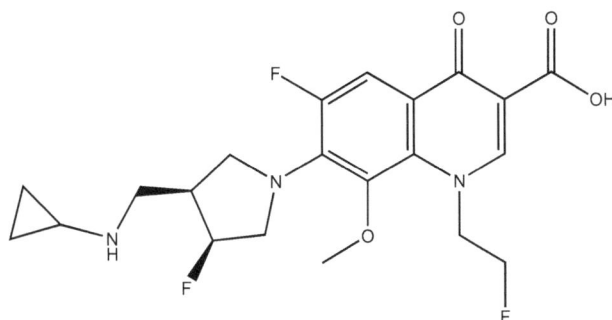

It is a novel fluoroquinolone antibacterial agent. *In vitro*, lascufloxacin was highly active against quinolone-resistant *S. aureus*, *S. pneumoniae*, and *E. coli* [35, 36]. It also illustrated inhibitory activity against target enzymes of wild-type and quinolone-resistant *S. aureus* were determined [35, 36]. A study was conducted to evaluate the intrapulmonary penetration of lascufloxacin in humans found that the lascufloxacin was rapidly distributed to the epithelial lining fluid with a time to maximum drug concentration of one hour [37]. Lascufloxacin is currently available as oral tablets in Japan.

Meropenem/Vaborbactam

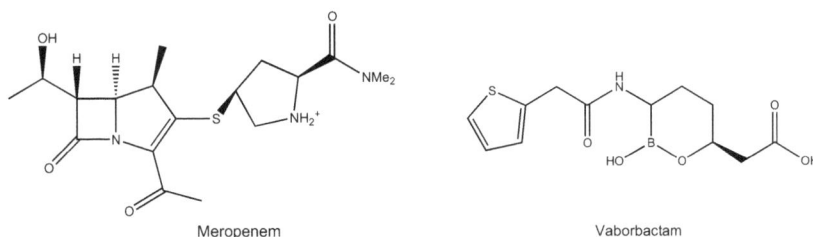

Meropenem

Vaborbactam

Meropenem/vaborbactam was approved in 2017. It is a combination of meropenem, a carbapenem, and vaborbactam, a carbapenemase inhibitor [38]. The addition of vaborbactam extends meropenem's antibacterial activity to cover KPC-producing Enterobacteriaceae and other Gram-negative bacilli, such as *P. aeruginosa* and *Acinetobacter* spp., but not against organisms producing metallo-β-lactamases (MBLs; such as NDM-1 and VIM) and oxacillinases (such as OXA-48) [39, 40]. Of note, vaborbactam also inhibits ESBL and *Amp*C β-lactamase. This combination was approved for the treatment of cUTI, including pyelonephritis. The most frequently reported adverse reactions were headache, phlebitis/infusion site reactions, and diarrhea [38]. It is available as a powder for IV infusion.

Obiltoxaximab

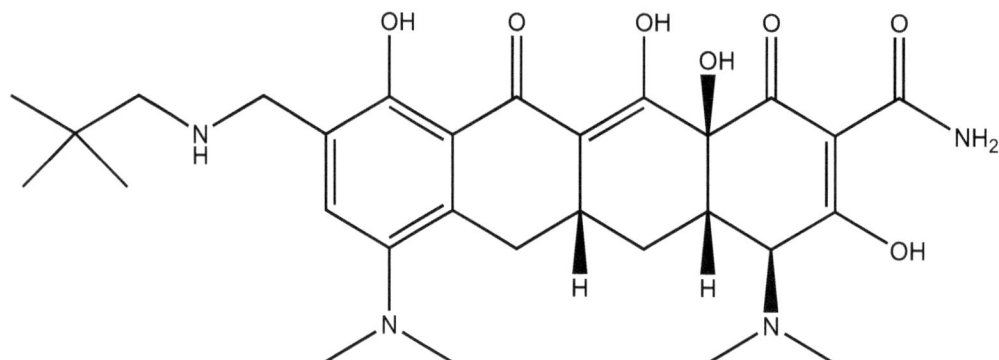

It is a monoclonal antibody against the toxin of *Bacillus anthracis*. It was approved by the U.S. FDA in 2016 for the treatment of inhalational anthrax in combination with antibiotics active against *B. anthracis* [41]. It can also be used as a prophylaxis when alternative therapies are not available or inappropriate [42]. Hypersensitivity reaction is the only adverse effect reported with this agent [43, 44]. Therefore, if obiltoxaximab is to be used for prophylaxis, it should be used only when the benefit for the prevention of inhalational anthrax outweighs the risk of hypersensitivity and anaphylaxis [44]. Obiltoxaximab is available as a solution for IV injection.

Omadacycline

It is a novel, aminomethyl tetracycline antibiotic for the treatment of community-acquired bacterial infections (CABP). Omadacycline is characterized by an aminomethyl substituent at the C9 position of the core 6-member ring. Modifications at this position result in an improved spectrum of antimicrobial activity by overcoming resistance known to affect older generation tetracyclines *via* ribosomal protection proteins and efflux pump mechanisms. *In vitro*, omadacycline has activity against Gram-positive and Gram-negative aerobes, anaerobes, and atypical pathogens including *Legionella* and *Chlamydia* spp. Omadacycline has potent activity against important skin and pneumonia pathogens, including community-acquired methicillin-resistant *S. aureus* (CA-MRSA), β-hemolytic *Streptococci*, penicillin-resistant *S. pneumoniae*, *H.*

influenzae, and *Legionella* spp [45]. Omadacycline was approved for CABP and ABSSSI in 2018 as a powder for IV injection and oral tablets [46].

Oritavancin

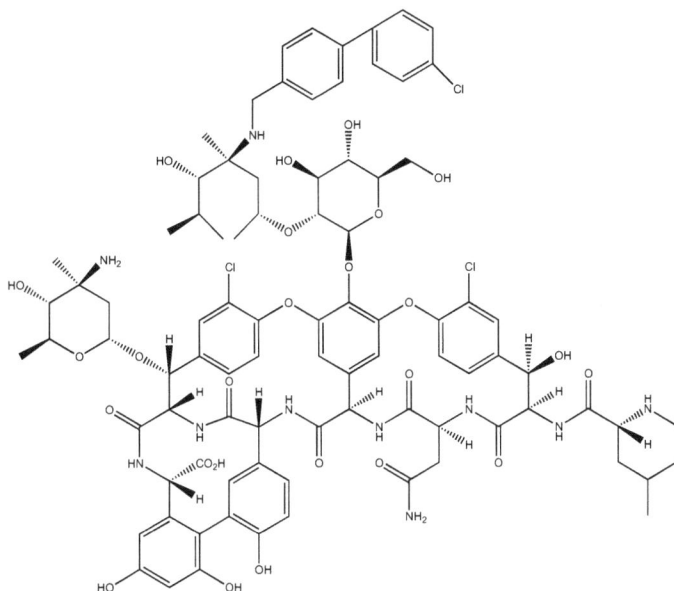

It is a semi-synthetic lipoglycopeptide that works similarly as dalbavancin. Similar to dalbavancin, oritavancin covers Gram-positive bacteria such as *S. aureus* (including MRSA), *S. pyogenes, S. agalactiae, S. anginosus, S. dysgalactiae* and *E. faecalis* (vancomycin-susceptible isolates only) [47]. Oritavancin was approved for ABSSSI as a single dose given over 3 hours [47]. The most common adverse effects are limb and subcutaneous abscesses, hypersensitivity reactions, and infusion-related reactions. Notably, prothrombin time (PT) and INR can be increased for up to 12 hours after dose administration; therefore, the drug should be used with caution with close monitoring in patients receiving warfarin [47]. The drug is available as a powder for IV infusion compatible with dextrose 5% in water (D5W) only.

Ozenoxacin

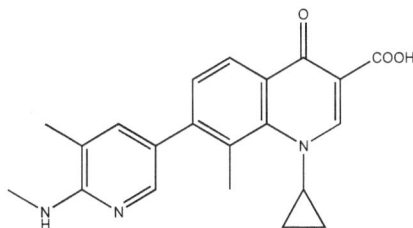

It is a topical quinolone antibiotic that works by inhibiting the bacterial DNA replication enzymes DNA gyrase A and topoisomerase IV [48]. It has activity against Gram-positive organisms, such as *S. aureus* and *Streptococcus pyogenes* [48]. Ozenoxacin was approved in 2017 to treat impetigo in patients aged 2 months and older. The most common adverse effects reported were rosacea and seborrheic dermatitis [48]. Ozenoxacin is available as a 1% topical cream.

Plazomicin

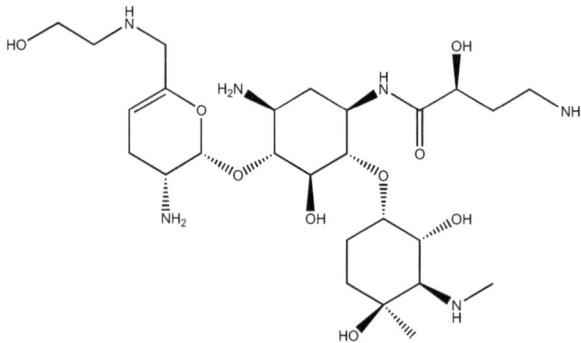

It is an aminoglycoside that was approved in 2018 and exhibits activity against pathogens including ESBL-producing and carbapenem-resistant Entero-bacteriaceae (CRE). Plazomicin is indicated for the treatment of patients 18 years of age or older with cUTI, including pyelonephritis [49]. The most common adverse reactions are decreased renal function, diarrhea, hypertension, headache, nausea, vomiting, and hypotension [49]. It was approved with boxed warnings of nephrotoxicity, ototoxicity, neuromuscular blockage, and fetal harm. To help mitigate nephrotoxicity risk, therapeutic drug monitoring is recommended for patients with creatinine clearance < 90 mL/min. Plazomicin is available as a solution for IV infusion.

Secnidazole

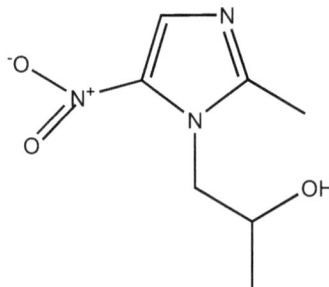

It is a second-generation 5-nitroimidazole antimicrobial that was approved in 2017 [50, 51]. Secnidazole is active against many anaerobic Gram-positive and Gram-negative bacteria and protozoa including *B. fragilis, Trichomonas vaginalis, Entamoeba histolytica*, and *Giardia lamblia*. Secnidazole is indicated for the treatment of bacterial vaginosis in adult women [51, 52]. An *in vitro* study comparing the activity of secnidazole with that of metronidazole against *T. vaginalis* showed that secnidazole had better activity (higher susceptibility rates) than its comparator [53]. The most common adverse reactions were vulvovaginal candidiasis and nausea [54]. Secnidazole is available as oral granules to be mixed with liquids or soft food.

Tedizolid

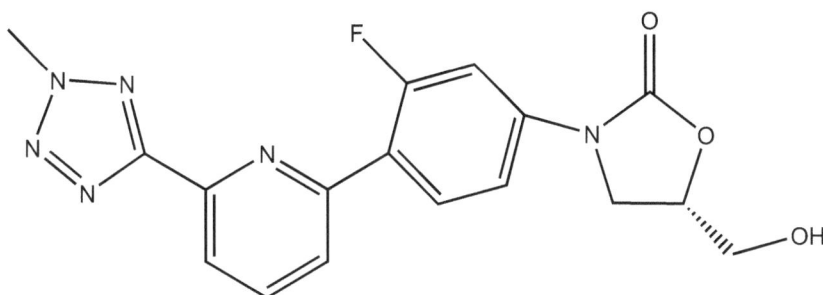

It is an oxazolidinone antibacterial (same class as linezolid) that exhibits its bacteriostatic properties *via* binding to 50S ribosomal subunit leading to inhibition of protein synthesis. Tedizolid covers aerobic and facultative Gram-positive bacteria such as *S. aureus* (including MRSA and MSSA), *S. pyogenes, S. agalactiae, S. anginosus*, and *E. faecalis*. Tedizolid was approved for acute bacterial skin and skin structure infections (ABSSSI) to be used for six days (compared with 10 days with linezolid) [55, 56]. The most common adverse effects are infusion-related reactions, increased hepatic transaminases, peripheral neuropathy, and neutropenia [57]. Animal studies have shown a lower probability of serotonin syndrome when tedizolid is given with selective serotonin reuptake inhibitors [58]. Phase III clinical trial in nosocomial pneumonia has been completed recently; however, FDA approval for this indication is still pending [59]. Tedizolid is available as a powder for IV infusion and oral tablets.

Antibacterial Agents Under Development

Aerucin (AR-105)

It is a fully human IgG-1 monoclonal antibody that targets cell surface polysaccharide that is widely distributed on *P. aeruginosa*, thus, it enhances compliment disposition and eventual killing of the organism. Phase II clinical trial for the use of aerucin as an adjunctive agent for the treatment of *P. aeruginosa* ventilator-associated pneumonia was initiated. Aerucin will be available as an IV formulation [60, 61].

AR-401

It is a fully human monoclonal antibody that is currently in phase II clinical trial to evaluate its efficacy for the treatment of acute pneumonia caused by *A. baumannii*. AR-401 will be available as an IV formulation [62].

Alalevonadifloxacin

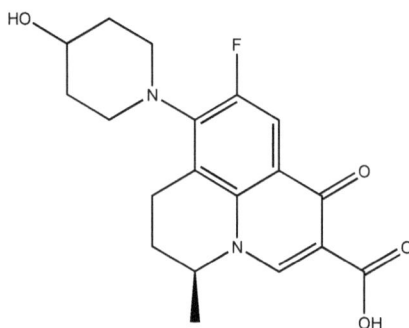

It is a pro-drug of levonadifloxacin being developed as an oral fluoroquinolone antibiotic [63]. Similar to fluoroquinolones, it works through the inhibition of DNA gyrase [64]. Phase II clinical trial demonstrated the efficacy of alalevonadifloxacin against MRSA infections [64]. Its efficacy in ABSSSI was demonstrated in phase III clinical trial [64]. Formulated for IV and oral administration.

Auriclosene (NVC-422)

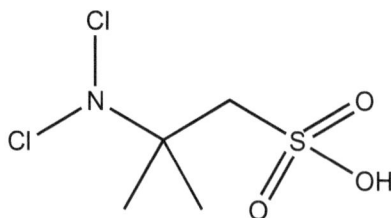

It is a fast-acting, broad-spectrum antimicrobial against multi-drug resistant bacteria, viruses, and fungi [65, 66]. Auriclosene has been studied for multiple indications, including in ophthalmology, dermatology, and urology. Auriclosene has been used in trials for the treatment of impetigo, adenoviral conjunctivitis, and the prevention of urinary catheter blockage and encrustation [66 - 69]. It is also effective topically against *S. aureus* biofilm, with dose-dependent efficacy in the animal model of sinusitis associated with biofilm [70].

Aztreonam/Avibactam

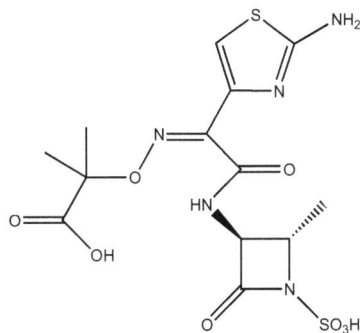

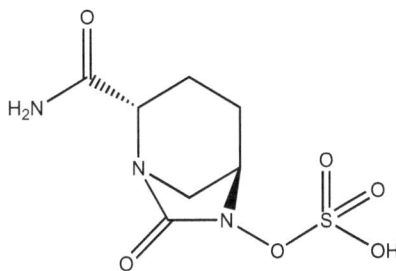

Aztreonam   Avibactam

This is a combination of the monobactam, aztreonam, and the non-β-lactam β-lactamase inhibitor, avibactam. While aztronam is refractory to hydrolysis by MBLs, it is inactivated by ESBLs, *Amp*C β-lactamase, and class A β-lactamases (KPC). On the other hand, avibactam inhibits class A, C, and some of class D β-lactamases. Aztreonam is a bactericidal agent that acts by inhibiting bacterial cell wall synthesis [71]. This combination is being developed to be used for the treatment of serious infections caused by MBL-producing Enterobacteriaceae [72]. Aztreonam/avibactam will be available as an IV formulation.

Brilacidin

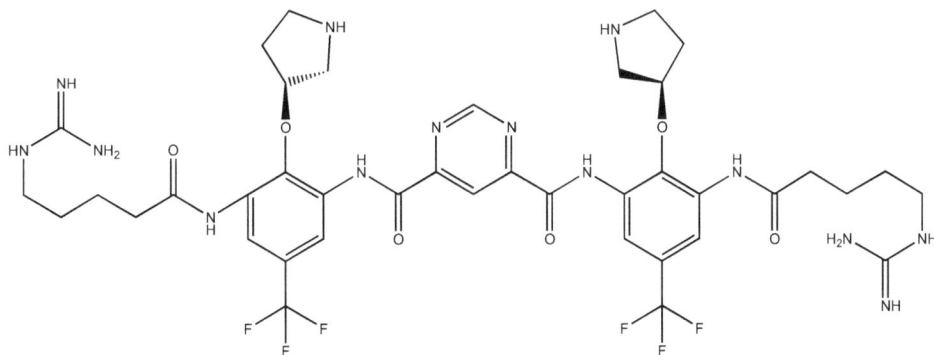

It is a novel defensin-mimetic (peptide) bactericidal antibiotic that works by disrupting the bacterial cell membrane. *In vitro*, brilacidin shows broad-spectrum activity against Gram-positive (including MRSA and *Enterococci*) and Gram-negative (including *E. coli* and *K. pneumoniae* including NDM-1-producing) organisms [73]. Phase II clinical trial in ABSSSIs has been completed recently [73, 74]. Brilacidin will be available as an IV formulation.

Cefilavancin (TD1792)

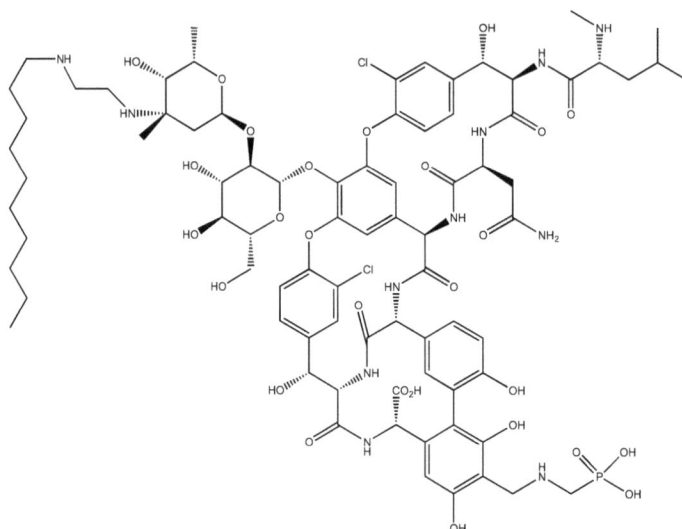

It is a novel glycopeptide-cephalosporin heterodimer bactericidal antibiotic that inhibits cell wall synthesis. Cefilavancin has antibacterial activity against Gram-positive bacteria, including MSSA and MRSA [75]. Phase III clinical trial for the treatment of complicated skin and skin-structure infections (cSSSI) was initiated [75]. Cefilavancin will be available as an IV formulation.

ETX0282-CPDP

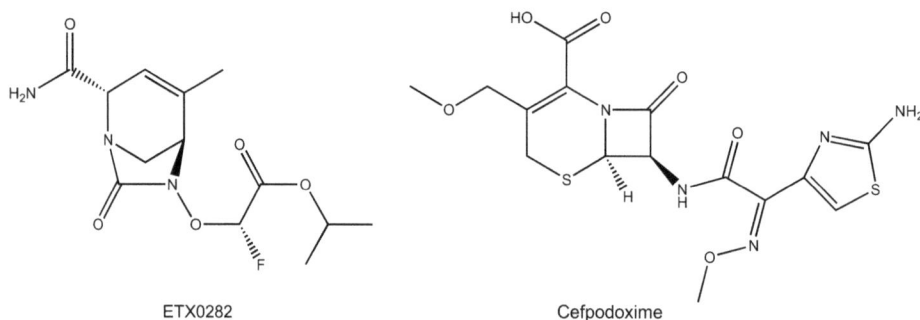

ETX0282   Cefpodoxime

ETX0282 is an oral β-lactamase inhibitor. ETX0282-CPDP is a combination of ETX0282 with cefpodoxime. ETX0282-CPDP is being developed as an oral therapy for infections caused by MDR Gram-negative bacteria including CRE, particularly in cUTI [76]. This combination will be available as an oral formulation.

Gepotidacin

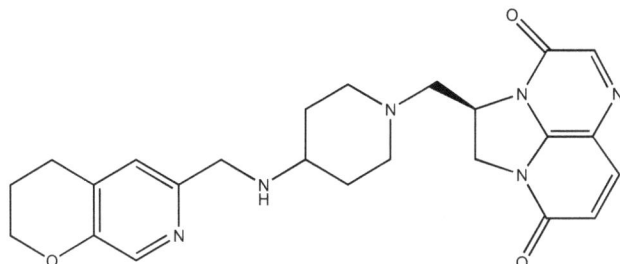

It is a novel triazaacenaphthylene bactericidal antibiotic that inhibits topoisomerase IV and DNA gyrase leading to the inhibition of DNA synthesis [77]. *In vitro*, gepotidacin showed activity against Gram-positive bacteria such as *S. aureus* (including MRSA), *S. pneumoniae* and Gram-negative bacteria such as *Neisseria gonorrhoeae* [78, 79]. It also has activity against ciprofloxacin-resistant strains. Geotidacin has just completed phase II clinical trial for uncomplicated urogenital gonorrhea caused by *N. gonorrhoeae* where the most common adverse effects reported in the trial were flatulence, hyperhidrosis, abdominal pain, and nausea [77]. Phase II clinical trial in ABSSSIs has just completed and phase II in acute cystitis was initiated, as well [77, 80]. Gepotidacin will be available as an IV formulation and oral tablets.

Iclaprim

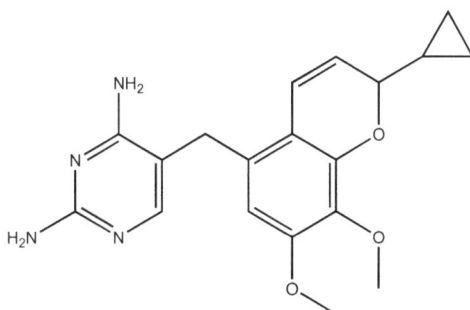

It is a novel investigational antibiotic of the diaminopyrimidine dihydrofolate reductase (DHFR)-inhibiting type targeting Gram-positive organisms [81, 82]. A study conducted to evaluate the efficacy of iclaprim *vs.* vancomycin for the treatment of ABSSSI due to Gram-positive pathogens showed iclaprim to be effective and safe [83]. Notably, iclaprim could also represent an alternative for the treatment of severe skin and pulmonary infections due to Gram-positive bacteria [82]. Iclaprim is currently in phase III clinical trial and it will be available as an IV infusion.

Lefamulin (BC-3781)

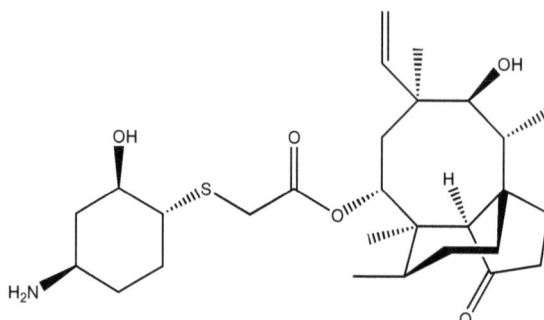

It is a novel pleuromutilin antibiotic currently undergoing phase III clinical trial for CABP [84]. It has a unique mode of action through inhibiting protein synthesis by binding to the peptidyl transferase center of the 50S bacterial ribosome [85]. Lefamulin displays activity against Gram-positive and atypical organisms associated with CABP, such as *S. pneumoniae, H. influenzae, Mycoplasma pneumoniae, Legionella pneumophila,* and *Chlamydophila pneumoniae* [84]. It also has an expanded Gram-positive spectrum of activity including activity against *S. aureus* (methicillin-resistant, vancomycin-intermediate, and heterogeneous strains) and vancomycin-resistant *Enterococcus faecium* [84, 85]. Lefamulin was also shown to retain activity against MDR *N. gonorrhoeae* and *Mycoplasma genitalium* [86]. Lefamulin exhibits time-dependent killing [86]. Lefamulin will be available in IV and oral formulations.

MEDI-3902

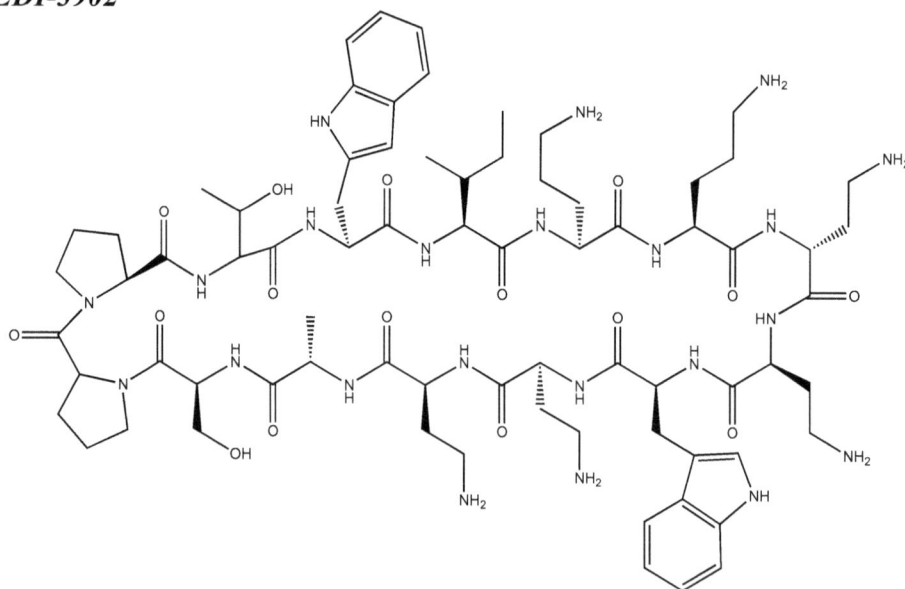

It is a bispecific monoclonal antibody that targets both PcrV and Psl exopolysaccharide of *P. aeruginosa* [87]. Phase II clinical trial for the prevention of nosocomial pneumonia caused by *P. aeruginosa* in mechanically ventilated patients was initiated [88]. The most common adverse effects reported in phase I trial were dyspepsia, rhinitis, infusion-related reaction, and pruritus [89]. MEDI-3902 will be available as an IV formulation.

Murepavadin

It is an antibacterial with a novel mechanism of action as it inhibits the lipopolysaccharide transport protein D [90]. *In vitro* and *in vivo* studies have shown high activity of murepavadin against carbapenemase-producing and colistin-resistant *P. aeruginosa*, as well as other Gram-negative and Gram-positive bacteria [90, 91]. It is currently being studied in phase III clinical trial for the treatment of HABP/VABP due to *P. aeruginosa* [91]. It will be available as an IV formulation.

Ridinilazole

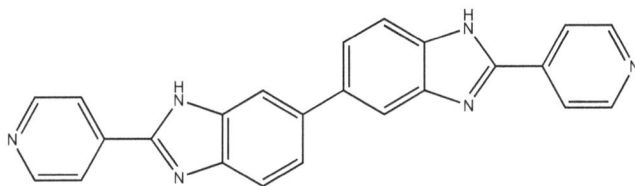

It is a narrow-spectrum antibiotic with activity against *C. difficile* [92]. Oral ridinilazole showed a good safety profile and was well-tolerated with minimal detectable plasma concentrations after it was administered in single and multiple doses in phase I clinical trial [92]. In phase II clinical trial, ridinilazole demonstrated a significant reduction in recurrent CDI rates [93]. As minimal disturbance of normal intestinal flora was observed, and the high selectivity of the compound was confirmed. These results further support the clinical development of ridinilazole as an oral therapy for CDI [93].

SER-109

It is a novel microbiome therapeutic made from 50 species of Firmicutes spores from healthy donors of stool specimens. Phase III clinical trial for the prevention of recurrent CDI was initiated [94]. The most common adverse effects reported were abdominal pain, nausea, and diarrhea. SER-109 will be available as oral tablets.

SER-262

It is a rationally-designed composition of commensal bacteria (in spore form) to be administered orally in a capsule form. It is manufactured using anaerobic fermentation and is developed for the prevention of recurrence of CDI in adult patients with primary CDI who are at risk for recurrence. SER-262 has just completed phase Ib trial [95].

Solithromycin

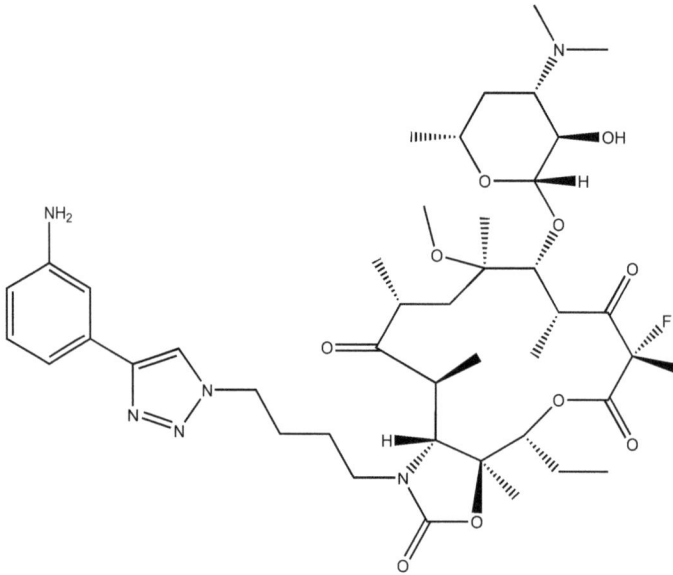

It is a next-generation macrolide antibiotic that inhibits bacterial translation and has antimicrobial properties which make it active against aerobic and anaerobic Gram-positive cocci. In phase II clinical trial comparing solithromycin *vs.* levofloxacin for CABP, solithromycin showed comparable success rates [96]. Consequently, solithromycin is currently in phase III clinical trial for the treatment of moderately-severe CABP. The most common adverse reaction is hepatotoxicity [97]. Solithromycin will be available as an oral capsule.

Sulbactam/Durlobactam

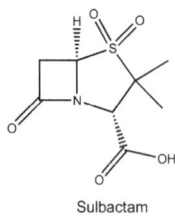

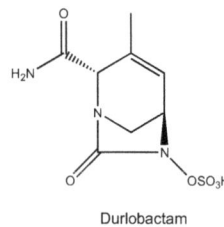

Sulbactam

Durlobactam

It is the first β-lactamase/β-lactamase inhibitor combination. Its strong antibacterial activity was demonstrated against MDR *A. baumannii* [98, 99]. It completed preclinical and phase I clinical trials and showed a good safety profile [98, 99]. Sulbactam-ETX2514 is being developed as an IV formulation.

Sulopenem

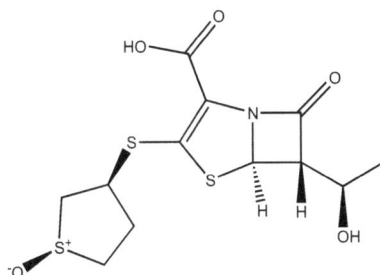

It is antimicrobial that acts as a cell wall synthesis inhibitor. Currently, it is in phase III clinical trial known as Sulopenem for Resistant Enterobacteriaceae (SURE) where oral sulopenem etzadroxil is combined with probenecid in a bilayer tablet. It is developed for the treatment of MDR Gram-negative infections, including UTI, cUTI, and cIAI [100]. Solupenem will be available in IV and oral formulations.

TP-271

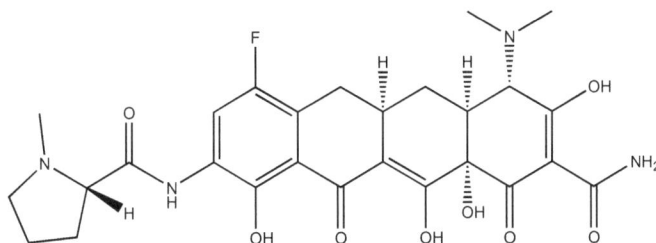

It is a synthetic fluorocycline (derivative of tetracycline) antibiotic in phase 1 clinical trial, for the treatment of CABP. TP-271 is active against Gram-positive and Gram-negative pathogens, including *S. pneumoniae*, *S. pyogenes*, MSSA, MRSA, *H. influenza,* and *Moraxella catarrhalis*. TP-271 demonstrated *in vitro* activity against the major pathogens associated with moderate to severe CABP. The site of action Tetracycline drug such as TP-271 is the 30S ribosomal subunit; drug binding interferes with the access of aminoacyl-tRNA to A-site on mRNA-ribosome complex, preventing new amino acid addition and peptide chain growth [101]. It will be available in oral and IV formulations.

TP-6076

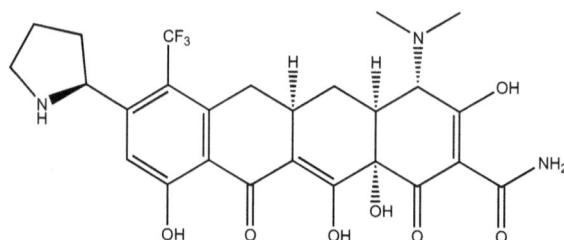

It is a synthetic fluorocycline antibiotic effective against carbapenem-resistant *A. baumannii* and currently undergoing phase I clinical trial. It works by inhibiting bacterial protein synthesis. In the randomized clinical trial, TP-6076 showed excellent *in vitro* activity and had lower MICs compared with other antibiotics against carbapenem-resistant *A. baumannii*. TP-6076 could be a promising candidate antibiotic for the treatment of patients with MDR *A. baumannii* infections [102]. TP-6076 will be developed as an IV formulation.

Zoliflodacin

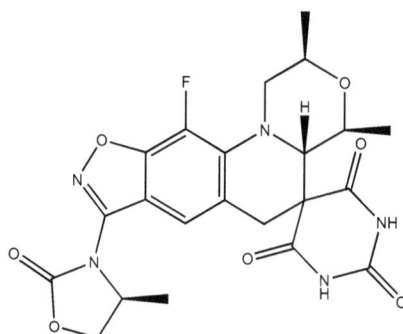

It is a novel spiropyrimidinetrione bactericidal antibiotic that inhibits topoisomerase and DNA gyrase leading to the inhibition of DNA synthesis. *In vitro*, zoliflodacin showed potent activity against fluoroquinolone-resistant bacteria, MDR Gram-positive bacteria including *S. aureus, Streptococci, E. faecalis*, and fastidious Gram-negative bacteria including *H. influenzae*, and *Neisseria gonorrhoeae* [103]. Recently, zoliflodacin completed phase II for uncomplicated urogenital gonorrhea where the most commonly reported adverse effects were diarrhea and headache [104]. Zoliflodacin will be available as oral tablets.

514G3 Antibody

It is a natural human monoclonal antibody against MRSA and MSSA bloodstream infections, targeting the cell wall moiety Protein A (SpA) [105]. Phase I and II clinical trials were completed in these infections with positive findings [106].

ANTIFUNGAL AGENTS

Albaconazole

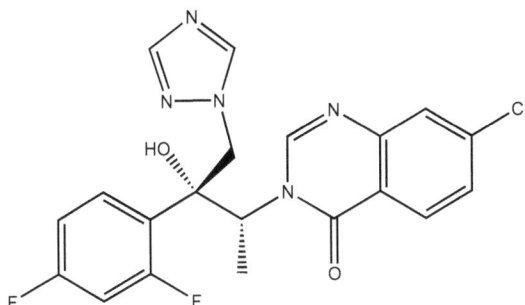

It is an azole antifungal that inhibits the synthesis of ergosterol leading to inhibition of the cell membrane. *In vitro*, albaconazole shows a broad-spectrum of activity against yeasts, filamentous fungi, and dermatophytes. Albaconazole has just completed phase II for distal subungual onychomycosis. The most common adverse effects were headache, elevated liver enzymes, and nausea. Albaconazole has a long half-life of 70.5 hours which may allow for weekly dosing [107]. Albaconazole will be available as oral capsules.

Amorolfine

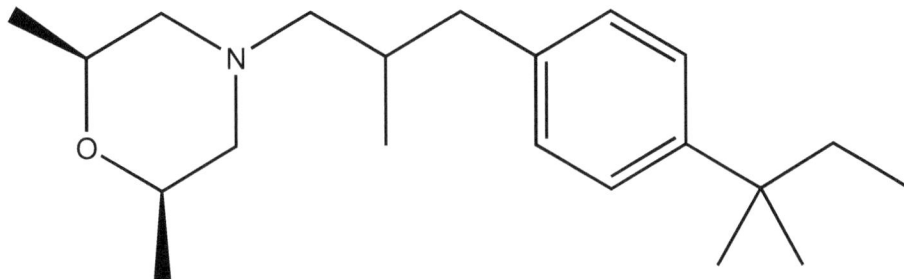

It is an antimycotic antifungal that inhibits cell membrane *via* inhibition of sterol synthesis. Amorolfine covers yeasts (including *Candida* and *Cryptococcus*), dermatophytes, molds, dematiacea, and dimorphic fungi. The most common adverse effects are itching, erythema, nail discoloration, and periungual scaling [108]. Amorolfine was approved for onychomycoses as a topical product.

Basifungin (aureobasidin)

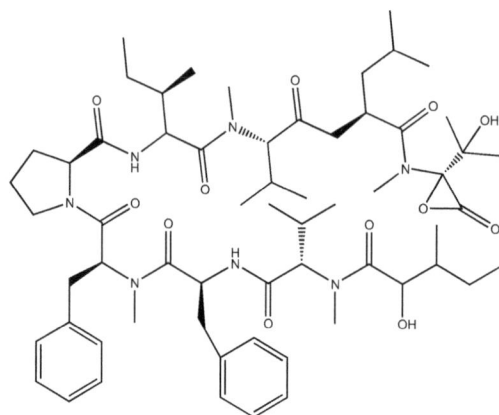

It is a natural antifungal produced by *Aureobasidium pullulans*. It exhibits its fungicidal properties *via* inhibition of inositol phosphorylceramide synthesis. Preclinical studies showed broad-spectrum activity against *Candida* spp., *Cryptococcus neoformans*, and *Aspergillus* species but not *A. fumigatus* [109, 110].

Rezafungin

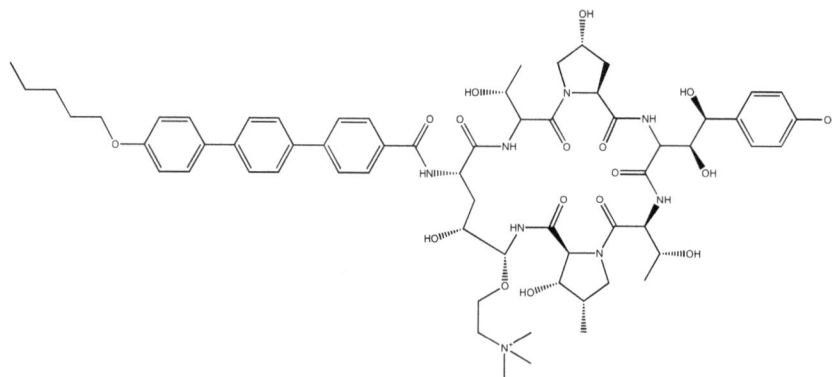

It is a novel echinocandin antifungal that inhibits the synthesis of the cell wall. *In vivo*, rezafungin showed broad-spectrum activity against *Candida* spp., *Aspergillus* spp., *Pneumocystis* spp., *Trichophyton mentagrophytes*, *Trichophyton rubrum*, and *Microsporum gypseum*. Rezafungin has just completed phase II clinical trial for candidemia and invasive candidiasis [111]. Rezafungin has a long half-life of 81 hours which may allow for once-weekly dosing [112]. It will be available in topical and IV formulations.

Encochleated amphotericin B

It is an orally administered formulation of amphotericin B that inhibits the synthesis of ergosterol leading to the inhibition of fungal cell membranes. It is a nanoparticle-based formulation where amphotericin B is encochleated within multi-layered lipid-based crystals of phosphatidylserine and calcium that are derived from soy. As known, amphotericin B has broad-spectrum activity against invasive candidiasis and aspergillosis. Encochleated amphotericin B demonstrated a good safety profile in phase I clinical trial without serious adverse effects [113]. It has just completed phase II for vulvovaginal candidiasis, and phase II in mucocutaneous candidiasis was initiated, as well [114, 115].

Haemofungin

It is an antifungal agent that produces its fungicidal by swelling and lysis of growing fungal cells. It primarily inhibits ferrochelatase (HemH) and the growth of *Aspergillus, Candida, Fusarium* and *Rhizopus* isolates [116].

Ibomycin

It is a potent antifungal agent that exhibits its activity by disturbing the membrane function. It has preferential activity against *Cryptococcus neoformans* due to its ability to selectively permeate its cell wall [117].

Isavuconazole (Isavuconazonium Sulfate)

Isavuconazonium sulfate is a prodrug that is converted into isavuconazole by the effect of plasma esterase. It is an azole antifungal that inhibits ergosterol synthesis leading to the inhibition of cell membrane synthesis. Isavuconazole covers *Aspergillus flavus*, *A. fumigatus*, *A. niger*, and Mucorales such as *Rhizopus oryzae* and *Mucormycetes* spp [118]. Isavuconazole was approved in 2015 for invasive aspergillosis and invasive mucormycosis [119]. In comparison with voriconazole, isavuconazole was non-inferior in all-cause mortality for the primary treatment of invasive mold disease [120]. The most common adverse effects are hepatotoxicity, infusion-related reactions, hypersensitivity reactions, and optic neuropathy. Isavuconazole administration is contradicted with all CYP3A4 inhibitors and inducers [121]. Phase III clinical trial in deep mycosis was initiated [122]. Additionally, phase I clinical trial in hematological malignancy pediatrics patient was also initiated [123]. Isavuconazole is available as oral capsules and powder for IV infusion.

Myriocin

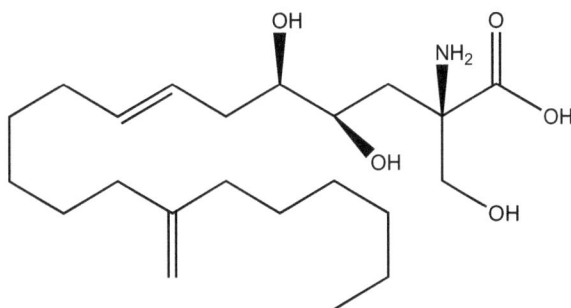

It is an inhibitor of de novo sphingolipid synthesis. Preclinical studies showed that myriocin has antifungal activity against *A. fumigatus* biofilm [124]. However, further studies with this agent are still ongoing.

Novamycin

It is an antifungal that rapidly kills both non-metabolically and metabolically active fungi through membrane perturbation and lysis [125]. Its spectrum of activity includes *Aspergillus* spp. and *Candida* spp. It also showed activity against pathogens that are resistant to conventional antifungals [126]. Novamycin is indicated for the treatment of fungal disease as inhaled, systemic, and mucocutaneous therapy. Clinical trials in respiratory aspergillosis and oral pharyngeal candidiasis have been initiated [127].

Sampangine

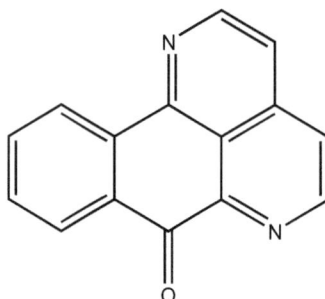

It is an azaoxoaporphine alkaloid natural antifungal that inhibits haem synthesis leading to the inhibition of ergosterol synthesis. In the preclinical phase, sampangine showed activity against *Cryptococcus neoformans*, *Candida* spp. and *Aspergillus* spp [128].

Tavaborole

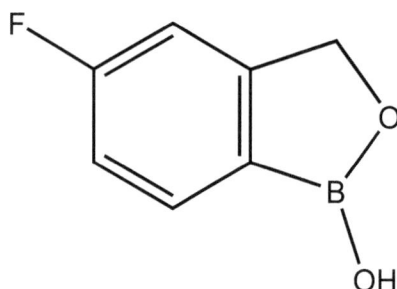

It is an antifungal that was approved in July 2014. It acts by inhibiting protein synthesis in the fungus, as well as inhibiting an enzyme known as cytosolic leucyl-transfer RNA synthetase [129]. It is indicated for the topical treatment of onychomycosis of the toenails due to *Trichophyton rubrum* or *T. mentagrophytes*. The most common adverse effect is skin exfoliation, erythema, dermatitis, and ingrown toenail [130].

PC945

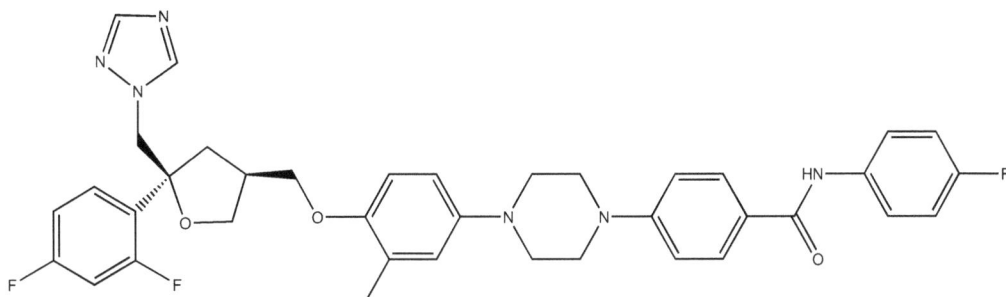

It is an azole antifungal that inhibits ergosterol synthesis leading to inhibition of the cell membrane. *In vitro*, PC945 showed broad-spectrum of activity against *A. fumigatus, A. terreus, Trichophyton rubrum, Candida albicans, Candida glabrata, Candida krusei, Cryptococcus gattii, Cryptococcus neoformans*, and *Rhizopus oryzae* [131]. Phase II clinical trial in cystic fibrosis patients and in lung transplant recipients who are infected by *A. fumigatus* was initiated [132, 133]. Phase II in asthma or other chronic respiratory diseases patients who are infected by *Aspergillus* spp. and *Candida* spp. was initiated, as well [134]. PC945 will be the first azole available as a once-daily inhaled formulation.

Quilseconazole (VT-1129) and VT-1598

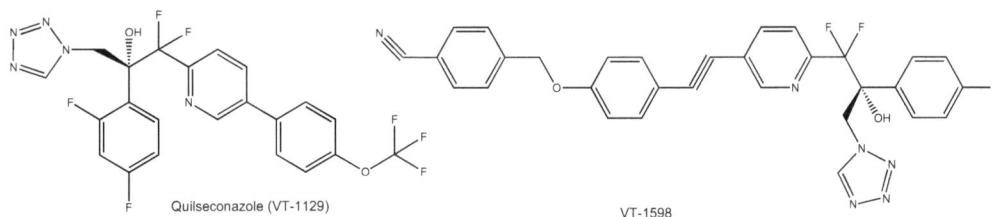

Quilseconazole (VT-1129)　　　　VT-1598

These belong to the novel class of metalloenzyme inhibitors which inhibit the fungal sterol 14α-demethylase (CYP51) enzyme leading to the inhibition of ergosterol synthesis. *In vitro*, quilseconazole shows activity against many *Cryptococcus* isolates, including *C. neoformans* and *C. gattii* [112]. Phase I for the treatment of coccidioidomycosis by VT-1598 was initiated [135]. Both will be available as oral formulations.

SCY-078 (MK-3118)

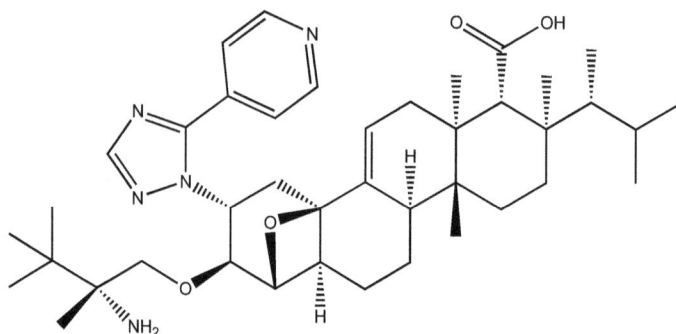

It is a potent antifungal against emerging non-*Aspergillus* molds that exhibits its activity *via* inhibiting fungal β-1,3-d-glucan synthases. It has preferential activity against *Paecilomyces variotii* and was the only compound displaying some activity against notoriously panresistant *Scedosporium prolificans* [136]. Phase II clinical trial in invasive mold infections was initiated [137]. SCY-078 (MK-3118) will be available as oral and IV formulations.

T-2307

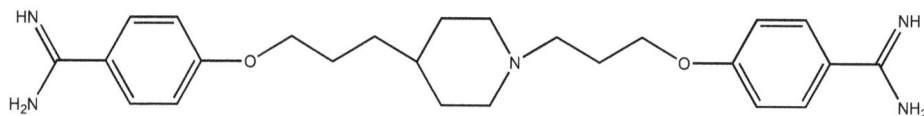

It is a novel arylamidine antifungal agent. Under both *in vitro* and *in vivo* conditions, T-2307 exhibited broad-spectrum of activity against the majority of fungal pathogens, including *Candida* spp., *Cryptococcus neoformans*, and *A. fumigatus*, with the most potent activity against *C. albicans*. T-2307 selectively disrupts yeast mitochondrial function by inhibiting respiratory chain complexes III and IV [138, 139].

VL-2397

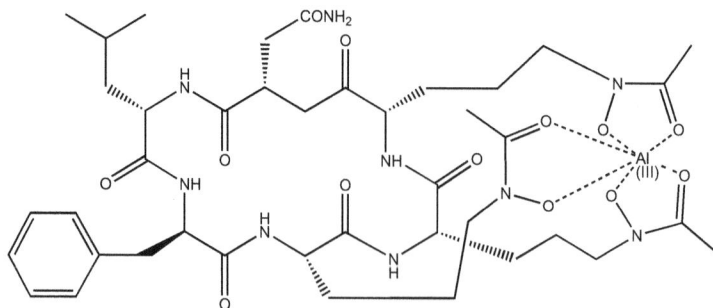

It is an antifungal, aluminum-chelating cyclic hexapeptide. It is structurally analogous to ferrichrome-type siderophores [140]. While it is active against *C. glabrata*, it was approved by the U.S. FDA in 2017 based on phase II clinical trial for invasive aspergillosis for patients with acute leukaemia and patients who have received an allogeneic haematopoietic cell transplant [140, 141].

Olorofim (F901318)

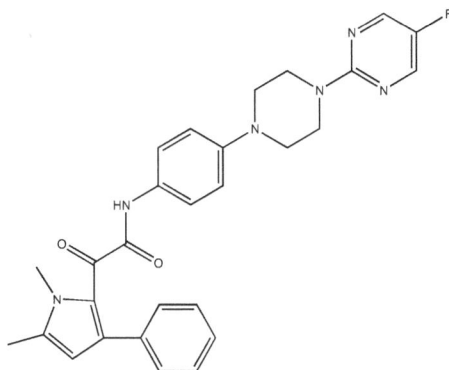

Olorfim belongs to a novel class of antifungals. It is an orotomide antifungal that inhibition of dihydroorotate dehydrogenase. It initially starts with a fungistatic effect; however, prolonged exposure results in fungicidal effect through hyphal swelling followed by cell lysis. Its activity was demonstrated against *A. fumigatus* [142, 143]. F901318 is currently in phase II clinical trial of invasive aspergillosis. It will be available as an oral formulation.

E1210

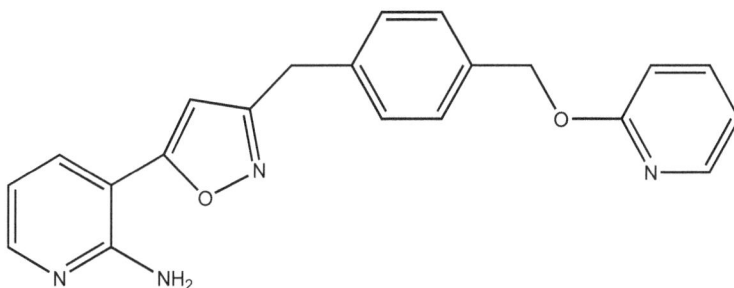

It is a potent antifungal that inhibits the inositol acylation of glycosylphosphatidylinositol (GPI) biosynthesis. It showed a broad-spectrum of activity against *Candida albicans* and *A. fumigatus*. Therefore, it is proposed for serious invasive fungal infections [144]. It will be available as an oral formulation.

ANTIPARASITIC AGENTS

Auranofin

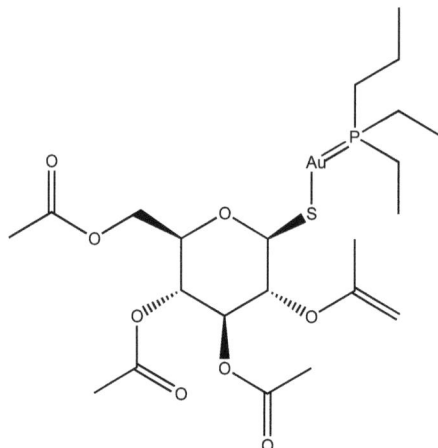

It is a gold-containing saccharide that is currently approved for use in rheumatoid arthritis. It has antiparasitic properties and is now in phase I clinical trial for the treatment of *E. histolytica* and *Giardia intestinalis* infections with particular activity against metronidazole-resistant strains [145, 146]. The main mechanism of action of auranofin is through the inhibition of reduction/oxidation enzymes that are essential for maintaining intracellular levels of reactive oxygen species. Inhibition of these enzymes leads to oxidative stress and apoptosis [147]. Common adverse effects include dermatologic and gastrointestinal reactions [148]. Auranofin will be available as oral capsules.

Benznidazole

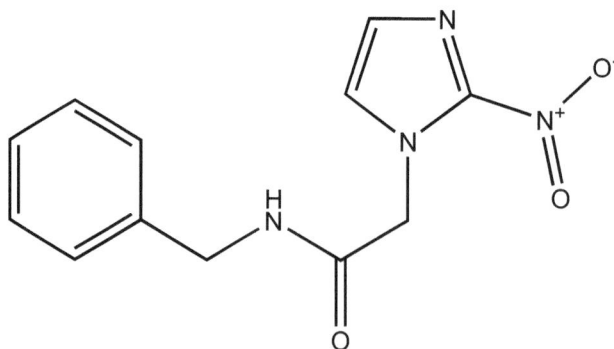

It is an antiparasitic agent that works by inhibiting the synthesis of DNA, RNA, and proteins within the *Trypanosoma cruzi* parasite [149]. It was approved by the

U.S. FDA in 2017 for the treatment of Chagas disease caused by *T. cruzi* in pediatric patients 2 to 12 years old [150, 151]. A study to assess whether the treatment with benzeneidazole previously given to women of childbearing age could prevent or reduce new cases of congenital Chagas disease was conducted and it was found that the agent did achieve this outcome [152]. Common adverse reactions include skin rash and lesions, weight loss, abdominal pain, and decreased appetite [153]. Benznidazole is available as oral tablets.

Encochleated Atovaquone (CATQ)

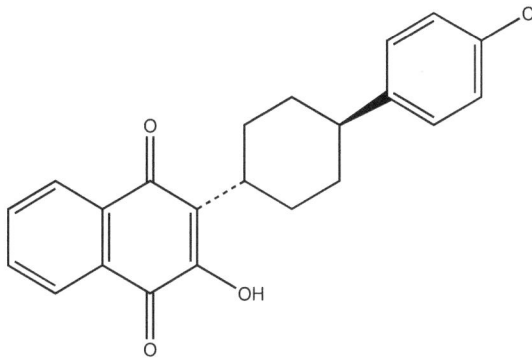

It is an alternative agent for the treatment and prevention of *Pneumocystis jirovecii* pneumonia (PJP; formerly *P. carinii* pneumonia [PCP]) and toxoplasmosis caused by *Toxoplasma gondii* and both are opportunistic infections that occur in immunocompromised patients, such as patients infected with human immunodeficiency virus (HIV) [154].

Miltefosine

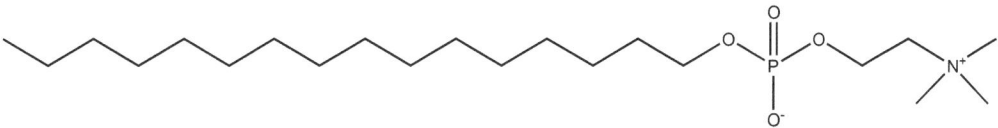

It is an antiparasitic agent. The exact mechanism of miltefosine is unknown; likely interaction with phospholipids and steroids in parasitic cell membranes, inhibition of cytochrome c oxidase, and eventually apoptosis-like cell death occur [155]. It was approved by the U.S. FDA in 2014 for the treatment of visceral (caused by *Leishmania donovani*), cutaneous (caused by *L. braziliensis*, *L. guyanensis*, and *L. panamensis*), and mucosal (caused by *L. braziliensis*) leishmaniasis in adults and adolescents [155, 156]. A case report showed miltefosine was also effective in the treatment of a patient infected with *Acanthamoeba* spp [157]. The efficacy of miltefosine was not evaluated in the treatment of other leishmaniasis species (*e.g.*, *L. infantum*). Common adverse reactions include headache, dizziness, and gastrointestinal upset [158]. Miltefosine is available as oral capsules.

CONCLUSION

In conclusion, it can be noticed that the discussed agents were not only synthesized or semi-synthesized chemical compounds, but rather many were biological products whether they are antibodies, peptide, or bacterial/microbiome products. This indicates that the development of new antimicrobials is taking a new dimension and indirect way of targeting the pathogens. The judicious use of these new antimicrobials after their release into the market is of utmost importance to preserve their potentials for tenacious infections caused by MDR organisms.

CONSENT FOR PUBLICATION

Not applicable.

CONFLICT OF INTEREST

The authors confirm that the contents of this chapter have no conflict of interest.

ACKNOWLEDGEMENTS

Declared none.

REFERENCES

[1]   Markham A. Bezlotoxumab: First global approval. Drugs 2016; 76(18): 1793-8.
        [http://dx.doi.org/10.1007/s40265-016-0673-1] [PMID: 27905086]

[2]   Lee Y, Lim WI, Bloom CI, Moore S, Chung E, Marzella N. Bezlotoxumab (Zinplava) for *Clostridium Difficile* infection: the first monoclonal antibody approved to prevent the recurrence of a bacterial infection. P&T 2017; 42(12): 735-8.
        [PMID: 29234211]

[3]   Orth P, Xiao L, Hernandez LD, *et al.* Mechanism of action and epitopes of *Clostridium difficile* toxin B-neutralizing antibody bezlotoxumab revealed by X-ray crystallography. J Biol Chem 2014; 289(26): 18008-21.
        [http://dx.doi.org/10.1074/jbc.M114.560748] [PMID: 24821719]

[4]   Wilcox MH, Gerding DN, Poxton IR, *et al.* MODIFY I and MODIFY II Investigators. Bezlotoxumab for prevention of recurrent *Clostridium difficile* infection. N Engl J Med 2017; 376(4): 305-17.
        [http://dx.doi.org/10.1056/NEJMoa1602615] [PMID: 28121498]

[5]   Product Information. FETROJA®, cefiderecol intravenous injection.. Osaka, Japan: Shionogi & Co., Ltd. 2019.

[6]   Bassetti M, Vena A, Castaldo N, Righi E, Peghin M. New antibiotics for ventilator-associated pneumonia. Curr Opin Infect Dis 2018; 31(2): 177-86.
        [http://dx.doi.org/10.1097/QCO.0000000000000438] [PMID: 29337703]

[7]   Study of S-649266 or Best Available Therapy for the Treatment of Severe Infections Caused by Carbapenem-resistant Gram-negative Pathogens (CREDIBLE - CR). 2018. Available at: https://www.clinicaltrials.gov/ct2/show/NCT02714595?cond=Cefiderocol&draw=1&rank=2 [Accessed 12 Sep 2018].

[8]   Deshpande D, Srivastava S, Chapagain ML, *et al.* The discovery of ceftazidime/avibactam as an anti-*Mycobacterium avium* agent. J Antimicrob Chemother 2017; 72 (suppl_2): i36-42. [http://dx.doi.org/10.1093/jac/dkx306] [PMID: 28922808]

[9]   Deshpande D, Srivastava S, Meek C, Leff R, Hall GS, Gumbo T. Moxifloxacin pharmacokinetics/pharmacodynamics and optimal dose and susceptibility breakpoint identification for treatment of disseminated *Mycobacterium avium* infection. Antimicrob Agents Chemother 2010; 54(6): 2534-9. [http://dx.doi.org/10.1128/AAC.01761-09] [PMID: 20385862]

[10]   Bensman TJ, Wang J, Jayne J, *et al.* Pharmacokinetic-pharmacodynamic target attainment analyses to determine optimal dosing of ceftazidime-avibactam for the treatment of acute pulmonary exacerbations in patients with cystic dibrosis. Antimicrob Agents Chemother 2017; 61. [http://dx.doi.org/10.1128/AAC.00988-17]

[11]   Chalhoub H, Tunney M, Elborn JS, *et al.* Avibactam confers susceptibility to a large proportion of ceftazidime-resistant *Pseudomonas aeruginosa* isolates recovered from cystic fibrosis patients. J Antimicrob Chemother 2015; 70(5): 1596-8. [http://dx.doi.org/10.1093/jac/dku551] [PMID: 25587996]

[12]   Zhanel GG, Lawson CD, Adam H, *et al.* Ceftazidime-avibactam: a novel cephalosporin/β-lactamase inhibitor combination. Drugs 2013; 73(2): 159-77. [http://dx.doi.org/10.1007/s40265-013-0013-7] [PMID: 23371303]

[13]   Lucasti C, Popescu I, Ramesh MK, Lipka J, Sable C. Comparative study of the efficacy and safety of ceftazidime/avibactam plus metronidazole *versus* meropenem in the treatment of complicated intra-abdominal infections in hospitalized adults: results of a randomized, double-blind, Phase II trial. J Antimicrob Chemother 2013; 68(5): 1183-92. [http://dx.doi.org/10.1093/jac/dks523] [PMID: 23391714]

[14]   El Solh A. Ceftobiprole: a new broad spectrum cephalosporin. Expert Opin Pharmacother 2009; 10(10): 1675-86. [http://dx.doi.org/10.1517/14656560903048967] [PMID: 19527192]

[15]   Liapikou A, Cillóniz C, Torres A. Ceftobiprole for the treatment of pneumonia: a European perspective. Drug Des Devel Ther 2015; 9: 4565-72. [PMID: 26316697]

[16]   Product Information. ZERBAXA®, ceftolozane and tazobactam for intravenous injection.. Whitehouse Station, NJ: Merck & Co. 2015.

[17]   Merck & Co. Safety and Efficacy Study of Ceftolozane/Tazobactam to Treat Ventilated Nosocomial Pneumonia 2018.

[18]   Product Information. DALVANCE®, dalbavancin intravenous injection.. Chicago, IL: Durata Therapeutics, Inc. 2014.

[19]   Study on the safety and efficacy of dalbavancin *versus* active comparator in adult subjects with osteomyelitis. 2017. Available at: https://www.clinicaltrials.gov/ct2/show/NCT02685033?cond= Dalbavancin&rank=4 .

[20]   Righi E, Carnelutti A, Vena A, Bassetti M. Emerging treatment options for acute bacterial skin and skin structure infections: focus on intravenous delafloxacin. Infect Drug Resist 2018; 11: 479-88. [http://dx.doi.org/10.2147/IDR.S142140] [PMID: 29670380]

[21]   Kingsley J, Mehra P, Lawrence LE, *et al.* A randomized, double-blind, Phase 2 study to evaluate subjective and objective outcomes in patients with acute bacterial skin and skin structure infections

treated with delafloxacin, linezolid or vancomycin. J Antimicrob Chemother 2016; 71(3): 821-9.
[http://dx.doi.org/10.1093/jac/dkv411] [PMID: 26679243]

[22]   Van Bambeke F. Delafloxacin, a non-zwitterionic fluoroquinolone in Phase III of clinical development: evaluation of its pharmacology, pharmacokinetics, pharmacodynamics and clinical efficacy. Future Microbiol 2015; 10(7): 1111-23.
[http://dx.doi.org/10.2217/fmb.15.39] [PMID: 26119479]

[23]   Thabit AK, Crandon JL, Nicolau DP. Pharmacodynamic and pharmacokinetic profiling of delafloxacin in a murine lung model against community-acquired respiratory tract pathogens. Int J Antimicrob Agents 2016; 48(5): 535-41.
[http://dx.doi.org/10.1016/j.ijantimicag.2016.08.012] [PMID: 27742208]

[24]   Bassetti M, Della Siega P, Pecori D, Scarparo C, Righi E. Delafloxacin for the treatment of respiratory and skin infections. Expert Opin Investig Drugs 2015; 24(3): 433-42.
[http://dx.doi.org/10.1517/13543784.2015.1005205] [PMID: 25604710]

[25]   Sutcliffe JA, O'Brien W, Fyfe C, Grossman TH. Antibacterial activity of eravacycline (TP-434), a novel fluorocycline, against hospital and community pathogens. Antimicrob Agents Chemother 2013; 57(11): 5548-58.
[http://dx.doi.org/10.1128/AAC.01288-13] [PMID: 23979750]

[26]   Monogue ML, Thabit AK, Hamada Y, Nicolau DP. Antibacterial efficacy of eravacycline *in vivo* against Gram-positive and Gram-negative organisms. Antimicrob Agents Chemother 2016; 60(8): 5001-5.
[http://dx.doi.org/10.1128/AAC.00366-16] [PMID: 27353265]

[27]   Thabit AK, Monogue ML, Newman JV, Nicolau DP. Assessment of *in vivo* efficacy of eravacycline against Enterobacteriaceae exhibiting various resistance mechanisms: A dose-ranging study and PK/PD analysis. Int J Antimicrob Agents 2018.
[http://dx.doi.org/10.1016/j.ijantimicag.2018.01.001]

[28]   Product Information. XERAVA®, eravacycline for intravenous injection.. Watertown, MA: Tetraphase Pharmaceuticals, Inc. 2018.

[29]   Tetraphase pharmaceuticals. Tetraphase announces top-line results from ignite3 phase 3 clinical trial of eravacycline in complicated urinary tract infections (cUTI). Watertown, MA2018.

[30]   McKeage K. Finafloxacin: first global approval. Drugs 2015; 75(6): 687-93.
[http://dx.doi.org/10.1007/s40265-015-0384-z] [PMID: 25808831]

[31]   Wagenlehner F, Nowicki M, Bentley C, *et al.* Explorative randomized Phase II clinical study of the efficacy and safety of finafloxacin *versus* ciprofloxacin for treatment of complicated urinary tract infections. Antimicrob Agents Chemother 2018; 62(4): 62.
[http://dx.doi.org/10.1128/AAC.02317-17] [PMID: 29339395]

[32]   Rhee EG, Rizk ML, Calder N, Nefliu M, Warrington SJ, Schwartz MS, *et al.* Pharmacokinetics, safety, and tolerability of single and multiple doses of relebactam, a β-Lactamase inhibitor, in combination with imipenem and cilastatin in healthy participants. Antimicrob Agents Chemother 2018; 62(9): e00280-18.
[http://dx.doi.org/10.1128/AAC.00280-18] [PMID: 29914955]

[33]   Product Information. RECARBRIO®, imipenem, cilastatin, and relebactam intravenous injection. Whitehouse Station, NJ: Merck & Co., Inc 2019.

[34]   Efficacy and Safety of Imipenem+Cilastatin/Relebactam (MK-7655 A) Versus Colistimethate Sodium + Imipenem+Cilastatin in Imipenem- Resistant Bacterial Infection (MK-7655 A-013) (RESTORE-IMI 1). 2017. Available at: https://www.clinicaltrials.gov/ct2/show/NCT02452047?cond=Imipenem+%2 BCilastatin%2FRelebactam&rank=2 [Accessed 20 Aug 2018].

[35]   Kishii R, Yamaguchi Y, Takei M. Activities and spectrum of the novel fluoroquinolone sascufloxacin (KRP-AM1977). Antimicrob Agents Chemother 2017; 61(6): e00120-17.

[http://dx.doi.org/10.1128/AAC.00120-17] [PMID: 28320717]

[36]   Murata M, Kosai K, Yamauchi S, *et al.* Activity of Lascufloxacin against *Streptococcus pneumoniae* with mutations in the quinolone resistance-determining regions. Antimicrob Agents Chemother 2018; 62(4): 62.
[http://dx.doi.org/10.1128/AAC.01971-17] [PMID: 29439959]

[37]   Furuie H, Tanioka S, Shimizu K, Manita S, Nishimura M, Yoshida H. Intrapulmonary pharmacokinetics of lascufloxacin in healthy adult volunteers. Antimicrob Agents Chemother 2018; 62(4): 62.
[http://dx.doi.org/10.1128/AAC.02169-17] [PMID: 29339391]

[38]   Product Information. VABOMERE®, meropenem and vaborbactam for intravenous injection.. Lincolnshire, IL: Melinta Therapeutics, Inc. 2018.

[39]   Cho JCZM, Zmarlicka MT, Shaeer KM, Pardo J. Meropenem/vaborbactam, the first carbapenem/β-lactamase inhibitor combination. Ann Pharmacother 2018; 52(8): 769-79.
[http://dx.doi.org/10.1177/1060028018763288] [PMID: 29514462]

[40]   Castanheira M, Huband MD, Mendes RE, Flamm RK. Meropenem-vaborbactam tested against contemporary Gram-negative isolates collected worldwide during 2014, including carbapenem-resistant, KPC-producing, multidrug-resistant, and extensively drug-resistant Enterobacteriaceae. Antimicrob Agents Chemother 2017; 61(9): e00567-17.
[http://dx.doi.org/10.1128/AAC.00567-17] [PMID: 28652234]

[41]   Yamamoto BJ, Shadiack AM, Carpenter S, *et al.* Obiltoxaximab Prevents Disseminated *Bacillus anthracis* Infection and Improves Survival during Pre- and Postexposure Prophylaxis in Animal Models of Inhalational Anthrax. Antimicrob Agents Chemother 2016; 60(10): 5796-805.
[http://dx.doi.org/10.1128/AAC.01102-16] [PMID: 27431219]

[42]   Hou AW, Morrill AM. Obiltoxaximab: Adding to the treatment arsenal for *Bacillus anthracis* infection. Ann Pharmacother 2017; 51(10): 908-13.
[http://dx.doi.org/10.1177/1060028017713029] [PMID: 28573869]

[43]   Head BM, Rubinstein E, Meyers AF. Alternative pre-approved and novel therapies for the treatment of anthrax. BMC Infect Dis 2016; 16(1): 621.
[http://dx.doi.org/10.1186/s12879-016-1951-y] [PMID: 27809794]

[44]   Product Information. ANTHIM®, obiltoxaximab for intravenous injection.. Pine Brook, NJ: Elusys Therapeutics, Inc. 2016.

[45]   Draper MP, Weir S, Macone A, *et al.* Mechanism of action of the novel aminomethylcycline antibiotic omadacycline. Antimicrob Agents Chemother 2014; 58(3): 1279-83.
[http://dx.doi.org/10.1128/AAC.01066-13] [PMID: 24041885]

[46]   Product Information. NUZYRA®, omadacycline injection and tablets.. Boston, MA: Paratek Pharmaceuticals, Inc. 2018.

[47]   Product Information. ORBACTIV®, oritavancin intravenous injection lyophilized powder.. Parsippany, NJ: The Medicines Company 2014.

[48]   Product Information. XEPTIM®, ozenoxacin topical cream.. Fairfield, NJ: Medimetriks Pharmaceuticals, Inc. 2017.

[49]   Product Information. ZEMDRI®, plazomicin for intravenous injection.. South San Francisco, CA: Achaogen, Inc. 2018.

[50]   Kaufman MB. Pharmaceutical approval update. P&T 2017; 42(12): 733-55.
[PMID: 29234210]

[51]   Product Information. SOLOSEC®, secnidazole oral granules.. Newark, NJ: Symbiomix Therapeutics, LLC 2017.

[52]   Nyirjesy P, Schwebke JR. Secnidazole: next-generation antimicrobial agent for bacterial vaginosis

treatment. Future Microbiol 2018; 13: 507-24.
[http://dx.doi.org/10.2217/fmb-2017-0270] [PMID: 29327947]

[53]   Ghosh AP, Aycock C, Schwebke JR. Study of the susceptibility of clinical Isolates of *trichomonas vaginalis* to metronidazole and secnidazole. Antimicrob Agents Chemother 2018; 62(4): 62.
[http://dx.doi.org/10.1128/AAC.02329-17] [PMID: 29439963]

[54]   Chavoustie SE, Gersten JK, Samuel MJ, Schwebke JR. A Phase 3, multicenter, prospective, open-label study to evaluate the safety of a single dose of secnidazole 2 g for the treatment of women and postmenarchal adolescent girls with bacterial vaginosis. J Womens Health (Larchmt) 2018; 27(4): 492-7.
[http://dx.doi.org/10.1089/jwh.2017.6500] [PMID: 29323627]

[55]   Hall RG II, Smith WJ, Putnam WC, Pass SE. An evaluation of tedizolid for the treatment of MRSA infections. Expert Opin Pharmacother 2018; 19(13): 1489-94.
[http://dx.doi.org/10.1080/14656566.2018.1519021] [PMID: 30200779]

[56]   Moran GJ, De Anda C, Das AF, Green S, Mehra P, Prokocimer P. Efficacy and safety of tedizolid and linezolid for the treatment of acute bacterial skin and skin structure infections in injection drug users: Analysis of two clinical trials. Infect Dis Ther 2018; 7(4): 509-22.
[http://dx.doi.org/10.1007/s40121-018-0211-4] [PMID: 30242736]

[57]   Product Information. SIVEXTRO®, tedizolid phosphate lyophilized powder for intravenous injection, oral tablets.. Lexington, MA: Cubist Pharmaceuticals 2014.

[58]   Rybak JM, Roberts K. Tedizolid Phosphate: A next-generation oxazolidinone. Infect Dis Ther 2015.
[http://dx.doi.org/10.1007/s40121-015-0060-3] [PMID: 25708156]

[59]   Tedizolid phosphate (TR-701 FA) *vs* linezolid for the treatment of nosocomial pneumonia (MK-198--002). 2018. Available at: https://clinicaltrials.gov/ct2/show/NCT02019420 [Accessed 15 Sep 2018].

[60]   Rello J, Perez A. Precision medicine for the treatment of severe pneumonia in intensive care. Expert Rev Respir Med 2016; 10(3): 297-316.
[http://dx.doi.org/10.1586/17476348.2016.1144477] [PMID: 26789703]

[61]   Adjunctive Therapeutic Treatment With Human Monoclonal Antibody AR-105 (Aerucin®) in *P. aeruginosa* Pneumonia. 2018. Available at: https://www.clinicaltrials.gov/ct2/show/NCT03027609?cond=Aerucin&rank=1 [Accessed 17 Sep 2018].

[62]   Aridis Pharmaceuticals | AR-401. 2018. Available at: https://aridispharma.com/ar-401 [Accessed 15 Oct 2018].

[63]   Rodvold KAGM, Gotfried MH, Chugh R, *et al.* Intrapulmonary pharmacokinetics of levonadifloxacin following oral administration of alalevonadifloxacin to healthy adult subjects. Antimicrob Agents Chemother 2018; 62(3): 02297-17.
[PMID: 29263070]

[64]   Alalevonadifloxacin-Wockhardt-AdisInsight. 2018. Available from https://adisinsight.springer.com/drugs/800038027.

[65]   Efficacy Study of Auriclosene Irrigation Solution on Urinary Catheter Patency. 2018. Available at: https://clinicaltrials.gov/ct2/show/NCT02130518 [Accessed 15 Sep 2018].

[66]   First Phase II milestone reached for NovaBay's 3-in-1 antimicrobial auriclosene. 2018. Available at: https://medtech.pharmaintelligence.informa.com/SC022789/First-Phase-II-milestone-reache--for-NovaBays-3in1-antimicrobial-auriclosene [Accessed 31 Aug 2018].

[67]   Iovino SM, Krantz KD, Blanco DM, *et al.* NVC-422 topical gel for the treatment of impetigo. Int J Clin Exp Pathol 2011; 4(6): 587-95.
[PMID: 21904634]

[68]   Jekle A, Abdul Rani S, Celeri C, *et al.* Broad-spectrum virucidal activity of (NVC-422) N,N-dichlor-

-2,2-dimethyltaurine against viral ocular pathogens *in vitro.* Invest Ophthalmol Vis Sci 2013; 54(2): 1244-51.
[http://dx.doi.org/10.1167/iovs.12-10700] [PMID: 23341010]

[69]   Yoon J, Jekle A, Najafi R, *et al.* Virucidal mechanism of action of NVC-422, a novel antimicrobial drug for the treatment of adenoviral conjunctivitis. Antiviral Res 2011; 92(3): 470-8.
[http://dx.doi.org/10.1016/j.antiviral.2011.10.009] [PMID: 22024427]

[70]   Singhal D, Jekle A, Debabov D, *et al.* Efficacy of NVC-422 against *Staphylococcus aureus* biofilms in a sheep biofilm model of sinusitis. Int Forum Allergy Rhinol 2012; 2(4): 309-15.
[http://dx.doi.org/10.1002/alr.21038] [PMID: 22434724]

[71]   Karlowsky JA, Kazmierczak KM, de Jonge BLM, Hackel MA, Sahm DF, Bradford PA. Activity of aztreonam-avibactam against Enterobacteriaceae and *Pseudomonas aeruginosa* isolated by clinical;aboratories in 40 countries from 2012 to 2015. Antimicrob Agents Chemother 2017; 61(9): 61.
[http://dx.doi.org/10.1128/AAC.00472-17] [PMID: 28630192]

[72]   Sader HSMR, Mendes RE, Pfaller MA, Shortridge D, Flamm RK, Castanheira M. Antimicrobial activities of aztreonam-avibactam and comparator agents against contemporary (2016) clinical Enterobacteriaceae isolates. Antimicrob Agents Chemother 2017; 62(1): 1856-7.
[http://dx.doi.org/10.1128/AAC.01856-17] [PMID: 29061754]

[73]   PolyMedix I Brilacidin (PMX-30063) Antibiotic Fact Sheet. Radnor, PA: PolyMedix, Inc. 2013.

[74]   Mensa B, Howell GL, Scott R, DeGrado WF. Comparative mechanistic studies of brilacidin, daptomycin, and the antimicrobial peptide LL16. Antimicrob Agents Chemother 2014; 58(9): 5136-45.
[http://dx.doi.org/10.1128/AAC.02955-14] [PMID: 24936592]

[75]   Stryjewski ME, Potgieter PD, Li YP, *et al.* TD-1792 Investigators Group. TD-1792 *versus* vancomycin for treatment of complicated skin and skin structure infections. Antimicrob Agents Chemother 2012; 56(11): 5476-83.
[http://dx.doi.org/10.1128/AAC.00712-12] [PMID: 22869571]

[76]   Entasis begins Phase I trial of ETX0282 and ETX0282CPDP to treat infections. 2018. Available at: https://www.drugdevelopment-technology.com/news/entasis-begins-phase-trial-etx0282-etx02-2cpdp-treat-infections [Accessed 31 Aug 2018].

[77]   Taylor SN, Morris DH, Avery AK, *et al.* Gepotidacin for the treatment of uncomplicated urogenital gonorrhea: A Phase 2, randomized, dose-ranging, single-oral dose evaluation. Clin Infect Dis 2018; 67(4): 504-12.
[http://dx.doi.org/10.1093/cid/ciy145] [PMID: 29617982]

[78]   Flamm RK, Farrell DJ, Rhomberg PR, Scangarella-Oman NE, Sader HS. Gepotidacin (GSK2140944). Antimicrob Agents Chemother 2017; 61(7): 61.
[PMID: 28483959]

[79]   Jacobsson S, Golparian D, Scangarella-Oman N, Unemo M. *In vitro* activity of the novel triazaacenaphthylene gepotidacin (GSK2140944) against MDR *Neisseria gonorrhoeae.* J Antimicrob Chemother 2018; 73(8): 2072-7.
[http://dx.doi.org/10.1093/jac/dky162] [PMID: 29796611]

[80]   O'Riordan W, Tiffany C, Scangarella-Oman N, *et al.* Efficacy, safety, and tolerability of gepotidacin (GSK2140944) in the treatment of patients with suspected or confirmed Gram-positive acute bacterial skin and skin structure infections. Antimicrob Agents Chemother 2017; 61(6): 61.
[http://dx.doi.org/10.1128/AAC.02095-16] [PMID: 28373199]

[81]   Aliouat EM, Dei-Cas E, Gantois N, *et al. In vitro* and *in vivo* activity of iclaprim, a diaminopyrimidine compound and potential therapeutic alternative against Pneumocystis pneumonia. Eur J Clin Microbiol Infect Dis 2018; 37(3): 409-15.
[http://dx.doi.org/10.1007/s10096-018-3184-z] [PMID: 29330709]

[82] Huang DB, Dryden M. Iclaprim, a dihydrofolate reductase inhibitor antibiotic in Phase III of clinical development: a review of its pharmacology, microbiology and clinical efficacy and safety. Future Microbiol 2018; 13: 957-69.
[http://dx.doi.org/10.2217/fmb-2018-0061] [PMID: 29742926]

[83] Holland TL, O'Riordan W, McManus A, *et al.* A Phase 3, randomized, double-blind, multicenter study to evaluate the safety and efficacy of intravenous iclaprim *versus* vancomycin for treatment of acute bacterial skin and skin structure infections suspected or confirmed to be due to Gram-positive pathogens (REVIVE-2 study). Antimicrob Agents Chemother 2018; 62(5): 62.
[http://dx.doi.org/10.1128/AAC.02580-17] [PMID: 29530858]

[84] Paukner S, Sader HS, Ivezic-Schoenfeld Z, Jones RN. Antimicrobial activity of the pleuromutilin antibiotic BC-3781 against bacterial pathogens isolated in the SENTRY antimicrobial surveillance program in 2010. Antimicrob Agents Chemother 2013; 57(9): 4489-95.
[http://dx.doi.org/10.1128/AAC.00358-13] [PMID: 23836172]

[85] Eyal Z, Matzov D, Krupkin M, *et al.* A novel pleuromutilin antibacterial compound, its binding mode and selectivity mechanism. Sci Rep 2016; 6: 39004.
[http://dx.doi.org/10.1038/srep39004] [PMID: 27958389]

[86] Veve MP, Wagner JL. Lefamulin: Review of a promising novel pleuromutilin antibiotic. Pharmacotherapy 2018; 38(9): 935-46.
[http://dx.doi.org/10.1002/phar.2166] [PMID: 30019769]

[87] Le HN, Quetz JS, Tran VG, *et al.* MEDI3902 correlates of protection against severe *Pseudomonas aeruginosa* pneumonia in a rabbit acute pneumonia model. Antimicrob Agents Chemother 2018; 62(5): 62.
[http://dx.doi.org/10.1128/AAC.02565-17] [PMID: 29483116]

[88] Effort to Prevent Nosocomial Pneumonia Caused by. *Pseudomonas aeruginosa* in mechanically ventilated subjects. EVADE 2018. Available from: https://www.clinicaltrials.gov/ct2/show/NCT02696902?cond=MEDI-3902&draw=1&rank=2

[89] Phase 1 randomized double-blind placebo controlled study to evaluate safety and PK of MEDI3902 in healthy adults. 2018. Available at: https://www.clinicaltrials.gov/ct2/show/results/NCT022 55760?cond=MEDI-3902&rank=1§=X43870156#othr [Accessed 18 Aug 2018].

[90] Sader HS, Flamm RK, Dale GE, Rhomberg PR, Castanheira M. Murepavadin activity tested against contemporary (2016-17) clinical isolates of XDR *Pseudomonas aeruginosa.* J Antimicrob Chemother 2018; 73(9): 2400-4.
[http://dx.doi.org/10.1093/jac/dky227] [PMID: 29901750]

[91] Martin-Loeches I, Dale GE, Torres A. Murepavadin: a new antibiotic class in the pipeline. Expert Rev Anti Infect Ther 2018; 16(4): 259-68.
[http://dx.doi.org/10.1080/14787210.2018.1441024] [PMID: 29451043]

[92] Bassères E, Endres BT, Khaleduzzaman M, *et al.* Impact on toxin production and cell morphology in *Clostridium difficile* by ridinilazole (SMT19969), a novel treatment for *C. difficile* infection. J Antimicrob Chemother 2016; 71(5): 1245-51.
[http://dx.doi.org/10.1093/jac/dkv498] [PMID: 26895772]

[93] Vickers R, Robinson N, Best E, Echols R, Tillotson G, Wilcox M. A randomised phase 1 study to investigate safety, pharmacokinetics and impact on gut microbiota following single and multiple oral doses in healthy male subjects of SMT19969, a novel agent for *Clostridium difficile* infections. BMC Infect Dis 2015; 15: 91.
[http://dx.doi.org/10.1186/s12879-015-0759-5] [PMID: 25880933]

[94] Khanna S, Pardi DS, Kelly CR, *et al.* A Novel microbiome therapeutic increases gut microbial diversity and prevents recurrent *Clostridium difficile* infection. J Infect Dis 2016; 214(2): 173-81.
[http://dx.doi.org/10.1093/infdis/jiv766] [PMID: 26908752]

[95]   Wortman JR, Lachey J, Lombardo M-J, Litcofsky KD, Button JE. Design and evaluation of SER-262: a fermentation-derived microbiome therapeutic for the prevention of recurrence in patients with primary clostridium difficile infection. ASM Microbe 2016. Boston, MA 2016.

[96]   Oldach D, Clark K, Schranz J, *et al.* Randomized, double-blind, multicenter phase 2 study comparing the efficacy and safety of oral solithromycin (CEM-101) to those of oral levofloxacin in the treatment of patients with community-acquired bacterial pneumonia. Antimicrob Agents Chemother 2013; 57(6): 2526-34.
[http://dx.doi.org/10.1128/AAC.00197-13] [PMID: 23507282]

[97]   Donald BJ, Surani S, Deol HS, Mbadugha UJ, Udeani G. Spotlight on solithromycin in the treatment of community-acquired bacterial pneumonia: design, development, and potential place in therapy. Drug Des Devel Ther 2017; 11: 3559-66.
[http://dx.doi.org/10.2147/DDDT.S119545] [PMID: 29263651]

[98]   McLeod SM, Shapiro AB, Moussa SH, *et al.* Frequency and mechanism of spontaneous resistance to sulbactam combined with the novel β-lactamase inhibitor ETX2514 in clinical isolates of *Acinetobacter baumannii.* Antimicrob Agents Chemother 2018; 62(2): 62.
[PMID: 29133555]

[99]   Evaluation of safety and efficacy of intravenous sulbactam-ETX2514 in the treatment of hospitalized adults with complicated urinary tract infections. 2018. Available at: https://www.clinicaltrials.gov/ct2/show/NCT03445195 [Accessed 31 Aug 2018].

[100]   Komoto A, Otsuki M, Nishino T. *In vitro* and *in vivo* antibacterial activities of sulopenem, a new penem antibiotic. Jpn J Antibiot 1996; 49(4): 352-66.
[PMID: 8786626]

[101]   Grossman TH, Fyfe C, O'Brien W, *et al.* Fluorocycline TP-271 Is Potent against Complicated Community-Acquired Bacterial Pneumonia Pathogens. MSphere 2017; 2(1): 2.
[http://dx.doi.org/10.1128/mSphere.00004-17] [PMID: 28251179]

[102]   Falagas ME, Skalidis T, Vardakas KZ, Voulgaris GL, Papanikolaou G, Legakis N. Hellenic TP-6076 Study Group. Activity of TP-6076 against carbapenem-resistant *Acinetobacter baumannii* isolates collected from inpatients in Greek hospitals. Int J Antimicrob Agents 2018; 52(2): 269-71.
[http://dx.doi.org/10.1016/j.ijantimicag.2018.03.009] [PMID: 29559273]

[103]   Giacobbe RA, Huband MD, deJonge BL, Bradford PA. Effect of susceptibility testing conditions on the *in vitro* antibacterial activity of ETX0914. Diagn Microbiol Infect Dis 2017; 87(2): 139-42.
[http://dx.doi.org/10.1016/j.diagmicrobio.2016.03.007] [PMID: 27856046]

[104]   Randomized, Open-label Phase 2 Study of Oral AZD0914 in the Treatment of Gonorrhea. 2017. Available at: https://www.clinicaltrials.gov/ct2/show/results/NCT02257918?cond=Zoliflodacin&ra [Accessed 20 Aug 2018].

[105]   Varshney AK, Kuzmicheva GA, Lin J, *et al.* A natural human monoclonal antibody targeting *Staphylococcus* Protein A protects against *Staphylococcus aureus* bacteremia. PLoS One 2018; 13(1): e0190537.
[http://dx.doi.org/10.1371/journal.pone.0190537] [PMID: 29364906]

[106]   XBiotech I. *S. aureus* Antibody Therapy by Xbiotech S. aureus therapeutic antibody. 2018. Available at: http://www.xbiotech.com/clinical/s-aureus.php [Accessed 15 Oct 2018].

[107]   Sigurgeirsson B, van Rossem K, Malahias S, Raterink K. A phase II, randomized, double-blind, placebo-controlled, parallel group, dose-ranging study to investigate the efficacy and safety of 4 dose regimens of oral albaconazole in patients with distal subungual onychomycosis. J Am Acad Dermatol 2013; 69(3): 416-25.
[http://dx.doi.org/10.1016/j.jaad.2013.03.021] [PMID: 23706639]

[108]   Product Information. LOCERYL NAIL LACQUER®, amorolfine nail lacquer.. Belrose, Australia: Galderma Australia, Pty, Ltd. 2011.

[109] Perfect JR. The antifungal pipeline: a reality check. Nat Rev Drug Discov 2017; 16(9): 603-16.
[http://dx.doi.org/10.1038/nrd.2017.46] [PMID: 28496146]

[110] Zhong W, Jeffries MW, Georgopapadakou NH. Inhibition of inositol phosphorylceramide synthase by aureobasidin A in *Candida* and *Aspergillus* species. Antimicrob Agents Chemother 2000; 44(3): 651-3.
[http://dx.doi.org/10.1128/AAC.44.3.651-653.2000] [PMID: 10681333]

[111] Cidara Therapeutics I. Rezafungin (Formerly CD101 IV). 2018. Available at: https://www.cidara.com/rezafungin/#overview [Accessed 15 Oct 2018].

[112] Pianalto KMAJ, Alspaugh JA. New horizons in antifungal therapy. J Fungi (Basel) 2016; 2(4): 26.
[http://dx.doi.org/10.3390/jof2040026] [PMID: 29376943]

[113] Gonzalez-Lara MFS-OJ, Sifuentes-Osornio J, Ostrosky-Zeichner L. Drugs in clinical development for fungal infections. Drugs 2017; 77(14): 1505-18.
[http://dx.doi.org/10.1007/s40265-017-0805-2] [PMID: 28840541]

[114] Safety and efficacy of oral encochleated amphotericin B (CAMB/MAT2203) in the treatment of vulvovaginal candidiasis (VVC). 2017. Available at: https://clinicaltrials.gov/ ct2/show/NCT02971007 [Accessed 20 Aug 2018].

[115] CAMB/MAT2203 in Patients With Mucocutaneous Candidiasis (CAMB). 2016.

[116] Ben Yaakov D, Rivkin A, Mircus G, *et al.* Identification and characterization of haemofungin, a novel antifungal compound that inhibits the final step of haem biosynthesis. J Antimicrob Chemother 2016; 71(4): 946-52.
[http://dx.doi.org/10.1093/jac/dkv446] [PMID: 26747101]

[117] Robbins N, Spitzer M, Wang W, *et al.* Discovery of ibomycin, a complex macrolactone that exerts antifungal activity by impeding endocytic trafficking and membrane function. Cell Chem Biol 2016; 23(11): 1383-94.
[http://dx.doi.org/10.1016/j.chembiol.2016.08.015] [PMID: 27746129]

[118] Product Information. CRESEMBA®, isavuconazonium sulfate intravenous injection and oral capsules.. Northbrook, IL: Astellas Pharma, Inc. 2015.

[119] Shirley M, Scott LJ. Isavuconazole: A Review in invasive aspergillosis and mucormycosis. Drugs 2016; 76(17): 1647-57.
[http://dx.doi.org/10.1007/s40265-016-0652-6] [PMID: 27766566]

[120] Horn D, Goff D, Khandelwal N, *et al.* Hospital resource use of patients receiving isavuconazole *vs* voriconazole for invasive mold infections in the phase III SECURE trial. J Med Econ 2016; 19(7): 728-34.
[http://dx.doi.org/10.3111/13696998.2016.1164175] [PMID: 26960060]

[121] Townsend R, Dietz A, Hale C, *et al.* Pharmacokinetic evaluation of CYP3A4-mediated drug-drug interactions of isavuconazole with rifampin, ketoconazole, midazolam, and ethinyl estradiol/norethindrone in healthy adults. Clin Pharmacol Drug Dev 2017; 6(1): 44-53.
[http://dx.doi.org/10.1002/cpdd.285] [PMID: 27273461]

[122] Clinical study of AK1820 (Isavuconazonium Sulfate) for the treatment of deep mycosis. 2017. Available at: https://clinicaltrials.gov/ct2/show/NCT03241550 [Accessed 12 Sep 2018].

[123] A study of intravenous and oral isavuconazonium sulfate in pediatric patients. 2017. Available at: https://clinicaltrials.gov/ct2/show/NCT03241550 [Accessed 12 Sep 2018].

[124] Perdoni F, Signorelli P, Cirasola D, *et al.* Antifungal activity of Myriocin on clinically relevant *Aspergillus fumigatus* strains producing biofilm. BMC Microbiol 2015; 15: 248.
[http://dx.doi.org/10.1186/s12866-015-0588-0] [PMID: 26519193]

[125] Novabiotics L. Novamycin NP339-novabiotics. 2018. Available at: https://www.novabiotics.co.uk/ pipeline/novamycin-np339 [Accessed 8 Sep 2018].

[126] Katvars LK, Smith D, Duncan VMS, *et al.* Novamycin®(NP339) as a novel approach against respiratory fungal infections. 27th European Congress of Clinical Microbiology and Infectious Diseases, abstract Vienna, Austria 2017.

[127] The Aspergillus Website. Novamycin (NP339) | Aspergillus & Aspergillosis Website. 2017. Available at: https://www.aspergillus.org.uk/content/novamycin-np339 [Accessed 8 Sep 2018].

[128] Agarwal AK, Xu T, Jacob MR, *et al.* Role of heme in the antifungal activity of the azaoxoaporphine alkaloid sampangine. Eukaryot Cell 2008; 7(2): 387-400.
[http://dx.doi.org/10.1128/EC.00323-07] [PMID: 18156292]

[129] Sharma N, Sharma D. An upcoming drug for onychomycosis: Tavaborole. J Pharmacol Pharmacother 2015; 6(4): 236-9.
[http://dx.doi.org/10.4103/0976-500X.171870] [PMID: 26816482]

[130] Product Information. KERYDIN®, tavaborole topical solution, 5.. Palo Alto, CA: Anacor Pharmaceuticals, Inc. 2014.

[131] Colley T, Alanio A, Kelly SL, *et al. In Vitro* and *In Vivo* Antifungal Profile of a Novel and Long-Acting Inhaled Azole, PC945, on Aspergillus fumigatus Infection. Antimicrob Agents Chemother 2017; 61(5): 61.
[http://dx.doi.org/10.1128/AAC.02280-16] [PMID: 28223388]

[132] The effect of PC945 on *aspergillus fumigatus*. Lung Infection in Patients With Cystic Fibrosis 2019. Available at: https://clinicaltrials.gov/ct2/show/NCT03870841 [Accessed 1 Apr 2020].

[133] The effect of early treatment of PC945 on *Aspergillus fumigatus*. Lung infection in lung transplant patients 2019. Available at: https://clinicaltrials.gov/ct2/show/NCT03905447 [1 Apr 2020].

[134] The effect of PC945 on *Aspergillus* or *Candida*. Lung infections in patients with asthma or chronic respiratory diseases 2018. Available at: https://clinicaltrials.gov/ct2/show/NCT03745196 [Accessed 1 Apr 2020].

[135] Safety and pharmacokinetics of VT-1598. 2019. Available at: https://clinicaltrials.gov/ct2/show/NCT04208321.

[136] Lamoth F, Alexander BD. Antifungal activities of SCY-078 (MK-3118) and standard antifungal agents against clinical non-*Aspergillus* mold isolates. Antimicrob Agents Chemother 2015; 59(7): 4308-11.
[http://dx.doi.org/10.1128/AAC.00234-15] [PMID: 25896696]

[137] Aspergillus & Aspergillosis Website. A prospective, phase 2, multicentre, open-label, randomized, comparative study to estimate the safety, tolerability, pharmacokinetics, and efficacy of oral SCY-078 vsstandard-of-care following initial intravenous echinocandin therapy. 2017. Available at: https://www.aspergillus.org.uk/content/prospective-phase-2-multicentre-open--abel-randomized-comparative-study-estimate-safety-0.

[138] Yamashita K, Miyazaki T, Fukuda Y, *et al.* The novel arylamidine t-2307 selectively disrupts yeast mitochondrial function by inhibiting respiratory chain complexes. Antimicrob Agents Chemother 2019; 63(8): 63.
[http://dx.doi.org/10.1128/AAC.00374-19] [PMID: 31182539]

[139] Shibata T, Takahashi T, Yamada E, *et al.* T-2307 causes collapse of mitochondrial membrane potential in yeast. Antimicrob Agents Chemother 2012; 56(11): 5892-7.
[http://dx.doi.org/10.1128/AAC.05954-11] [PMID: 22948882]

[140] Dietl AM, Misslinger M, Aguiar MM, *et al.* The siderophore transporter sit1 determines susceptibility to the antifungal VL-2397. Antimicrob Agents Chemother 2019; 63(10): 63.
[http://dx.doi.org/10.1128/AAC.00807-19] [PMID: 31405865]

[141] Aspergillus & Aspergillosis Website. Vical announces Phase 2 efficacy trial for antifungal VL-2397 2017. Available at: https://www.aspergillus.org.uk/blog/vical-announces-phase-2-efficacy--

rial-antifungal-vl-2397.

[142] du Pré S, Beckmann N, Almeida MC, *et al.* Effect of the novel antifungal drug F901318 (olorofim) on growth and viability of *Aspergillus fumigatus*. Antimicrob Agents Chemother 2018; 62(8): 62.
[http://dx.doi.org/10.1128/AAC.00231-18] [PMID: 29891595]

[143] Oliver JD, Sibley GEM, Beckmann N, *et al.* F901318 represents a novel class of antifungal drug that inhibits dihydroorotate dehydrogenase. Proc Natl Acad Sci USA 2016; 113(45): 12809-14.
[http://dx.doi.org/10.1073/pnas.1608304113] [PMID: 27791100]

[144] Watanabe NA, Miyazaki M, Horii T, Sagane K, Tsukahara K, Hata K. E1210, a new broad-spectrum antifungal, suppresses *Candida albicans* hyphal growth through inhibition of glycosylphosphatidylinositol biosynthesis. Antimicrob Agents Chemother 2012; 56(2): 960-71.
[http://dx.doi.org/10.1128/AAC.00731-11] [PMID: 22143530]

[145] Capparelli EV, Bricker-Ford R, Rogers MJ, McKerrow JH, Reed SL. Phase I clinical trial results of auranofin, a novel antiparasitic agent. Antimicrob Agents Chemother 2016; 61(1): 61.
[PMID: 27821451]

[146] Tejman-Yarden N, Miyamoto Y, Leitsch D, *et al.* A reprofiled drug, auranofin, is effective against metronidazole-resistant *Giardia lamblia*. Antimicrob Agents Chemother 2013; 57(5): 2029-35.
[http://dx.doi.org/10.1128/AAC.01675-12] [PMID: 23403423]

[147] Roder C, Thomson MJ. Auranofin: repurposing an old drug for a golden new age. Drugs R D 2015; 15(1): 13-20.
[http://dx.doi.org/10.1007/s40268-015-0083-y] [PMID: 25698589]

[148] Product Information. RIDAURA®, auranofin oral capsules.. San Diego, CA: Prometheus Laboratories, Inc. 2016.

[149] Rajão MA, Furtado C, Alves CL, *et al.* Unveiling benznidazole's mechanism of action through overexpression of DNA repair proteins in *Trypanosoma cruzi*. Environ Mol Mutagen 2014; 55(4): 309-21.
[http://dx.doi.org/10.1002/em.21839] [PMID: 24347026]

[150] Torrico F, Gascon J, Ortiz L, *et al.* E1224 Study Group. Treatment of adult chronic indeterminate Chagas disease with benznidazole and three E1224 dosing regimens: a proof-of-concept, randomised, placebo-controlled trial. Lancet Infect Dis 2018; 18(4): 419-30.
[http://dx.doi.org/10.1016/S1473-3099(17)30538-8] [PMID: 29352704]

[151] Molina I, Gómez i Prat J, Salvador F, *et al.* Randomized trial of posaconazole and benznidazole for chronic Chagas' disease. N Engl J Med 2014; 370(20): 1899-908.
[http://dx.doi.org/10.1056/NEJMoa1313122] [PMID: 24827034]

[152] Álvarez MG, Vigliano C, Lococo B, Bertocchi G, Viotti R. Prevention of congenital Chagas disease by Benznidazole treatment in reproductive-age women. An observational study. Acta Trop 2017; 174: 149-52.
[http://dx.doi.org/10.1016/j.actatropica.2017.07.004] [PMID: 28720492]

[153] Product Information. BENZIDAZOLE tablets. Florham Park, NJ: Exeltis USA, Inc. 2017.

[154] Kumar P, Cushion MT, Lu R, *et al.* a novel encochleated atovaquone formulation is active in a murine model of pneumocystis pneumonia, abstract 3673. ASM Microbe 2018. Atlanta, GA 2018.

[155] Sundar S, Jha TK, Thakur CP, Bhattacharya SK, Rai M. Oral miltefosine for the treatment of Indian visceral leishmaniasis. Trans R Soc Trop Med Hyg 2006; 100 (Suppl. 1): S26-33.
[http://dx.doi.org/10.1016/j.trstmh.2006.02.011] [PMID: 16730038]

[156] Centers for Disease Control and Prevention. NIOSH list of antineoplastic and other hazardous drugs in healthcare settings 2016 US Department of Health and Human Services; Centers for Disease Control and Prevention. National Institute for Occupational Safety and Health 2016.

[157] Aichelburg AC, Walochnik J, Assadian O, *et al.* Successful treatment of disseminated *Acanthamoeba*

sp. infection with miltefosine. Emerg Infect Dis 2008; 14(11): 1743-6.
[http://dx.doi.org/10.3201/eid1411.070854] [PMID: 18976559]

[158] Product Information. IMPAVIDO®, miltefosine capsules.. Wilmington, DE: Paladin Therapeutics, Inc. 2014.

CHAPTER 11

Global Initiatives to Combat Antimicrobial Resistance

Jonathan C. Cho[1], Rebecca L. Dunn[2] and Takova D. Wallace-Gay[2,*]

[1] *Mountain View Hospital, Las Vegas, NV, USA*

[2] *Fisch College of Pharmacy, The University of Texas at Tyler, Tyler, TX, USA*

Abstract: Antimicrobial resistance (AMR) remains one of the major global public health threats today. Infections due to multi-drug resistant organisms have been shown to not only increase healthcare costs but also be a significant cause of morbidity and mortality in patients. Global efforts have been employed to combat the issue of AMR. Specifically, the World Health Organization's global action plan on antimicrobial resistance recognizes key areas to be addressed including: increased awareness and understanding of AMR, infection prevention and control, enhanced structure with the use of antimicrobials in animals, research, and economic investment in intervention methods. Several approaches exist to help mitigate this issue such as the development of antimicrobial stewardship programs (ASPs), clinician education, improved infection control practices and judicious antibiotic use in animals. This chapter will outline many of the current strategies proposed to counter and prevent the global concern of AMR.

Keywords: Agriculture, Animals, Antimicrobial Stewardship, Infection Control, Infection Prevention.

BACKGROUND

One of the major global public health threats, today, is the development of antimicrobial resistance (AMR). Antimicrobial resistance impacts the prevention and treatment of infections caused by bacteria, parasites, viruses and fungi. As resistance to effective treatments develop, organisms called superbugs or multidrug-resistant organisms (MDRO) are created [1]. Healthcare-associated infections (HAI) due to MDRO are associated with increased healthcare costs and have been shown to be a significant cause of morbidity and mortality [2, 3]. In the United States alone, the Centers for Disease Control and Prevention (CDC) estimates that approximately 35,000 deaths occur annually due to infections caused by MDRO [4].

---

* **Corresponding author Takova D. Wallace-Gay:** Fisch College of Pharmacy, The University of Texas at Tyler, Tyler, TX, USA; Fax 903-565-5598; Tel: 903-566-6140; E-mail: twallacegay@uttyler.edu

Islam M. Ghazi & Michael J. Cawley (Eds.)

Globally, it is estimated that the European Union sustains 25,000 deaths per year, India loses over 58,000 babies, annually, and Thailand has more than 38,000 deaths, per year, due to resistant organisms [5].

To this end, in 2015, the World Health Assembly, in conjunction with the World Health Organization, developed and endorsed a global action plan to address AMR. The intent of this plan is to ensure the ability to successfully prevent and treat infectious diseases. While many national organizations and governing bodies have similar initiatives and guidelines to combat AMR, the WHO used much of this information to inform the development of their objectives: 1) improve awareness and understanding of AMR, 2) strengthen knowledge through surveillance and research, 3) reduce the incidence of infection, 4) optimize the use of antimicrobial agents, and 5) create an economic framework, beneficial to all counties, that supports the development of new medicines, diagnostic agents, vaccines and more [1].

The objective of this chapter is to discuss many of the initiatives, endorsed by the global action plan and other guidelines that help combat AMR. One pivotal approach to help curb this issue is through the development and implementation of antimicrobial stewardship programs (ASPs). These programs have the goal of optimizing antimicrobial use to improve patient and healthcare outcomes. In addition to ASPs, optimal infection prevention and control practices serve as foundational principles to combat AMR. Finally, judicious antimicrobial use in animals and agricultural, while often overlooked, must be considered as a necessary initiative to mitigate the development of AMR.

ANTIMICROBIAL STEWARDSHIP PROGRAMS

A major cause of resistance is the inappropriate use of antimicrobials. Estimates show up to 50% of antimicrobial use is unnecessary in hospitals [6]. The goal of ASPs is to improve patient care and health-care outcomes and reduce healthcare costs through the optimization of antimicrobial selection and use. This optimization includes selecting the appropriate dose, route, and duration of therapy while minimizing the unintended consequences such as the emergence of AMR and associated adverse effects [6]. Evidence exists showing that ASPs achieve this intended purpose and have significant benefits in reducing mortality, length of stay (LOS), and healthcare costs. The need for enhancing antimicrobial stewardship as a means to combat AMR is highlighted in the executive order issued by United States President, Barack Obama [7]. In tandem with the executive order, a report by the Executive Office of the President of the United States stated that Centers for Medicare and Medicaid Services (CMS) should use reimbursement incentives to drive antibiotic stewardship [8]. The state of

California recognized the importance of ASP early on. Since 2008, California required acute care facilities to develop a process for monitoring judicious use of antibiotics, and recently signed Senate Bill 1311 which further requires hospitals to adopt and implement antimicrobial stewardship in accordance with guidelines established by the federal government and professional organizations [9]. California remains the first and only state to enact legislation related to antimicrobial stewardship practices [9]. The Department of Veterans Affairs (VA) also issued a national directive (VHA Directive 1031) to establish a policy for the implementation and maintenance of ASPs at all VA medical facilities [10]. State and national legislations make clear the need and importance for combating resistance through antimicrobial stewardship.

Multidisciplinary Members of Antimicrobial Stewardship Programs

An infectious diseases (ID) physician and a clinical pharmacist with ID training are recognized as core members of a multidisciplinary antimicrobial stewardship team [6]. The CDC published a document, "Core Elements of Hospital Antibiotic Stewardship Programs", and suggests having both a physician leader, who is responsible for program outcomes, and a pharmacist leader, who is responsible for working to improve antibiotic use [11]. The American Society of Health-System Pharmacists (ASHP) also released a statement detailing the responsibility pharmacists must take in their prominent roles in ASPs and participation in infection prevention and control programs. This responsibility stemmed from pharmacists' understanding and influence on antimicrobial use within an institution [12]. Although national guidelines recommend a pharmacist with ID training sufficient to cultivate and maintain expert knowledge on the appropriate use of antimicrobials to be a core member of ASP, this is not always feasible. Many institutions have pharmacists without specialized ID training participating in successful stewardship activities [6, 13]. As there continues to be a limited number of formally trained ID pharmacists, adequate training from professional societies, including certificate programs, are critical to the continued success of ASPs.

Other members of an ASP team, according to the Infectious Diseases Society of America (IDSA) and the Society for Healthcare Epidemiology of America (SHEA) guidelines, include a clinical microbiologist, hospital epidemiologist, infection preventionist, and information system specialist [6]. A clinical microbiologist can provide surveillance data needed to create tools such as an antibiogram (an institution-specific profile of microorganism susceptibility to various antimicrobials) and also play an integral role in obtaining new rapid diagnostic testing needed to identify organisms and related antimicrobial susceptibilities. Hospital epidemiologists and infection preventionists can aid with surveillance through monitoring and reporting of MDRO trends, ensure compliance with hand hygiene and appropriate isolation for patients carrying MDROs. They can also educate clinicians on the prudent and appropriate use of antibiotics [14]. Information system specialists are also essential members of ASPs as many of the ASP initiatives can be facilitated through the use of electronic medical records and computerized physician order entry [15 - 17]. Information technology can assist with implementation of clinical pathways or institutional guidelines, enforce formulary restriction (limiting the use of specific formulary medications to certain physicians based on a number of considerations such as ID expertise or patient population) and preauthorization, and provide data needed to analyze and measure outcomes of ASP related initiatives.

Antimicrobial Stewardship Models and Strategies

In the guidelines released by the IDSA/SHEA on developing an institutional program to enhance antimicrobial stewardship, two core strategies were recognized: (1) prospective audit with intervention and feedback and (2) formulary restriction and preauthorization [6]. In the prospective audit with intervention and feedback model, a review of appropriateness of a prescriber's order for antimicrobials occurs when they are initially ordered. If the order for an antimicrobial agent is inappropriate, the prescriber is contacted with a recommendation for alternative therapy. The advantages with this method include maintenance of prescriber autonomy, opportunity for educational dialogue to influence future prescribing, and avoidance of any potential delays in initiation of appropriate antimicrobial therapy. Some of the potential barriers include difficulty contacting and communicating with prescribers, providers that dispute or decline stewardship recommendations, and identifying patients that are on inappropriate therapy who may benefit from intervention. The use of computerized support systems can help decrease these barriers.

The formulary restriction and preauthorization method encompasses many different strategies to help limit the use of certain antimicrobial agents. One way to accomplish this is through the pharmacy and therapeutics (P & T) committee, or an equivalent group, where a decision is made on which antimicrobial agents to keep on a hospital formulary. Antimicrobial agents can also be restricted to specific physician services or based on treatment indications. Formulary restriction and preauthorization has been shown to immediately reduce targeted antimicrobial use and associated costs. A shift to prescribing of alternative antimicrobials may be seen. This method decreases prescriber autonomy and has the potential to cause delays in initiation of antimicrobial therapy while obtaining approval from an authorized prescriber. Several institutions have allowed first dose dispensing of antimicrobial agents to be excluded from the requirement of formulary restriction and preauthorization in order to prevent delays in therapy. Although each method has advantages and disadvantages, both prospective audit with intervention and feedback and formulary restriction and preauthorization strategies have shown to be beneficial in reducing the amount of antimicrobial use and associated costs. Several institutions use a combination of the two strategies, but there are also other ASP strategies that are used. Some examples of successful ASPs are shown in Table **1**.

Table 1. Antimicrobial stewardship programs and related outcomes.

Study	Primary ASP Strategy	Outcomes
Carling P *et al.* 2003 [18]	Prospective audit and intervention	22% decrease in use of parenteral broad-spectrum ABX (p<0.0001) Significant decrease in nosocomial infections caused by *Clostridium difficile* and Enterobacteriaceae (p=0.02)
Sanders J *et al.* 2014 [19]	Multifaceted, multidisciplinary stewardship efforts	Number of medication errors significantly decreased from 50% to 34% (p<0.001) ID consultant resulted in higher error resolution rate from 32% to 68% (p=0.002)
Benson JM 2014 [20]	Pharmacy students daily monitoring of all infection-related patient problems	The mean (± SD) antimicrobial costs per patient day were $75.37 ± $11.85 in the baseline period *versus* $64.13 ± $13.78 in the intervention period (p=0.022) Represents cost savings of $261,630 during the two-year intervention period
Reed EE *et al.* 2013 [21]	Formulary restriction with prior authorization	Significant decrease in anti-pseudomonal carbapenem use (11 antimicrobial days/1,000 patient days *vs.* 27 antimicrobial days/1,000 patient days; p=0.0008)
Liew YX *et al.* 2015 [22]	Prospective audit and feedback within 48 hours of antibiotic prescription	Culture-directed treatment: shorter mean DOT in recommendation accepted group *versus* rejected group (2.26 days *vs.* 5.56 days; p<0.001) Empiric treatment: shorter DOT (3.61 days *vs.* 6.25 days; p<0.001); decreased 30-day all-cause mortality (p=0.003); decreased infection-related mortality (p=0.002) were observed in accepted group *versus* rejected group

Abbreviations: ABX, antibiotics; DOT, duration of therapy; SD, standard deviation

Education is another important component to an ASP. Education of medicine, nursing, pharmacy staff, and other personnel, is important regarding general antimicrobial stewardship concepts, the goals of the ASP, as well as, the specific metrics being implemented. Examples of antimicrobial stewardship educational endeavors include updates on antibiotic prescribing trends, antibiogram education and review of de-identified cases from the local institution. Additionally, education is a vital component of other supplemental antimicrobial stewardship strategies [6]. A large academic medical center used an educational approach to decrease unnecessary antimicrobial use for the treatment of asymptomatic bacteriuria (ASB) [23]. Education, delivered by APS members, was conducted *via* in-services to targeted physicians and pharmacists; notifications in physician offices, conference rooms and mailboxes; a pocket card with an algorithm on ASB diagnosis; electronic communication to hospitalists with recommendations for ASB management; pharmacist rounding with emergency and internal medicine teams; and daily review of common antimicrobials for the treatment of urinary tract infections (UTI). The educational initiative was deemed to be successful with 62% of patients (66/107) receiving unnecessary antibiotics prior to the education *versus* 26% (28/107), p<0.0001, after education [23]. The success of this program is likely due to the significant time invested by the ASP team and the multifaceted approach.

The development and use of standard treatment guidelines, in the management of infectious diseases, has been cited as an effective strategy for combating AMR. While inappropriate use of antimicrobials is a global problem and a major contributor to the development of resistance, a large percentage of patients, especially in developing countries, still are not treated per standard treatment guidelines [24, 25]. While treatment guidelines may vary from one region or country to the next, guidelines can be useful in optimizing antibiotic selection, dosing, route of administration, duration of therapy and in maintaining antimicrobial effectiveness [1, 24]. Guidelines and clinical pathways are one component of an ASP that can be implemented in the community setting or at an institution without a large number of personnel dedicated to the ASP. Most guideline implementations do not require an extensive implementation period. The majority of time invested is in the planning and approval phases. An evaluation is needed, after implementation of the guideline/pathway, to assure adherence and success. Education improves uptake and adherence to the guideline/pathway. Many institutions implement guidelines and clinical pathways specific to a disease state. Electronic medical records systems and/or clinical decision support systems (CDSS) can be utilized to streamline the implementation of clinical pathways and measure provider adherence. Education in the form of in-services, posters and pocket guides assist in increasing adherence to newly implemented pathways. Implementation of an electronic UTI order set, in conjunction with, prospective audit and feedback at a large academic medical center emergency department was evaluated in a prospective review [26]. Adherence to the guideline, antimicrobial use, and diagnostic accuracy were evaluated at baseline, after implementation of the order set (period 1) and after implementation of audit and feedback (period 2). Adherence to the guideline increased from 44% to 68% to 82% from baseline through phase 2 (p<0.015 for each successive period). This shows the value of both guideline implementation and the addition of prospective audit and feedback [26]. Additionally, prescription of fluoroquinolones (FQs) for uncomplicated cystitis and unnecessary antibiotic days also decreased in each period from baseline.

Antimicrobial cycling, another stewardship strategy, is the sequential use of antimicrobials that ideally do not share a common resistance mechanism. The intention is to reverse or prevent development of AMR within the institution. Antimicrobial cycling is the weakest recommendation of the IDSA antimicrobial guidelines (C-II; not routinely recommended) [6]. Cycling of antibiotics may transiently reduce resistance to the agent not in use, but the eventual reintroduction of an agent will likely lead to recurrence of the original resistance. An example of antimicrobial cycling would be using cefepime as the anti-pseudomonal antibiotic of choice in an institution for three months and then switching to piperacillin/tazobactam for the next three months. The cycle is then repeated, or a third anti-pseudomonal could be added to the cycle. Adherence to the protocol and education are also difficult and time consuming with this strategy as they must be repeated with each new cycle. Furthermore, the widespread use of antibiotics has led to incorporation of antibiotic resistant genes on plasmids within the bacterial cell. Genes that lead to resistance to different antibiotics are commonly found on the same plasmid and plasmids may transfer to other bacteria. This means that one antibiotic may select for all antibiotic resistance mechanisms since they are linked on one plasmid. This is known as co-selection of resistance genes and could reduce the intended efficacy of antimicrobial cycling.

Combination therapy is an important strategy in the management of difficult to treat infections due to MDRO. Combination therapy may be employed in effort to achieve synergy, allow broad spectrum empiric coverage or prevent development of resistance. For example, colistin in combination therapy with rifampicin has been shown to be more effective than colistin alone for the treatment of MDR *Acinetobacter baumannii* [27]. Combination therapy may be appropriate in the empiric antimicrobial selection for treatment of patients with sepsis. Due to the increased mortality associated with inadequate treatment of sepsis, broad-spectrum coverage of Gram-negative organisms, with combination therapy, is appropriate. While de-escalation is a large focus of many ASPs, it is equally important for programs to have strategies in place to ensure that adequate empiric therapy is selected for patients with suspected sepsis or other serious infections. Recently, interest has also increased in the area of combination therapy for the treatment of Gram-positive infections. While combination therapy is not routinely employed for the treatment of Gram-positive infections, it may be used on a case-by-case basis for difficult to treat blood stream, complicated intra-abdominal, and ventilator-acquired pneumonia infections, among others requiring intensive care measures. Goals of combination therapy for Gram-positive infections include enhancing clinical success rates, treating pathogens that may be non-susceptible to standard regimens, and minimizing the risk of emerging resistance. Research in this area is currently limited, with β-lactam antimicrobials, in conjunction with daptomycin, as the most common combination [28, 29].

Dose optimization is another strategy that can be used by ASPs to ensure that maximal antibiotic exposure is obtained by capitalizing on pharmacokinetic and pharmacodynamic principles. The two most common examples are extended interval aminoglycoside dosing and extended infusion β-lactam administration. Aminoglycoside usage is increasing in some institutions due to increasing spread of MDR Gram-negative organisms and increasing resistance to alternative agents such as FQs. Optimization of aminoglycoside dosing by administering a large dose once daily increases the chances of a positive outcome without increasing the risk of nephrotoxicity. Recent work has also emphasized the importance of limiting the duration of aminoglycoside therapy [30]. In a group of critically ill patients receiving treatment for *P. aeruginosa,* the cohort receiving extended infusion piperacillin-tazobactam had improved clinical outcomes (mortality and duration of infection related hospital stay) compared to a similar cohort of patients receiving intermittent infusions of piperacillin-tazobactam [31]. In a similar evaluation, extended infusion of cefepime, for the treatment of *P. aeruginosa* (bacteremia and/or pneumonia), was compared to standard doses of cefepime [32]. Decreased mortality, length of stay and hospital costs were seen in the extended infusion group. While implementation of extended infusion protocols needs extensive planning and education of pharmacy and nursing staff to ensure success, they may be an effective stewardship approach.

De-escalation of antimicrobial therapy is considered the core of antimicrobial stewardship by many clinicians. Due to the increased use of empiric combinations and broad-spectrum therapy for the treatment of critically ill and septic patients, appropriate streamlining of therapy after culture and susceptibility data is known is important to decrease the risk of promoting resistance in pathogens, exposure to adverse effects, and collateral damage such as *C. difficile*-associated diarrhea (CDAD). De-escalation is the stewardship approach that attempts to balance the two competing priorities of appropriate initial therapy and narrowing definitive therapy. Due to the complexities associated with evaluation of individual patients and ensuring appropriateness of de-escalation, dedicated personnel, with appropriate training and time, are necessary to be effective with this stewardship initiative. De-escalation is most often completed as part of an ASP conducting prospective audit and feedback. Recent work has focused on the use of electronic decision support to effectively identify which patients should be evaluated for de-escalation to decrease the time needed to review reports [33]. Data from a community hospital-based ASP focused on appropriate use of eight antimicrobials. Stewardship personnel made recommendations five days per week, including recommendations to discontinue, de-escalate or consult ID physician. Review of the first-year outcomes showed reduced utilization of the targeted antimicrobials, reduced odds of *C. difficile* development and reduced antimicrobial costs. No difference was noted in mortality or readmission rates [34].

Intravenous (IV) to oral (PO) conversion programs are often part of an institution's ASP, and have been in place at many institutions prior to the formal implementation of an ASP. Benefits of these programs include institutional economic benefits and positive clinical outcomes such as reduction in IV antibiotic use and shortened length of hospital stay. Most patients admitted to the hospital with severe infections will be initiated on IV medications since this provides the best likelihood of achieving optimal concentrations at the site of infection for many antibiotics. However, once patients have improved, typically within two to three days, IV medications may not be merited. Broadly, IV to PO programs can be categorized as sequential, switch, and step-down. Conversion of an IV medication to a therapeutically equivalent PO medication is considered sequential. Switch therapy is when an IV medication is converted to a PO medication in the same class. Finally, step-down therapy is a conversion to a PO medication in a different class from the original IV medication or in the same class but with a different spectrum of activity. Medications selected for IV to PO conversion usually have high bioavailability and are well tolerated. Other criteria must be in place for an IV to PO program. Such criteria may include a functioning gastrointestinal tract, improving clinical signs and symptoms of infection, and tolerating other PO medications. IV to PO conversion has been referred to as a type of "low hanging fruit" owing to the relative ease of implementation compared to other stewardship initiatives [35]. A recent review evaluated the trends and impact of IV to PO conversion as a part of ASPs. The majority of studies evaluated showed improvement in cost savings, reduced length of stay, reduced duration of IV therapy and comparable clinical efficacy rates. An increasing involvement of pharmacists in IV to PO conversion programs was also noted [36].

Rapid diagnostic testing, an important tool in the management of infections, is expanding as many instruments have recently been approved by the Food and Drug Administration (FDA) for use in the clinical setting. One important and common use for rapid microbial identification instruments are for identifying bloodstream pathogens. Prompt pathogen identification is critical to ensure antimicrobials are optimized in these patients, as the timely initiation of appropriate antimicrobials is associated with improved outcomes [37, 38].

Currently, there are a number of different commercial tests available for blood samples that can be classified as MALDI-TOF MS, DNA microarray, multiplex PCR, real time PCR, and peptide nucleic acid-fluorescence *in situ* hybridization (PNA-FISH) [39]. Most of the outcome data currently available is with the use of MALDI-TOF MS, and although not all studies show a mortality benefit, time to active therapy or optimal therapy (depending on the outcome measured) was always significantly shorter when using the rapid diagnostic test in combination with active antimicrobial stewardship efforts. In order to determine the exact clinical impact of newer tests, future studies combining rapid diagnostics, in combination with antimicrobial stewardship, are warranted. Rapid diagnostics is also advancing in the area of identification of respiratory pathogens [13]. For the routine evaluation and diagnosis of patients with suspected respiratory infections, we continue to rely on older methods that include microscopy and culture of respiratory tract and blood specimens, as well as, detection of antigens in the urine [40]. A number of multiplex PCR systems have been developed for use on various types of respiratory samples. Panels may include different strains of influenza and atypical bacterial pathogens with therapeutic options that can be initiated upon detection [41]. Within this testing, if viral infections are identified, this can be useful in de-escalation of antimicrobial therapy, implementing infection control isolation precautions, tracking disease outbreaks for epidemiological purposes, and reduction in unnecessary antibiotic use.

Potential Challenges in Antimicrobial Stewardship

Several barriers have been identified for successful implementation of various antimicrobial stewardship strategies. Culture of an institution and availability of resources are important factors to consider. Creating a culture of inclusiveness with subcommittees and face-to-face recommendations may be of benefit in order to reduce potential conflict and foster cohesive interprofessional ASP networks. Additionally, lack of dedicated ASP personnel, physician engagement, and IT systems equipped to track interventions and outcomes also pose a significant barrier [42]. Other barriers in acceptance of stewardship recommendations can include unique patient presentations and/or inconclusive clinical evidence that results in physician prescribing that may deviate from guideline recommendations. One example of this would be the empiric use of daptomycin or linezolid (*versus* vancomycin) as a first choice in a patient with suspected methicillin-resistant *Staphylococcus aureus* (MRSA) infection who is deemed "high risk" for nephrotoxicity. The physician makes the clinical judgment that the patient is "high risk" but may not have an objective value, such as a screening/risk assessment tool. However, the avoidance of a nephrotoxic medication, such as vancomycin, is feasible in a person who is more likely to be at risk. Another barrier to acceptance of stewardship recommendations would be the reluctance to change a patient from an IV to a PO antibiotic even when there is high bioavailability. This is mainly attributed to the "serious infection" the patient originally presented with; although, there is not a clear definition of what constitutes a serious infection. Duration of therapy can also be inconclusive when it comes to discontinuing antibiotics, specifically if it requires a few days for the patient to respond to therapy. An example of this would be a patient with hospital acquired pneumonia as a result of *H. influenzae*. In this case, evidence and guidelines recommend that eight (8) days of antibiotics is equivalent to fifteen (15) days of initial antibiotic selection, except for non-fermenting Gram-negative bacilli [43, 44]. However, when considering patient specific factors, even if the patient has been afebrile for more than 48 hours and appears to be clinically improving, a slow initial response to therapy could prompt a physician to extend treatment beyond the recommended 8 days. Further research is needed to elucidate the potential challenges in antimicrobial stewardship and practical and effective ways to overcome them.

INFECTION PREVENTION AND CONTROL

While not unique to combating AMR, infection prevention and control is critical in helping prevent or stop the spread of infections, in general. Notably, infection control practices and standards differ based on the healthcare setting, region and country. There are various tenants to proper infection prevention and control, including: standard precautions, transmission-based precautions, environmental controls and hand hygiene [24]. Additionally, infection control and prevention strategies can help combat the development of AMR at the patient, community, hospital, national and international levels [24].

Standard Precautions

Standard precautions include strategies such as properly using personal protective equipment as dictated by the setting, type of infection or possible exposure; properly handling, cleaning and disinfecting patient care environments, equipment and devices; following safe injection practices and proper handling and disposal of sharps [43]. Standard precautions serve as a minimum necessary practice, and should be used across all patient care settings.

Transmission-Based Precautions

As indicated by the CDC, transmission-based precautions are the "second-tier" of basic infection control. These should be used, in combination with standard precautions, for patients who are potentially colonized or infected with certain organisms that require additional measures to prevent transmission. Transmission-based precautions include contact, droplet and airborne precautions, as well as, appropriate placement of patients (*e.g.* isolation or negative pressure rooms), source control, use of specialized personal protective equipment, limiting transport of patients to decrease exposure, use of patient-specific and disposable patient-care equipment, proper cleaning and disinfection of patient rooms and immunizing susceptible persons against vaccine-preventable diseases, if exposure has occurred [43].

Hand Hygiene

It is well-known that skin is colonized with normal bacterial flora, and that various anatomical sites differ in number and type of bacteria present. Bacteria may either be transient or resident. While both types of bacteria may result in infection, transient bacteria are usually responsible for the transmission of infections, and are more susceptible to good hand hygiene practices. These bacteria, acquired from patients or inanimate objects in the care environment, can lead to colonization or infection, and can lead to increased morbidity, mortality and healthcare costs [44, 45].

Appropriate hand hygiene can prevent the spread of microbes from patients to healthcare workers and to other patients, and is aimed at limiting the incidence of HAIs. Hand hygiene also refers to personal hygiene practices that can limit the spread of infections at the community and patient level. Hand hygiene is multimodal, including: handwashing with soap (non-antimicrobial or antimicrobial) and water, antiseptic hand washes, antiseptic hand rubs, surgical hand antisepsis, and use of gloves and appropriate skin/nail care. Notably, infections related to spore-forming bacteria (*e.g. Clostridioides difficile, Bacillus anthracis*) are not susceptible to antiseptic hand washes or antiseptic hand-rubs, and healthcare workers should be encouraged to wear gloves and wash their hands with non-antimicrobial or antimicrobial soap when caring for patients infected with these bacteria. In addition to selecting the correct hygiene product, the indications for performing hand hygiene and correct techniques must also be observed [44, 45]. The simple practice of proper hand hygiene using alcohol-based hand sanitizer, when appropriate, or washing hands is a proven way to prevent infection and the spread of infection, including those from resistant bacteria. This alone can limit the development and spread of AMR [24]. According to the World Health Organization (WHO), alcohol-based hand rubs are the gold standard for hand hygiene in healthcare. The selection of alcohol-based hand rubs as the gold standard was based on a number of factors: effectiveness, fast-acting, low likelihood of producing resistance, suitability for resource-limited and remote areas, convenience, accessibility, cost effectiveness and association with fewer skin intolerances than other products. While WHO states that commercially available, alcohol-based hand rubs are acceptable, to foster adoption of the gold standard globally, WHO has identified two formulations that can be locally prepared. Preparation methods are thoroughly described in the WHO Guidelines on Hand Hygiene in Health Care. These were developed with consideration for logistics, economics, safety and cultural and religious factors [45].

Adherence to appropriate hand hygiene is variable and reasons for lack of adherence are multifactorial. Possible strategies to enhance hand hygiene include: ease of access to hand hygiene materials (*e.g.* alcohol-based hand rubs, sinks, soaps, *etc.*), education regarding hand hygiene practices, optimizing workload/avoiding understaffing, and the use of written guidelines and administrative leadership for these practices [44, 45]. Although there is lack of strong scientific evidence to quantify the impact of hand hygiene, there is evidence to support that proper hand antisepsis reduces the transmission and incidence of HAIs and prevents the spread of resistant organisms, including bacteria [44, 45].

Patient, Community & Hospital

At the patient and community level, many techniques are valuable in preventing AMR, and are often overlooked. Use of fastidious aseptic protocol for all patient procedures, breaking the chain of infectivity (*e.g.* covering mouths while coughing, patient isolation, staying home when sick and washing hands), effective diagnosis and treatment of infections, rational antimicrobial use, and patient adherence to antimicrobial regimens are key elements to infection prevention and control [24, 46]. Unfortunately, patient adherence to antimicrobial treatment regimens is approximately 50% worldwide, indicating a need for improvement [25].

Proper microbiology practices, within institutions, are key in fighting AMR. This includes accurate collection and handling of specimens, expeditious reporting, complying with national and international testing standards [24]. Surveillance programs, which collect data on antimicrobial use and resistance patterns, can facilitate the identification and containment of resistance. Additionally, it can aid in the development of antibiograms, guide appropriate antimicrobial selection and inform policy and guideline development [24]. Furthermore, establishing a committee, within healthcare facilities, to oversee all aspects infection prevention and control measures may be warranted [24]. There are other infection prevention and control measures that may be unique to specific healthcare settings. For example, in the CDC's campaign to prevent AMR in healthcare settings, they list measures such as using IV lines and catheters only when necessary, and removing lines and catheters expeditiously [46]. Additional preventative measures to consider based on the setting and patient are the prevention of aspiration, pressure ulcers and other conditions that may lead to infection [46].

National and International

Finally, infection prevention is at the forefront of global action plans to combat AMR since it eliminates infections that require treatment, is cost effective, and can be implemented even in environments where resources are limited [1]. Proper vaccination practices should also be considered as an important infection prevention measure, at all levels. Vaccines can help in several ways: by eliminating the need for antimicrobials, reducing the prevalence of viral infections which are often incorrectly treated with antibiotics, preventing illnesses that can result in secondary bacterial infections that require antibiotic treatment, and by preventing diseases that are untreatable or difficult to treat secondary to AMR [1].

ANTIMICROBIAL USE IN ANIMALS AND AGRICULTURE

In addition to human medicine, antimicrobial agents have been widely utilized in veterinary medicine. Penicillin was introduced in the early 1900s, and was initially used to treat animals with illnesses, as well as, to prevent infection. This made it possible to perform procedures such as caesarian sections in cattle. As time progressed, antimicrobials, such as penicillin, were used in animals for prophylaxis and treatment on infection, and for growth promotion purposes in "food producing animals". Currently, animals in the United States consume more than twice as many medically important antibiotics (Table **2**) as compared to humans [47]. Food producing animals refer to any terrestrial or aquatic animal bred to produce food [48]. For over 50 years, antibiotics have been used to enhance growth and reduce mortality in broilers. The use of growth promoting antibiotics (GPA) has been defined as providing antibiotics, through feed, to healthy animals in low doses for greater than 14 days [49]. This differs from prophylactic or treatment dosing with antibiotics which are typically administered at higher doses in water or feed. Although many countries are making efforts to limit the use of antimicrobials, their continued use for prophylaxis, treatment and growth promotion is pertinent to the discussion of global initiatives to combat AMR. Because of continued use, livestock and other animals have begun to develop resistance to antimicrobial agents. If MRSA is present in farm livestock, farmers and other workers managing these livestock may be at a higher risk of acquiring this resistant bacterium. This resistance also affects typical veterinary practice by challenging the effectiveness of antimicrobials used for infection treatment and prevention.

Unfortunately, resistance to the general public may also be at risk since up to 90% of antimicrobials used in food animals may be excreted unmetabolized in water and animal waste used for fertilization of crops [50]. This mode of distribution of antimicrobials subsequently spreads to the environment and the recipients of plant and meat products for consumption. There are various proposed mechanisms by which humans may be contaminated; however, three main mechanisms include 1) direct contact with livestock or ingestion of bacteria through food or water, 2) human-to-human transmission after initial contact or ingestion from contaminated food or water, 3) horizontal transmission of resistance genes originating from livestock [51]. Certain bacteria that are at a higher risk for transmission from animal producers to human consumers, whether pathogenic or symbiotic, may also lead to AMR. Examples of this is are non-typhoidal *Salmonella* spp. and *Escherichia coli*. Resistance to these commonly encountered bacterial infections may have more severe consequences such as treatment failure, prolonged hospitalization and sustained ailment for the infected human. For example, studies have hypothesized that following FQ use in cattle, the incidence of *Campylobacter jejuni* infection complicated by FQ failure may have risen from contaminated ground beef. In this example, it is predicted that in less than 10 years, the occurrence of FQ failure following *Campylobacter jejuni* infection will amount to approximately 40 cases and at least one death. Additional data shows a profound burden of over 400,000 excess days of illness in the United States each year due to FQ-resistant *Campylobacter* infections because of FQ use in animals, particularly poultry. Although there is still a gap in our understanding and knowledge related to transmission of resistant organisms, it is known that following exposure of humans to resistant organisms from agriculture, further spread from human to human may occur in the general population. Additionally, it is important to consider the potential transmission from human to livestock and possibly back to human and the role that this may play in AMR. Lastly, bacteria may also transfer resistant genes between strains of the same species or between different species. Although this mechanism exists, it is extremely difficult to trace and quantify, and determine if there has been a transfer of the resistant organism, in whole, or of specific genes, alone [51]. Due to this rising issue, WHO released guidelines in 2017 on the use of medically important antimicrobials in food-producing animals. They highlight four main recommendations [48]:

1. An overall reduction in the use of all classes of medically important antimicrobials in food-producing animals.
2. Completely restricted use of all classes of medically important antimicrobials in food-producing animals for growth promotion.
3. Completely restricted use of all classes of medically important antimicrobials in food-producing animals for prevention of infectious diseases that have not yet been clinically diagnosed.
4. A) Antimicrobials classified as critically important (Table **2**) for human

medicine should not be used for control of the dissemination of a clinically diagnosed infectious disease identified within a group of food-producing animals. B) Antimicrobials classified as highest priority critically important for human medicine should not be used for treatment of food-producing animals with a clinically diagnoses infectious disease.

Table 2. Medically Important Antimicrobials.

Critically Important Antimicrobials	Highest Priority *Cephalosporins (3rd, 4th, and 5th generation)* *Glycopeptides* *Macrolides and Ketolides* *Polymyxins* *Quinolones*
	High Priority *Aminoglycosides* *Ansamycins* *Carbapenems and other penems* *Glycylcyclines* *Lipopeptides* *Monobactams* *Oxazolidinones* *Penicillins (natural, aminopenicillins, and antipseudomonal)* *Phosphonic acid derivatives* *Drugs used solely to treat tuberculosis or other mycobacterial diseases*
Highly Important Antimicrobials	*Amdinopenicillins* *Amphenicols* *Cephalosporins (1st and 2nd generation) and cephamycins* *Lincosamides* *Penicillins (anti-staphylococcal)* *Pseudomonic acids* *Riminofenazines* *Steroid antibacterials* *Streptogramins* *Sulfonamides, dihydrofolate reductase inhibitors and combinations* *Sulfones* *Tetracyclines*
Important Antimicrobials	*Aminocyclitols* *Cyclic polypeptides* *Nitrofurantoins* *Nitroimidazoles* *Pleuromutilins*

Modified from: WHO Critically Important Antimicrobials for Human Medicine 5th revision (October 2016) [52]

In addition to these four recommendations, the WHO introduced two "Best Practice Statements" in order to highlight the importance of these points that were not pertinent enough for a formal recommendation. In these statements, they mention that all new classes of antimicrobials, and new combinations of antimicrobials, will be considered critically important for human medicine until otherwise classified by the WHO. Furthermore, any medically important antimicrobials that are not currently being utilized in food production should not be used in future food production, including food-producing animals or plants [48] It is important to note that antimicrobial use varies tremendously among regions of the world, where Spain and Italy use about 300 mg/kg of antibiotics, the United States, Portugal, and Germany use approximately 175 mg/kg and Australia and Sweden use about 25 mg/kg of antibiotics. Additionally, although this is a widespread issue, the animal industry has been working on ways to reduce resistance such as developing animal-only antibiotics and vaccinations, using supplements to boost animal immune health, and adopting the WHO Global Action Plan [47, 53].

Agriculture

Antimicrobials are also widely used for certain crops; although, the extent is estimated to be much lower when compared to livestock. Therefore, placing restrictions on this use is not a major priority. Fungal diseases tend to be more prevalent in crops, especially cereals and grapes, leading to use of antifungals or fungicides. Subsequently, antifungal use in humans is becoming more relevant as medicine evolves and patients with weakened immune systems are living longer. This increased use in humans and the use of fungicides in crops has led to increased problems with resistance overtime. Specifically, azole-based fungicides are widely used, and azole-based therapies are extremely relevant in order to address infections such as *Aspergillus*. Human fungal-resistance to these therapies is likely to worsen over time. Because fungicides are important for world food production, placing a ban on these agents is less likely. However, it may be reasonable to ban all newly developed classes of clinical antifungals and place restrictions on the certain azoles. Lastly, it appears that fungicide use varies widely among global regions. For example, the United States uses about a tenth the amount of fungicide as Europe; however, the reasons for this are unknown [47].

ALTERNATIVES TO ANTIMICROBIALS FOR GROWTH PROMOTION AND TREATMENT

A number of alternative agents have been proposed in order to assist with the reduction of AMR, as well as, the unintended impact of increased infection and decreased animal production in the animal industry. Some of these alternatives include, probiotics and prebiotics, in-feed enzymes, vaccines, and immune modulators [54, 55]. These alternatives may be used for prevention, treatment or growth promotion. The measurement of efficacy for these alternatives varies widely among the literature, and not all products in a category have equal efficacy.

Probiotics and Prebiotics

Probiotics are agents that may be added to the diet in order to improve gastrointestinal balance. The probiotic product may be defined, meaning that the exact composition of the product is described, or undefined. Undefined probiotics typically have better efficacy for disease prevention and treatment which may lead to better performance and growth promotion. Probiotics have been shown to be beneficial as growth promoters in swine, and they may also help to prevent diarrhea and reduce infection-related mortality in this species. Additionally, probiotics have shown some benefits for improving productivity through growth promotion and preventing disease in cattle. Conversely, prebiotics, compounds that when added to the diet are indigestible by animals but broken down by certain micro-organisms in the gut, may promote immune function and have shown some anti-viral activity. Prebiotics have shown benefit in growth promotion in swine, cattle, chickens, and turkeys; however, disease prevention data is variable across these species. Specifically, after prebiotics are administered to pigs, there could be up to an 8% increase in average daily gains. In young cattle who were given liquid feed, not from their mothers, that included the prebiotic galactosyl-lactose, average body gains were significantly higher than in cattle nursed by their mothers. The variability in probiotic and prebiotic products makes it difficult to fully assess their efficacy for growth promotion and disease prevention [54, 55].

In-feed Enzymes

Certain enzymes may be added to animal feed in order to help them digest plant materials. The exact mechanism behind using in-feed enzymes (*e.g.*, xylanses, amylases, lipases and beta-glucanases) as growth promoters is not fully understood; however, they may be reliably used for chicken and turkey. Results for in-feed enzymes in swine and cattle are variable due to enzyme inactivation upon ingestion [55]. In general, swine and poultry have issues with digestion of feed because the ingredients may contain undegradable products, or the animal may not contain sufficient levels of enzyme needed to digest the feed. Enzymes are proteins used to help with chemical reactions, such as digestion, in the body. Enzyme supplementation may help improve long-term health of livestock by allowing more of the nutrients from the feed be digested and accessible. In-feed enzymes may assist with the breakdown of undegradable products that could hinder meat or egg production and may enhance digestive tract health. The type of in-feed enzyme used will depend on the substrate by which it acts upon. For example, amylases act on starches while lipases act on lipids. In livestock, most feed consists of fiber, protein, starches and phytates, so enzymes will be selected for these substrates. Although enzyme use can be beneficial, there are a few factors that may affect their optimal response including: 1) digestive physiology and location of enzyme digestion; 2) duration of time needed in the digestive tract for optimal degradation; 3) pH of the feed, enzymes, and digestive tract; and 4) digestive proteases that threaten the enzyme activity [56]. Despite these factors, in-feed enzymes are well-accepted options to improve digestive performance, increase nutrient uptake, boost weight, increase egg production and promote overall long-term health.

Vaccines

For years vaccines have been used to prevent viral and bacterial diseases in veterinary medicine. Evidence suggests that some vaccines may provide positive outcomes related to growth rates and overall animal performance. However, this use may not be supported by all governing bodies due to questions related to cost-effectiveness and practicality. By using vaccinations for both bacterial and viral infection prevention, there may be fewer infections and a reduced need for antibiotic use in veterinary medicine. As with humans, vaccines are among one of the most promising mechanisms for disease prevention, but challenges such as increased labor cost, reduced immune response caused by stress due to increased handling of the animal, and narrow range of effectiveness for many bacterial or viral strains exist [54, 55].

Immune Modulators

Immune modulators, defined as "the transfer of antibodies to elicit passive immune responses", particularly immunostimulants, may lead to enhanced innate immune functions. This can improve the host's resistance to diseases. These agents stimulate the immune system just as vaccinations do, but they are less dependent on the pathogen causing infection. These characteristics allow them to broaden the range of pathogenic effectiveness. The majority of data with these agents is around disease prevention in chickens, swine, and cattle, and the United States has approved to immune modulators for safe and efficacious use in cattle. While they have been shown to be effective at preventing disease in these species, the efficacy of immunostimulants depends on the animal having a developed and functioning immune system; therefore, younger and severely stressed animals, who are prone to infection, may not benefit. Additionally, the fact that they have a non-linear, dose-effect relationship may pose a challenge for developing consistent dosing regimens [54, 55].

In general, the topic of antibiotic use in livestock is controversial, and several agencies have adopted guidelines in order to regulate and reduce use. Consequently, recent survey statistics suggest that the utilization of GPAs for production purposes has reduced overtime, and many European countries have ceased use of GPAs, altogether. Specifically, one new European legislation bans the use of antibiotic for animals if they are deemed important for human use. It also prohibits the use of any antimicrobial in livestock unless there is a prescription from the veterinarian. The Food and Drug Administration (FDA) has a five-year plan (2019-2023) which is meant to support antimicrobial stewardship in veterinary settings and move towards elimination of "medically important" antimicrobials unless there is oversight by a licensed veterinarian. With an increase in consumer desire for non-GPA raised meats, reduction in producer use, regulations on which antibiotics may be utilized, and inclusion of alternative agents, the issue of agriculturally induced AMR may be a much smaller issue than originally anticipated.

CONCLUSION

The issue of AMR impacts health of the individual patient and the global population. Even more, AMR goes beyond the obvious impact on health. It adversely affects personal and global economic development, food sustainability, and more. One of the most important factors in the development of AMR is inappropriate antimicrobial use. In addition to potential suboptimal treatment of infections at the patient level, inappropriate use also poses a significant threat to global antimicrobial effectiveness. This is a major public and global health concern since there are few antibiotics in the development pipeline. Research and development of new antimicrobials is lacking due to limited profitability. The WHO calls for a revitalization of this market, or infections from MDRO will soon supersede the ability to treat them [1].

It is critical that strategies are employed to prevent development of resistance and ensure that medically important agents maintain effectiveness for as long as possible. To this end, various practices, can aid in this endeavor. Antimicrobial stewardship programs, composed of interdisciplinary teams using a variety of models and strategies, have proved essential, and are a seminal element in supporting appropriate antimicrobial use and preventing development and spread of resistance. Additionally, the foundation of combating infection, including those from MDRO, includes infection prevention and control practices. Without these basic measures, all other strategies are futile. These must be implemented through the entire scope of healthcare (*i.e.* patient, system, global) and carried out with diligence and consistency. Finally, judicious antimicrobial practices in animals and agricultural, and the adoption of alternative practices to spare medically important antimicrobials cannot be ignored. Beyond the impact on AMR, improvements in this arena will help maintain effectiveness of current antimicrobials, sustain new antimicrobial development, promote global health and promote food security [1]. While each strategy has its utility, they cannot be used in partial measures. The adoption of all the initiatives suggested by the WHO and other guiding bodies, in entirety and at a global level, will give the best chance at successfully combating AMR.

CONSENT FOR PUBLICATION

Not applicable.

CONFLICT OF INTEREST

The authors confirm that the contents of this chapter have no conflict of interest.

ACKNOWLEDGEMENTS

Declared none.

REFERENCES

[1] World Health Organization. Global Action Plan on Antimicrobial Resistance. https://apps.who.int/iris/bitstream/handle/10665/193736/9789241509763_eng.pdf?sequence=1

[2] Mauldin PD, Salgado CD, Hansen IS, Durup DT, Bosso JA. Attributable hospital cost and length of stay associated with health care-associated infections caused by antibiotic-resistant gram-negative bacteria. Antimicrob Agents Chemother 2010; 54(1): 109-15.
[http://dx.doi.org/10.1128/AAC.01041-09] [PMID: 19841152]

[3] Maragakis LL, Perencevich EN, Cosgrove SE. Clinical and economic burden of antimicrobial resistance. Expert Rev Anti Infect Ther 2008; 6(5): 751-63.
[http://dx.doi.org/10.1586/14787210.6.5.751] [PMID: 18847410]

[4] Center for Disease Control and Prevention. Antibiotic resistance threats in the United States 2019. https://www.cdc.gov/drugresistance/pdf/threats-report/2019-ar-threats-report-508.pdf

[5] Centers for Disease Control and Prevention, National Center for Emerging and Zoonotic Infectious Diseases. 2018. https://www.cdc.gov/drugresistance/solutions-initiative/stories/ar-global-threat.html

[6] Dellit TH, Owens RC, McGowan JE Jr, *et al.* Infectious diseases society of America; Society for healthcare epidemiology of America. Infectious diseases society of America and the society for healthcare epidemiology of america guidelines for developing an institutional program to enhance antimicrobial stewardship. Clin Infect Dis 2007; 44(2): 159-77.
[http://dx.doi.org/10.1086/510393] [PMID: 17173212]

[7] The White House. Executive order on combating antimicrobial resistance 2014. https://obamawhitehouse.archives.gov/the-press-office/2014/ 09/18/e xecutive-order-combati-g-antibiotic-resistant-bacteria

[8] https://www.cdc.gov/drugresistance/pdf/report-to-the-president-on-combating-antibiotic-resistance.pdf

[9]   The California Antimicrobial Stewardship Program Initiative. 2018. https://www.cdph.ca.gov/ Programs/CHCQ/HAI/Pages/CA_AntimicrobialSteward shipProgramInitiative.aspx

[10]   Veterans Health Administration Directive 1031 – Antimicrobial Stewardship Programs (ASP) In: Affairs DoV. 2014., 2019.

[11]   Pollack LA, Srinivasan A. Core elements of hospital antibiotic stewardship programs from the Centers for Disease Control and Prevention. Clin Infect Dis 2014; 59 (Suppl. 3): S97-S100.
        [http://dx.doi.org/10.1093/cid/ciu542] [PMID: 25261548]

[12]   ASHP statement on the pharmacist's role in antimicrobial stewardship and infection prevention and control. Am J Health Syst Pharm 2010; 67(7): 575-7.
        [http://dx.doi.org/10.2146/sp100001] [PMID: 20237387]

[13]   Cosgrove SE, Hermsen ED, Rybak MJ, File TM Jr, Parker SK, Barlam TF. Society for healthcare epidemiology of America; Infectious diseases society of America; Making-a-difference in infectious diseases; National foundation of infectious diseases; Pediatric infectious diseases society; Society of infectious disease pharmacists. Guidance for the knowledge and skills required for antimicrobial stewardship leaders. Infect Control Hosp Epidemiol 2014; 35(12): 1444-51.
        [http://dx.doi.org/10.1086/678592] [PMID: 25419765]

[14]   Moody J, Cosgrove SE, Olmsted R, *et al.* Antimicrobial stewardship: a collaborative partnership between infection preventionists and healthcare epidemiologists. Infect Control Hosp Epidemiol 2012; 33(4): 328-30.
        [http://dx.doi.org/10.1086/665037] [PMID: 22418626]

[15]   Pogue JM, Potoski BA, Postelnick M, *et al.* Bringing the "power" to Cerner's PowerChart for antimicrobial stewardship. Clin Infect Dis 2014; 59(3): 416-24.
        [http://dx.doi.org/10.1093/cid/ciu271] [PMID: 24748518]

[16]   Kullar R, Goff DA, Schulz LT, Fox BC, Rose WE. The "epic" challenge of optimizing antimicrobial stewardship: the role of electronic medical records and technology. Clin Infect Dis 2013; 57(7): 1005-13.
        [http://dx.doi.org/10.1093/cid/cit318] [PMID: 23667260]

[17]   Forrest GN, Van Schooneveld TC, Kullar R, Schulz LT, Duong P, Postelnick M. Use of electronic health records and clinical decision support systems for antimicrobial stewardship. Clin Infect Dis 2014; 59 (Suppl. 3): S122-33.
        [http://dx.doi.org/10.1093/cid/ciu565] [PMID: 25261539]

[18]   Carling P, Fung T, Killion A, Terrin N, Barza M. Favorable impact of a multidisciplinary antibiotic management program conducted during 7 years. Infect Control Hosp Epidemiol 2003; 24(9): 699-706.
        [http://dx.doi.org/10.1086/502278] [PMID: 14510254]

[19]   Sanders J, Pallotta A, Bauer S, *et al.* Antimicrobial stewardship program to reduce antiretroviral medication errors in hospitalized patients with human immunodeficiency virus infection. Infect Control Hosp Epidemiol 2014; 35(3): 272-7.
        [http://dx.doi.org/10.1086/675287] [PMID: 24521593]

[20]   Benson JM. Incorporating pharmacy student activities into an antimicrobial stewardship program in a long-term acute care hospital. Am J Health Syst Pharm 2014; 71(3): 227-30.
        [http://dx.doi.org/10.2146/ajhp130321] [PMID: 24429017]

[21]   Reed EE, Stevenson KB, West JE, Bauer KA, Goff DA. Impact of formulary restriction with prior authorization by an antimicrobial stewardship program. Virulence 2013; 4(2): 158-62.
        [http://dx.doi.org/10.4161/viru.21657] [PMID: 23154323]

[22]   Liew YX, Lee W, Tay D, *et al.* Prospective audit and feedback in antimicrobial stewardship: is there value in early reviewing within 48 h of antibiotic prescription? Int J Antimicrob Agents 2015; 45(2): 168-73.
        [http://dx.doi.org/10.1016/j.ijantimicag.2014.10.018] [PMID: 25511192]

[23]   Kelley D, Aaronson P, Poon E, McCarter YS, Bato B, Jankowski CA. Evaluation of an antimicrobial stewardship approach to minimize overuse of antibiotics in patients with asymptomatic bacteriuria. Infect Control Hosp Epidemiol 2014; 35(2): 193-5.
        [http://dx.doi.org/10.1086/674848] [PMID: 24442085]

[24]   Uchil RR, Kohli GS, Katekhaye VM, Swami OC. Strategies to combat antimicrobial resistance. J Clin Diagn Res 2014; 8(7): ME01-4.
        [PMID: 25177596]

[25]   The World Medicines Situation 2011: Rational Use of Medicines 2011.

[26]   Hecker MT, Fox CJ, Son AH, *et al.* Effect of a stewardship intervention on adherence to uncomplicated cystitis and pyelonephritis guidelines in an emergency department setting. PLoS One 2014; 9(2): e87899.
        [http://dx.doi.org/10.1371/journal.pone.0087899] [PMID: 24498394]

[27]   Durante-Mangoni E, Signoriello G, Andini R, *et al.* Colistin and rifampicin compared with colistin alone for the treatment of serious infections due to extensively drug-resistant Acinetobacter baumannii: a multicenter, randomized clinical trial. Clin Infect Dis 2013; 57(3): 349-58.
        [http://dx.doi.org/10.1093/cid/cit253] [PMID: 23616495]

[28]   Barber KE, Werth BJ, Rybak MJ. The combination of ceftaroline plus daptomycin allows for therapeutic de-escalation and daptomycin sparing against MRSA. J Antimicrob Chemother 2015; 70(2): 505-9.
        [http://dx.doi.org/10.1093/jac/dku378] [PMID: 25246437]

[29]   Rose WE, Schulz LT, Andes D, *et al.* Addition of ceftaroline to daptomycin after emergence of daptomycin-nonsusceptible *Staphylococcus aureus* during therapy improves antibacterial activity. Antimicrob Agents Chemother 2012; 56(10): 5296-302.
        [http://dx.doi.org/10.1128/AAC.00797-12] [PMID: 22869564]

[30]   Drusano GL, Louie A. Optimization of aminoglycoside therapy. Antimicrob Agents Chemother 2011; 55(6): 2528-31.
        [http://dx.doi.org/10.1128/AAC.01314-10] [PMID: 21402835]

[31]   Lodise TP Jr, Lomaestro B, Drusano GL. Piperacillin-tazobactam for Pseudomonas aeruginosa infection: clinical implications of an extended-infusion dosing strategy. Clin Infect Dis 2007; 44(3): 357-63.
        [http://dx.doi.org/10.1086/510590] [PMID: 17205441]

[32]   Bauer KA, West JE, O'Brien JM, Goff DA. Extended-infusion cefepime reduces mortality in patients with Pseudomonas aeruginosa infections. Antimicrob Agents Chemother 2013; 57(7): 2907-12.
        [http://dx.doi.org/10.1128/AAC.02365-12] [PMID: 23571547]

[33]   Schulz L, Osterby K, Fox B. The use of best practice alerts with the development of an antimicrobial stewardship navigator to promote antibiotic de-escalation in the electronic medical record. Infect Control Hosp Epidemiol 2013; 34(12): 1259-65.
        [http://dx.doi.org/10.1086/673977] [PMID: 24225610]

[34]   Malani AN, Richards PG, Kapila S, Otto MH, Czerwinski J, Singal B. Clinical and economic outcomes from a community hospital's antimicrobial stewardship program. Am J Infect Control 2013; 41(2): 145-8.
        [http://dx.doi.org/10.1016/j.ajic.2012.02.021] [PMID: 22579261]

[35]   Goff DA, Bauer KA, Reed EE, Stevenson KB, Taylor JJ, West JE. Is the "low-hanging fruit" worth picking for antimicrobial stewardship programs? Clin Infect Dis 2012; 55(4): 587-92.
        [http://dx.doi.org/10.1093/cid/cis494] [PMID: 22615329]

[36]   Sallach-Ruma R, Phan C, Sankaranarayanan J. Evaluation of outcomes of intravenous to oral antimicrobial conversion initiatives: a literature review. Expert Rev Clin Pharmacol 2013; 6(6): 703-29.

[http://dx.doi.org/10.1586/17512433.2013.844647] [PMID: 24164616]

[37]   Lodise TP, McKinnon PS, Swiderski L, Rybak MJ. Outcomes analysis of delayed antibiotic treatment for hospital-acquired *Staphylococcus aureus* bacteremia. Clin Infect Dis 2003; 36(11): 1418-23.
[http://dx.doi.org/10.1086/375057] [PMID: 12766837]

[38]   Kang CI, Kim SH, Park WB, *et al*. Bloodstream infections caused by antibiotic-resistant gram-negative bacilli: risk factors for mortality and impact of inappropriate initial antimicrobial therapy on outcome. Antimicrob Agents Chemother 2005; 49(2): 760-6.
[http://dx.doi.org/10.1128/AAC.49.2.760-766.2005] [PMID: 15673761]

[39]   Kothari A, Morgan M, Haake DA. Emerging technologies for rapid identification of bloodstream pathogens. Clin Infect Dis 2014; 59(2): 272-8.
[http://dx.doi.org/10.1093/cid/ciu292] [PMID: 24771332]

[40]   Murdoch DR, Jennings LC, Bhat N, Anderson TP. Emerging advances in rapid diagnostics of respiratory infections. Infect Dis Clin North Am 2010; 24(3): 791-807.
[http://dx.doi.org/10.1016/j.idc.2010.04.006] [PMID: 20674804]

[41]   Babady NE. The FilmArray® respiratory panel: an automated, broadly multiplexed molecular test for the rapid and accurate detection of respiratory pathogens. Expert Rev Mol Diagn 2013; 13(8): 779-88.
[http://dx.doi.org/10.1586/14737159.2013.848794] [PMID: 24151847]

[42]   Pakyz AL, Moczygemba LR, VanderWielen LM, Edmond MB, Stevens MP, Kuzel AJ. Facilitators and barriers to implementing antimicrobial stewardship strategies: Results from a qualitative study. Am J Infect Control 2014; 42(10) (Suppl.): S257-63.
[http://dx.doi.org/10.1016/j.ajic.2014.04.023] [PMID: 25239719]

[43]   Center for Disease Control and Prevention. https://www.cdc.gov/infectioncontrol/index.html

[44]   Boyce JM, Pittet D. Healthcare infection control practices advisory committee. society for healthcare epidemiology of America. association for professionals in infection control. infectious diseases society of America. hand hygiene task force. Guideline for hand hygiene in health-care settings: recommendations of the healthcare infection control practices advisory committee and the HICPAC/SHEA/APIC/IDSA hand hygiene task force. Infect Control Hosp Epidemiol 2002; 23(12) (Suppl.): S3-S40.
[http://dx.doi.org/10.1086/503164] [PMID: 12515399]

[45]   WHO. Guidelines on hand hygiene in health care: first global patient safety challenge clean care is safer care.

[46]   Department of Health and Human Services Centers for Disease Control and Prevention. 2004. https://portal.ct.gov/-/media/Departments-a-d-Agencies/DPH/dph/HAI/PDF/12StepsPrevAntimicrobResistinLTCFpdf.pdf?la=en

[47]   The review on antimicrobial resistance. Antimicrobials in agriculture and the environment: reducing unnecessary use and waste 2015. https://amr-review.org/sites/default/files/Antimicrobials%20in%20agriculture%20and%20the%20environment%20-%20Reducing%20unnecessary%20use%20and%20waste.pdf

[48]   WHO guidelines on use of medically important antimicrobials in food-producing animals. 2017. https://apps.who.int/iris/bitstream/handle/10665/258970/9789241550130-eng.pdf?sequence=1

[49]   Graham JP, Boland JJ, Silbergeld E. Growth promoting antibiotics in food animal production: an economic analysis. Public Health Rep 2007; 122(1): 79-87.
[http://dx.doi.org/10.1177/003335490712200111] [PMID: 17236612]

[50]   Marshall BM, Levy SB. Food animals and antimicrobials: impacts on human health. Clin Microbiol Rev 2011; 24(4): 718-33.
[http://dx.doi.org/10.1128/CMR.00002-11] [PMID: 21976606]

[51]   Chang Q, Wang W, Regev-Yochay G, Lipsitch M, Hanage WP. Antibiotics in agriculture and the risk to human health: how worried should we be? Evol Appl 2015; 8(3): 240-7.

[http://dx.doi.org/10.1111/eva.12185] [PMID: 25861382]

[52] https://apps.who.int/iris/bitstream/handle/10665/312266/9789241515528-eng.pdf?ua=1

[53] Health for animals: global animal health association five ways the animal health industry is tackling AMR https://healthf oranimals.org/resources-and-events/newsletter-repository/6-respons-ble-antibiotic-use.html?q=20 Available from

[54] Cheng G, Hao H, Xie S, *et al.* Antibiotic alternatives: the substitution of antibiotics in animal husbandry? Front Microbiol 2014; 5: 217.
[http://dx.doi.org/10.3389/fmicb.2014.00217] [PMID: 24860564]

[55] Alternatives to Antibiotics in Animal Agriculture. Vaccines, probiotics, immune modulators, and more can help maintain healthy herds and reduce the need for antibiotics 2017. https://www.pewtrusts.org/en/research-an--analysis/reports/2017/07/alternatives-to-antibiotics-in-animal-agriculture

[56] Ojha B, Singh P, Shrivastava B. Enzymes in the animal feed industry enzymes in food biotechnology. Elsevier 2019.

CHAPTER 12

Antimicrobials Dosing Strategies in Patients Receiving Renal Replacement Therapy and Extracorporeal Membrane Oxygenation

Wasim S. El Nekidy[1,*], **Janise Philllips**[2] and **Nizar Attallah**[3]

[1] *Department of Pharmacy Services, Cleveland Clinic Abu Dhabi, Abu Dhabi, UAE*

[2] *Department of Pharmacy Services, Houston Methodist Willowbrook, Houston, Texas, USA*

[3] *Department of Nephrology, Cleveland Clinic Abu Dhabi, Abu Dhabi, UAE*

Abstract: Antimicrobial dosing in patients with acute kidney injury requiring renal replacement therapies is challenging. Generally, renal replacement therapy is either diffusive or convective. The most commonly used modalities are: Intermittent Hemodialysis (IHD), Continuous Renal Replacement Therapy - CRRT (continuous venovenous hemofiltration (CVVH), continuous venovenous hemodialysis (CVVHD), and continuous venovenous hemodiafiltration (CVVHDF)), Prolonged Intermittent Renal Replacement Therapies (PIRRT), and Peritoneal Dialysis (PD). Several factors affect the transport of the drugs in these dialysis modalities, such as; the drug's molecular weight, membrane properties (high-flux or low-flux), protein binding, blood flow rate, and dialysate flow rate, and dialyzer surface area. The Food and Drug Administration (FDA) does not mandate manufacturers to provide dosing in different renal replacement therapy modalities, which overwhelmingly complicate the dosing strategies of antimicrobials in this population. Furthermore, different CRRT modalities complicate the dosing with variable prescriptions in which the blood flow rate, dialysate flow rate, and effluent flow rate might significantly differ based on patients' needs. Additionally, extrapolation of pharmacokinetics (PK) from normal patient population and extending it to patients utilizing RRT is a questionable practice. In addition, the situation gets more complicated when those patients require extracorporeal membrane oxygenation (ECMO). Predicting the plasma concentrations of drugs during ECMO is difficult because many factors simultaneously impact the PK and because inconsistent results have been obtained in PK studies and the significant heterogeneity of data including medical and surgical patients or patients under venovenous and venoarterial ECMO in variable proportion. In conclusion, dosing of antimicrobials in patients receiving RRT or ECMO would require comprehensive understanding of the antimicrobials' PK/PD as well as thorough understanding of the RRT and ECMO techniques and their effects on PK/PD.

* **Corresponding author Wasim S. El Nekidy:** Department of Pharmacy Services, Cleveland Clinic Abu Dhabi, Abu Dhabi, UAE; Tel: +971 2 6590200, Ext: 47969; Fax: +971 2 4108223; E-mail: elneiw@clevelandclinicabudhabi.ae

Islam M. Ghazi & Michael J. Cawley (Eds.)

ACUTE KIDNEY INJURY AND RENAL REPLACEMENT THERAPY

Acute kidney injury (AKI) is denoted by an abrupt decline in glomerular filtration rate (GFR) sufficient to decrease the elimination of nitrogenous waste products and other uremic toxins [1, 2]. This has traditionally been referred to as *acute kidney injury (AKI).* Standardized definitions of AKI have been developed (Table 1) [2]. Staging criteria have been developed based on the magnitude of the rise in serum creatinine and changes in the volume of urine output over 1 week [2]. Although AKI is defined by reduced GFR, the underlying cause of renal impairment is most frequently tubular and vascular factors. AKI can be caused by a broad range of etiologies, and the differential diagnosis must be considered in a systematic fashion. The traditional paradigm divides AKI into prerenal, renal, and postrenal causes [2]. Prerenal causes are usually related to hypovolemia or a decreased effective arterial volume. Postrenal kidney failure is usually due to obstruction. Intrinsic renal causes of AKI should be considered under different anatomic components of the kidney (vascular supply, glomerular, tubular, and interstitial disease) [2]. Major extrarenal artery or venous occlusion must be considered in the differential diagnosis.

Among outpatients, prerenal causes commonly contribute to AKI. On the other hand, in the inpatient's settings, prerenal azotemia and acute tubular necrosis (ATN) account for the majority of AKI cases, often in the setting of AKI superimposed on chronic kidney disease (CKD) [2]. Prerenal AKI is usually related to decreased perfusion to the kidneys, mainly related to hypovolemia, decreased cardiac output, or third spacing. It is usually reversible once the etiology is reversed [2]. ATN normally happens due to trauma, vascular and cardiac surgery, severe burns, pancreatitis, sepsis, and chronic liver disease. In the intensive care unit, two-thirds of cases of AKI are due to the combination of impaired renal perfusion, sepsis, and nephrotoxic agents [2]. The typical course of uncomplicated ATN is recovery over 2 to 3 weeks period; however, superimposed renal insults or multiple comorbidities often alter this pattern.

Development of AKI (especially when it is severe and causing dialysis dependence) increases the risk of development of CKD and mortality. Lo and colleagues showed that dialysis-requiring AKI was independently associated with a 28-fold increase in the risk of developing stage 4 or worse CKD (adjusted HR 28.1) (95% CI 21.1-37.6) [3]. Similarly, Bucolic and fellows showed that patients who recovered from AKI in the hospital are still at increased risk of death over the following 6 years when compared with patients who were hospitalized during the same period and did not develop AKI [4].

Several drugs can affect the kidney at multiple levels and cause AKI. Medications affecting the renin-angiotensin-aldosterone system like angiotensin-converting enzyme inhibitors and angiotensin receptor blockers can affect renal hemodynamics and cause prerenal AKI [1, 2]. Non-steroidal anti-inflammatory drugs (NSAIDs), whether they are non-selective or COX- 2 specific commonly cause AKI in the community because of the large amounts of these drugs either prescribed or purchased over the counter [1, 2]. NSAIDs-related AKI is most often due to a hemodynamically mediated reduction in GFR that occurs in patients who are particularly dependent on vasodilatory prostaglandins to maintain renal perfusion. These include elderly patients with atherosclerotic disease, volume-depleted patients, and those in sodium-avid states such as cirrhosis, nephrotic syndrome, and congestive heart failure. This type of AKI is usually reversible on discontinuation of the offending drug and rarely occurs in otherwise healthy individuals. Less frequently, NSAIDs induce ATN or even more rarely papillary necrosis. NSAIDs also may cause acute interstitial nephritis, often with significant proteinuria [2]. Very rarely, they can contribute to glomerular diseases like membranous nephropathy. Calcineurin inhibitors can also cause afferent arteriolar vasoconstriction (prerenal AKI) and also thrombotic microangiopathy (TMA) [2]. Other drugs like Gemcitabine, Vascular endothelial growth factor (VEGF) inhibitors, and Mitomycin C can also cause TMA. Hydralazine and Propylthiouracil can cause rapidly progressive glomerulonephritis. Amphotericin, Aminoglycosides, Foscarnet, Tenofovir, Cisplatin, and Ifosfamide can cause acute tubular necrosis [2, 5 - 8]. Acyclovir, Atazanavir, Ethylene glycol and Methotrexate can cause crystal formation and intra-tubular obstruction [2, 9]. Multiple antimicrobials and other drugs, such as (penicillins, cephalosporins, rifampicin, sulfamethoxazole, ciprofloxacin), Allopurinol, Cimetidine and Proton pump inhibitors can cause acute interstitial nephritis. A lot of those effects are reversible (partially or completely) once the drug is stopped.

Biomarkers to diagnose AKI early are still not well developed. The most commonly used marker is serum creatinine. Creatinine is filtered by the glomerular basement membrane, but it is also secreted in the proximal tubules. It has to be adjusted to sex, race, age, and muscle mass. Unfortunately, it rises late after AKI and sometimes may take 24 hours before it rises. Cystatin C, a cysteine protease inhibitor, is secreted by all nucleated cells and filtered through the kidney with minimal metabolism in the tubules. It may be a better marker of kidney function as compared to serum creatinine but still rises a little later after AKI. Other molecules like urinary neutrophil gelatinase-associated lipocalin (NGAL) and kidney injury molecule-1 (KIM-1) can differentiate **AKI from urinary tract infection (UTI)** and CKD but only in small studies especially when the timing of the injury is known [10]. It might be better to combine some of those markers like

NGAL, KIM-1, and serum creatinine to be able to diagnose AKI early and be able to intervene in a timely fashion.

Therapy relies on early diagnosis and volume resuscitation to maintain a euvolemic state. All nephrotoxic agents need to be stopped, and in the case of sepsis-induced AKI, source control and early antibiotics administration play a very important role [2]. In severe cases of ATN and cortical necrosis, uremic toxins accumulate, and the patient may develop hypervolemia, hyperkalemia or severe acidosis that are resistant to medical therapy. Also, a mental status change may occur. In those cases, some form of dialysis might be needed to help control electrolyte disturbances, improve volume status, and reverse some of the AKI complications [11].

In general, renal replacement therapy, that is needed to manage complications of AKI, is either diffusive (which relies on concentration gradient across the membrane for solutes to move) or convective (which relies on pressure gradient across the membrane and that makes fluid moves across the membrane and drag solutes with it through large membrane pore sizes) [11]. Regular dialysis (mainly hemodialysis which is mainly diffusive) or continuous renal replacement therapy (CRRT) (can be diffusive or convective or a combination of both) could be performed [11]. The choice mainly depends on the center's experience, stability of the patient, and availability of different machines. There are different methods to perform CRRT. Continuous venovenous hemodialysis (CVVHD – urea clearance is 30 mL/min) and slow low efficiency dialysis (SLED – urea clearance is 70-80 mL/min) are mainly diffusive [11 - 13]. Continuous venovenous hemofiltration (CVVH) is mainly convective (urea clearance is 17 mL/min). Continuous venovenous hemodiafiltration (CVVHDF) combines both diffusion and convection (urea clearance is 30 mL/min) [11 - 14].

Intermittent hemodialysis (IHD) is the most commonly used dialysis modality worldwide. This modality relies on diffusion based on the concentration gradient between blood and dialysate. Several factors affect the transport of the drugs in this modality such as; drug molecular weight, membrane properties (high-flux or low-flux), protein binding, blood flow rate, and dialysate flow rate, and dialyzer surface area [15]. For example, drugs with molecular weight > 500 Da such as vancomycin (1500 Da) will not be freely removed by low-flux dialysis membranes as compared with high-flux dialysis membrane, which could remove drugs with molecular weights up to 12,000 Da. A common practice in dialysis units is to administer antibiotics in the last hour of dialysis. However, these antibiotics doses need to be higher than the regularly administered after the complete end of dialysis, to compensate for the portion removed by dialysis.

Peritoneal dialysis (PD) is another ambulatory care dialysis modality. In this modality, the patients use their peritoneal membrane as the dialysis membrane where they instil approximately 2 L of dialysate solution into their peritoneal cavity, leave it to dwell and they repeat this process 4 to 5 times daily. There are two main PD modalities, continuous ambulatory peritoneal dialysis (CAPD) and automated peritoneal dialysis (APD). Antibiotics can be used in the dialysis solution and left to dwell during the PD process.

The three CRRT modalities do not provide any tubular secretion and /or reabsorption found in patients with normal kidney function (*e.g.* Beta-lactams are actively secreted in the proximal tubules through an active transport system). The main advantages of CRRT *vs.* IHD is better hemodynamic stability because of the gradual fluid and toxin removal. This method can lead to less ischemia in different organs. However, there was no mortality benefit once the patients are hemodynamically stable. Continuous renal replacement therapy is usually employed to help hemodynamically unstable patients with acute kidney injury (AKI) to receive renal replacement therapy while maintaining over 24 hours daily. The Food and Drug Administration (FDA) does not mandate manufacturers to provide dosing in different renal replacement therapy modalities which overwhelmingly complicate the dosing strategies of antimicrobials in this population. Further, the different CRRT modalities (CVVH, CVVHD, and CVVHDF) complicate the dosing with variable prescriptions in which the blood flow rate, dialysate flow rate, and effluent flow rate might significantly differ depending on patients' needs. Scarce published data in this population led several researchers to develop dosing equations based on the pharmacokinetics of drugs. However, these equations led to wide variability in drug dosing and its implementation is questionable secondary to that [16, 17].

Hemofiltration (CVVH) can remove drugs *via* convection, which is usually independent on molecular size and can remove substantially large drugs such as vancomycin (1500 Da). Replacement fluids could be added before the filter (predilution) or after the filter (post dilution) or mixed. The choice for pre or post-dilution is dependent on the use of anticoagulation. For instance, patients who experience filter clotting and cannot use anticoagulation, will usually be prescribed pre-filter fluid replacement. The pre-filter replacement, will dilute the plasma. This will make the expected drug removal lower than post-filter fluid replacement (given all other variables are constant). Hemodialysis removes drugs *via* a diffusion process from high concentration to low concentration. Several factors affect the equilibrium across the filtration membrane as listed earlier in the text. In CVVHD the dialysate flow rate is lower than the blood flow rate which makes the dialysate flow rate the rate limiting step of drug and toxin removal. Multiple experts recommend using the dialysate flow rate in lieu of the glomerular flow rate. Hemodiafiltration is a hybrid technique combining both convection and diffusion to eliminate toxins and drugs. When combining both removal techniques together, the net result of solute and/or drug removal is less than the sum of both because they interact and reduce the efficiency of each other [15 - 17]. Prolonged Intermittent Renal Replacement Therapies (PIRRT) such as Slow Low-Efficiency Daily Dialysis (SLEDD) combine both IHD and CRRT features. This method would be performed on a daily basis at a lower blood pump speed and low dialysate flow rate and will last for 6 to 12 hours [15].

Table 1. Stages of acute kidney injury according to the Kidney Disease Improving Global Outcomes (KDIGO) working group [2].

Stage	Serum Creatinine	Urine Output
1	Increase in serum creatinine by 1.5–1.9 times baseline OR Increase ≥ 0.3 mg/dl (≥ 26.5 μmol/l)	< 0.5 mL/kg/h for 6–12 hours
2	Increase of serum creatinine by 2 –2.9 times baseline	< 0.5 mL/kg/h for ≥12 hours
3	Increase of serum creatinine 3 times baseline OR Increase in serum creatinine to ≥ 4.0 mg/dl (≥ 353.6 μmol/L) OR Initiation of renal replacement therapy OR In patients younger than 18 years, decrease in eGFR to < 35 ml/min per 1.73 m^2	< 0.3 mL/kg/h for ≥ 24 hours OR Anuria for ≥12 hours

DOSING CONSIDERATIONS IN PATIENTS UTILIZING RRT

The current dosing recommendations of antimicrobials in patients on RRT have wider variability and mostly based on assumptions and weight-based calculations while keeping the effluent rates constant, ignoring wide variability in CRRT prescriptions (blood flow rate, dialysate flow rate, replacement fluids rate, and effluent flow rate). There is no sufficient data on pharmacokinetics modelling in this population. The best model for drug dosing, should be based on therapeutic drug monitoring in each individual [16].

Pharmacokinetics of each drug should be taken into consideration when trying to dose it in patients on RRT. For instance, patients with AKI who are critically ill patients in septic shock, the volume of distribution (Vd) is increased secondary to extensive fluids resuscitation. In addition, in mechanically ventilated patients, the Vd of trimethoprim and sulfamethoxazole are 1.6 L/kg and 0.5 L/kg as compared to 1.4 L/kg and 0.4 L/kg in non-ventilated patients respectively. Typically, Vd affects the loading doses of antimicrobials while the clearance affects the maintenance dose. The clearance in RRT is dependent on the drug dose, CRRT mode, sieving or saturation coefficient of the drug. The sieving coefficient and saturation coefficient are dependent on the plasma protein binding, which could be affected by AKI status [18, 19].

Patients with chronic renal disease (CKD), may have nausea, vomiting, diabetic gastroparesis, and intestinal edema. These factors decrease oral drugs' absorption. The use of alkalinizing agents such as sodium bicarbonate tablets in this population may also decrease the absorption of drugs, which require acidic medium such as some azoles antifungals. Moreover, the use of phosphate binders will chelate fluoroquinolones and tetracyclines, reducing their systemic effects. Finally, acidosis paired with reduced plasma protein, may lead to increase in free drug levels in the blood [17].

The Pharmacokinetic / Pharmacodynamic Relationships (PK/PD) must be taken in consideration while dosing antimicrobials in patients utilizing RRT. The time dependant killing is dependent on free drug concentration to stay above the Minimum Inhibitory Concentration (MIC) for most of the dosing interval (*e.g.* beta lactams fT/MIC between 40% and 100% of dosing interval), however, such duration is not well clearly defined or studied in critically ill patients on renal replacement therapy. The current evidence suggests maintaining the free drug concentration above the MIC for the whole dosing interval which is associated with better mortality data. Continuous drug infusion or extended infusion could help to maximize the time above MIC; however, this practice is not well studied in patients utilizing RRT. The compromised kidney function in critically ill population acts as a prolonged infusion in this population by default. For drugs that exhibit concentration dependent killing, Cmax/MIC is the main predictor of outcomes (*e.g.* aminoglycosides). In other drugs, the 24 hours area under the curve AUC:MIC ratio (*e.g.* fluoroquinolones) is more important. In those models of drugs, keeping the same doses and extending the intervals is recommended [15, 18].

Inappropriate dosing of antibiotics in patients with patients with CKD-5D, can result in either overdosing and toxicity or under dosing and therapy failure. The main toxicity is neurologic such as visual and auditory hallucinations, myoclonus, and seizures. Those side effects were mainly reported with beta-lactams, acyclovir, and fluoroquinolones. Those side effects are usually reversible upon discontinuation of the offending agent. Sulfamethoxazole was found to stimulate insulin secretion and can displace oral hypoglycemic agents from their protein binding sites leading to hypoglycemia. Penicillins can exacerbate platelet dysfunction and augment the anticoagulants actions. Fluoroquinolones overdose can cause spontaneous Achilles tendon rupture. Tetracyclines should be avoided in patients with kidney failure since they can cause hepatotoxicity [15, 20].

The initial dosing of antibacterial agents relies on the volume of distribution. This important criterion should be considered while selecting initial dosing of antimicrobials. For example, several antibacterial agents have shown to exhibit larger Vd in critically ill patients such as ciprofloxacin, meropenem, ceftazidime, and aminoglycosides. Drugs with a large volume of distribution will exhibit less elimination because of their wide distribution all over the body. Maintenance doses are determined by antibacterial clearance through the RRT modality. As a result, maintenance doses of each antimicrobial should be adjusted according to the removal of the used RRT modality. Residual kidney function should be considered as well while dosing antimicrobials [15, 18, 20, 21].

Several publications and review articles aimed to address the drug dosing in patients in different RRT modalities, especially the CRRT ones (Table **2**) [15 - 29]. Multiple variables must be considered while dosing antimicrobials in patients on CRRT. The dosing in separate studies might widely vary because of the different CRRT prescriptions (fluid removal rate, blood flow rate, dialysate flow rate, ...*etc*). In addition, several older data were driven from CRRT where arteriovenous hemofiltration modalities were used, which is no longer available. Previously published data suggested to use the average daily effluent rate and substitute it for the estimated glomerular filtration rate [20, 21].

Table 2. Dosing recommendations of antimicrobials utilizing different renal replacement therapy modalities [15 - 29].

Drug	CVVH	CVVHD	CVVHDF	IHD	PIRRT
Acyclovir	5–10 mg/kg q24h	5–10 mg/kg q12–24h	5–10 mg/kg q12–24h	2.5–5 mg/kg q24h	
Amikacin	LD: 10-15 mg/kg MD: 7.5 mg/kg q24–48h	LD: 10 mg/kg MD: 7.5 mg/kg q24–48h	LD: 10-15 mg/kg MD: 7.5 mg/kg q24–48h	5–7.5 mg/kg q48–72hg (post dialysis)	
Amoxicillin	1.0 g q12h	1.0 g q12h	1.0 g q12h	500 mg Q24h after dialysis	
Amphotericin B deoxycholate	0.5–1 mg/kg q24h	0.5–1 mg/kg q24h	0.5–1 mg/kg q24h	0.5–1 mg/kg q24h	
Amphotericin B Lipid complex (Liposomal)	3–5 mg/kg q24h	3–5 mg/kg q24h	3–5 mg/kg q24h	3–5 mg/kg q24h	
Ampicillin	1–2 g q8–12h	1–2 g q8h	1–2 g q6–8h	1–2 g q12–24h	

(Table 2) cont.....

Drug	CVVH	CVVHD	CVVHDF	IHD	PIRRT
Ampicillin/Sulbactam	1.5–3 g q8–12h	1.5–3 g q8h	1.5–3 g q8h	1.5–3 g q12–24h	3 g (2/1 g) (single dose) q24h
Azithromycin	250–500 mg q24h	250–500 mg q24h	250–500 mg q24h	250–500 mg q24h	
Aztreonam	1–2 g q 8-12h	1 -2 g q8 -12 h	1 -2 g q8 -12 h	500 mg q12h	
Caspofungin	70 mg then 50 mg q24h	70 mg then 50 mg q24h	70 mg then 50 mg q24h	70 mg then 50 mg q24h	
Cefazolin	1–2 g q12h	1 -2 g q8 to 12h	1 -2 g q8 to 12h	1 g daily or 2 g post dialysis (TIW)	
Cefepime	1–2 g q12h	1 to 2 g q8 to 12 h	1 to 2 g q8 to 12 h	500–1000 mg q24h or 1 to 2 g post dialysis (TIW)	1 g q 6 h
Cefotaxime	1–2 g q8–12h	1–2 g q8h	1–2 g q 8h	1–2 g q24 h	
Ceftazidime	1 g q 8-12 h	1 g q8h or 2 g q12h	1 g q8h or 2 g q12h	500–1000 mg q24h or 2 g post dialysis (TIW)	2 g q 12 h
Ceftriaxone	1–2 g q12–24h	1–2 g q12–24h	1–2 g q12–24h	1–2 g q24h	
Cefuroxime	750 to 1500 mg q24h	750 to 1500mg q12h	750 to 1500 mg q12h	(0.75–1.5 g q24h) post dialysis	
Cephalexin	0.5 g q12h	0.5 g q12h	0.5 g q12h	(250–500 mg q12h) post dialysis	
Ciprofloxacin	200–400 mg q8–12h	600–900 mg q8h	600–900 mg q8h	600–900 mg q8h	
Daptomycin	4–6 mg/kg q48h	4–6 mg/kg q24-48h	4–6 mg/kg q24 to 48h	4–6 mg/kg q48–72h post dialysis (TIW) HD)	6mg/kg q8h
Ertapenem	1 g 24H	1 g 24H	1 g 24H	500 mg daily	1 g q24h
Ethambutol	10-15 mg/kg q24-48 h	10-15 mg/kg q24-48 h	10-15 mg/kg q24-48 h		
Fluconazole	200–400 mg q24h	400–800 mg q24h	400 - 800 mg q24h	200–400 mg q48–72h or 100–200 mg q24h	

(Table 2) cont.....

Drug	CVVH	CVVHD	CVVHDF	IHD	PIRRT
Flucytosine	37.5 mg/kg q12h	37.5 mg/kg q12h	37.5 mg/kg q12h		
Ganciclovir (CMV infection)	I: 2.5 mg/kg q24h M: 1.25 mg/kg q24h	I: 2.5 mg/kg q12h M: 2.5 - 5mg/kg q24h to 48h	I: 2.5 mg/kg q12h M: 2.5 - 5mg/kg q24h to 48h	I: 1.25 mg/kg q48–72h M: 0.625 mg/kg q48–72h	
Gentamicin	1 to 3 mg/kg q24h (depending on infection) re-dose once serum conc < 2 mg/L	2.0 mg/kg q24h	2.0 mg/kg q24h	2–3 mg/kg load x 1,then 1 to 1.5 mg/kg post dialysis (TIW)	3-7mg/kg before SLEDD or 0.6mg/kg post dialysis
Imipenem-Cilastatin	0.5 g 6–8H	0.5 g 6–8H	0.5 g 6–8H	250–500 mg q12h	750 to 1000 mg q6 y to 8h
Isoniazid	300 mg q24h	300 mg q24h	300 mg q24h		
Itraconazole	100-200 mg q12 to 24h	100-200 mg q12 to 24h	100-200 mg q12 to 24h		
Levofloxacin	250–500 mg q24h	250–500 mg q24h	250–750 mg q24h	250–500 mg q48h	250 or 500mg q 12h
Linezolid	600 mg q12h	600 mg q12h	600 mg q12h	600 mg q12h	0.6 g 12H
Meropenem	0.5 to 1 g q8 to 12h	0.5 to 1 g q8 to 12h	0.5 to 1 g q8 to 12h	250–500 mg q24h post dialysis	1 g every 12 h
Metronidazole	500 mg q6–12h	500 mg q6–12h	500 mg q6–12h	500 mg q8–12h	
Moxifloxacin	400 mg q24h	400 mg q24h	400 mg q24h	400 mg q24h	400mg q24h
Nafcillin	2 g q4–6h	2 g q4–6h	2 g q4–6h	2 g q4–6h	
Penicillin G	LD: 4 MU 2 MU q4–6h	2–3 MU q4–6h	2–4 MU q4–6h	LD: 4 MU then 25–50% normal dose q4–6h or 50–100% normal dose q8–12h	
Piperacillin/tazobactam	3.375 - 4.5 g q6–8h	3.375 - 4.5 g q6–8h	3.375 - 4.5 g q6–8h	2.25 g q8–12h	4.5 g q 6 to 8 h
Rifampin	300–600 mg q12–24h	300–600 mg q12–24h	300–600 mg q12–24h	300–600 mg q12–24h	

(Table 2) cont.....

Drug	CVVH	CVVHD	CVVHDF	IHD	PIRRT
Ticarcillin-Clavulanate	2 g q6–8h	3.1 g q6–8h	3.1 g q 8-6h	2 g q12h	
Tigecycline	100 mg then 50 mg q12h	100 mg then 50 mg q12h	100 mg then 50 mg q12h	100 mg then 50 mg q12h	
Tobramycin	LD: 1.5 to 2.5 mg/kg q24h	LD: 2.0 mg/kg q24h	LD: 2.0 mg/kg q24h	LD: 1–1.7 mg/kg post dialysis	
Trimethoprim (TMP) and sulfamethoxazole (SMX)	2.5–7.5 mg/kg (TMP) q12h	2.5–7.5 mg/kg (TMP) q12h	2.5–7.5 mg/kg (TMP) q12h	2.5–10 mg/kg (TMP) q24h or 5–20 mg/kg 3 times/wk post dialysis	
Vancomycin	LD: 15–25 mg/kg 10–15 mg/kg q24–48h	10–15 mg/kg q24h	7.5–10 mg/kg q12h	LD 15–25 mg/kg MD: 5–10 mg/kg after HD	LD: 20 mg/kg MD: 15 mg/kg daily (after PIRRT)
Voriconazole Oral)	LD: 400 mg q12h x 2 MD: 200 mg q12h	LD: 400 mg q12h x 2 MD: 200 mg q12h	LD: 400 mg q12h x 2 MD: 200 mg q12h	200 mg q12h	

h=hour, I=induction, LD=Loading dose, MD=Maintenance dose, M=Maintenance, MU= million units, TIW=three times weekly (References 15 to 29).

Cephalosporins are significantly removed by RRT and approximately 50% of ceftazidime and cefepime are removed. Published data suggest doses of 4 to 8 g (ceftazidime) and 2 to 6 g (cefepime) daily in patients utilizing CRRT. These suggested doses are based on the MICs of 8 mg/L. Clinical monitoring during cephalosporins administration is the commonly used technique, but therapeutic drug monitoring *via* serum concentration is not commonly available. Penicillins are highly bound to protein (flucloxacillin 90% and piperacillin 30%). As a result, only around 10% of flucloxacillin is removed by CRRT, while up to 42% of piperacillin would be removed. Piperacillin dosing in CRRT range from 8/1 g up to 16/2 g daily. The high dose of 16 /2 g would exceed the MIC of 16 mg/L but will lead to accumulation of tazobactam. Ampicillin is 87% removed by PIRRT. Carbapenems removal depends on the CRRT prescription. Meropenem can be removed up to 50% with high CRRT and PIRRT doses and it is recommended to give 2 to 3 g daily to maintain free drug concentration above the MIC in patients utilizing CRRT. Similarly, imipenem and doripenem are reported to be removed between 20 and 30%. Ertapenem is also significantly removed by different RRT modalities. Fluoroquinolones (levofloxacin and ciprofloxacin) are removed by

CRRT and PIRRT up to 40% and 20% respectively [20 - 23]. Glycopeptides such as vancomycin volume of distribution is reported to be between 0.7 to 0.9 mg/L in patients on RRT. Vancomycin removal is affected by effluent flow rate (CVVH) and could be significantly removed when this rate increases. Daptomycin was found to be removed up to 30% in CVVHD. A dose of 4 to 6 mg/kg/day is advocated for in patients utilizing CRRT. Linezolid (Oxazolidinones) is reported to be removed between 8 and 40% depending on the modality. Colistin has limited data in patients on RRT. Loading doses are still needed in this population [20, 21].

ANTIMICROBIAL DOSING CONSIDERATIONS IN ADULTS RECEIVING EXTRACORPOREAL MEMBRANE OXYGENATION

Extracorporeal membrane oxygenation (ECMO) is a mechanical circulatory support device used for patients with severe respiratory and/or cardiac failure refractory to standard therapies. ECMO provides temporary life support until organ function recovers, or more commonly as a bridge to transplant or a long-term cardiac assist device [30]. Venovenous ECMO (VV ECMO) supports the lung by extracting blood from a vein, oxygenating the blood through an oxygenator, and returning the blood back into the large central veins or right atrium [31]. VV ECMO is indicated in patients with acute respiratory failure, most commonly due to acute respiratory distress syndrome, pneumonia, trauma, or primary graft failure post-lung transplantation. Venoarterial ECMO (VA ECMO) supports both the heart and lung by returning the blood back into the aorta after oxygenation [31]. VA ECMO is indicated for patients with cardiogenic shock, most commonly due to open heart surgery, post-heart transplant, acute coronary syndromes, cardiomyopathy, or myocarditis.

Historically, ECMO was used primarily in neonates, however, its use in critically ill adults worldwide has increased exponentially since the H1N1 influenza pandemic in 2009 [32 - 34]. Additionally, the Conventional Ventilator or ECMO for Severe Adult Respiratory Failure (CESAR) trial showed improved survival rates without severe disability with ECMO [32, 33]. Although survival rates are increasing, more than 60% of adult patients receiving ECMO will develop nosocomial infections [34]. The mortality of patients on ECMO with reported infections ranges from 56–68% [32]. Therefore, optimizing antimicrobial regimens is essential to improve outcomes.

There are considerable pharmacokinetic (PK) changes in patients requiring ECMO assistance, making antimicrobial dosing challenging in this population. In general, ECMO has been shown to impact PK in three primary ways: 1) increased volume of distribution (Vt), 2) decreased clearance (CL), and 3) drug sequestration by the circuit [33 - 35]. Drugs with high lipophilicity and high protein binding are more likely to be sequestered in ECMO circuits, which results in a higher loss of the drugs [33]. The type of circuit also influences the degree of drug binding. More drugs were isolated in silicone membrane oxygenators than in newer hollow-fiber microporous membrane oxygenators [33]. Decreased pulmonary blood flows during VA ECMO could affect the metabolism of drugs in the lungs [33].

The majority of the PK data on antimicrobials used on ECMO come from neonatal studies, with vancomycin being the most commonly studied drug [35]. The effects of ECMO are drug-specific, and the results from adult studies do not always correlate with pediatric studies. A recent review article concluded that the PK of vancomycin, piperacillin-tazobactam, meropenem, azithromycin, amikacin and spongin did not change significantly in adult patients receiving ECMO, suggesting minimal effect on Veda in adults. However, there were significant changes in the PK of imipenem, oseltamivir, rifampicin and voriconazole. The trough concentrations of imipenem were highly variable, oseltamivir had a decreased CL and increased Vt and rifampicin concentrations were below therapeutic levels, even when the dose was increased. Voriconazole exhibited high mean peak concentrations during ECMO [33]. Additionally, ECMO technology changes over time, and it is unknown whether dosing recommendations derived from trials using the older technology can be extrapolated to patients supported with modern ECMO circuits [35].

Compounding the problem, a large percentage of critically ill patients on ECMO require renal replacement therapy (RRT) due to acute kidney injury. The reported rate of RRT during ECMO use in adults has been reported as 50% and 41% for VV and VA ECMO, respectively [33]. A retrospective study found that the percentage of patients achieving a target vancomycin concentration of 10-20 mcg/mL was significantly lower in patients receiving ECMO and continuous renal replacement therapy (CRRT) concurrently, compared to CRRT alone [36]. Three patients had subtherapeutic levels, while 2 patients had supratherapeutic levels. Of note, these patients received CRRT by on-line hemofiltration through the ECMO circuit. Alternatively, Donadello and colleagues showed that ECMO had no significant impact on vancomycin pharmacokinetics when CRRT was administered using independent vascular access [37].

Predicting the plasma concentrations of drugs during ECMO is difficult because many factors simultaneously impact the PK and because inconsistent results have been obtained in PK studies [33]. Available antibiotic PK studies have significant heterogeneity, including medical and surgical patients or patients under VV- and VA ECMO in variable proportion [34]. Table **1** provides adult dosing recommendations based on the available literature, primarily pharmacokinetic studies of small sample size [35]. However, therapeutic drug monitoring is recommended when possible to optimize PK targets due to considerable inter-patient variability and lack of high-quality studies. More studies are needed to provide guidance on optimal dosing, particularly with appropriate critically ill control groups and clinical outcome data (Table **3**).

The pharmacist plays a pivotal role in managing critically ill patients with AKI especially in the ICU and/or if they are requiring some form of dialysis and/or ECMO [39]. Medications, especially antibiotics will need to be adjusted according to urea/creatinine clearance. Also, controlling the volume of different infusions and total parenteral nutrition prescriptions will need cooperation between the pharmacists, the nephrologists, and the primary teams [30].

Table 3. Anti-infective dosing recommendations in adults utilizing ECMO [35].

Antimicrobial Agent	Standard Dosing in Critically Ill Patients	Dosing Recommendations for Patients on ECMO
Amphotericin B (Liposomal)	3–5 mg/kg q24h	Standard dosing
Azithromycin	500 mg q24h or 500 mg × 1 then 250 mg q24h	Standard dosing
Caspofungin	70 mg on day 1 then 50 mg q24h	Definitive dosing recommendations cannot be made
Ethambutol	Weight 40–55 kg: 800 mg q24hWeight 56–75 kg: 1200 mg q24hWeight 76–90 kg: 1600 mg q24h	50% increase over standard dosing
Ganciclovir	6 mg/kg q12h	Standard dosing
Imipenem	500–1000 mg q6–8h	Standard dosing unless treating resistant organism
Levofloxacin	500–1000 mg q24h	Standard dosing
Linezolid	600 mg IV q12h	Standard dosing unless MRSA MIC is >1mg/L
Meropenem	General: 500 mg q6h or 1 g q8h Meningitis/Cystic Fibrosis: 2 g q8h	1 g q8h for susceptible organisms (MIC≤2) 2 g q8h for resistant organisms (MIC >2 to 8)
Oseltamivir	75 mg or 150 mg enterally BID for severe illness	Standard dosing unless impaired renal function or enteral absorption
Piperacillin/tazobactam	3.375 g q6h- 4.5 g q6–8h	Standard dosing may be adequate for susceptible organisms

(Table 3) cont.....

Pyrazinamide	Weight 40–55 kg: 1000 mg q24hWeight 56–75 kg: 1500 mg q24hWeight 76–90 kg: 2000 mg q24h	50% increase over standard dosing
Rifampin	Tuberculosis treatment: 10 mg/kg q24h	20 mg/kg q24h
Tigecycline	100 mg once then 50 mg q12h	Standard dosing
Vancomycin	15–20 mg/kg/dose q8–12h	Standard dosing
Voriconazole	6 mg/kg q12h × 2 doses then 4 mg/kg q12h	Definitive dosing recommendations cannot be made

CONCLUSION

Several pharmacokinetic studies tried to address the different antimicrobials dosing in patients on RRT and ECMO. However, most of these studies had significant shortcomings such as; small sample size, lack of RRT prescription details (such as dialysate flow rate, effluent flow rate, blood flow rate, and duration of RRT and/or interruptions secondary to filter clotting), lack of drug concentration if the effluent or urine, lack of protein binding in this population. All of these variables made robust and standard dosing recommendations difficult. In Summary, in order to appropriately dose antimicrobials in patients on renal replacement therapies, the pharmacokinetics data of these drugs in this specific population is needed (residual kidney function, PB, Vd, nonrenal clearance) as well as the knowledge of the RRT modality and its prescription which may widely vary between patients. Moreover, there might be variability between prescribed and administered doses of CRRT (due to interruptions RRT). Outcome studies are scarce in this population. Controlled studies are highly needed to evaluate these dosing recommendations in this particular population.

CONSENT FOR PUBLICATION

Not applicable.

CONFLICT OF INTEREST

The authors confirm that the contents of this chapter have no conflict of interest.

ACKNOWLEDGEMENTS

Declared none.

REFERENCES

[1]   Nash K, Hafeez A, Hou S. Hospital-acquired renal insufficiency. Am J Kidney Dis 2002; 39(5): 930-6.

[http://dx.doi.org/10.1053/ajkd.2002.32766] [PMID: 11979336]

[2]   KDIGO clinical practice guideline for acute kidney injury. Kidney Int Suppl 2012; 2(1): 1-138.

[3]   Lo LJ, Go AS, Chertow GM, *et al*. Dialysis-requiring acute renal failure increases the risk of progressive chronic kidney disease. Kidney Int 2009; 76(8): 893-9.
[http://dx.doi.org/10.1038/ki.2009.289] [PMID: 19641480]

[4]   Bucaloiu ID, Kirchner HL, Norfolk ER, Hartle JE II, Perkins RM. Increased risk of death and de novo chronic kidney disease following reversible acute kidney injury. Kidney Int 2012; 81(5): 477-85.
[http://dx.doi.org/10.1038/ki.2011.405] [PMID: 22157656]

[5]   Lopez-Novoa JM, Quiros Y, Vicente L, Morales AI, Lopez-Hernandez FJ. New insights into the mechanism of aminoglycoside nephrotoxicity: an integrative point of view. Kidney Int 2011; 79(1): 33-45.
[http://dx.doi.org/10.1038/ki.2010.337] [PMID: 20861826]

[6]   Safdar A, Ma J, Saliba F, *et al*. Drug-induced nephrotoxicity caused by amphotericin B lipid complex and liposomal amphotericin B: a review and meta-analysis. Medicine (Baltimore) 2010; 89(4): 236-44.
[http://dx.doi.org/10.1097/MD.0b013e3181e9441b] [PMID: 20616663]

[7]   Tourret J, Deray G, Isnard-Bagnis C. Tenofovir effect on the kidneys of HIV-infected patients: a double-edged sword? J Am Soc Nephrol 2013; 24(10): 1519-27.
[http://dx.doi.org/10.1681/ASN.2012080857] [PMID: 24052632]

[8]   Wohl D, Oka S, Clumeck N, *et al*. Brief Report: A randomized, double-blind comparison of tenofovir alafenamide versus tenofovir disoproxil fumarate, each coformulated with elvitegravir, cobicistat, and emtricitabine for initial HIV-1 treatment: week 96 results. J Acquir Immune Defic Syndr 2016; 72(1): 58-64.
[http://dx.doi.org/10.1097/QAI.0000000000000940] [PMID: 26829661]

[9]   Hara M, Suganuma A, Yanagisawa N, Imamura A, Hishima T, Ando M. Atazanavir nephrotoxicity. Clin Kidney J 2015; 8(2): 137-42.
[http://dx.doi.org/10.1093/ckj/sfv015] [PMID: 25815168]

[10]   McIlroy DR, Wagener G, Lee HT. Biomarkers of acute kidney injury: an evolving domain. Anesthesiology 2010; 112(4): 998-1004.
[http://dx.doi.org/10.1097/ALN.0b013e3181cded3f] [PMID: 20216399]

[11]   Wang AY, Bellomo R. Renal replacement therapy in the ICU: intermittent hemodialysis, sustained low-efficiency dialysis or continuous renal replacement therapy? Curr Opin Crit Care 2018; 24(6): 437-42.
[http://dx.doi.org/10.1097/MCC.0000000000000541] [PMID: 30247213]

[12]   Palevsky PM, Zhang JH, O'Connor TZ, *et al*. Intensity of renal support in critically ill patients with acute kidney injury. N Engl J Med 2008; 359(1): 7-20.
[http://dx.doi.org/10.1056/NEJMoa0802639] [PMID: 18492867]

[13]   Bellomo R, Cass A, Cole L, *et al*. Intensity of continuous renal-replacement therapy in critically ill patients. N Engl J Med 2009; 361(17): 1627-38.
[http://dx.doi.org/10.1056/NEJMoa0902413] [PMID: 19846848]

[14]   Ronco C, Bellomo R, Homel P, *et al*. Effects of different doses in continuous veno-venous haemofiltration on outcomes of acute renal failure: a prospective randomised trial. Lancet 2000; 356(9223): 26-30.
[http://dx.doi.org/10.1016/S0140-6736(00)02430-2] [PMID: 10892761]

[15]   John S, Eckardt KU. Renal replacement strategies in the ICU. Chest 2007; 132(4): 1379-88.
[http://dx.doi.org/10.1378/chest.07-0167] [PMID: 17934125]

[16]   Kempke AP, Leino AS, Daneshvar F, Lee JA, Mueller BA. Antimicrobial doses in continuous renal replacement therapy: a comparison of dosing strategies. Crit Care Res Pract 2016; 3235765.
[http://dx.doi.org/10.1155/2016/3235765] [PMID: 27433357]

[17]   Gilbert B, Robbins P, Livornese LL Jr. Use of antibacterial agents in renal failure. Infect Dis Clin North Am 2009; 23(4): 899-924, viii.
[http://dx.doi.org/10.1016/j.idc.2009.06.009] [PMID: 19909890]

[18]   Choi G, Gomersall CD, Tian Q, Joynt GM, Freebairn R, Lipman J. Principles of antibacterial dosing in continuous renal replacement therapy. Crit Care Med 2009; 37(7): 2268-82.
[http://dx.doi.org/10.1097/CCM.0b013e3181aab3d0] [PMID: 19487930]

[19]   Brown GR. Cotrimoxazole - optimal dosing in the critically ill. Ann Intensive Care 2014; 4: 13.
[http://dx.doi.org/10.1186/2110-5820-4-13] [PMID: 24910807]

[20]   Heintz BH, Matzke GR, Dager WE. Antimicrobial dosing concepts and recommendations for critically ill adult patients receiving continuous renal replacement therapy or intermittent hemodialysis. Pharmacotherapy 2009; 29(5): 562-77.
[http://dx.doi.org/10.1592/phco.29.5.562] [PMID: 19397464]

[21]   Jamal JA, Economou CJ, Lipman J, Roberts JA. Improving antibiotic dosing in special situations in the ICU: burns, renal replacement therapy and extracorporeal membrane oxygenation. Curr Opin Crit Care 2012; 18(5): 460-71.
[http://dx.doi.org/10.1097/MCC.0b013e32835685ad] [PMID: 22820155]

[22]   Shaw AR, Mueller BA. Antibiotic dosing in continuous renal replacement therapy. Adv Chronic Kidney Dis 2017; 24(4): 219-27.
[http://dx.doi.org/10.1053/j.ackd.2017.05.004] [PMID: 28778361]

[23]   Lewis S J, Kays M B, Mueller B A. 2016.Use of Monte Carlo simulations to determine optimal carbapenem dosing in critically ill patients receiving prolonged

[24]   Wong WT, Choi G, Gomersall CD, Lipman J. To increase or decrease dosage of antimicrobials in septic patients during continuous renal replacement therapy: the eternal doubt. Curr Opin Pharmacol 2015; 24: 68-78.
[http://dx.doi.org/10.1016/j.coph.2015.07.003] [PMID: 26667969]

[25]   Ulldemolins M, Vaquer S, Llauradó-Serra M, *et al.* Beta-lactam dosing in critically ill patients with septic shock and continuous renal replacement therapy. Crit Care 2014; 18(3): 227.
[http://dx.doi.org/10.1186/cc13938] [PMID: 25042938]

[26]   König C, Braune S, Roberts JA, *et al.* Population pharmacokinetics and dosing simulations of ceftazidime in critically ill patients receiving sustained low-efficiency dialysis. J Antimicrob Chemother 2017; 72(5): 1433-40.
[http://dx.doi.org/10.1093/jac/dkw592] [PMID: 28175308]

[27]   Jang SM, Gharibian KN, Lewis SJ, Fissell WH, Tolwani AJ, Mueller BA. A monte carlo simulation approach for beta-lactam dosing in critically Ill patients receiving prolonged intermittent renal replacement therapy. J Clin Pharmacol 2018; 58(10): 1254-65.
[http://dx.doi.org/10.1002/jcph.1137] [PMID: 29746711]

[28]   Lewis SJ, Mueller BA. Development of a vancomycin dosing approach for critically ill patients receiving hybrid hemodialysis using Monte Carlo simulation. SAGE Open Med 2018; 6: 2050312118773257.
[http://dx.doi.org/10.1177/2050312118773257] [PMID: 29780587]

[29]   Moriyama B, Henning SA, Neuhauser MM, Danner RL, Walsh TJ. Continuous-infusion β-lactam antibiotics during continuous venovenous hemofiltration for the treatment of resistant gram-negative bacteria. Ann Pharmacother 2009; 43(7): 1324-37.
[http://dx.doi.org/10.1345/aph.1L638] [PMID: 19584386]

[30]   Marasco SF, Lukas G, McDonald M, McMillan J, Ihle B. Review of ECMO (extra corporeal membrane oxygenation) support in critically ill adult patients. Heart Lung Circ 2008; 17 (Suppl. 4): S41-7.
[http://dx.doi.org/10.1016/j.hlc.2008.08.009] [PMID: 18964254]

[31]   Pillai AK, Bhatti Z, Bosserman AJ, Mathew MC, Vaidehi K, Kalva SP. Management of vascular complications of extra-corporeal membrane oxygenation. Cardiovasc Diagn Ther 2018; 8(3): 372-7.
[http://dx.doi.org/10.21037/cdt.2018.01.11] [PMID: 30057883]

[32]   Extracorporeal Life Support Organization Registry Report: International Summary. January 2016. ASAIO J 2017; 63(1): 60-7.
[http://dx.doi.org/10.1097/MAT.0000000000000475] [PMID: 27984321]

[33]   Hahn J, Choi JH, Chang MJ. Pharmacokinetic changes of antibiotic, antiviral, antituberculosis and antifungal agents during extracorporeal membrane oxygenation in critically ill adult patients. J Clin Pharm Ther 2017; 42(6): 661-71.
[http://dx.doi.org/10.1111/jcpt.12636] [PMID: 28948652]

[34]   Bouglé A, Dujardin O, Lepère V, *et al.* PHARMECMO: Therapeutic drug monitoring and adequacy of current dosing regimens of antibiotics in patients on Extracorporeal Life Support. Anaesth Crit Care Pain Med 2019; 38(5): 493-7.
[http://dx.doi.org/10.1016/j.accpm.2019.02.015] [PMID: 30831307]

[35]   Sherwin J, Heath T, Watt K. Pharmacokinetics and dosing of anti-infective drugs in patients on extracorporeal membrane oxygenation: a review of the current literature. Clin Ther 2016; 38(9): 1976-94.
[http://dx.doi.org/10.1016/j.clinthera.2016.07.169] [PMID: 27553752]

[36]   Yang CJ, Wu CW, Wu CC. Effect of extracorporeal membrane oxygenation on the new vancomycin dosing regimen in critically ill patients receiving continuous venovenous hemofiltration. Ther Drug Monit 2018; 40(3): 310-4.
[http://dx.doi.org/10.1097/FTD.0000000000000495] [PMID: 29746432]

[37]   Donadello K, Roberts JA, Cristallini S, *et al.* Vancomycin population pharmacokinetics during extracorporeal membrane oxygenation therapy: a matched cohort study. Crit Care 2014; 18(6): 632.
[http://dx.doi.org/10.1186/s13054-014-0632-8] [PMID: 25416535]

[38]   Extracorporeal Life Support Organization Registry Report: International Summary. 2017 January; https://www.elso.org/Portals/0/Files/Reports/2017/International%20Summary%20January%202017.pdf

[39]   Joannes-Boyau O, Velly L, Ichai C. Optimizing continuous renal replacement therapy in the ICU: a team strategy. Curr Opin Crit Care 2018; 24(6): 476-82.
[http://dx.doi.org/10.1097/MCC.0000000000000564] [PMID: 30308541]

CHAPTER 13

Practice and Impact of Antimicrobial Stewardship

Elisa Morgan[1], **Lucia Rose**[2] and **Madeline King**[3,*]

[1] *Doylestown Hospital, 595 W State St, Doylestown, PA 18901, USA*

[2] *Cooper University Hospital, Camden, NJ 08103, USA*

[3] *Phialdelphia College of Pharmacy, Univeristy of the Sciences, Philadelphia, PA 19104, USA*

Abstract: Antimicrobial stewardship in inpatient, as well as outpatient settings, is crucial for preserving antimicrobial susceptibility, combating antibiotic resistance, and reducing unnecessary antibiotic use. The Centers for Disease Control and Prevention, as well as the World Health Organization, and various infectious diseases and government organizations have developed guidance on how to implement stewardship in different settings. A wide variety of practices are in place depending on the setting. Examples include educational activities, antibiotic recommendations and restriction, and facility guidelines. Stewardship practices are mandated in most healthcare settings, and tracking of antibiotic use is important in maintaining good practices.

Keywords: Antibiotic resistance, Antibiotic use, Antimicrobial stewardship, Centers for Disease Control and Prevention, Days of therapy, Defined daily doses, Metrics, Regulatory, Regulatory measures, Stewardship programs, World Health Organization.

INTRODUCTION

Antimicrobial stewardship programs (ASP) originated in Hartford, Connecticut in the 1970s. Since then, programs have evolved, and are now required in hospitals throughout the United States. Additionally, antimicrobial stewardship (AS) is becoming more prevalent in outpatient settings as the number of antibiotic prescriptions from outpatient clinics increases. The Centers for Disease Control and Prevention (CDC) and Society for Healthcare Epidemiology of America (SHEA) have developed guidelines for implementing and deploying ASP [1]. The appropriate use of antibiotics is essential for preventing antibiotic-associated complications such as *Clostridioides difficile* infection (CDI), other adverse effects, or multi-drug resistant (MDR) bacteria. The SHEA guideline states that

---

* **Corresponding authors Madeline King:** Philadelphia College of Pharmacy, Univeristy of the Sciences, Philadelphia, PA 19104, USA; Tel: 215-593-8831; E-mail: m.king@usciences.edu

Islam M. Ghazi & Michael J. Cawley (Eds.)

appropriately managing antimicrobials is fundamental in reducing the incidence of resistant organisms, therefore, improving the health of patients [1]. There are a variety of methods which have been successful in reducing the inappropriate use of antimicrobials, both in the inpatient and outpatient settings. Programs often include education to providers or institutions, review of antimicrobial prescriptions at the time of order entry or retrospectively, and protocols which specify the duration of treatment for different infections. Providers should be cautious when discriminating between signs and symptoms of an infection versus other processes. Additionally, ordering cultures should be restricted to patients showing signs of an infection, rather than routine cultures (*e.g.* preoperative urine cultures).

Regulatory Measures

The U.S. regulatory requirements for AS have drastically changed over the last few years. While many inpatient stewardship programs have been established for decades, the implementation requirements have taken much longer. The 2019 CDC report, "Antibiotic Resistance Threats in the United States" highlights the large burden of antibiotic resistance in our country [2]. This document classified urgent and serious threats to help prioritize concerns, and aid in identification methods and infection prevention practices. The most notable changes to the 2019 report versus the 2013 report are the addition of *Candida auris*, relisting carbapenem-resistant *Acinetobacter* as urgent instead of serious, and the removal of vancomycin resistant *staphylococcus aureus* [2]. In addition, the CDC created tracking platforms for antibiotic resistance and began requiring the submission of data to the national healthcare safety network (NHSN) [3].

In September of 2014, President Obama signed Executive Order 13676 to establish a task force comprised of key stakeholders charged to develop a 5-year national action plan to combat antibiotic resistance. This accompanied the President's Council of Advisors on Science and Technology (PCAST) report that outlined in detail various veterinary and human based recommendations aimed towards reduction of resistance, growth of antibiotic research, and antibiotic development. The PCAST report also included economic incentives to support antibiotic development, in addition to several recommendations for Centers for Medicaid & Medicare Services (CMS) to help enforce the adoption of antibiotic stewardship programs across all hospital settings [4].

The National Action Plan released by the White House in March 2015 outlines specific targets and steps to achieve a reduction in antimicrobial resistance by 2020. Table **1** outlines these national targets. Many objectives are discussed throughout the document but one of the main objectives (objective 1.1) is to strengthen antibiotic stewardship in inpatient, outpatient and long-term care settings [5].

Table 1. Combating Antibiotic Resistant Bacteria (adapted from "National Action Plan for Combating Antibiotic-Resistant Bacteria") [6].

National Targets to Combat Antibiotic-Resistant Bacteria, by 2020
For CDC Recognized Urgent Threats:
• Reduce by 50% the incidence of overall *Clostridium difficile* infection compared to estimates from 2011. • Reduce by 60% carbapenem-resistant Enterobacteriaceae infections acquired during hospitalization compared to estimates. • Maintain the prevalence of ceftriaxone-resistant *Neisseria gonorrhoeae* below 2% compared to estimates from 2013.
For CDC Recognized Serious Threats:
• Reduce by 35% multidrug-resistant *Pseudomonas* spp. infections acquired during hospitalization compared to estimates from 2011. • Reduce by at least 50% overall methicillin-resistant *staphylococcus aureus* (MRSA) bloodstream infections by 2020 as compared to 2011. • Reduce by 25% multidrug-resistant non-typhoidal *Salmonella* infections compared to estimates from 2010-2012. • Reduce by 15% the number of multidrug-resistant TB infections. • Reduce by at least 25% the rate of antibiotic-resistant invasive pneumococcal disease among <5 year-olds compared to estimates from 2008. • Reduce by at least 25% the rate of antibiotic-resistant invasive pneumococcal disease among >65 year-olds compared to estimates from 2008.

The World Health Organization (WHO) also developed a Global Action Plan on antimicrobial resistance, adopted in May 2015. This involved coordination of human and veterinary sectors along with agricultural, financial, and environmental partners. Although the plan had no regulatory requirements, it provided expectations for each country to adopt their own national action plan. Some countries have a more targeted focus on sanitation and infection prevention while others (*i.e.* U.S.) have resources to optimize antimicrobial usage. In addition to the action plan, the WHO developed a Global Priority List of multi-drug resistant (MDR) bacteria that should be utilized to guide research, discovery, and development of new antibiotics [5]. The criteria for MDR bacteria inclusion included health care burden, prevalence of resistance, and attributable mortality. The list is categorized into critical, high, and medium priorities.

In response to these recommendations, two Federal acts were passed: the 21st Century Cures Act ("Cures Act") of 2016 and Generating Antibiotic Incentives Now Act of 2011 ("GAIN Act"). The antibiotic section of the Cures Act is intended to accelerate drug development and monitor resistance across federal institutions. Another important section of this Act creates an easier pathway for antibiotics and antifungals that are seeking approval by the FDA for serious infections in specific populations. Lastly, section 3044 was developed to expedite recognition of antimicrobial susceptibility test interpretive criteria (STIC) also known as "breakpoints" and provide up-to-date information to the healthcare community in a more streamlined manner. The GAIN Act, provides additional market exclusivity to pharmaceutical companies that developed new antibiotics for treatment of specific MDR bacteria. Antibiotics that met this criteria would be designated a qualified infectious disease product (QIDP). Incentives to develop drugs that would meet QIDP designation included fast track review and market exclusivity for five additional years [6].

The Joint Commission (TJC) developed a critical medication management standard for antibiotic stewardship that became effective January 1, 2017. This standard applied to all acute care and critical access hospitals as well as nursing care centers. There are eight elements of performance within this standard that essentially enforce the initiation or continuation of antibiotic stewardship programs at every acute care hospital in the U.S. that is TJC accredited. The standard also emphasized the need to have antibiotic stewardship as an organizational priority. Staff education and organization approved protocols were also included in the elements of performance. In addition, a lead pharmacist and physician (both preferably with infectious disease training) are required for continued TJC accreditation [7].

CMS is in the process of finalizing various Conditions of participation (CoP) for acute care hospitals, long-term care facilities and outpatient clinics to encourage antibiotic stewardship. CMS CoP already exists for infection prevention and the idea is to mirror a similar process.

Various guidelines and/or guidance documents have been published, notably the CDC "Core Elements of Hospital Antibiotic Stewardship Programs" [8]. and the Infectious Diseases Society of America (IDSA) guidelines on "Implementing an ASP" [1]. The CDC also has Core Elements documents for nursing homes and outpatient practices.

Tracking and Reporting

Tracking and reporting is a recommended component of all ASP. Tracking can help evaluate effectiveness of interventions and identify areas of intervention [8, 9]. Reporting to other departments and committees throughout the hospital can help provide education and support for the program's initiatives. With the increased regulatory focus on AS, standardized metrics are needed to show the effectiveness of programs. Additionally, most metrics are unable to distinguish appropriate use from inappropriate use and distinguish the impact of stewardship on patient outcomes due to confounders [9].

The most common metrics utilized by antimicrobial stewardship in the inpatient setting are those that track antibiotic consumption. Metrics of antibiotic consumption should be normalized to patient volume (*i.e.* 1,000 patient days or 1,000 days present) [8, 9]. Defined daily doses (DDD) is the metric recommended by the WHO and is calculated utilizing standard dose definitions available on the WHO website. Interpretation of DDD can be limited with reductions in dosing for pediatrics and organ impairment [8 - 10]. More information on calculations of DDD is available on the WHO website [10]. In the United States., the recommended metric of antibiotic consumption is days of therapy (DOT). DOT is calculated by aggregating the number of days a patient is on antibiotics [8, 9]. More information on calculating DOT is available in the National Healthcare Safety Network (NHSN) Antibiotic Use and Resistance (AUR) module (available at: https://www.cdc.gov/nhsn/PDFs/pscManual/11pscAURcurrent.pdf). Addition-ally, NHSN provides a database that tracks antibiotic utilization and resistance trends among institutions. Currently, reporting to NHSN is voluntary. NHSN has established the Standardized Antimicrobial Administration Ratio (SAAR). The SAAR can provide benchmarking among similar institutions and calculates a ratio based on actual antimicrobial utilization compared to expected utilization to help identify potential areas of overuse and underuse [3, 8, 9]. Length of therapy (LOT) has had limited study with ASP but may be useful in evaluating de-escalation and duration of therapy interventions. Unfortunately, all of the antibiotic consumption metrics are limited by their inability to distinguish appropriate use from inappropriate use [9].

Inpatient programs can also track a variety of other measures. Antimicrobial costs are relatively simple to track as most pharmacies are easily able to access purchasing data. Antimicrobial resistance trends should be tracked with antibiograms but it can be difficult to measure the impact of AMS interventions on changes in patterns of resistance. Linking interventions to length of stay (LOS) trends may provide further support for ASP. More research is needed to define the optimum metrics to evaluate the effectiveness of ASP [9].

Audit and feedback is a common method of tracking and reporting antibiotic utilization in the outpatient setting. Programs should determine the level at which to track (*i.e.* clinician level versus facility level). Whenever possible, the individual clinician level is preferred, as peer-to-peer comparison and individualized feedback have been shown to improve adherence to guidelines [11]. Programs can also track appropriateness of prescribing for targeted high-priority conditions. For example, programs may evaluate the percentage of visits for acute bronchitis that each clinician prescribed antibiotics and provide peer comparison. Programs should be cautious with this targeted approach as it may lead to diagnosis shifting (altering of the diagnostic code to a different indication that validates an antibiotic prescription). Including a comparison of overall rate of antibiotic prescriptions for all visits may help capture data missed when tracking by a high-priority condition alone if diagnosis shifting occurs. Programs should attempt to account or compare for each clinicians' patient population as some populations (such has a higher HIV population) may lead to higher rates of antibiotic prescribing. Complications of antibiotic use (*C. difficile* infections, drug interactions and adverse drug events) can provide valuable outcomes data but may be difficult to track for most facilities at this time [12].

To improve AS in nursing home and long-term care facilities (LTCFs), the CDC also created guidance for tracking and reporting of antimicrobial use in those settings. The three methods recommended for evaluating are: process measures, antibiotic use measures, and antibiotic outcomes measures. Documented clinical assessment and need for antibiotics, as well as appropriate antibiotic selection are important for improving the antimicrobial use process. Point prevalence surveys and antibiotic start tracking are valuable tools for determining antimicrobial use. Antibiotic days of therapy (DOT) is also a useful measurement of the overall use of antibiotics (the sum of all antibiotic days for all residents in the facility during a given time frame. Lastly, assessing adverse events (*e.g. C. difficile*) and antibiotic costs are helpful ways to measure antibiotic outcomes. Based on a study in LTCFs, the CDC suggests using education and feedback to providers to improve antibiotic use [13].

ANTIMICROBIAL STEWARDSHIP IN THE INPATIENT SETTING

ASP in the inpatient setting are tasked with optimizing antibiotic regimens and reducing the spread of resistance in an acutely ill population. Increased regulatory focus on ASP emphasizes the importance of these programs in preventing a public health crisis but pressures facilities to implement the required programs in an effective manner. Core components of a successful ASP include a multidisciplinary team, formulary restriction, prospective audit and feedback and education. Ideally, teams should incorporate feedback from the facility's prescribers [1, 8, 14, 15].

In an ideal setting, physicians and pharmacists trained in infectious diseases (ID) offer accountability and drug expertise as leaders of the program. However, this may not be feasible in acute care facilities with limited resources. In these situations, generalists can successfully fulfill these roles [1, 8, 14]. Two professional societies, the Society of Infectious Diseases Pharmacists (SIDP) and

Making a Difference in Infectious Diseases (MAD-ID), offer training programs to help participants develop the practice skills needed in AMS practice [16, 17]. The CDC also now offers its own AS training program for all levels of providers and practitioners, available at https://www.train.org/cdctrain/course/1075730.

Optimizing antimicrobial regimens reduces antimicrobial consumption, antibiotic resistance, and costs while improving clinical outcomes (*i.e.* reduction in *C. difficile*, length of stay) [1, 8, 15, 18, 19]. A variety of strategies exist to develop ASP initiatives and not a single template fits all facilities. Programs should implement initiatives one at a time, focusing on those of highest priority first [8]. This section of the chapter seeks to evaluate intervention strategies with a focus on their pros, cons, and implementation considerations.

Formulary Management Strategies

Antimicrobial stewardship committees should work with their hospital's or medical center's pharmacy and therapeutics committee to optimize the antimicrobial formulary for the organization. Considerations for formulary management include formulary status, antibiotic cycling or mixing strategies and shortage management [1, 14]. Programs should review their current antimicrobial formulary and any newly FDA-approved antimicrobials to determine any prescribing restrictions by designating agents as formulary, non-formulary or restricted [14].

Preauthorization

Formulary restriction, also referred to as preauthorization or prior authorization, confines prescriptions for targeted antimicrobials to pre-defined criteria to decrease their use [1, 8, 14]. Implementation strategies involve restricting the agent to an approval process or to infectious diseases consultation [14]. Reasons for restricting an agent include cost, potential toxicities, and resistance patterns.

Preauthorization can optimize antimicrobial therapy through improved empiric antimicrobial selection and reduction of unnecessary antibiotics in patients without an infection [1, 8, 14, 20]. Additionally, restriction can help maintain supply during antimicrobial shortages. For instance, during a cefotaxime shortage, hospitals may opt to restrict this agent to neonatal populations only to reduce the potential for hyperbilirubinemia seen with ceftriaxone in this population [21]. The exact implementation and targeted agents vary by the institution. Programs may either require authorization prior to dispensing or require authorization within a certain timeframe (such as 24 hours).

Unfortunately, preauthorization may have unintended consequences. Restriction may drive the use of alternative, unrestricted agents, potentially leading to increased resistance of these agents (*i.e.* "squeezing the balloon") [1, 14, 20]. Limitation of provider autonomy through restriction can lead to a negative perception of the ASP [1]. Processes must be in place to prevent delays in care, and programs will need to determine their hours of coverage (*i.e.* 24-hour approval process vs. off-hours process). Programs with 24-hour processes may experience variability in appropriateness of approvals during off-hour coverage while programs without 24-hour coverage may have clinicians delay treatment initiation until off-hours. Additional workarounds include misrepresentation or manipulation of data to gain approval [15, 22].

Computerized decision support software (CDSS) or electronic approval systems may reduce the workload of a pre-authorization initiative. One program that created an electronic approval system that manages 250-300 approvals per month found a sustained reduction on their utilization of targeted antimicrobials [23].

Regardless of the initial approval method, programs should determine when, if at all feasible, approved requests will be reevaluated for continued appropriateness. Programs should periodically track their data for impact and review appropriateness of the initiative [15].

Antibiotic Cycling and Antibiotic Mixing

Antibiotic cycling and antibiotic mixing attempt to introduce heterogeneity to reduce selective ecological pressures that contribute to resistance.

Antibiotic cycling is the process of a scheduled rotation of the preferred antibiotic for a designated indication in a particular unit or facility. Typically, antibiotics are cycled from different classes that have a comparable spectrum of activity but different mechanisms of resistance. This process is most commonly evaluated with gram-negative resistance [1, 14, 24]. The idea for antibiotic cycling stems from studies in the 1980's that rotated the preferred aminoglycoside to reduce the development of resistance to each agent. In theory, resistance should decline when an agent is not active in the rotation as the selective pressures that lead to resistance should be reduced [14, 24].

Antibiotic mixing is similar in concept to cycling but the targeted antibiotics are alternated with each patient rather than by period of time [1, 14, 24, 25]. Antibiotic mixing theoretically reduces selective pressure by maximizing heterogeneity [24].

Most studies evaluating these two strategies have several limitations and provide conflicting results. A multicenter, international study in eight European ICUs compared the two strategies and found that neither strategy reduced acquisition of antibiotic-resistant, gram-negative bacteria more than the other nor compared to baseline (baseline resistance 28%, cycling resistance 23%, and mixing resistance 22%) [24].

In addition to a lack of data to support the use of either of these stewardship strategies at this time, both are labor intensive processes to maintain compliance and develop contingency plans in patients with contraindications to their assigned agent [1, 14, 24, 25].

Prospective Audit and Feedback

Prospective audit and feedback (PAF) is the process of external review of the antibiotic regimen for appropriateness with recommendations made to the treating team to optimize therapy [1, 8]. Potential benefits of PAF initiatives include increased appropriateness of antimicrobial regimen, decreased antibiotic utilization, decreased antibiotic resistance, decreased *C. difficile* rates, decreased length of stay and decreased mortality. Benefits may vary by the type of initiative and the implementation strategy [1, 14, 26]. PAF can be labor-intensive and prescriber compliance with recommendations is often voluntary [1, 18, 20].

There are several potential targets for PAF initiatives, including but not limited to empiric selection, de-escalation, mismatches in culture results and current therapy (*i.e.* drug/bug mismatch), positive blood culture review, positive culture and not on antimicrobials, duplicate coverage, targeted antimicrobials, and duration of therapy. While programs typically wait to review patients for 48-96 hours when additional clinical data is available, early interventions (< 48 H) have been shown to reduce antibiotic utilization without compromising patient safety [27]. Implementation strategies depend on the available resources of the facility. CDSS or other information technology support provides assistance in identifying patients that have potential for intervention to optimize therapy [1, 28]. Whenever possible, the availability of a clinical team that involves the prescriber in the development of the PAF initiative can lead to more sustained effects [15]. ID physician support improves the acceptance of the program [29]. Programs with dedicated ID pharmacist support are associated with a greater degree of impact than programs utilizing other clinical pharmacists; however, clinical pharmacists still provide an impact on optimizing antimicrobial regimens through PAF, especially with training specific to that initiative. Clinical pharmacists can provide added support to a program with an infectious diseases pharmacist or serve as the steward in critical access facilities [30, 31]. Since PAF can be labor-intensive, programs should give due consideration to the frequency of PAF review. For programs with limited resources where daily review is not feasible, benefit was shown with thrice-weekly review [1, 32]. Programs with enhanced infrastructure and resources should consider coverage for holiday and weekends. A program found that lack of weekends and holiday coverage led to significant increases in time to optimization of therapy (approximately 132 hours versus 41 hours during the week) and delayed reevaluation of restricted antimicrobials leading to an average of 3.775 additional days of restricted antimicrobials [33]. Utilizing specially trained pharmacy residents (pharmacy residents in infectious diseases or critical care specialties) to perform PAF on weekends resulted in a decrease in antibiotic utilization and assisted with review of restrictions, PAF initiatives and rapid diagnostics [34].

Restricted Antimicrobials versus Prospective Audit and Feedback

Limited strong data exists comparing the two stewardship initiatives. Contradictory data exists as some studies have shown improved antibiotic consumption with switch from preauthorization to PAF and other studies have shown worse outcomes with the switch [14, 35]. Preauthorization is thought to work faster than PAF and is more effective when the need is urgent (*i.e.* shortages or outbreaks of resistance) (Table **2**) [15].

Table 2. Preauthorization vs Prospective Audit and Feedback.

	Preauthorization	Prospective Audit and Feedback
Provider autonomy	Loss of prescriber autonomy	Autonomy maintained and can promote collegial relationship
Resource utilization	Labor-intensive in real-time	Labor-intensive review
Impact on empiric/initial regimens	Improves initial selection Concern for "squeezing the balloon" effect on unrestricted agents Reduced initiation of unnecessary starts of targeted agents	Usually does not address
Impact on de-escalation	Usually does not address but some programs may have an approval duration limit to prompt re-evaluation	May address
Compliance	Required	Voluntary
Timing of Review	Needs to be available at all times or have an off-hours process in place to prevent delays in care	Flexible Enhanced impact with daily review but still beneficial with limited review

(Table 2) cont.....

	Preauthorization	**Prospective Audit and Feedback**
Availability of microbiological data	Usually not available at time of initial review Can ensure proper cultures are ordered at initiation for targeted drugs	Increased evidence-based review based on available microbiological and clinical data
Success dependent on	Skills of reviewer Potential for "gaming the system"	Delivery method of feedback

Behavioral Change

Currently data is limited in utilizing behavioral change initiatives to improve antimicrobial prescribing; however, for sustained improvements to antimicrobial prescribing, changes in the behavior and culture of antimicrobial prescribing are necessary [37]. Behaviors behind antimicrobial prescribing are complex and multifactorial, consisting of choosing the right antibiotic for the indication, assessing the benefits and risks of treatment, and choosing the appropriate route, dose and duration. Many external factors influence prescribing behavior, such as time pressures, competing priorities, and fear of treatment failure [36, 37]. One program found a sustained increase in antimicrobial appropriateness after working with seven departments to develop their own interventions to improve their antibiotic utilization [38]. Further study is needed determine the optimal implementation of behavioral change techniques.

Peer Comparison

Peer comparison is a retrospective form of audit and feedback that compares providers to their fellow prescribers. Peer comparison is an effective intervention for the outpatient setting and may also be beneficial in the inpatient setting. One study evaluated utilizing DOT per 100 service days as a metric to identify outliers in the inpatient setting but did not analyze the impact of feedback on prescribing rates. While this metric would help account for prompt de-escalation (rather than just evaluating initial prescriptions) there are some potential biases. Service days do not account for patient volume or continued use for appropriate indications [39]. Peer comparison of pharmacists' vancomycin dose order verification was found to be effective in improving adherence to an institution's dosing guidelines [40]. More data is needed to validate an appropriate metric and the impact of this feedback in the inpatient setting.

Education

Despite the recognition of problems associated with antimicrobial resistance, concern for contributing to antimicrobial resistance is often not a major consideration during antimicrobial prescribing. One study found providers often ranked "contributing to antimicrobial resistance" the lowest of 7 factors influencing selection of antibiotics in patients with community-acquired pneumonia (CAP) [41]. Education on antimicrobial resistance and optimization of antibiotics is a fundamental concept of AS; however, programs should not rely on education alone, as the effect wanes over time and likely has minimal sustained effects on prescribing behavior [1, 36, 42]. Educational strategies include didactic lectures or in-services and distribution of educational pamphlets, posters, and other materials. Active education is likely more effective at eliciting change than passive education [1, 14]. Education and especially targeted education is more likely to be effective when combined with corresponding initiatives [1, 8].

Clinical Practice Guidelines

Clinical practice guidelines and order sets for common infectious diseases can standardize empiric antibiotic prescribing and increase utilization of preferred therapy. Guidelines should be maintained and updated periodically and programs should monitor usage and provide education to increase adherence with facility-specific guidelines [1, 8]. Incorporating guidelines into order sets increases the impact of the guidelines. More drastic improvements in appropriateness of surgical prophylaxis were found with requiring the use of an antibiotic order form versus providing a handbook. The handbook arm increased compliance from 11% to 18% (p=0.06]. compared to an increase from 17% to 78% (p < 0.01]. in the order set group. Guideline compliance may be low on its own. One study found adding restrictions to enforce their guidelines for third-generation cephalosporin utilization increased compliance from 24% to 85%. Including provider champions and local input into development of institutional guidelines can help improve acceptance rates. This promotes a feeling of collaboration among the providers and the stewardship committee and promotes ownership. Additionally, this may be important in teaching facilities to influence the senior attending physicians on trainees' prescribing habits [14].

Targeting Specific Infectious Diseases Syndromes

The combination of multiple strategies targeting a specific disease state can improve antibiotic use. Implementation often includes utilization of bundles including multiple interventions such as treatment algorithms, electronic order sets, provider champions, and periodic feedback to providers on compliance. Common disease states that have been targeted are skin and soft tissue infections (SSTI's), asymptomatic bacteriuria (ASB), CAP, *C. difficile*, and positive blood cultures with specific pathogens. Goals of such program include decreasing inappropriate diagnostics, decreasing unnecessary antibiotics in patients who are not actively infected, decreasing antibiotic DOT, decreasing duration of treatment, increasing IV to PO conversion, and increasing de-escalation rates [1, 8].

Reduce Use of Drugs with High Risk for CDI

Restriction of antibiotics associated with a high-risk for CDI has been shown to reduce hospital-onset CDI. Commonly targeted agents include clindamycin, broad-spectrum cephalosporins and fluoroquinolones. Interventions to reduce usage of these agents include treatment guidelines, prospective audit and feedback, reduction in duration of therapy or formulary restriction [1]. While any antibiotic use can be associated with CDI onset, variation of risk exist among different classes. Clindamycin consistently is found to have the strongest association with CDI risk; however, fluoroquinolones, cephalosporins, carbapenems and monobactams have also demonstrated higher risks than other antibiotic classes [1, 43, 44]. Conversely, the tetracyclines consistently demonstrate no increased risk of CDI. Penicillin's, macrolides and trimethoprim/sulfamethoxazole have a moderate risk for CDI [43, 44]. The implementation of ASP is associated with reductions in CDI rates. Additionally, programs can specifically target agents associated with high risk for CDI. Restriction of clindamycin to ID consultation reduced CDI rates from 11.5 cases/month to 3.33 cases per month in one facility with a CDI outbreak [45]. Restrictions of cephalosporins and fluoroquinolones have also been associated with decreased CDI rates [46]. Success with reducing CDI rates has also been found with a bundle of initiatives that included facility-specific guidelines and PAF to reduce the use of second and third-generation cephalosporins, ciprofloxacin, clindamycin and macrolides [47].

Strategies to Encourage Prescriber-led Review of Antibiotic Regimens

The goals of these initiatives are to encourage clinicians to reevaluate antibiotic regimens for continued appropriateness without added prompting from the stewardship team [1, 8, 49]. There is currently a paucity of data evaluating strategies to prompt prescriber self-stewardship and limited guidance exists for implementation [1]. These strategies include antibiotic time outs and antibiotic stop orders. It is important with both of these strategies to have processes in place to prevent inappropriate discontinuations that could lead to patient harm and damage the collegial relationship between the clinicians and the ASP.

Antibiotic Time Out (ATO)

An antibiotic time out serves to reevaluate the antibiotic regimen for continued appropriateness [1, 8, 48, 49]. Key questions to consider when performing an antibiotic time out are: (a) does the patient have an infection that will respond to antibiotics?, (b) if so, is the patient on the right antibiotic(s), dose and route of administration?, (c) can a more targeted antibiotic be used to treat the infection?, and (d) how long should the patient receive antibiotics [49]. It is not apparent that ATOs reduce overall antibiotic consumption, but some programs have found success when targeting specific agents, such as vancomycin and fluoroquinolones. Implementation strategies investigated in the literature include pharmacist driven prompts on rounds, twice-weekly checklist completed by a medical resident, optional questionnaires, and one program developed an electronic template to evaluate continued utilization of vancomycin and piperacillin/tazobactam beyond 3 days [50 - 55]. As the utilization of electronic health records (EHR) and computerized decision support systems (CDSS) in stewardship continues to grow, this will likely become an interesting avenue for antibiotic time out programs that will require further study.

Automatic Stop Orders

Automatic stop dates have a limited duration of use before the orders expire. As with ATO's, limited data exists on utilizing automatic stop orders [1, 8]. One area of use is with surgical prophylaxis to prevent durations exceeding the recommended 24 hours for most procedures as this can be associated with increased risk for adverse events, such as *C. difficile* infection [8, 56]. Potential future utilization may focus on establishing defined durations based on the specified indication in the EHR.

Dose Optimization

ASP should implement initiatives to optimize antimicrobial dosing as dosing can impact efficacy and toxicity [57, 58]. Hospitals often have renal dosing guidelines so that dosing is standardized and has been reviewed by someone with infectious diseases expertise. Pharmacists can also provide expert dosing recommendations either while rounding with multidisciplinary teams, or upon order verification.

Dose Adjustments for Organ Impairment

ASP should consider providing initiatives that help optimize dosing in patients with organ impairment to reduce potential for adverse effects [8, 59, 60]. Programs should ideally consider including a process for adjusting doses in patients with improving renal function to prevent under-dosing as well. Often, this is a pharmacy-driven process with either automatic dose adjustments based on a protocol or recommendations based on review [57, 60, 61]. Incorporation of recommended doses into order sets and empiric treatment guidelines can assist providers with initial dosing [57].

Pharmacokinetic (PK) Monitoring and Adjustment

Individualized PK monitoring and adjustment of aminoglycosides and vancomycin can lead to increased likelihood of obtaining therapeutic levels, decreased costs, decreased nephrotoxicity, decreased length of stay and decreased mortality [1]. A variety of approaches to optimize PK dosing and monitoring are possible depending on the resources of the facility. Dedicated PK dosing services or PAF programs for vancomycin and aminoglycosides have been shown to increase the number of patients achieving targeted levels, decrease toxicity, decrease duration of therapy and decrease the number of levels obtained [62 - 64]. Programs with limited resources can consider providing dosing calculators or nomograms to assist initial prescribing [65, 67].

PK/PD Dose Optimization

β-lactam efficacy is dependent on the time the drug concentration exceeds the MIC. Traditionally, β-lactams are administered by intermittent dosing, which leads to high peak concentrations but rapid drops in drug levels due to their short half-lives. Time above the MIC can be increased either by shortening the dosing interval or prolonging the infusion [67 - 69]. Theoretically, strategies that optimize the time-dependent properties of β-lactams may improve efficacy and reduce the development of resistance. Currently, data is conflicting among published systematic reviews and meta-analysis. In general, there exists few randomized controlled-trials and most studies on the subject are at risk for bias. Despite conflicting outcomes data for benefit, there have not been any reports of increased adverse events with these strategies and there exists the potential cost savings with strategies utilizing a decreased total daily dose [8, 67, 69]. Logistical concerns with implementation include education, provider buy-in, smart-pump utilization, and IV compatibilities given longer durations of infusion [8, 57, 69].

Duration of Therapy

For many infections, shorter courses of therapy are associated with similar efficacy outcomes as longer courses and can reduce the risk for adverse effects and *C. difficile* acquisition [70]. A combination of efforts including treatment guidelines, education and PAF can reduce durations [1]. It was traditionally thought that discontinuing antibiotics too early may lead to the development of resistant organisms; however, longer durations of therapy may be more likely to lead to the development of resistant organisms due to the more prolonged impact on the microbiome. Increasing evidence from randomized controlled trials continues to support that shortened courses of antibiotics are equally effective of longer course for a number of indications, including pneumonia, SSTI's, uncomplicated urinary tract infections and intra-abdominal infections. A recent review summarized several of those trials and discussed benefits of short antibiotic courses [71].

IV to PO Conversion

Early IV to PO conversion can reduce costs and improve patient outcomes [1, 8, 72 - 78]. The conversion of an IV medication to its PO counterpart is often referred to as sequential therapy. In contrast, step-down therapy refers to change from an IV antibiotic to an oral agent that may not be therapeutically equivalent (*i.e.* ceftriaxone to oral cefpodoxime) [72]. Increasing the number of patients that are appropriately converted to oral antibiotics is associated with a decrease for both direct costs (drug acquisition cost) and indirect cost (including preparation and administration time and cost of IV tubing) [72 - 78]. In fluid-restricted patients, conversion to the oral route is associated with improved patient safety due to a decreased risk for catheter-related infections, infiltration and fluid overload [1, 72]. Additional benefits include decreased risk of needle-stick injury to healthcare works and a potential decrease in patient length of stay [1, 71, 72].

The CDC recommends automatic sequential conversion as a recommended pharmacy-driven intervention to improve antibiotic use [8]. This intervention should be targeted towards antimicrobials with oral bioavailability that can achieve similar systemic concentrations to their IV counterparts [71, 76, 77]. Studies demonstrate decrease in time to conversion and decrease costs without causing patient harm with automatic conversion [73 - 77]. Facilities should work with provider champions (including infectious diseases physicians) and their Pharmacy and Therapeutics committee to establish criteria for identifying appropriate patients for IV to PO conversion. Typical criteria should encompass signs that the patient can tolerate oral intake, is improving clinically and has an indication than can be treated by the oral route [72 - 77].

One study demonstrated an increase in step-down IV to PO conversion therapy through the utilization of a checklist. For all patients receiving any IV antibiotic, a checklist was included in each patient's chart on day three of therapy for the primary physician to complete, resulting in a reduction of days of IV treatment by 19% [1, 74]. The impact of initiatives to improve step-down therapy with IV agents that do not have an oral equivalent or have low oral bioavailability requires further study.

β-lactam Allergy

The treatment of choice for empiric and definitive treatment of many infections consist of β-lactams due to their efficacy and safety profiles [78 - 80]. Approximately 10% of the population and up to 18-25% of hospitalized patients report penicillin allergy [1, 78, 79]. However, more than 90% of patients reporting allergies are not truly allergic and 80% of patients that experienced true allergic reactions lose their IgE sensitivity after 10 years [78, 80, 81]. Furthermore, true anaphylaxis rates to penicillin are low, only 0.01-0.05% [82]. Despite the low incidence of true allergies, these allergies often are not challenged due to fear of anaphylaxis or legal liability. Cross-reactivity rates are likely lower than initially thought between β-lactams and are more likely due to similarities in side chains than the β-lactam ring [80]. Unfortunately, unnecessary avoidance of β-lactams can lead to inferior outcomes in patients with all edged penicillin allergies. Unfortunately, unnecessary avoidance of β-lactams leads to worse outcomes for patients with penicillin allergy labels including increased risk of VRE, *C. difficile*, MRSA, surgical site infections, adverse drug events and clinical treatment failures due to the use of alternative agents [1, 78 - 82]. Limitations of alternative agents include increased adverse effects, increased cost, inferior spectrum of activity, and increased resistance rates [78, 83, 84].

ASP can target a variety of approaches to improve antibiotic use in patients with allergy labels. Obtaining appropriate allergy histories, graded challenges (also known as test doses) and penicillin-skin tests are approaches that can help improve utilization of β-lactams through allergy de-labeling or identification of agents the patient tolerates [78, 80, 85]. Considerations for implementation of these initiatives include creation of algorithms to define criteria to define populations to receive challenges or skin tests, processes to prevent allergy from being added back in future visits, education of staff and patients and collaboration with allergists, when possible [78, 86].

Microbiology Data

The lack of available microbiology data or misinterpretation of the results often contributes to the continued use of inappropriate or unnecessarily broad antibiotic regimens. Collaboration with the microbiology laboratory is an important component of successful antimicrobial stewardship teams to optimize antibiotic utilization and optimize utilization and interpretation of microbiology data [19]. It is important that hospital staff involved in acquiring and transporting culture samples are aware of the importance of proper technique. Misplaced samples and inappropriately drawn blood cultures contribute to diagnostic complications by delaying microbiology results or introducing contamination to samples. A positive and synergistic relationship between the microbiology lab and infectious diseases clinicians is vital for ensuring up to date technology is available and results are reported in a clinically meaningful way.

Antibiogram

Programs should work closely with the microbiology laboratory to develop institutional antibiograms. Antibiograms allow institutions to trend resistance patterns and assist in the development of empiric treatment and surgical prophylaxis guidelines based on local resistance patterns. Antibiograms can assist with empiric selection of antibiotics based on suspected or confirmed organisms [1, 19]. Stratified guidelines by location (such as ICU vs non-ICU) or culture site (urine vs non-urine) has limited evidence to support use but can help identify key differences in susceptibility to provide additional information to optimize empiric therapy [1]. Further information on the construction and reporting of antibiograms is available through the Clinical and Laboratory Standards Institute guidelines.

Susceptibility Reporting

Both selective and cascade reporting of susceptibility results help optimize utilization of preferred antibiotics. Selective reporting lists results for a limited number of selected antibiotics instead of all antibiotics tested. Cascade reporting is an algorithm-based type of selective reporting in which antibiotics are ranked and susceptibilities are released only up to the lowest ranking agents that are susceptible. Rankings can be performed on a variety of criteria such as cost, adverse event profile, and spectrum. An example of cascade reporting would be the following: cefazolin is susceptible to a given organism, later generation cephalosporins (such as ceftriaxone) are not reported. For either method, suppressed results should be released upon clinician request [1, 19]. It is important to also consider the impact of these strategies on the development of an antibiogram in cases where data from suppressed results may not be available for the antibiogram development [1]. Programs should reevaluate their reporting structure periodically to ensure optimal quality of reporting [19].

Carefully worded comments of negative results and flora can assist with AS de-escalation strategies. One program changed their reporting of respiratory cultures isolating flora from "Commensal respiratory flora" to "commensal respiratory flora only: No *S. aureus*/MRSA or *P. aeruginosa*". This change resulted in more frequent de-escalation and discontinuations in the intervention group (73% vs 39% in the control) and resulted in a reduction in acute kidney injury rates (14% vs 31%) [85].

Biomarkers

Procalcitonin (PCT), which is secreted by organs in response to bacterial infections, is the most commonly utilized biomarker in AS. A variety of algorithms and protocols have been evaluated for the utilization of PCT from reducing durations, initiating therapy, broadening therapy, and avoiding initiation of antibiotics [1, 19]. While results have been varied, there have been successful implementations of PCT when combined with AS team efforts to reduce antimicrobial durations without affecting mortality [1, 19, 74].

Rapid Diagnostics

Rapid diagnostic testing (RDT) appears to be a promising avenue to assist with AS strategies as delays in in microbiology results hinder recommendations to optimize antimicrobial regimens [1, 19]. A variety of technologies are emerging and AS teams should work closely with the microbiology laboratory to determine which method would be appropriate for the institution based on cost, speed, burden of samples to test, and types of results available [19]. Success with these programs is most commonly seen when they are instituted in conjunction with stewardship efforts to ensure the results are acted upon in a timely manner. Studies that evaluated RDT without stewardship support or rapid notification of results did not find significant improvements in antibiotic use [1, 19]. AS teams and the microbiology laboratory should determine an agreement for the indications of use and determine how results will display. Additionally, clinicians should receive training on the technology itself, appropriate indications for ordering, limitations of the RDT, turnaround time, and interpretation of results [19].

Computerized Decision Support System (CDSS) and Electronic Health Records

Electronic health records (EHR) and computerized decision support system (CDSS) can assist ASP with the implementation of initiatives to optimize antibiotic utilization by quickly identifying patients for review [14, 23, 28, 43]. A variety of EHR vendors and CDSS platforms exists and each system has pros and cons. Overall, most programs can assist with generating lists of patients to review for various PAF initiatives, incorporating evidence-based treatment guidelines, monitoring for drug dosing in organ impairment, assisting with identifying potential IV-to-PO conversions and alerting ASP team members or clinicians to test results. Most EHRs can also provide methods for programs to require indications on antibiotic orders, and create order sets to assist adherence to institutional specific guidelines [28]. Some programs have even developed tools in their EHR or CDSS to assist with pre authorization requests by having prescribers select specific criteria before allowing targeted agents to be prescribed or dispensed [23, 28]. The largest limitation with the lists of patients created by CDSS or EHR reports is alert fatigue. Real-time alerts can be useful for quickly identifying patients that can benefit from intervention; however, the volume of alerts may be impractical to review in a timely manner. One program found that approximately 76% of their alerts were non-actionable and that it took approximately 2-3 hours per day to review [28]. Additional considerations for implementation include costs and appropriate information technology support [14, 28].

Antibiotic Stewardship in Pediatrics

The untoward effects of antibiotics such as promoting resistance and causing adverse effects have clearly been established. In addition, pediatric specific literature has suggested that early exposure to antibiotics is linked to obesity and greater chance of childhood atopy [87, 88]. With this growing body of literature, many studies have been performed to limit duration or usage of antibiotics, particularly in the outpatient pediatric environment. Pediatric antibiotic prescribing during ambulatory visits accounts for more than 20% of visits [89]. therefore, this has been an interest for years. Efforts to reduce unnecessary antibiotic prescribing in pediatrics have been far more successful than in adults. Pediatric outpatient prescribing has decreased by 13% whereas adult prescriptions have remained the same [90].

A great opportunity exists for improvement in all populations, including pediatrics. The National Action Plan for Combating Antibiotic-Resistant Bacteria set a goal to reduce inappropriate outpatient antibiotic use by 50% by 2020 [6]. The challenge is that although there have been many successful interventions previously shown, the sustainability is questionable. Gerber and colleagues conducted an outpatient pediatric ambulatory study with interventions including provider education and commitment posters [91]. They showed a significant reduction in antibiotic prescribing for acute respiratory tract infections (ARTIs), however, when the education ceased, antibiotic prescribing resumed at a normal rate again. Programs aimed at reducing antibiotic prescribing with lasting effects need to be widely implemented. In addition to reduction of antibiotic usage, pediatric programs have had to focus on the many antibiotic dosing errors that exist in this population which makes it unique in terms of needs [92, 93]. Pediatric specific treatment guidelines have being developed on a national level in conjunction with various national infectious diseases and pediatric organizations in order to streamline overall management of various infections in this patient population. In addition, the CDC has pediatric specific treatment recommendations for acute sinusitis, acute otitis media, pharyngitis, common cold, and other common upper respiratory illnesses [90]. In terms of methodology for inpatient practice, it is recommended to have prior approval/formulary restriction in addition to audit and feedback (Magsarili H) [94]. Prompt de-escalation, dosing optimization, and limiting duration if possible are key components for pediatric patients.

Antibiotic Stewardship in Hematologic Malignancy

The oncology population is quite vulnerable to antibiotic associated adverse effects and are particularly susceptible to superinfection such as *C.difficile*. In our era of worsening antibiotic resistance, limiting unnecessary antibiotic usage in this population, is more critical than ever. This population is often difficult to assess due to atypical clinical presentations and laboratory studies coupled with high susceptibility to infections and long differentials for fevers. Prophylaxis against viral and fungal infections have been established, however, antibacterial prophylaxis remains somewhat controversial. Many cancer centers have stopped recommending fluoroquinolone prophylaxis due to the growing rate of resistance as well as antibiotic related toxicity. Although efficacy of quinolone prophylaxis in reducing Gram-negative infections has been previously established [95]. it has also been shown to drive Gram-negative resistance [96, 97]. Caution must be made when initiating any antimicrobial, particularly in this patient population.

While inpatient guidelines for management of febrile neutropenia do exist, many of the recommendations are grey in terms of discontinuation of Gram-negative coverage. The guidelines specify appropriate usage of vancomycin (or other MRSA active therapy), both for initiation and prompt de-escalation, intravenous catheter management, and the importance of de-escalation when a bacterial isolate is recovered from a clinical specimen [98]. Limited data exists on specific durations for documented infections in the oncology population. However, a growing body of literature is being published on evidence for more rapid de-escalation in patients admitted with febrile neutropenia. Aguilar-Guisado and colleagues performed an investigator-driven, superiority, open-label randomized controlled phase 4 trial to evaluate whether discontinuation of empiric antimicrobial therapy by clinical evaluation versus neutrophil count was safe and effective at reducing unnecessary antibiotic exposure. A total of 157 episodes (78 in experimental group; 79 in control group) were evaluated. Overall, this study, albeit small, found that antimicrobials can be safely discontinued in high risk patients with hematologic malignancy once they have been afebrile for 72 hours and have clinically recovered. Many more studies are ongoing in order to establish safety with early discontinuation of antimicrobials in this population. In May of 2018, IDSA and American Society of Clinical Oncology (ASCO) published guidelines on outpatient management of febrile neutropenia in conjunction with IDSA [99]. These should be reviewed when managing an oncologic patient with febrile neutropenia in the outpatient setting.

Antibiotic Stewardship in the Intensive Care Unit (ICU)

Patients in the intensive care unit are particularly vulnerable to developing multi-drug resistant infections. The causes for acquisition of MDR pathogens are multifactorial including but not limited to necessitating central lines, endotracheal tubes, urinary catheters, feeding tubes, *etc.* as well as receipt of broad-spectrum antibiotics for a variety of indications. Properly diagnosing infections in many of these patients can be challenging as they often have multiple comorbidities alongside the acute problems rendering imaging and laboratory work potentially less useful than in non-ICU patients. Appropriate antibiotic prescribing is essential to help avoid further development of antibiotic resistant infections and while this concept is not specific to the ICU, it is of utmost importance here. Diagnostic uncertainty in patients with fever and multiple potential sources of infection often leads to multiple antibiotic courses throughout their stay. The concern that many clinicians have in performing antibiotic stewardship (AS) activities in the ICU is worse outcomes. However, a systematic review evaluating 11 studies that used mortality as an endpoint did not identify a change in mortality associated with active AS in the ICU [100]. Key items to focus on when conducting AS is the ICU include appropriate empiric selection, prompt de-escalation when culture data is available, limiting duration to what is necessary, and ensuring need for antibiotics. These activities need to be conducted in conjunction with the primary ICU team who is closely evaluating the patient [101]. Utilizing published guidelines and new evidence-based recommendations to guide duration is critical in the ICU. In addition, various tools and strategies to assist with de-escalation have been evaluated in the ICU setting and all have a role, albeit, not without their own limitations.

MRSA nasal screening has been shown to have a high specificity and negative predictive value for ruling out MRSA pneumonia thereby allowing for earlier de-escalation of anti- MRSA active agents such as vancomycin [102]. However, in certain cases, it may be difficult to de-escalate vancomycin regardless of the absence of MRSA colonization in the nares. For example, necrotizing or cavitary pneumonias may require continuation of vancomycin until definitive confirmation that MRSA is not involved. As with any test, clinical correlation and careful evaluation is warranted when using MRSA nasal screens in ICU patients. Another tool that can assist with earlier de-escalation is use of procalcitonin (PCT), a biomarker that is upregulated in many bacterial infections. It is considered much more specific for bacterial infection than C-reactive protein or other inflammatory markers. Systemic response to infection often leads to progressive elevation of PCT. Many studies have evaluated its utility for a variety of infections, both in the inpatient and outpatient setting. Many of the studies focused on its use in sepsis and in respiratory infections. Data on its use in distinguishing bacterial vs viral meningitis is also ample. Studies have shown conflicting data in terms of clinical outcomes and mortality [103]. However, when used correctly and it the right setting, it undoubtedly reduces antibiotic duration which can be incredibly useful for antibiotic stewardship [104 - 106]. Ultimately appropriate de-escalation in the ICU is critical but careful considerations are necessary. Use of guidelines, biomarkers, and other tools can be helpful in assisting the clinician with assessment of infection.

OUTPATIENT STEWARDSHIP

In 2016, 273 million antibiotic prescriptions were dispensed from outpatient settings in the US, with the highest number prescribed per 1000 residents in Kentucky [107]. It is unclear why some states have significantly higher antibiotic prescribing rates than others, but patients in southern states typically get more antibiotics (*e.g.* acute respiratory tract infections). The CDC evaluates trends in antibiotic prescribing and found that from 2011 to 2015 there were decreases overall in outpatient antibiotic prescribing nationwide, but mostly driven by a reduction in pediatric prescriptions with minimal change seen in adult prescriptions. Overall, it appears that over 30% of outpatient prescriptions are unnecessary [108]. Additionally, many patients don't receive first line therapy when antibiotics are indicated [109]. For example, patients may receive amoxicillin/clavulanate for acute otitis media or sinusitis when amoxicillin is first line. This results in unnecessary broad spectrum antibiotic use, putting patients at risk of developing resistance to amoxicillin/clavulanate, or diarrheal illness.

Diagnoses that often result in outpatient antibiotic prescriptions are respiratory and urinary tract infections. One of the antibiotic classes of most concern and most in need of stewardship initiatives is fluoroquinolones. With concerning adverse events including *C. difficile* infection and aortic aneurysm, they should be prescribed with caution [110]. Those areas can be targets for AS. Additionally, providers who prescribe a significant proportion of antibiotics include nurse practitioners, physician assistants, and dentists. ASP can also target these providers in addition to physicians. Sociology research shows that often providers in outpatient settings feel rushed, feel pressured by patients, or fear "under treating" their patients. The CDC provides guidance on outpatient antibiotic stewardship and a new proposal from the Joint Commission states that they plan to require antimicrobial stewardship in ambulatory care settings in the future [7]. Public education and awareness are ways to start reducing the demand for antibiotic prescriptions by patients. Using the "watch and wait" method to delay antibiotic prescriptions for likely viral infections can also be useful. Additionally, using diagnostic testing can help by allowing providers to test for viral illnesses or receive rapid bacterial results in some cases.

Emergency Departments and Urgent Care Clinics

When patients present to the emergency department (ED) or urgent care (UC), they are often feeling very ill and may specifically request antibiotics. Culture and laboratory results are not often readily available while the patient is in the UC or ED. A nationwide survey has demonstrated that UC facilities prescribe a significant amount of antibiotics in the outpatient setting, compared to other types of facilities. An analysis of outpatient practices found that while physician offices had the highest visit volume, UC and retail clinics (*e.g.* Minute Clinic) had higher rates of antibiotic prescriptions than ED and physician offices, and that UC clinics provided the most inappropriate antibiotic prescriptions [111].

Physicians may often interpret patient complaints as antibiotic-seeking, however one survey has found this not to be consistently accurate. Patients may just be seeking more information or looking for symptom resolution, rather than specifically for antibiotics [36, 112, 113]. Often, providers may feel rushed and lack the ability to perform viral tests to rule out bacterial infection promptly. This can also lead to inappropriate antibiotic use.

The appropriateness of antibiotic prescribing in an emergency department in Australia has also been evaluated. In their study, antibiotics were inappropriate over 30% of the time in children and adults, and patients were more likely to get inappropriate antibiotics if they were deemed to be septic. They found that excessively broad spectrum antibiotics made up the majority of inappropriate antibiotics [114]. These are all indicators of the need for stewardship practices in the ED and UC settings.

To implement stewardship practices, some clinics have added posters stating that the providers are committed to safe antibiotic practices [115]. Other ideas would include providing flyers or education to patients in outpatient offices stating that not every infection is bacterial or requires antibiotics. With a thorough explanation as to why antibiotics are not appropriate for a specific patient, patients may be more understanding of provider decisions not to provide antibiotics, which can result in a decrease in inappropriate antibiotic usage. This requires education to providers of all levels (*e.g.* nurse practitioners and physician assistants) about the appropriate prescribing of antibiotics.

Dental

Dentists frequently prescribe antibiotics to patients who have evidence of an infection, or patients who may be at risk of developing a post-procedural infection. Antibiotic prescriptions by dentists are increasing; approximately 10% of antibiotic prescriptions written in the outpatient setting are from dentists [107,

116]. The average defined daily doses (DDD) prescribed by dentists was near that of physicians and surgeons [116]. The American Dental Association (ADA) provides guidance to dentists on AS. They state that patients with a history of prosthetic joints do not require antibiotics prior to dental procedures due to a low risk of joint infection. Guidelines from the American Heart Association (AHA) provide guidance for patients who may be at a higher risk for infections after dental procedures. They explain that daily dental hygiene presents a greater risk for transient bacteremia episodes, simply due to the sheer number of times people typically brush their teeth compared to the number of dental visits the average person has per year. Patients who have a history of joint arthroplasty are also not at a greater risk for developing infections after dental procedures, and therefore they typically do not need any antibiotic prophylaxis [117]. Additionally, patients with prosthetic joints who do receive antibiotics prior to dental procedures do not have a decreased risk of joint infections. The ADA recommends that the orthopedic surgeon, rather than the dentist, be the one to prescribe antibiotics for patients in whom the risk of an infection outweighs the risks of antibiotics.

For the prevention of endocarditis after dental procedures, there are certain circumstances (see Fig. **1**) which may necessitate antibiotic prophylaxis, however it is not required for all patients [118, 119]. Only patients at a high risk of developing an infection, or a high risk of complications from endocarditis (*e.g.* history of IE or prosthetic valves) should be considered as candidates for antibiotic prophylaxis [119].

❖ prosthetic cardiac valves, including transcatheter-implanted prostheses and homografts
❖ prosthetic material used for cardiac valve repair, such as annuloplasty rings and chords
❖ history of infective endocarditis
❖ cardiac transplant with valve regurgitation due to a structurally abnormal valve
❖ congenital heart disease:
   ➤ unrepaired cyanotic congenital heart disease, including palliative shunts and conduits
   ➤ repaired congenital heart defect with residual shunts, or valvular regurgitation at the site of or adjacent to the site of a prosthetic patch or a prosthetic device

---

Fig. (1). Prevention of endocarditis in dental procedures - Criteria for antibiotic use.

Antibiotics are not without risk in any population. In 2017 a study specifically evaluated the link between dentist prescribed antibiotics and *C. difficile* infection in Minnesota [120]. Of all community acquired CDI over 6 years, 15% of the confirmed antibiotic associated cases were from dental antibiotic prescriptions [121]. It is crucial to include dentists and the dental community in outpatient AS efforts. High quality studies that link antibiotics to harm and don't show increases in dental infections are needed to persuade dentists to decrease antibiotic prescribing.

The American Dental Association (ADA) developed guidelines for appropriate antibiotic prescribing [122]. Antibiotics that target oral flora are often used for treatment or prophylaxis of dental infections. Clindamycin is commonly used as it covers many of these bacteria [121]. It also carries the highest risk of *C. difficile* among oral antibiotics [123]. The ADA guidelines list examples of narrow and broad spectrum antibiotics as a reference for dentists. Clindamycin has been listed as a narrow spectrum antibiotic, despite having a relatively wide spectrum of activity. Others listed in this category include metronidazole and penicillin. Several other β-lactams, along with macrolides and tetracyclines are listed as broad spectrum. Based on these guidelines, clindamycin likely gets unnecessarily overused [122].

Dentists must be included in AS discussions and to make sure patients who are having dental procedures performed understand their risk of infection, or lack thereof. In general, most dental procedures do not require an antibiotic, and when they do, the most narrow spectrum antibiotic should be chosen (*e.g.* amoxicillin). For patients who state that they have an allergy to penicillins, the dentist and pharmacist should determine whether or not this is a true allergy. Avoiding amoxicillin in favor of a more broad, non-β-lactam option is not ideal when the patient doesn't have a true allergy.

Lastly, while dental abscesses can often be drained without receipt of antibiotics, one condition, Ludwig's angina, is an emergency that requires prompt attention in an emergency room and antibiotics [121, 124]. Aside from this condition, antibiotics are not frequently necessary in the dental setting. Education to dentists and other dental professionals, as well as to patients at the time of their visits is important in reducing the number of antibiotic prescriptions written by dentists. Asking patients about their antibiotic allergies or obtaining medical records prior to prescribing clindamycin can also reduce the number of unnecessarily broad spectrum antibiotics prescribed.

Dialysis Centers

As with other outpatient settings, many patients receiving chronic hemodialysis are often prescribed unnecessary antibiotics. Reducing the number of prescriptions provided to hemodialysis patients is key, and education to providers in this setting may decrease inappropriate prescribing. Over 30% of antibiotics prescribed to patients in hemodialysis centers are deemed inappropriate [125]. Interventions targeting this population have shown some reduction in antimicrobial prescriptions, but no significant changes in patient outcomes.

Important methods for reducing inappropriate use of antibiotics in dialysis centers can focus on using the most narrow spectrum antibiotic, when a true infection is present, and no antibiotic when no infection is present. For example, there is literature stating that vancomycin is often used to treat MSSA bacteremia in this setting, but there is significant evidence that β-lactams should be used for MSSA in patients who do not have a true penicillin allergy. Education to providers regarding the most narrow and specific regimen could help them make more educated decisions regarding antimicrobial choice. Additionally, choosing oral agents over intravenous (IV) agents can cut down on the number of lines a patient requires, or the frequency with which they are accessed, reducing the possibility of catheter-related infections [126].

Patients who receive regular hemodialysis are not necessarily at a higher risk for MDRO than other patients, and may not need broad spectrum antibiotics. It is also important to rule out other causes of illness. For example, patients complaining of shortness of breath may be fluid overloaded rather than have a respiratory illness.

Patients receiving dialysis are at risk for bloodstream infections as well as SSTI's. In 2014 there were over 29,000 bloodstream infections reported from dialysis centers nationwide, and *Staph. aureus* was the predominant organism isolated. The CDC has created The Making Dialysis Safer for Patients Coalition to reduce dialysis related infections and improve patient outcomes. They use evidence-based literature to provide guidance for infection prevention measures [127, 128,]. Infection prevention through proper hygiene practices is crucial to preventing infections in the dialysis setting. All providers and staff in dialysis centers should be practicing hand hygiene when working directly with patients.

Nursing Homes and Long Term Care Facilities

Despite a great need for antimicrobial agents, overuse of them has led to increasing antibiotic resistance and the need for stricter control of their use. Patients in nursing homes or long-term care facilities often get prescribed antibiotics without even being seen by a provider. Since elderly patients are at a higher risk for adverse events, antibiotics should be prescribed to them with caution. The CDC statement on AS in nursing homes cites that 40-75% of antibiotics prescribed in nursing homes may be inappropriate, similar to rates seen in the hospital setting [13]. Often, antibiotic associated adverse events occur more frequently in the elderly population, or are more severe [129]. This includes *C. difficile* infection, which can be detrimental to the elderly [130]. As with other healthcare settings, appropriate use of antibiotics in nursing facilities is vital to avoid complications.

The CDC and Association for Health Research and Quality (AHRQ) have developed guidance specifically for nursing homes and other long-term care facilities on implementation of AS. The Centers for Medicare and Medicaid services (CMS) mandated that nursing homes have a stewardship program by the end of 2017. New guidelines were developd by SHEA and the Association for Professionals in Infection Control and Epidemiology (APIC) to provide guidance for nursing homes and LTCF [133]. Performing AS in NH and LTCF presents a challenge, but is an important task since there are so many nursing home residents [131]. There are approximately 1.4 million residents in NHs within the USA, and 2-5% of the developed world's older population is in a LTCF [132]. With one report of 5.3% infection prevalence among LTCF residents [132]., treating these patients for infections is a concern especially since there are not always physicians or laboratory facilities on-site. Nursing staff are frequently the front-line healthcare workers who evaluate the patients and make recommendations for starting antimicrobial therapy. One study reported that non-physician providers more often prescribe antibiotics for suspected infections than physicians do. Point prevalence studies have reported 7-10% antibiotic usage within LTCF [132].

Reports of high rates of UTIs and treatment of UTIs and ASB in LTCFs demonstrate the need for stewardship and proper assessment of patients. Inappropriate assessment of ASB as a UTI can lead to unnecessary antibiotic use. There are also reports of patients with urinary catheters in LTCFs who have higher rates of antibiotic use than those without urinary catheters [134]. Patient assessment by a provider is key, rather than having a nurse or staff member describe patient symptoms to an off-site provider. All nurses and providers in LTCFs should have some type of AS education to ensure appropriate antibiotic use.

Stewardship practices that have been documented in LTCFs include education to nurses and providers, facility specific algorithms and guidelines, and assessments with feedback of antibiotic prescribing that were provided to prescribers [135]. It can be helpful to have a consultant pharmacist who is educated in AS on staff or available at these facilities to work with the nursing staff and coordinate with off-site providers to ensure unnecessary antibiotics are avoided and the most appropriate ones are used when indicated.

Telemedicine

Many studies that have evaluated AS have evaluated programs with robust infectious diseases departments, or dedicated antimicrobial stewardship clinicians. However, there are community and more rural hospitals that may not have infectious diseases clinicians on site to provide these services regularly. The

Infectious Diseases Society of America supports telemedicine or telehealth practices for institutions that don't have their own infectious diseases or stewardship clinicians [136]. They offer suggestions such as providing education via technology, or consultation with providers at the institution on specific cases. One multicenter trial of remote AS practices at 15 community hospitals suggests that more intensive interventions may be necessary versus passive monitoring, to achieve optimal antimicrobial stewardship practices [137]. They divided up the small hospitals to receive one of 3 models. The first included basic AS education and tools, access to an infectious disease hotline, and antibiotic utilization data. The hospitals in the 2nd model received those interventions plus advanced education, audit and feedback for select antibiotics, and locally controlled antibiotic restrictions. Hospitals in the 3rd group received program 2 interventions plus audit and feedback on the majority of antibiotics, and an infectious diseases-trained clinician approved restricted antibiotics and reviewed microbiology results. Hospitals in the first 2 models did not show a significant reduction in antibiotic use during the study period, whereas hospitals in group 3 did.

A quasi-experimental study in a 220-bed hospital in Brazil aimed to evaluate the impact of a telemedicine ASP on antimicrobial resistance and consumption. Infectious diseases physicians were available by phone, email, or text 7 days per week, and providers could accept or reject ID recommendations. They used post-prescription audit and feedback to intervene. They saw an increased rate of appropriate antibiotic prescribing from 2014 to 2016, a reduction in hospital-acquired CDI, an overall reduction in antimicrobial resistance (particularly in *Acinetobacter*), and a significant cost reduction over the study period. Overall, they found the program to be effective, and received quick responses from remote ID providers [138].

Lastly, a telehealth-based ASP was implemented in 2 community hospitals (part of a large health system network) in Pennsylvania that aimed to evaluate and improve treatment of LRTI and SSTI, as well as reduce use of select antimicrobial agents. Pharmacists from the remote hospitals were trained to perform AS and communicated with ID physicians, and AS clinicians at another site who remotely reviewed patients. They found a high acceptance rate of recommendations, increased rates of ID consultation, significant reductions in selected antimicrobials during the 6-month study period, and significant cost savings [139].

For institutions in which infectious diseases clinicians are not available on site, telemedicine stewardship is an effective tool that should be considered. Small hospitals that are part of a larger health system likely have access to ID clinicians at their larger counterparts, whereas small independent community hospitals may have to employ private practice ID physicians from urban areas, or collaborate with larger institutions to share AS resources.

SUMMARY

- Tracking and reporting of antimicrobial use within a variety of healthcare settings is vital for improving the appropriateness of antimicrobial use. This is mandated in most settings, and there is guidance on what metrics to track.
- Programs should review their current antimicrobial formulary and any newly FDA-approved antimicrobials and modifications to package inserts to determine any prescribing restrictions by designating agents as formulary, non-formulary or restricted.
  - Formulary restriction confines prescriptions for targeted antimicrobials to pre-defined criteria to decrease their use for reasons of cost, potential toxicities, and resistance trends.
  - Prospective audit and feedback (PAF) is the process of external review of the antibiotic regimen for appropriateness with recommendations made to the treating team to optimize therapy.
- Stewardship practices in the outpatient setting and LTCFs are increasing, as antibiotics are prescribed in all outpatient settings, and there will soon be more guidance on requirements for AS in outpatient settings (Table **3**).

Table 3. Summary of Stewardship Interventions.

Intervention	Recommended Setting	Potential Benefits	Potential Cons/Obstacles	Example
Allergy Management	All	• Improve patient outcomes • ↓cost • ↓VRE, *C. difficile*, MRSA	• Labor intensive	• Optimize allergy histories • Test dose/challenges • Penicillin skin tests
Antibiogram	Inpatient, LTCF, ED	More appropriate empiric antimicrobial choices	• Labor intensive to develop • Most useful if different floors/areas are separated (*e.g.* ICU vs ED)	Choosing cefepime over meropenem for hospital-acquired pneumonia if *Pseudomonas* susceptibility is high for cefepime.
Antibiotic Cycling or Mixing	Not recommended	↓ development of resistance	High resource utilization	Antibiotic cycling every 6 weeks between 3rd or 4th generation cephalosporins, piperacillin/tazobactam and carbapenems

(Table 3) cont.....

Intervention	Recommended Setting	Potential Benefits	Potential Cons/Obstacles	Example
Antibiotic Time Out	Inpatient LTCF	• ↓ DOT • ↓ cost • ↓ Duration	• Alert fatigue • IT support	• Pop-up in EHR on day 3 of antibiotic • Pharmacist prompt on rounds to question if antibiotics are still needed.
Automatic IV to PO Conversion	Inpatient, possibly LTCF	• ↓cost • ↓length of stay • ↑patient safety • ↓ nursing and pharmacy workload	• Dedicated time and staff to review • Conversion criteria should be easily identifiable in the chart	Automatic conversion by a pharmacist of IV to PO levofloxacin in patients meeting established criteria (*i.e.* oral intake, signs of clinical improvement, indication that can be treated by oral route)
Automatic Stop Orders	Inpatient, LTCF	• ↓ Duration	Antibiotics could "drop off" without someone realizing	• 10 day stop date on all antibiotic orders • 5 day stop date on azithromycin for pneumonia • 24 H duration for surgical prophylaxis
Behavioral Change	All	• Optimize antimicrobial prescribing • Promotes collegial intervention • Sustained impact on prescribing habits	• Limited data on implementation techniques	Have prescribers/departments select their own goal for improvement each quarter/year (or other designated time frame)
Biomarkers and Rapid Diagnostics	All	• ↓overall costs • ↓ DOT • ↓ duration	• Initial high costs (acquisition of new technology) • Education to lab staff on new technology	• Procalcitonin algorithm to reduce antibiotic durations for CAP • Rapid diagnostics to identify coagulase negative staphylococcus in the blood
Clinical Practice Guidelines	All	• Standardize empiric prescribing by indication	• Require period maintenance	• Facility-specific guidelines for empiric treatment of pneumonia • Internal antimicrobial prophylaxis guidelines for surgery

(Table 3) cont.....

Intervention	Recommended Setting	Potential Benefits	Potential Cons/Obstacles	Example
Computerized decision support systems	All	● More rapid identification of patients for stewardship review	● Alert fatigue ● IT resources ● Acquisition cost of software	● Identification of patients for IV to PO conversion ● Requiring indications on antibiotic orders ● Electronic order sets for empiric treatment
Dose Optimization	Inpatient, LTCF	● Optimize therapeutic drug monitoring ● ↓ cost ● ↓ nephrotoxicity/adverse events ● +/- ↑ efficacy ● +/- ↓ resistance (optimization of PK/PD) ● +/- optimize outcomes (LOS and mortality)	● High initial burden with protocol development, training and technology implementation ● Low maintenance resource utilization ● Pharmacist time	● Extended infusion of piperacillin/tazobactam ● Vancomycin dosing and monitoring by pharmacy protocol ● Automatic dose adjustment by pharmacy for select antibiotics based on renal function
Duration of therapy	All	● ↓ DOT ● ↓ cost ● ↓ adverse events/CDI	● Labor time ● +/- IT resources	● PAF review of all antibiotics at day 5 of therapy ● Restriction of meropenem requiring justification for continued use beyond 72 hours
Education	All	● ↑ appropriateness of antibiotic prescribing ● ↑ recognition of the problem of antimicrobial resistance	● can be labor intensive to develop and distribute materials ● Minimal sustained effects on prescribing behavior	● In-service on new initiative targeted community-acquired pneumonia ● Emailed monthly brief educational tip
Peer comparison	All	● ↓ inappropriate antibiotic prescribing	● Limited data outside the outpatient setting ● Potential for misrepresentation of data to "game" the system	Report card comparing providers to their peers for rate of antibiotic prescriptions for diagnosis of bronchitis

(Table 3) cont.....

Intervention	Recommended Setting	Potential Benefits	Potential Cons/Obstacles	Example
Preauthorization (aka Restriction)	Inpatient, LTCF	• ↓ utilization of targeted agents • ↓ Resistance • ± ↑ appropriateness of initial cultures	• ↓ provider autonomy • Labor intensive • May not address de-escalation • May lead to ↑ utilization of unrestricted agents • Requires off-hours process or 24H approval process • Potential for misrepresentation of data to "game" the system	• Restriction of Ceftazidime/avibactam to infectious diseases consult only • Restricting Meropenem to approval by antimicrobial stewardship team member
Prospective audit and feedback	Inpatient (other settings if staffing permits)	• ↑ de-escalation • ↓ DOT • ↓ Cost • Promotes collegial relationship • ± improved patient outcomes	• Alert fatigue • Labor intensive • Usually does not address appropriateness of empiric regimens • Compliance is voluntary	• Drug-bug mismatches • Duplicate coverage • Duration of therapy • De-escalation
Reduce Use of Antibiotics with High Risk of CDI	All	• ↓incidence CDI and associated morbidity	• Labor time • ± cons associated with preauthorization or PAF depending on methods utilized	Restriction of broad spectrum antibiotics to ID consult
Susceptibility Reporting	All	• ↑ utilization of preferred antimicrobials	• Consider impact of suppressed results on antibiogram development • Method to allow suppressed results to be released upon clinician request	• Selective reporting • Cascade reporting

(Table 3) cont.....

Intervention	Recommended Setting	Potential Benefits	Potential Cons/Obstacles	Example
Targeting Specific Syndromes	All	• Optimize antibiotic regimens for select indications • ↓ durations • ↓ antibiotic utilization • Improve patient outcomes • Optimize diagnostics	• Labor time to build bundles and monitor compliance and outcomes with bundles	• Bundles of initiatives to optimize empiric treatment and reduce antibiotic durations for CAP • Initiative bundles to improve treatment of *staphylococcus aureus* bacteremia
Tracking and Reporting	All	• ↑awareness and support for the program and it's initiatives • Identify areas for improvement	• Labor intensive to perform data collection or to develop tools to for compiling and analyzing data • Optimal metrics not yet elucidated and difficult to measure impact on outcomes	• DOT • SAAR • Antibiotic expenditures • Prescription rates for high-priority conditions (*i.e.* bronchitis)

CONSENT FOR PUBLICATION

Not applicable.

CONFLICT OF INTEREST

Lucia Rose is on the speakers' bureau for Allergan. Madeline King is on the speaker's bureau for Tetraphase.

ACKNOWLEDGEMENTS

Declared none.

REFERENCES

[1]   Barlam TF, Cosgrove SE, Abbo LM, *et al.* Implementing an antibiotic stewardship program: guidelines by the infectious diseases society of america and the society for healthcare epidemiology of America. Clin Infect Dis 2016; 62(10): e51-77.
[http://dx.doi.org/10.1093/cid/ciw118] [PMID: 27080992]

[2]   Centers for Disease Control and Prevention. Antibiotic resistance threats in the United States [Internet] 2013. [cited 2018 Nov 27].   https://www.cdc.gov/drugresistance/threat-report-2013/pdf/ar-thre-ts-2013-508.pdf

[3]   ACH surveillance for antimicrobial use and antimicrobial resistance options | NHSN | CDC [Internet] , 2018 [cited 2018 Dec 21]; https://www.cdc.gov/nhsn/acute-care-hospital/aur/index.html

[4]   President's Council of Advisors on Science and Technology [Internet]. The White House , [cited 2019 Feb 19.];https://obamawhitehouse.archives.gov/node/8490

[5]   World Health Organization. Global Action Plan on Antimicrobial Resistance 2015.

[6]   Centers for Disease Control and Prevention. National action plan for combating antibiotic-resistant bacteria 2015; 63.

[7]   The joint commission. Proposed New Requirements for Antimicrobial Stewardship [Internet] 2018. [cited 2019 Feb 18]. https://jointcommission.az1.qualtrics.com/WRQualtricsControlPanel/File.php? F=F_eJ88Q1VIj0hLKjr

[8]   Centers for Disease Control and Prevention. Core Elements of Hospital Antibiotic Stewardship Programs. Atlanta, GA: US Department of Health and Human Services, CDC 2019.

[9]   Bennett N, Schulz L, Boyd S, Newland JG. Understanding inpatient antimicrobial stewardship metrics. Am J Health-Syst Pharm AJHP Off J Am Soc Health-Syst Pharm 2018; 15;75(4): 230-8.
        [http://dx.doi.org/10.2146/ajhp160335]

[10]   WHOCC - Definition and general considerations [Internet]. WHOCC 2018. [cited 2018 Dec 20]. https://www.whocc.no/ddd/definition_and_general_considera/

[11]   Meeker D, Linder JA, Fox CR, *et al.* Effect of behavioral interventions on inappropriate antibiotic prescribing among primary care practices: a randomized clinical trial. JAMA 2016; 315(6): 562-70.
        [http://dx.doi.org/10.1001/jama.2016.0275] [PMID: 26864410]

[12]   Sanchez GV, Fleming-Dutra KE, Roberts RM, Hicks LA. Core elements of outpatient antibiotic stewardship. MMWR Recomm Rep 2016; 65(No. RR-6): 1-12.
        [http://dx.doi.org/10.15585/mmwr.rr6506a1]

[13]   Centers for disease control and prevention. The Core Elements of Antibiotic Stewardship for Nursing Homes. Atlanta, GA: US Department of Health and Human Services, CDC 2015.

[14]   MacDougall C, Polk RE. Antimicrobial stewardship programs in health care systems. Clin Microbiol Rev 2005; 18(4): 638-56.
        [http://dx.doi.org/10.1128/CMR.18.4.638-656.2005] [PMID: 16223951]

[15]   Davey P, Brown E, Charani E, *et al.* Interventions to improve antibiotic prescribing practices for hospital inpatients. Cochrane Database Syst Rev [Internet] 2013. [cited 2018 Dec 20]. https://www.readcube.com/articles/10.1002/14651858.CD003543.pub3
        [http://dx.doi.org/10.1002/14651858.CD003543.pub3]

[16]   https://sidp.org/StewardshipCertificate

[17]   https://mad-id.org/antimicrobial-stewardship-programs/

[18]   Davey P, Marwick CA, Scott CL, Charani E, McNeil K, Brown E, *et al.* Interventions to improve antibiotic prescribing practices for hospital inpatients. Cochrane Database Syst Rev 2017; 09: 2-CD003543.
        [http://dx.doi.org/10.1002/14651858.CD003543.pub4]

[19]   Morency-Potvin P, Schwartz DN, Weinstein RA. Antimicrobial stewardship: how the microbiology laboratory can right the ship. Clin Microbiol Rev 2016; 30(1): 381-407.
        [http://dx.doi.org/10.1128/CMR.00066-16] [PMID: 27974411]

[20]   Tamma PD, Avdic E, Keenan JF, *et al.* What is the more effective antibiotic stewardship intervention: preprescription authorization or postprescription review with feedback? Clin Infect Dis 2017; 64(5): 537-43.
        [PMID: 27927861]

[21]   Bradley JS. Alternatives to consider during cefotaxime shortage. AAP News 2015; E150225-1.

[22]   Linkin DR, Fishman NO, Landis JR, *et al.* Effect of communication errors during calls to an antimicrobial stewardship program. Infect Control Hosp Epidemiol 2007; 28(12): 1374-81.

[http://dx.doi.org/10.1086/523861] [PMID: 17994518]

[23]   Buising KL, Thursky KA, Robertson MB, *et al.* Electronic antibiotic stewardship--reduced consumption of broad-spectrum antibiotics using a computerized antimicrobial approval system in a hospital setting. J Antimicrob Chemother 2008; 62(3): 608-16.
[http://dx.doi.org/10.1093/jac/dkn218] [PMID: 18550680]

[24]   van Duijn PJ, Verbrugghe W, Jorens PG, *et al.* The effects of antibiotic cycling and mixing on antibiotic resistance in intensive care units: a cluster-randomised crossover trial. Lancet Infect Dis 2018; 18(4): 401-9.
[http://dx.doi.org/10.1016/S1473-3099(18)30056-2] [PMID: 29396000]

[25]   Beardmore RE, Peña-Miller R, Gori F, Iredell J. Antibiotic cycling and antibiotic mixing: which one best mitigates antibiotic resistance? Mol Biol Evol 2017; 34(4): 802-17.
[http://dx.doi.org/10.1093/molbev/msw292] [PMID: 28096304]

[26]   Camins BC, King MD, Wells JB, *et al.* Impact of an antimicrobial utilization program on antimicrobial use at a large teaching hospital: a randomized controlled trial. Infect Control Hosp Epidemiol 2009; 30(10): 931-8.
[http://dx.doi.org/10.1086/605924] [PMID: 19712032]

[27]   Liew YX, Lee W, Tay D, *et al.* Prospective audit and feedback in antimicrobial stewardship: is there value in early reviewing within 48 h of antibiotic prescription? Int J Antimicrob Agents 2015; 45(2): 168-73.
[http://dx.doi.org/10.1016/j.ijantimicag.2014.10.018] [PMID: 25511192]

[28]   Forrest GN, Van Schooneveld TC, Kullar R, Schulz LT, Duong P, Postelnick M. Use of electronic health records and clinical decision support systems for antimicrobial stewardship. Clin Infect Dis 2014; 59 (Suppl. 3): S122-33.
[http://dx.doi.org/10.1093/cid/ciu565] [PMID: 25261539]

[29]   DiazGranados CA. Prospective audit for antimicrobial stewardship in intensive care: impact on resistance and clinical outcomes. Am J Infect Control 2012; 40(6): 526-9.
[http://dx.doi.org/10.1016/j.ajic.2011.07.011] [PMID: 21937145]

[30]   Bessesen MT, Ma A, Clegg D, *et al.* Antimicrobial stewardship programs: comparison of a program with infectious diseases pharmacist support to a program with a geographic pharmacist staffing model. Hosp Pharm 2015; 50(6): 477-83.
[http://dx.doi.org/10.1310/hpj5006-477] [PMID: 26405339]

[31]   Carreno JJ, Kenney RM, Bloome M, *et al.* Evaluation of pharmacy generalists performing antimicrobial stewardship services. Am J Health Syst Pharm 2015; 72(15): 1298-303.
[http://dx.doi.org/10.2146/ajhp140619] [PMID: 26195656]

[32]   LaRocco A Jr. Concurrent antibiotic review programs--a role for infectious diseases specialists at small community hospitals. Clin Infect Dis 2003; 37(5): 742-3.
[http://dx.doi.org/10.1086/377286] [PMID: 12942418]

[33]   Freeman T, Eschenauer G, Patel T, *et al.* Evaluating the need for antibiotic stewardship prospective audit and feedback on weekends. Infect Control Hosp Epidemiol 2017; 38(10): 1262-3.
[http://dx.doi.org/10.1017/ice.2017.174] [PMID: 28826421]

[34]   Siegfried J, Merchan C, Scipione MR, Papadopoulos J, Dabestani A, Dubrovskaya Y. Role of postgraduate year 2 pharmacy residents in providing weekend antimicrobial stewardship coverage in an academic medical center. Am J Health Syst Pharm 2017; 74(6): 417-23.
[http://dx.doi.org/10.2146/ajhp160133] [PMID: 28274985]

[35]   Mehta JM, Haynes K, Wileyto EP, *et al.* Centers for disease control and prevention epicenter program. Comparison of prior authorization and prospective audit with feedback for antimicrobial stewardship. Infect Control Hosp Epidemiol 2014; 35(9): 1092-9.
[http://dx.doi.org/10.1086/677624] [PMID: 25111916]

[36] Szymczak J. Towards a more "human stewardship": leverage social sciences in antimicrobial stewardship research. ID Week 2016. 2016 Oct 30; New Orleans, LA.

[37] Davey P, Peden C, Charani E, Marwick C, Michie S. Time for action-Improving the design and reporting of behaviour change interventions for antimicrobial stewardship in hospitals: Early findings from a systematic review. Int J Antimicrob Agents 2015; 45(3): 203-12.
[http://dx.doi.org/10.1016/j.ijantimicag.2014.11.014] [PMID: 25630430]

[38] Sikkens JJ, van Agtmael MA, Peters EJG, *et al.* Behavioral approach to appropriate antimicrobial prescribing in hospitals: the dutch unique method for antimicrobial stewardship (dumas) participatory intervention study. JAMA Intern Med 2017; 177(8): 1130-8.
[http://dx.doi.org/10.1001/jamainternmed.2017.0946] [PMID: 28459929]

[39] Bork JT, Morgan DJ, Heil EL, Pineles L, Kleinberg M. Peer comparison of anti-mrsa agent prescription in the inpatient setting. Infect Control Hosp Epidemiol 2017; 38(12): 1506-8.
[http://dx.doi.org/10.1017/ice.2017.219] [PMID: 29067897]

[40] Nguyen CT, Davis KA. Evaluating the impact of peer comparison on vancomycin dose order verification among pharmacists. J Am Coll Clin Pharm 2018; pp. 1-6.

[41] Metlay JP, Shea JA, Crossette LB, Asch DA. Tensions in antibiotic prescribing: pitting social concerns against the interests of individual patients. J Gen Intern Med 2002; 17(2): 87-94.
[http://dx.doi.org/10.1046/j.1525-1497.2002.10711.x] [PMID: 11841523]

[42] Mertz D, Brooks A, Irfan N, Sung M. Antimicrobial stewardship in the intensive care setting--a review and critical appraisal of the literature. Swiss Med Wkly 2015; 145: w14220.
[http://dx.doi.org/10.4414/smw.2015.14220] [PMID: 26692020]

[43] Brown KA, Khanafer N, Daneman N, Fisman DN. Meta-analysis of antibiotics and the risk of community-associated *Clostridium difficile* infection. Antimicrob Agents Chemother 2013; 57(5): 2326-32.
[http://dx.doi.org/10.1128/AAC.02176-12] [PMID: 23478961]

[44] Deshpande A, Pasupuleti V, Thota P, *et al.* Community-associated *Clostridium difficile* infection and antibiotics: a meta-analysis. J Antimicrob Chemother 2013; 68(9): 1951-61.
[http://dx.doi.org/10.1093/jac/dkt129] [PMID: 23620467]

[45] Climo MW. Hospital-wide Restriction of Clindamycin: Effect on the Incidence of *Clostridium difficile*-Associated Diarrhea and Cost. Ann Intern Med 1998; 128(12_Part_1): 989.

[46] Price J, Cheek E, Lippett S, *et al.* Impact of an intervention to control *Clostridium difficile* infection on hospital- and community-onset disease; an interrupted time series analysis. Clin Microbiol Infect 2010; 16(8): 1297-302.
[http://dx.doi.org/10.1111/j.1469-0691.2009.03077.x] [PMID: 19832710]

[47] Valiquette L, Cossette B, Garant M-P, Diab H, Pépin J. Impact of a Reduction in the Use of High-Risk Antibiotics on the Course of an Epidemic of *Clostridium difficile*-Associated Disease Caused by the Hypervirulent NAP1/027 Strain. Clin Infect Dis 2007; 45(Supplement_2): S112-21.

[48] Thom KA, Tamma PD, Harris AD, *et al.* Impact of a prescriber-driven antibiotic time-out on antibiotic use in hospitalized patients. Clin Infect Dis 2019; 68(9): 1581-4.
[http://dx.doi.org/10.1093/cid/ciy852] [PMID: 30517592]

[49] https://med.stanford.edu/cme/courses/online/optimizing-antimicrobial-therapy.html

[50] Schooneveld V. 2016. https://idsa.confex.com/idsa/2016/webprogram/Paper58320.html

[51] Polisetty RS, Borkowski J, Jochum E, Delacruz J, Lewis S, Manam B, *et al.* Multicenter study to evaluate the impact of antibiotic time out in four community hospitals 2016.
https://academic.oup.com/ofid/article/3/suppl_1/988/2637225
[http://dx.doi.org/10.1093/ofid/ofw172.691]

[52] Vasina L, Dehner M, Wong A, *et al.* The impact of a pharmacist driven 48-hour antibiotic time out

during multi-disciplinary rounds on antibiotic utilization in a community non-teaching hospital. Open Forum Infect Dis 2017; 4(Suppl 1): S272-3.

[53]   Graber CJ, Jones MM, Glassman PA, *et al.* Taking an antibiotic time-out: utilization and usability of a self-stewardship time-out program for renewal of vancomycin and piperacillin-tazobactam. Hosp Pharm 2015; 50(11): 1011-24.
[http://dx.doi.org/10.1310/hpj5011-1011] [PMID: 27621509]

[54]   Lee TC, Frenette C, Jayaraman D, Green L, Pilote L. Antibiotic self-stewardship: trainee-led structured antibiotic time-outs to improve antimicrobial use. Ann Intern Med 2014; 161(10 Suppl): S53-58.
[http://dx.doi.org/10.7326/M13-3016]

[55]   Senn L, Burnand B, Francioli P, Zanetti G. Improving appropriateness of antibiotic therapy: randomized trial of an intervention to foster reassessment of prescription after 3 days. J Antimicrob Chemother 2004; 53(6): 1062-7.
[http://dx.doi.org/10.1093/jac/dkh236] [PMID: 15128726]

[56]   Balch A, Wendelboe AM, Vesely SK, Bratzler DW. Antibiotic prophylaxis for surgical site infections as a risk factor for infection with Clostridium difficile. PLoS One 2017; 12(6): e0179117.
https://www.ncbi.nlm.nih.gov/pmc/articles/PMC5473553/

[57]   2019.
https://www.publichealthontario.ca/en/BrowseByTopic/InfectiousDiseases/AntimicrobialStewardship Program/Pages/ASP-Strategies.aspx

[58]   Dellit TH, Owens RC, McGowan JE Jr, *et al.* Infectious diseases society of America; Society for healthcare epidemiology of America. Infectious diseases society of america and the society for healthcare epidemiology of America guidelines for developing an institutional program to enhance antimicrobial stewardship. Clin Infect Dis 2007; 44(2): 159-77.
[http://dx.doi.org/10.1086/510393] [PMID: 17173212]

[59]   Evans RS, Pestotnik SL, Classen DC, Burke JP. Evaluation of a computer-assisted antibiotic-dose monitor. Ann Pharmacother 1999; 33(10): 1026-31.
[http://dx.doi.org/10.1345/aph.18391] [PMID: 10534212]

[60]   Falconnier AD, Haefeli WE, Schoenenberger RA, Surber C, Martin-Facklam M. Drug dosage in patients with renal failure optimized by immediate concurrent feedback. J Gen Intern Med 2001; 16(6): 369-75.
[http://dx.doi.org/10.1046/j.1525-1497.2001.016006369.x] [PMID: 11422633]

[61]   Jiang S-P, Zhu Z-Y, Ma K-F, Zheng X, Lu X-Y. Impact of pharmacist antimicrobial dosing adjustments in septic patients on continuous renal replacement therapy in an intensive care unit. Scand J Infect Dis 2013; 45(12): 891-9.
[http://dx.doi.org/10.3109/00365548.2013.827338] [PMID: 24024759]

[62]   Han Z, Pettit NN, Landon EM, Brielmaier BD. Impact of pharmacy practice model expansion on pharmacokinetic services: optimization of vancomycin dosing and improved patient safety. Hosp Pharm 2017; 52(4): 273-9.
[http://dx.doi.org/10.1310/hpx5204-273] [PMID: 28515506]

[63]   Truong J, Smith SR, Veillette JJ, Forland SC. Individualized pharmacokinetic dosing of vancomycin reduces time to therapeutic trough concentrations in critically ill patients. J Clin Pharmacol 2018; 58(9): 1123-30.
[http://dx.doi.org/10.1002/jcph.1273] [PMID: 29957824]

[64]   Kaplun O, Monteforte M, Tirmizi S, Abate M, Psevdos G, Go R. The role of antimicrobial stewardship program on appropriate use, dose and duration of vancomycin treatment. Poster presented at: ID Week. San Francisco, CA.

[65]   Hamad A, Cavell G, Hinton J, Wade P, Whittlesea C. A pre-postintervention study to evaluate the impact of dose calculators on the accuracy of gentamicin and vancomycin initial doses. BMJ Open

2015; 5(6): e006610.
[http://dx.doi.org/10.1136/bmjopen-2014-006610] [PMID: 26044758]

[66] McCluggage L, Lee K, Potter T, Dugger R, Pakyz A. Implementation and evaluation of vancomycin nomogram guidelines in a computerized prescriber-order-entry system. Am J Health Syst Pharm 2010; 67(1): 70-5.
[http://dx.doi.org/10.2146/ajhp080625] [PMID: 20044371]

[67] Tamma PD, Putcha N, Suh YD, Van Arendonk KJ, Rinke ML. Does prolonged β-lactam infusions improve clinical outcomes compared to intermittent infusions? A meta-analysis and systematic review of randomized, controlled trials. BMC Infect Dis 2011; 11: 181.
[http://dx.doi.org/10.1186/1471-2334-11-181] [PMID: 21696619]

[68] Falagas ME, Tansarli GS, Ikawa K, Vardakas KZ. Clinical outcomes with extended or continuous versus short-term intravenous infusion of carbapenems and piperacillin/tazobactam: a systematic review and meta-analysis. Clin Infect Dis 2013; 56(2): 272-82.
[http://dx.doi.org/10.1093/cid/cis857] [PMID: 23074314]

[69] Shiu J, Wang E, Tejani AM, Wasdell M. Continuous versus intermittent infusions of antibiotics for the treatment of severe acute infections. Cochrane Database Syst Rev 2013; (3): CD008481.
[http://dx.doi.org/10.1002/14651858.CD008481.pub2] [PMID: 23543565]

[70] Hanretty AM, Gallagher JC. Shortened courses of antibiotics for bacterial infections: a systematic review of randomized controlled trials. Pharmacotherapy 2018; 38(6): 674-87.
[http://dx.doi.org/10.1002/phar.2118] [PMID: 29679383]

[71] Béïque L, Zvonar R. Addressing concerns about changing the route of antimicrobial administration from intravenous to oral in adult inpatients. Can J Hosp Pharm 2015; 68(4): 318-26.
[http://dx.doi.org/10.4212/cjhp.v68i4.1472] [PMID: 26327706]

[72] McLaughlin CM, Bodasing N, Boyter AC, Fenelon C, Fox JG, Seaton RA. Pharmacy-implemented guidelines on switching from intravenous to oral antibiotics: an intervention study. QJM 2005; 98(10): 745-52.
[http://dx.doi.org/10.1093/qjmed/hci114] [PMID: 16126741]

[73] Goff DA, Bauer KA, Reed EE, Stevenson KB, Taylor JJ, West JE. Is the "low-hanging fruit" worth picking for antimicrobial stewardship programs? Clin Infect Dis 2012; 55(4): 587-92.
[http://dx.doi.org/10.1093/cid/cis494] [PMID: 22615329]

[74] Mertz D, Koller M, Haller P, *et al.* Outcomes of early switching from intravenous to oral antibiotics on medical wards. J Antimicrob Chemother 2009; 64(1): 188-99.
[http://dx.doi.org/10.1093/jac/dkp131] [PMID: 19401304]

[75] Davis SL, Delgado G Jr, McKinnon PS. Pharmacoeconomic considerations associated with the use of intravenous-to-oral moxifloxacin for community-acquired pneumonia. Clin Infect Dis 2005; 41 (Suppl. 2): S136-43.
[http://dx.doi.org/10.1086/428054] [PMID: 15942880]

[76] Kuti JL, Le TN, Nightingale CH, Nicolau DP, Quintiliani R. Pharmacoeconomics of a pharmacist-managed program for automatically converting levofloxacin route from i.v. to oral. Am J Health Syst Pharm 2002; 59(22): 2209-15.
[http://dx.doi.org/10.1093/ajhp/59.22.2209] [PMID: 12455304]

[77] Wong-Beringer A, Nguyen KH, Razeghi J. Implementing a program for switching from i.v. to oral antimicrobial therapy. Am J Health Syst Pharm 2001; 58(12): 1146-9.
[http://dx.doi.org/10.1093/ajhp/58.12.1146] [PMID: 11449860]

[78] Blumenthal KG, Shenoy ES, Varughese CA, Hurwitz S, Hooper DC, Banerji A. Impact of a clinical guideline for prescribing antibiotics to inpatients reporting penicillin or cephalosporin allergy. Ann Allergy Asthma Immunol 2015; 115(4): 294-300.e2.
[http://dx.doi.org/10.1016/j.anai.2015.05.011] [PMID: 26070805]

[79]   Trubiano JA, Thursky KA, Stewardson AJ, *et al*. Impact of an integrated antibiotic allergy testing program on antimicrobial stewardship: a multicenter evaluation. Clin Infect Dis 2017; 65(1): 166-74.
        [http://dx.doi.org/10.1093/cid/cix244] [PMID: 28520865]

[80]   Solensky R, Khan DA. Joint task force on practice parameters; American academy of allergy, asthma and immunology; American college of allergy, asthma and immunology; Joint council of allergy, asthma and immunology. Drug allergy: an updated practice parameter. Ann Allergy Asthma Immunol 2010; 105(4): 259-73.
        [http://dx.doi.org/10.1016/j.anai.2010.08.002] [PMID: 20934625]

[81]   Solensky R. Penicillin allergy and the law. Ann Allergy Asthma Immunol 2018; 121(5): 517-8.
        [http://dx.doi.org/10.1016/j.anai.2018.09.451] [PMID: 30389082]

[82]   Puchner TC Jr, Zacharisen MC. A survey of antibiotic prescribing and knowledge of penicillin allergy. Ann Allergy Asthma Immunol 2002; 88(1): 24-9.
        [http://dx.doi.org/10.1016/S1081-1206(10)63589-2] [PMID: 11814274]

[83]   Jeffres MN, Narayanan PP, Shuster JE, Schramm GE. Consequences of avoiding β-lactams in patients with β-lactam allergies. J Allergy Clin Immunol 2016; 137(4): 1148-53.
        [http://dx.doi.org/10.1016/j.jaci.2015.10.026] [PMID: 26688516]

[84]   Blumenthal KG, Lu N, Zhang Y, Li Y, Walensky RP, Choi HK. Risk of meticillin resistant *staphylococcus aureus* and *Clostridium difficile* in patients with a documented penicillin allergy: population based matched cohort study. BMJ 2018; 361: k2400.
        [http://dx.doi.org/10.1136/bmj.k2400] [PMID: 29950489]

[85]   Musgrove MA, Kenney RM, Kendall RE, *et al*. Microbiology comment nudge improves pneumonia prescribing. Open Forum Infect Dis 2018; 5(7): ofy162.
        [http://dx.doi.org/10.1093/ofid/ofy162] [PMID: 30057928]

[86]   Chen JR, Tarver SA, Alvarez KS, Tran T, Khan DA. A proactive approach to penicillin allergy testing in hospitalized patients. J Allergy Clin Immunol Pract 2017; 5(3): 686-93.
        [http://dx.doi.org/10.1016/j.jaip.2016.09.045] [PMID: 27888034]

[87]   Mbakwa CA, Scheres L, Penders J, Mommers M, Thijs C, Arts ICW. Early life antibiotic exposure and weight development in children. J Pediatr 2016; 176: 105-113.e2.
        [http://dx.doi.org/10.1016/j.jpeds.2016.06.015] [PMID: 27402330]

[88]   Gerber JS, Bryan M, Ross RK, *et al*. Antibiotic exposure during the first 6 months of life and weight gain during childhood. JAMA 2016; 315(12): 1258-65.
        [http://dx.doi.org/10.1001/jama.2016.2395] [PMID: 27002447]

[89]   Hersh AL, Shapiro DJ, Pavia AT, Shah SS. Antibiotic prescribing in ambulatory pediatrics in the United States. Pediatrics 2011; 128(6): 1053-61.
        [http://dx.doi.org/10.1542/peds.2011-1337] [PMID: 22065263]

[90]   https://www.cdc.gov/antibiotic-use/community/for-hcp/outpatient-hcp/pediatric-treatment-rec.html

[91]   Gerber JS, Prasad PA, Fiks AG, *et al*. Effect of an outpatient antimicrobial stewardship intervention on broad-spectrum antibiotic prescribing by primary care pediatricians: a randomized trial. JAMA 2013; 309(22): 2345-52.
        [http://dx.doi.org/10.1001/jama.2013.6287] [PMID: 23757082]

[92]   Bielicki J, Lundin R, Patel S, Paulus S. Antimicrobial stewardship for neonates and children: a global approach. Pediatr Infect Dis J 2015; 34(3): 311-3.
        [http://dx.doi.org/10.1097/INF.0000000000000621] [PMID: 25584443]

[93]   Di Pentima MC, Chan S, Eppes SC, Klein JD. Antimicrobial prescription errors in hospitalized children: role of antimicrobial stewardship program in detection and intervention. Clin Pediatr (Phila) 2009; 48(5): 505-12.
        [http://dx.doi.org/10.1177/0009922808330774] [PMID: 19224865]

[94]   Magsarili HK, Girotto JE, Bennett NJ, Nicolau DP. Making a Case for Pediatric Antimicrobial Stewardship Programs. Pharmacotherapy 2015; 35(11): 1026-36.
[http://dx.doi.org/10.1002/phar.1647] [PMID: 26598095]

[95]   Bucaneve G, Micozzi A, Menichetti F, *et al.* Gruppo Italiano Malattie Ematologiche dell'Adulto (GIMEMA) Infection Program. Levofloxacin to prevent bacterial infection in patients with cancer and neutropenia. N Engl J Med 2005; 353(10): 977-87.
[http://dx.doi.org/10.1056/NEJMoa044097] [PMID: 16148283]

[96]   De Rosa FG, Motta I, Audisio E, *et al.* Epidemiology of bloodstream infections in patients with acute myeloid leukemia undergoing levofloxacin prophylaxis. BMC Infect Dis 2013; 13: 563.
[http://dx.doi.org/10.1186/1471-2334-13-563]

[97]   Bow EJ. Fluoroquinolones, antimicrobial resistance and neutropenic cancer patients. Curr Opin Infect Dis 2011; 24(6): 545-53.
[http://dx.doi.org/10.1097/QCO.0b013e32834cf054] [PMID: 22001945]

[98]   Freifeld AG, Bow EJ, Sepkowitz KA, *et al.* Clinical practice guideline for the use of antimicrobial agents in neutropenic patients with cancer: 2010 update by the infectious diseases society of america. Clin Infect Dis 2011; 52(4): e56-93.
[http://dx.doi.org/10.1093/cid/cir073] [PMID: 21258094]

[99]   Taplitz RA, Kennedy EB, Bow EJ, *et al.* Outpatient Management of Fever and Neutropenia in Adults Treated for Malignancy: American Society of Clinical Oncology and Infectious Diseases Society of America Clinical Practice Guideline Update. J Clin Oncol 2018; 36(14): 1443-53.
[http://dx.doi.org/10.1200/JCO.2017.77.6211] [PMID: 29461916]

[100]   Lindsay PJ, Rohailla S, Taggart LR, *et al.* Antimicrobial stewardship and intensive care unit mortality: a systematic review. Clin Infect Dis 2019; 68(5): 748-56.
[http://dx.doi.org/10.1093/cid/ciy550] [PMID: 29982376]

[101]   Álvarez-Lerma F, Grau S, Echeverría-Esnal D, *et al.* A before-and-after study of the effectiveness of an antimicrobial stewardship program in critical care. Antimicrob Agents Chemother 2018; 62(4): e01825-17. https://www.ncbi.nlm.nih.gov/pmc/articles/PMC5913992/
[http://dx.doi.org/10.1128/AAC.01825-17]

[102]   Parente DM, Cunha CB, Mylonakis E, Timbrook TT. The clinical utility of methicillin-resistant *staphylococcus aureus* (MRSA) nasal screening to rule out mrsa pneumonia: a diagnostic meta-analysis with antimicrobial stewardship implications. Clin Infect Dis 2018; 67(1): 1-7.
[http://dx.doi.org/10.1093/cid/ciy024] [PMID: 29340593]

[103]   Charles PE, Ladoire S, Snauwaert A, *et al.* Impact of previous sepsis on the accuracy of procalcitonin for the early diagnosis of blood stream infection in critically ill patients. BMC Infect Dis 2008; 8: 163.
[http://dx.doi.org/10.1186/1471-2334-8-163] [PMID: 19055740]

[104]   Wirz Y, Meier MA, Bouadma L, *et al.* Effect of procalcitonin-guided antibiotic treatment on clinical outcomes in intensive care unit patients with infection and sepsis patients: a patient-level meta-analysis of randomized trials. Crit Care 2018; 22(1): 191. https://www.ncbi.nlm.nih.gov/pmc/articles/PMC6092799/
[http://dx.doi.org/10.1186/s13054-018-2125-7]

[105]   Lisboa T, Salluh J, Povoa P. Do we need new trials of procalcitonin-guided antibiotic therapy? Crit Care 2018; 22: 17. https://www.ncbi.nlm.nih.gov/pmc/articles/PMC5787295/
[http://dx.doi.org/10.1186/s13054-018-1948-6]

[106]   Bouadma L, Luyt C-E, Tubach F, Cracco C, Alvarez A, Schwebel C, *et al.* Use of procalcitonin to reduce patients' exposure to antibiotics in intensive care units (PRORATA trial): a multicentre randomised controlled trial 2010; 375: 12.

[107]   Hicks LA, Bartoces MG, Roberts RM, *et al.* US outpatient antibiotic prescribing variation according to geography, patient population, and provider specialty in 2011. Clin Infect Dis 2011; 60(9): 1308-6.

https://academic.oup.com/cid/article-lookup/doi/10.1093/cid/civ076

[108] Fleming-Dutra KE, Hersh AL, Shapiro DJ, *et al.* Prevalence of Inappropriate Antibiotic Prescriptions Among US Ambulatory Care Visits, 2010-2011. JAMA 2016; 315(17): 1864-73.
[http://dx.doi.org/10.1001/jama.2016.4151] [PMID: 27139059]

[109] Hersh AL, Fleming-Dutra KE, Shapiro DJ, Hyun DY, Hicks LA. Outpatient antibiotic use target-setting workgroup. Frequency of first-line antibiotic selection among us ambulatory care visits for otitis media, sinusitis, and pharyngitis. JAMA Intern Med 2016; 176(12): 1870-2.
[http://dx.doi.org/10.1001/jamainternmed.2016.6625] [PMID: 27775770]

[110] Pasternak B, Inghammar M, Svanström H. Fluoroquinolone use and risk of aortic aneurysm and dissection: nationwide cohort study. BMJ 2018; 360: k678.
[http://dx.doi.org/10.1136/bmj.k678] [PMID: 29519881]

[111] Palms DL, Hicks LA, Bartoces M, *et al.* Comparison of antibiotic prescribing in retail clinics, urgent care centers, emergency departments, and traditional ambulatory care settings in the United States. JAMA Intern Med 2018; 178(9): 1267-9.
[http://dx.doi.org/10.1001/jamainternmed.2018.1632] [PMID: 30014128]

[112] Szymczak JE. What parents think about antibiotics for their child's acute respiratory tract infection. Journal of the Pediatric Infectious Diseases Society 2018; 7(4): 303-9. https://idsa.confex.com/idsa/2015/webprogram/Paper51903.html
[http://dx.doi.org/10.1093/ofid/ofv133.83]

[113] Szymczak J, Feemster K, Zaoutis T, Gerber J. Pediatrician perceptions of an outpatient antimicrobial stewardship intervention. Infect Control Hosp Epidemiol 2014; 35(s3).
[http://dx.doi.org/10.1086/677826]

[114] Denny KJ, Gartside JG, Alcorn K, Cross JW, Maloney S, Keijzers G. Appropriateness of antibiotic prescribing in the Emergency Department. J Antimicrob Chemother 2019; 74(2): 515-20.
[http://dx.doi.org/10.1093/jac/dky447] [PMID: 30445465]

[115] Meeker D, Knight TK, Friedberg MW, *et al.* Nudging guideline-concordant antibiotic prescribing: a randomized clinical trial. JAMA Intern Med 2014; 174(3): 425-31.
[http://dx.doi.org/10.1001/jamainternmed.2013.14191] [PMID: 24474434]

[116] Marra F, George D, Chong M, Sutherland S, Patrick DM. Antibiotic prescribing by dentists has increased: Why? J Am Dent Assoc 2016; 147(5): 320-7.
[http://dx.doi.org/10.1016/j.adaj.2015.12.014] [PMID: 26857041]

[117] Sollecito TP, Abt E, Lockhart PB, *et al.* The use of prophylactic antibiotics prior to dental procedures in patients with prosthetic joints: Evidence-based clinical practice guideline for dental practitioners--a report of the American Dental Association Council on Scientific Affairs. J Am Dent Assoc 2015; 146(1): 11-16.e8.
[http://dx.doi.org/10.1016/j.adaj.2014.11.012] [PMID: 25569493]

[118] Wilson W, Taubert KA, Gewitz M, *et al.* Prevention of infective endocarditis: Guidelines from the American Heart Association. J Am Dent Assoc 2008; 139 (Suppl.): 3S-24S.
[http://dx.doi.org/10.14219/jada.archive.2008.0346] [PMID: 18167394]

[119] Thornhill MH, Dayer M, Lockhart PB, Prendergast B. Antibiotic prophylaxis of infective endocarditis. Curr Infect Dis Rep 2017; 19(2): 9. https://www.ncbi.nlm.nih.gov/pmc/articles/PMC5323496/
[http://dx.doi.org/10.1007/s11908-017-0564-y]

[120] Bye M, Whitten T, Holzbauer S. Antibiotic prescribing for dental procedures in community-associated clostridium difficile cases, minnesota, 2009-2015. 2017. https://idsa.confex.com/idsa/2017/webprogram/Paper66373.html

[121] https://www.ada.org/en/member-center/oral-health-topics/antibiotic-stewardship

[122] https://www.wolterskluwercdi.com/blog/understanding-antibiotic-prescribing-and-steward-hip-general-dentists/

[123] Vardakas KZ, Trigkidis KK, Boukouvala E, Falagas ME. *Clostridium difficile* infection following systemic antibiotic administration in randomised controlled trials: a systematic review and meta-analysis. Int J Antimicrob Agents 2016; 48(1): 1-10.
[http://dx.doi.org/10.1016/j.ijantimicag.2016.03.008] [PMID: 27216385]

[124] Candamourty R, Venkatachalam S, Babu MRR, Kumar GS. Ludwig's Angina - An emergency: A case report with literature review. J Nat Sci Biol Med 2012; 3(2): 206-8.
[http://dx.doi.org/10.4103/0976-9668.101932] [PMID: 23225990]

[125] Hui K, Nalder M, Buising K, *et al.* Patterns of use and appropriateness of antibiotics prescribed to patients receiving haemodialysis: an observational study. BMC Nephrol 2017; 18: 156.
https://www.ncbi.nlm.nih.gov/pmc/articles/PMC5427537/
[http://dx.doi.org/10.1186/s12882-017-0575-9]

[126] Cunha CB, D'Agata EMC. Implementing an antimicrobial stewardship program in out-patient dialysis units. Curr Opin Nephrol Hypertens 2016; 25(6): 551-5.
[http://dx.doi.org/10.1097/MNH.0000000000000281] [PMID: 27636769]

[127] Nguyen DB, Shugart A, Lines C, *et al.* National healthcare safety network (NHSN) dialysis event surveillance report for 2014. Clin J Am Soc Nephrol 2017; 12(7): 1139-46.
[http://dx.doi.org/10.2215/CJN.11411116] [PMID: 28663227]

[128] Patel PR, Brinsley-Rainisch K. The making dialysis safer for patients coalition: a new partnership to prevent hemodialysis-related infections. Clin J Am Soc Nephrol 2017; 13(1): 175-81.
[http://dx.doi.org/10.2215/CJN.02730317] [PMID: 28794000]

[129] Daneman N, Bronskill SE, Gruneir A, *et al.* Variability in antibiotic use across nursing homes and the risk of antibiotic-related adverse outcomes for individual residents. JAMA Intern Med 2015; 175(8): 1331-9.
[http://dx.doi.org/10.1001/jamainternmed.2015.2770] [PMID: 26121537]

[130] Chopra T, Goldstein EJC. *Clostridium difficile* Infection in Long-term Care Facilities: A Call to Action for Antimicrobial Stewardship. Clin Infect Dis 2015; 60(suppl_2): S72-6.
[http://dx.doi.org/10.1093/cid/civ053]

[131] Mody L. Optimizing antimicrobial use in nursing homes: no longer optional. J Am Geriatr Soc 2007; 55(8): 1301-2.
[http://dx.doi.org/10.1111/j.1532-5415.2007.01253.x] [PMID: 17661973]

[132] Rhee SM, Stone ND. Antimicrobial stewardship in long-term care facilities. Infect Dis Clin North Am 2014; 28(2): 237-46.
[http://dx.doi.org/10.1016/j.idc.2014.01.001] [PMID: 24857390]

[133] Smith PW, Bennett G, Bradley S, *et al.* SHEA/APIC Guideline: Infection prevention and control in the long-term care facility. Am J Infect Control 2008; 36(7): 504-35.
[http://dx.doi.org/10.1016/j.ajic.2008.06.001] [PMID: 18786461]

[134] Sundvall P-D, Stuart B, Davis M, Roderick P, Moore M. Antibiotic use in the care home setting: a retrospective cohort study analysing routine data. BMC Geriatr 2015; 15: 71. http://bmcgeriatr.biomed central.com/articles/10.1186/s12877-015-0073-5
[http://dx.doi.org/10.1186/s12877-015-0073-5]

[135] Nicolle LE. Antimicrobial stewardship in long term care facilities: what is effective? Antimicrob Resist Infect Control 2014; 3(1): 6.
[http://dx.doi.org/10.1186/2047-2994-3-6] [PMID: 24521205]

[136] Young JD, Abdel-Massih R, Herchline T, *et al.* Infectious diseases society of America position statement on telehealth and telemedicine as applied to the practice of infectious diseases. Clin Infect Dis 2019; 68(9): 1437-43.
[http://dx.doi.org/10.1093/cid/ciy907] [PMID: 30851042]

[137] Stenehjem E, Hersh AL, Buckel WR, *et al.* Impact of implementing antibiotic stewardship programs in

15 small hospitals: a cluster-randomized intervention. Clin Infect Dis 2018; 67(4): 525-32.
[http://dx.doi.org/10.1093/cid/ciy155] [PMID: 29790913]

[138] Dos Santos RP, Dalmora CH, Lukasewicz SA, *et al.* Antimicrobial stewardship through telemedicine and its impact on multi-drug resistance. J Telemed Telecare 2019; 25(5): 294-300.
[http://dx.doi.org/10.1177/1357633X18767702] [PMID: 29720043]

[139] Shively NR, Moffa MA, Paul KT, *et al.* Impact of a telehealth-based antimicrobial stewardship program in a community hospital health system. Clinical Infectious Diseases 2019; 1-7.
[http://dx.doi.org/10.1093/cid/ciz878]

CHAPTER 14

Financial and Regulatory Roadblocks for Antimicrobial Development

Benjamin Georgiades[*] and **Sean Nguyen**

Shionogi Inc, Florham Park, NJ, USA

Abstract: • In the US, the Centers for Disease Control and Prevention has estimated that 2 million patients a year suffer from infections due to drug resistant bacteria and antimicrobial resistance is predicted to result in 10 million deaths worldwide by 2050.

• Growing antimicrobial resistance combined with a dry antibiotic pipeline has led clinicians to utilize older antibiotics that can be more toxic and/or ineffective.

• There has been development and regulatory progress made, but this is leading to an increasing number of antibiotics that will be reaching the market with limited datasets. Clinicians should understand how to best interpret and incorporate the data into clinical decision-making.

• Clinicians should understand the various challenges for the decline in antibiotic development and understand the initiatives that are currently in place to help fix the issues as well as further potential solutions.

Keywords: Antibiotic, Barriers, Clinical Development, Discovery, Pipeline, Research, Solutions.

INTRODUCTION

Antibiotics play a critical role in medicine and are exceptionally valuable to humanity as appropriate use of these drugs can cure disease and stop the spread of deadly bacterial infections. However, one of the unique qualities of antibiotics that separate this class of drugs from other therapeutic classes is that the more they are used, the less effective they can become over time. In addition, despite the numerous commercially available antibiotics, too many antibiotics are prescribed unnecessarily which can lead to the development of multi-drug resistant bacteria [1].

---

[*] **Corresponding author Benjamin Georgiades:** Shionogi Inc, Florham Park, NJ, USA; Tel: 908-812-2978; E-mail: BenjaminGeorgiades@gmail.com

When antibiotics are over utilized or used unnecessarily, healthcare providers are left with limited treatment options to treat multi-drug resistant infections and forced to use antibiotics that can potentially be more toxic and less effective than first-line agents. Without effective antibiotics, the practice of medicine would be drastically different. Bacterial infections that would normally be easy to treat would lead to high mortality rates and patients would be at an increased risk of fatal infections secondary to routine surgical procedures (*e.g.* knee replacement), as well as from organ transplantation or cancer chemotherapy [2].

Despite an increasing incidence and severity of antimicrobial resistance, the development of new anti-infective agents is threatened by the cessation of research by the pharmaceutical industry [3, 4]. The research and development of new antimicrobials is an expensive and time consuming process that requires a long-term commitment to maintain a substantial and sophisticated infrastructure and personnel [5]. Ensuring the continued availability of novel antibiotics that combat existing pathogens and pathogens expressing resistance to currently available therapies, is a critical global public health issue [6, 7].

To bring recognition to rising antimicrobial resistance and lack of antibacterial agents in clinical development, numerous agencies have called for public-private partnerships and innovative funding mechanisms. The Infectious Diseases Society of America (IDSA) established its 10x20' initiative, where they campaigned for the development and regulatory approval of ten novel, efficacious, and safe systemically administered antibiotics by 2020 [2]. In Europe, the Innovative Medicines Institute formed the New Drugs 4 Bad Bugs (ND4BB) campaign in 2012 which brought a partnership between industry, academia, and biotech organizations to combat antimicrobial resistance [8]. The ND4BB project's ultimate goal is to find solutions to the scientific, regulatory and business challenges that are hampering the development of new antibiotics. In 2015, the U.S. released a National Action Plan for Combating Antibiotic-Resistant Bacteria which was closely followed by the World Health Organization's Global Action Plan on Antimicrobial Resistance [9, 10]. The U.S. National Action Plan called for public–private partnerships to accelerate research, enhance innovation, and increase the number of antibiotics in the pipeline. In addition to governmental efforts, several non-governmental organizations including the Pew Charitable Trusts, the Brookings Institution, Chatham House, and the Wellcome Trust have concentrated efforts toward antimicrobial resistance research and development [11]. Between the different organizations, the initiatives have addressed various global challenges in antibiotic development, covering basic science and early stage drug development, clinical trials, and economics which have subsequently reinvigorated the antibiotic development pipeline.

OVERVIEW OF ANTIBIOTIC DISCOVERY AND ANTIBACTERIAL RESISTANCE

The discovery of antibiotics has saved millions of lives and has prolonged life expectancy by drastically changing the outcome of bacterial infections. Prior to the discovery of penicillin in 1928, there was no effective treatment for bacterial infections such as pneumonia, gonorrhea or rheumatic fever [12, 13]. However, by the late 1930s, mortality secondary to pneumonia declined approximately 30%. As for severe infections such as bacterial meningitis and endocarditis, mortality declined by 60-75% [6]. In 1945, penicillin was made available to the US public and by 1952, less than 95,000 Americans died from the same bacterial illnesses that killed over 250,000 people in 1936 (and 300,000 people in 1930) [14].

The introduction of penicillin marked the beginning of the "golden era" of antibiotic discovery. Between 1940 and 1962, antibiotic development skyrocketed and additional classes of antibiotics such as tetracyclines, macrolides, cephalosporins, aminoglycosides, sulfonamides and quinolones were discovered and introduced to the public. Consequently, with the advent of antibiotics, the rise of antibiotic resistance became a significant clinical problem as the first case of methicillin-resistant *Staphylococcus aureus* (MRSA) was identified in the 1960's [7, 13]. Vancomycin was introduced into clinical practice in 1972 for the treatment of MRSA infections; however, cases of vancomycin resistance were reported in coagulase-negative *Staphylococci* by 1979 [15]. Since then, cases of antibiotic resistance have been documented to nearly all antibiotics that have been developed, as seen in Fig. (**1**).

Antimicrobial resistance is also a rapidly growing global public health challenge, with estimates of up to 700,000 deaths per year [17]. New resistance mechanisms are evolving and spreading globally, threatening the ability to treat common infectious diseases in developing countries. Where antibiotics can be purchased for human or animal consumption without a prescription, the emergence and spread of resistance is worse. In countries without standard treatment guidelines, antibiotics are often over-prescribed by health care perscribers and antibiotics are generally over-utilized by the public [18, 19]. In a Lebanese study, it was shown that in 52% of cases, the prescription dose was inappropriate while 63.7% of physicians prescribed antibiotics with a wrong duration of treatment [20].

There are higher mortality rates in patients with resistant bacterial infections, while survivors have significantly longer hospital stays, increased healthcare costs, delayed recuperation, and long-term disability [21, 22]. The Centers for Disease Control and Prevention (CDC) estimated that at least 2 million patients a year in the US will acquire serious infections due to drug-resistant bacteria that are resistant to one or more of the antibiotics designed to treat those infections and that at least 23,000 people will die each year secondary to those infections [7]. Consequently, the 2 million infections a year within the US will cost the US health system $20 billion in excess costs per year and if continued on its current trajectory, antibiotic resistance is predicted to result in 10 million deaths by 2050 and cost up to $100 trillion, worldwide [7, 23, 24].

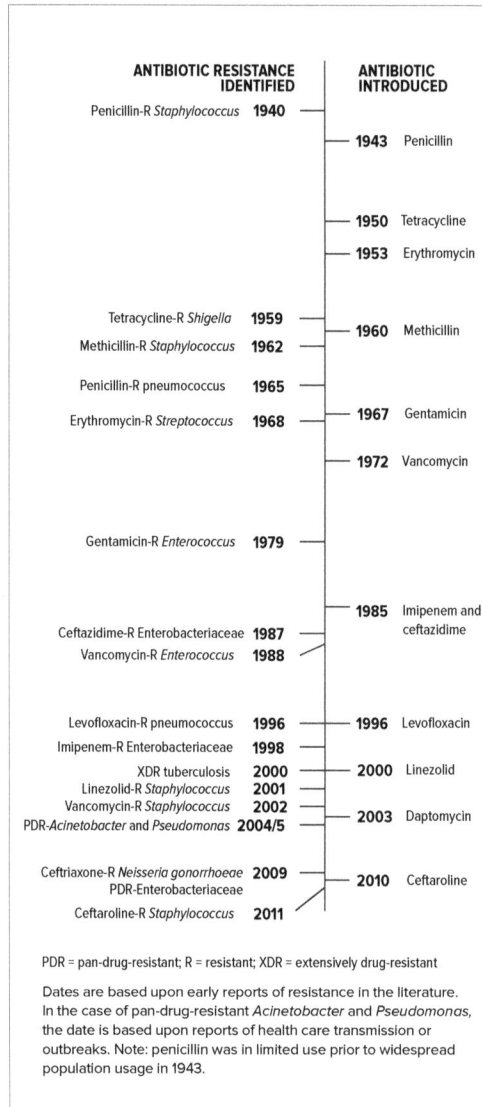

ANTIBIOTIC RESISTANCE IDENTIFIED		ANTIBIOTIC INTRODUCED	
Penicillin-R *Staphylococcus*	**1940**		
		1943	Penicillin
		1950	Tetracycline
		1953	Erythromycin
Tetracycline-R *Shigella*	**1959**	**1960**	Methicillin
Methicillin-R *Staphylococcus*	**1962**		
Penicillin-R pneumococcus	**1965**		
Erythromycin-R *Streptococcus*	**1968**	**1967**	Gentamicin
		1972	Vancomycin
Gentamicin-R *Enterococcus*	**1979**		
		1985	Imipenem and ceftazidime
Ceftazidime-R Enterobacteriaceae	**1987**		
Vancomycin-R *Enterococcus*	**1988**		
Levofloxacin-R pneumococcus	**1996**	**1996**	Levofloxacin
Imipenem-R Enterobacteriaceae	**1998**		
XDR tuberculosis	**2000**	**2000**	Linezolid
Linezolid-R *Staphylococcus*	**2001**		
Vancomycin-R *Staphylococcus*	**2002**	**2003**	Daptomycin
PDR-*Acinetobacter* and *Pseudomonas*	**2004/5**		
Ceftriaxone-R *Neisseria gonorrhoeae*	**2009**	**2010**	Ceftaroline
PDR-Enterobacteriaceae			
Ceftaroline-R *Staphylococcus*	**2011**		

PDR = pan-drug-resistant; R = resistant; XDR = extensively drug-resistant

Dates are based upon early reports of resistance in the literature. In the case of pan-drug-resistant *Acinetobacter* and *Pseudomonas*, the date is based upon reports of health care transmission or outbreaks. Note: penicillin was in limited use prior to widespread population usage in 1943.

Fig. (1). Timeline of Antibiotic Approval and time to documented Antibiotic Resistance. Figure adapted from the Center of Disease Control and Prevention [16].

As a result of increasing antibiotic resistance, several decades after the first patients were treated with antibiotics, bacterial infections have once more become a global health threat due to the lack of treatment alternatives for antibiotic-resistant infections [24, 25]. In the 2017 report from the World Health Organization's (WHO) Global Antimicrobial Resistance Surveillance System (GLASS), data from 22 countries and more than 500,000 isolates show that *Escherichia coli, Klebsiella pneumoniae, Staphylococcus aureus, Streptococcus pneumoniae*, and *Salmonella* spp are the most commonly reported resistant bacteria [26]. The WHO has also published a list of antibiotic-resistant "priority pathogens" which consists of 12 families of bacteria that pose the greatest threat to human health [27]. The list is categorized according to the urgency of need for new antibiotics: critical, high and medium. The most critical group consists of multidrug resistant bacteria that pose a threat in hospitals and nursing homes as well as in patients whose care requires devices such as ventilators and blood catheters. The critical list include carbapenem resistant *Acinetobacter, Pseudomonas aeruginosa* and Enterobacteriaceae (including ESBL producers). The high and medium priority categories consist of increasingly drug-resistant bacteria that cause more common diseases such as *Gonorrhoea* and food poisoning caused by *Salmonella*. In regards to the United States, the CDC has reported three classifications of antibiotic-resistant bacteria (urgent, serious, and concerning) that pose the greatestthreats [7]. Urgent threats are high-consequence, antibiotic-resistant threats because of the significant risks identified across several criteria. They include carbapenem-resistant Enterobacteriaceae, drug-resistant *Neisseria gonorrhoeae*, and *Clostridium difficile*. It was noted that *C. difficile* does not have true antibiotic resistance, but is rather a consequence of overuse of antibiotics. Serious threats are threats that have potential to worsen but may potentially become urgent without public health monitoring and preventative interventions. Pathogens include multidrug-resistant *Acinetobacter*, drug-resistant *Campylobacter*, fluconazole-resistant *Candida*, extended-spectrum ß-lactamas--producing Enterobacteriaceae, vancomycin-resistant *Enterococcus*, multidrug-resistant *P. aeruginosa*, drug-resistant non-typhoidal *Salmonella*, drug-resistant *Salmonella Typhimurium*, drug-resistant *Shigella*, methicillin-resistant *S. aureus*, drug-resistant *S. pneumoniae*, and drug-resistant tuberculosis. Lastly, concerning threats are bacteria for which the threat of antibiotic resistance is small, and/or there are various therapeutic options for treatment of the resistant infections. These bacterial pathogens include vancomycin-resistant *S. aureus*, erythromycin-resistant Group A *Streptococcus*, and clindamycin-resistant Group B *Streptococcus*.

CAUSES OF THE DRYING PIPELINE

In 1980, there were more than 25 international pharmaceutical companies with active antibiotic drug discovery programs, however despite the growing necessity for new agents there is a substantial gap in antibiotic discovery which has led to an inadequate development pipeline [4]. The pharmaceutical industry has tried to combat the issue of increasing antibiotic resistance with the introduction of several new antibiotics but historically, the success rate for clinical anti-infective development is low as only 1 out of 5 infectious disease drugs that reach the initial phase of testing in humans will receive approval from the US FDA [28].

The decline in the antimicrobial pipeline is a result of several disincentives which are driven primarily by scientific, economic, regulatory, and commercial challenges [29 - 31]. The various challenges have led pharmaceutical companies to divest resources from anti-infectives to focus on therapeutic areas that have a higher commercial return on investment, such as oncology [17]. This problem has persisted for several decades and has progressed to the point where antibiotics are losing effectiveness at a faster rate than they are being replaced by new agents [12].

Scientific Challenges

Antibiotic research and development poses several unique scientific challenges that makes development of antibiotics relatively riskier as compared to drugs from other therapeutic areas. The majority of antibiotic classes that are available today were discovered during the "golden era" of antibiotic development but there is a limited number of antibiotics developed since that possess a novel mechanism of action. The discovery of novel agents today has become exceedingly difficult and expensive [32, 33].

In order to discover a novel molecule, a lead candidate is typically identified by screening a library of whole cell assays or purified targets that were previously designed to inhibit a process that is required for bacterial survival. However, repetitive screening of the same libraries over time has produced molecules with few inherent differences from what is currently marketed. Since microbial resistance is continuously evolving, discovery of a compound that can withstand the resistance mechanisms while ensuring favorable pharmacokinetics, efficacy, and safety has proven to be extremely challenging [30, 34].

This scientific hurdle is also exacerbated by the decline in investment by industrial and public funders, as a move towards non-communicable diseases has been favored during the second half of the 20th century [17]. As a result, the traditional research and development approach no longer applies to the contemporary anti-bacterial landscape; companies and their respective funders have invested billions of dollars, yet no new class of antibiotic for gram-negative infections has reached approval in over 40 years [35].

Economic Challenges

The antimicrobial discovery industry is experiencing a market failure, which is a situation where supply and demand are not efficiently harmonized [36]. There are many factors that contribute to market failure in this instance, with the primary ones being externalities, imperfect information and an unwillingness to pay for public goods [17].

Externalities are the costs or benefits to a third party when the third party has no control over the use of a product, and they can have either positive or negative qualities. For example, antibiotic consumption fits into the category of possessing a negative externality because each individual patient who receives treatment may benefit from using antibiotics, but the resistance that emerges with increased use impacts all of society due to the transmissible nature of bacterial infections. Governments typically tax and regulate products that have negative externalities so as to discourage their use and development. Antibiotics can also be considered to possess positive externalities because when a patient uses them the infection is often cured, which inhibits it from being spread to other people. Governments typically subsidize products that have positive externalities. In the case of antibiotics the negative externalities most likely outweigh the positive ones, however in the current legislative and regulatory landscape, the negative externalities of antibiotic consumption are not regulated strongly which has led to overuse in human and animal populations [17].

Imperfect information scenarios arise when there are differences in data surrounding the same subject. This applies to antimicrobials in two separate ways- the first being that at the time of prescribing and antibiotic, the provider often does not know what the antimicrobial susceptibility of the infecting organism is and therefore may prescribe an antibiotic that may be ineffective. Consequently, there will be a delay in appropriate treatment, resulting in a longer duration of infection and higher risk of transmission to other patients. The same principle applies in the reverse as low-quality information may result in a clinician prescribing a second- or third-line agent when a first-line antibiotic would have been effective. Lack of viable information may also lead to antibiotics being prescribed for infections that are not of bacterial etiology, such as those caused by viruses [17, 37].

Lack of information also applies to antimicrobial resistance because it is difficult to predict how resistance trends will evolve in the future, making it challenging for pharmaceutical researchers to forecast the appropriate need to develop an antibiotic and justify its development. This uncertainty has led to companies to not invest resources into antimicrobial research and development until there is already an urgent need. Unfortunately, this model has led to the discovery of effective agents for urgent issues 10 to 15 years after the resistance arises. Imperfect information has contributed to inappropriate antimicrobial prescribing as well as a business model that is more reactive rather than proactive [17].

Public goods are those that may benefit many people, but are not paid for directly by those who benefit from it. This applies to antimicrobials because a large proportion of the healthcare industry relies on the ability for infections to be managed properly with relative ease. For example, if there were no effective treatments for bacterial infections, routine medical practices such as surgery, chemotherapy, and many other common procedures would not be able to be performed. If antibiotics were not available, the sales of products like artificial joints and chemotherapy drugs would be negatively impacted and subsequently lead to worse outcomes for patients. As with all public goods, there is a need for industry, government, and society to work collaboratively to correct the current model [17, 32, 38].

Regulatory Challenges

Clinical development of a lead candidate is extremely difficult as only 5 out of 5,000-10000 candidate molecules will reach phase 1 clinical trials [6]. In regards to infectious disease products, only 1 in 5 products that enter phase 1 clinical trials will actually receive FDA approval [28]. In oncology, for instance, there were close to 800 new products in the development pipeline in 2014, of which around 80 percent were potentially "first-in-class" as compared to an antibiotics pipeline today consisting of fewer than 50 products [17]. Products can fail to receive approval for various reasons, including lack of effectiveness or safety concerns. Rather than taking the calculated risk, pharmaceutical companies have generally opted to focus on slightly modifying or combining already existing compounds rather than attempting to identify novel antibacterial molecules.

When a lead candidate has been identified by a company, it must undergo a rigorous pre-clinical and clinical development program in order to achieve regulatory agency approval. Of the agents that progress to this stage, difficulties in clinical trial design and operations are quickly encountered [39]. There is the perception that pivotal trials for antimicrobials are an obstacle to overcome and that they offer little translatability to the clinical world [40], as illustrated by the large amount of off-label use of antibiotics once they are approved [41]. Modern development programs are typically centered on non-inferiority comparisons of the candidate compound *versus* a microbiologically-active comparator in the setting of patients with infections that are not caused by drug-resistant pathogens [39]. This may be in part due to the nature of antibiotics and treatment of bacterial infections since antibiotics are curative in nature and it is unethical to enroll patients into a trial where the infective pathogen may be resistant to the antibiotics used in the study [39]. The resulting dilemma is that most new antibiotics in clinical development are aimed at treating multi-drug-resistant infections, for which upon approval, there is no clinical data available to support their use. Essentially, many pivotal trials enroll patients who are clinically different than those patients who will actually be receiving the antibiotic in the clinical setting post approval [40]. Therefore, after the antibiotic is approved, there is a substantial amount of pressure from the medical community to invest more resources into investigating the new agent's safety and efficacy in a more clinically relevant patient population. This not only increases the additional expenses for the drug manufacturer but also results in a delay in clinically-meaningful data being available to clinicians to help guide use.

The developmental phase of a drug is a substantial investment as it is estimated to cost upwards of \$2.5 billion to bring a single drug to market [42]. In an antimicrobial development program, it may be difficult to enroll a large sample size of patients and the cost of clinical trial program can comprise up to 65% of total expenditures when adjusted for the risk of failure [17, 43]. In regards to an antibiotic, conducting a phase 3 study can be exceptionally expensive depending on the clinical indication; A phase 3 trial in acute bacterial skin and skin structure infections can cost anywhere between \$30 to 50 million while a study in hospital-acquired and ventilator-associated bacterial pneumonia can cost \$100-150 million [43]. When the cost of development is taken into account by pharmaceutical developers, the decision to move forward with a promising agent is often made only when there is a potential market large enough to recoup these expenses [44]. If the targeted pathogens are rare, the incurred expenses may be too high to justify development which creates a disparity between the societal impact of a new antimicrobial agent and the business opportunity that might be realized.

Commercial Challenges

Despite their high value to society, antibiotics have historically been priced relatively lower than other classes of medications (*e.g.* oncology). In fact, generic antibiotics are so inexpensive that many community pharmacies in the US offer to fill these prescriptions at no cost in an effort to drive traffic into their stores [45]. These types of practices are not only detrimental to profitability, but they are counter-productive to antimicrobial stewardship principles. The institutional setting is different because of the way which antibiotics are paid for, as they are included in bundled payments when a patient is admitted to a hospital [36]. Because hospitals will be reimbursed the same amount of money whether they use an expensive agent or not, they are incentivized to use less expensive agents and only use expensive alternatives when deemed absolutely necessary. This may seem like a practical approach, but in many cases the less expensive choices are often toxic and less efficacious than more expensive choices. This practice is illustrated by antibacterial agents accounting for 6.4% of prescriptions in the US, but only 2.6% of total cost of prescriptions in 2013 when compared against the 19 other most common categories of medications [43].

Once a new antibiotic agent is approved, hospital antimicrobial stewardship initiatives appropriately limit its use in an effort to preserve its efficacy and to control costs [46]. These results benefit the broader population, but do not account for the value that new antimicrobials bring to the public when they are in need. Further exacerbating the issue, cost reduction in antimicrobial stewardship programs leads to lower use of new agents, which has the unintended consequence of discouraging new antibiotic development. The principles of antimicrobial stewardship are entirely necessary to preserve the currently available treatment options, however these practices must be factored in when policies that affect antimicrobial development are being implemented [29].

The aforementioned commercial challenges have contributed to pharmaceutical companies finding small opportunities in terms of return-on-investment. To quantify these perceptions, the US Department of Health and Human Services sponsored a project to examine the net present value of private returns on antibiotics as well as the net present value of antimicrobials to society as a whole [43]. Of the six indications that were studied, none of them exceeded the $100 million net present value threshold necessary to justify development by a company. This stands in contrast to the societal value that these agents bring. For example, the private returns of a drug developed for hospital-acquired or ventilator-associated pneumonia range from -$23.5 million to $126.7 million with an average return of -$4.5 million, as opposed to the societal value that an antibiotic for the same indication being $1.068 billion to $161.355 billion with the average being $12.166 billion. This trend was upheld in all indications studied, which included acute bacterial otitis media, acute bacterial skin and skin structure, community-acquired pneumonia, and complicated urinary tract infections. These estimations contain a large degree of variability, however they are the most accurate available and they represent the enormous discrepancy between commercial returns on antimicrobials and the value that they bring to society [43].

Despite the many clinical, pharmacological, and societal differences that antibiotics possess relative to other new marketed pharmaceuticals, the business model for commercializing them remains remarkably similar. The current model of selling new antimicrobials is the same price to volume model that most other new drugs use. This model has a paradoxical effect when used for antibiotics because it encourages use of the new antimicrobial agents, which in turn drives resistance. Given the shortage of good choices and the difficulty in developing antibiotics that treat drug-resistant infections, the business model used to promote them should one which is more in harmony with antimicrobial stewardship efforts [47].

POTENTIAL SOLUTIONS FOR THE DRYING PIPELINE

Although several initiatives have been implemented to spur antimicrobial development, there is still room for improvement. If the problem is to be alleviated, the economic, regulatory, and commercial disincentives must be addressed.

The potential solutions that can be implemented can be categorized as either "push" or "pull" incentives. Push incentives aim to reduce the cost of antimicrobial research and development that is associated with bringing a new agent to market, while pull incentives establish a market for new products to ensure that return on investment is enough to incentivize development [36]. Since the reasons for the problem are multifactorial, there is not one push or pull incentive that will solve the entire problem, so a combination of incentives from both categories must be employed to reinstate balance into the antimicrobial market.

Thankfully there are many potential solutions available that can help drive the net present value of antimicrobials towards a threshold that is conducive to antimicrobial development. While having several treatment options for bacterial infections is ideal, there must be careful consideration to implement the strategies in a way that favors development of products that target an unmet medical need. Lessons from the recent past must be applied to avoid repeated failures as there were many antibiotics that were approved in the 1980s and 1990s that were not used clinically and subsequently withdrawn from the market due to a lack of significant differentiation from other marketed agents. This experience can be avoided by focusing incentives on discovery and development of antibiotics that address the largest bacterial threats [47, 48]. If executed properly, a combination of interventions may provide the required incentives for pharmaceutical developers to return to the field of infectious diseases.

Formation of Sustainable Clinical Trial Networks

A large problem facing clinical development of antimicrobials is the disparity between the high cost of pivotal trials and return-on-investment. This inefficiency can be reversed with a push incentive that has been proven effective in the oncology therapeutic area- the creation of global disease-specific Phase 2 and

Phase 3 non-inferiority clinical trial networks which target common bacterial infections [36, 39]. Biomedical Advanced Research and Development Authority (BARDA) has recently issued a request for more information to assess the feasibility of this approach [49]. While there are meaningful differences between the oncology and infectious diseases therapeutic areas, the proven nature of such networks are encouraging and are likely replicable in infectious diseases for new antibacterials, antifungals and diagnostic technologies [39].

Clinical trial networks can focus on common infections that have relatively predictable morbidity and mortality rates and be compared to a high-quality agent as a control. Example study indications include: complicated urinary tract, complicated intra-abdominal, and hospital-associated/ventilator-associated bacterial pneumonia. In these networks, master protocols would be applied to patients with a designated infection due to usual drug resistance profiles, who would be continuously enrolled and randomized [39, 49]. Since patients commonly present to hospitals with these infections, the pace of the trials would be predictable. In addition, global enrollment would be a possibility since many of the common antibiotic treatments are available around the world. Due to the continuous enrollment of patients, investigational drugs can be rotated in and out of the randomization process and several drugs can be investigated at one time [39].

There are several potential benefits that the implementation of clinical trial networks can provide to Phase 2 and Phase 3 studies. First, once a constant control arm has been established, assuming the clinical outcomes to the study designs are consistent, it is possible to share data from subjects enrolled in the control arm among the different clinical trials. For example, if several study drugs were being investigated at the same time, only one control arm would be required, which in turn would decrease the number of subjects required for enrollment by an estimated 33% therefore translating into an enormous cost-savings. Additionally, having a constantly on-going clinical trial would expedite the time it takes to complete the clinical trial. It is estimated that a mature clinical trial network could generate data equivalent to a stand-alone 700-patient clinical trial in the time required to enroll only 400 patients yielding a time and cost reduction of 43% [39].

Another benefit of sustainable clinical trial networks would be the elimination of "biocreep." If the progression of new pivotal trials is Drug A *vs* B, then B *vs* C, then C *vs* D, a situation may arise where each investigational drug is statistically non-inferior, but slight reductions in efficacy over time could lead to Drug D being inferior to Drug A. This is known as "biocreep," and clinical trial networks would eliminate this phenomenon because the control group would be consistent over time, meaning one investigational agent could essentially be compared to the same control arm as other investigational agents [39].

The formation of global clinical trial networks would also make clinical trial operations more efficient [39, 49]. There would be a lesser need for contract negotiations, ethical approval, and other startup processes that are time-consuming and costly. While these networks would not eliminate startup processes altogether (due to the need to include the investigational agents), they would be greatly reduced, resulting in an estimated increase in net present value of $55 million on a drug with total lifetime future revenue net present value of $1 billion [39].

The formation of sustainable global clinical trial networks can potentially reduce the size of clinical trials, improve the quality of the data generated, and decrease the amount of time it takes to generate the necessary data for regulatory approval. If implemented, these networks would address the economic and regulatory challenges of antimicrobial development by decreasing the cost of developing these public goods. If rapid diagnostics are incorporated into the standardized protocols, these networks would help address the imperfect information associated with using these agents. This intervention would result in not only cost savings but it would standardize the data in a way which leads to a better understanding of the investigational drugs.

Streamlined and Standardized Regulatory Frameworks

The regulatory guidelines in different jurisdictions around the world have led to a fractionated global antimicrobial market where even if an antimicrobial agent was available in one country, there is no guarantee that the same antibiotic would be available in another country where it may be needed. A way to alleviate this issue would be to establish a push incentive that would standardize a global regulatory framework which can lead to global regulatory approval based off of the same research data regardless of the geographic region.

One concept for a universal regulatory framework has been proposed which involves four tiers (tier A through tier D) of regulatory pathways and is based off of experience from the orphan drug regulatory pathway. The different tiers are shown in Fig. (**2**) and vary in requirements of data that would be needed for regulatory approval and range from standard non-inferiority development programs with robust clinical data to small programs with limited data. Moving from Tier A to Tier D requires increased reliance on human pharmacokinetic data combined with preclinical data [50, 51]. The data required for Tier A would be two well-controlled, adequately powered phase 3 clinical trials per body site; Tier B requirements would be one phase 3 clinical trial plus smaller comparative and descriptive studies; Tier C requirements would be small comparative and descriptive studies alone; Tier D requirements would be human safety studies and the "animal rule," which would apply when acquisition of clinical efficacy data is either unethical or not feasible [50]. As the tiers progress, the focus turns from body sites of infection (tier A) to pathogen-focused development (tiers B and C) to infectious agent focused (tier D) [51]. The tier that would be most applicable to pursue would be related to the extent of the unmet medical need of the compound being studied as well as the feasibility of completion of the required clinical data. This approach takes advantage of a unique characteristic of antibiotics; the clinical applicability of preclinical data for antibiotics is particularly high compared to other classes of drugs. As a result, clinical decision making can be made based off of well-understood *in vitro* and pharmacokinetic-pharmacodynamic data in a setting with a confirmed serious or life-threatening disease caused by a drug-resistant infection. This proposal will be most helpful in situations where a clinical trial examining the efficacy of an antibiotic in infections caused by resistant organisms is not feasible [50].

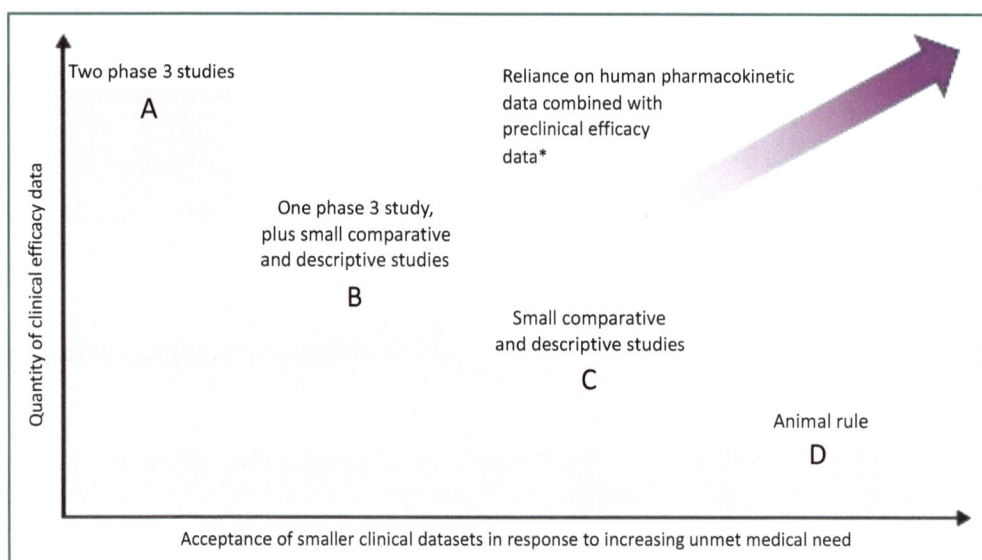

Fig. (2). Balance of quantity of clinical data with increasing unmet medical need. Figure adapted from the Lancet Infectious Diseases [50].

While these regulatory pathways would be beneficial in any single jurisdiction, and resemble those already in place at the FDA, if access to antimicrobials is going to be optimized, a similar approach towards regulatory approval must be recognized in as many countries as possible. The challenges that such frameworks would address would be economic and regulatory-related due to the streamlined nature of these global regulatory frameworks, which would impact access to new antimicrobial therapies. Because patients around the world would have increased access to new therapies, this type of intervention would decrease the effect that externalities affect the industry [50].

De-linked Return-on-Investment from Sales

The differences of antimicrobial agents to other therapeutic areas have been well described above. However, the return on investment of a new antimicrobial is similar to other therapeutic classes, and is based off of the volume that is used. Since the likelihood of antibiotic resistance is increased with high use of antibiotics, this business model is counter-productive towards antimicrobial stewardship principles. In an effort to recoup their return on investment, manufacturers in this model may encourage the use of new antibiotics which may lead to resistance to occur more rapidly. If companies can only generate a return on investment with a high sales volume, and if a high sales volume is more likely to lead to antibiotic resistance, this creates a paradox where companies are incentivized to cause resistance to their own agent in an effort to chase commercial returns. The current return on investment model combined with the paucity of new antimicrobials in development has the potential to exacerbate the public health crisis as described previously.

Hospitals are faced with a similar dilemma by being forced to balance cost-containment of new antimicrobials and rapid diagnostics with optimal patient care in the setting of limited treatment options. This has led to an ethical debate as to whether hospitals without extraordinary financial means should continue using less expensive, yet older, more toxic, and less efficacious agents in multidrug resistant infections, *versus* more expensive, newer, safer and more efficacious agents and make cuts elsewhere in their system to recoup the expense. To address this issue, a focus on a pull incentive affecting reimbursement of new antimicrobials is of upmost importance. If done correctly, alternative models can be implemented that encourage the commercialization of new antimicrobial agents without encouraging their use in a volume-to-sales model [17, 52].

One solution to this problem is to break the link between sales volume and return on investment, also known as "de-linkage," which means companies are paid to produce antimicrobial agents on some basis other than sales volume [52]. In June 2018, the FDA released a statement indicating that discussions are underway to address this by implementing a strategy to de-link antimicrobial use and profitability from sales. Under this approach, rather than institutions paying for antibiotics on a per-use basis, the model can change to a licensing model. Under such a model, the institutions that are most likely to prescribe these new agents would pay a fixed licensing fee for access to the drugs, which would provide them access to a certain number of annual doses. According to the FDA, there have been discussions with CMS to determine the feasibility of such a program as well as whether it might achieve the intended benefits. This model would provide a predictable return on investment and revenue stream for drug developers through more predictable licensing fees [53].

In January of 2019, the United Kingdom accounced that it is committing to a 20-year vision and initial 5-year plan to combat antimicrobial resistance [54, 55]. There are several actions included in the plan but one of the most important is finding a path to de-link volume of antibiotic purchased from sales. The plan states that "We will test a new model that will de-link the payments made to companies from the volumes of antibiotics sold, basing the payment on a NICE led assessment of the value of the medicines and supporting good stewardship [55]." This model would reimburse companies based off the value their antimicrobial brings to the National Health Service (NHS) rather than the volume sold which represents a radical change from the current model employed.

Another potential model to de-link return on investment from sales is the implementation of milestone payments, where payments could be predictable in size and duration after registration. Such payments would only be provided if the new agent targets an area of unmet need, which would decrease the likelihood of companies developing new but clinically-irrelevant antibiotics [52]. One model that has been developed assumes a net present value of $100 million at commencement of R&D and would cost $919 million in payments spread out over the entire development process per antimicrobial [56]. Another model assumes net present value of $300 million at commencement of R&D and would cost a total of $2.5 billion over the course of 5 years [5 payments of $500 million per year) [57]. One last model does not specify net present value at the start of R&D but estimates costs to be between $2-4 billion per antimicrobial, paid 3 years after registration [17].

While de-linking antimicrobial sales from volume sold may address some of the commercial challenges associated with antimicrobial development, the proposals are not without limitations. First, it is not reasonable to assign the same de-linked reward to all antibiotics. Deciding how much each individual agent should receive would be difficult and potentially arbitrary. Also, there would be no incentive to develop the drug beyond the minimum requirements to receive payment, which would impact the amount of information available to prescribing physicians and ultimately might affect patient outcomes [52]. Lastly, a stable form of funding would need to be secured through public funding. Some models suggest creating a world-wide authority to implement this fund, which may not be feasible [58, 59].

It is possible that some form of de-linked payments may prove useful in the future, such as the one proposed by the UK and FDA, however there must be additional work done in this area.

Non-Antimicrobial Interventions

The emergence of bacteria which develop resistance to antimicrobials is well known, documented, and nearly impossible to prevent. As long as there are new antimicrobials available and being used, bacteria will eventually devise ways to survive in their presence. For this reason, it is imperative to develop new ways of preventing and treating infections that are not conventional small molecule antibiotics but still a considered a pharmacological intervention. These new products may be able to prolong the amount of time that currently available agents retain antimicrobial activity which may come in the form of vaccines, probiotics, antibodies, bacteriophages, or lysins [17].

In addition to new non-antibiotic pharmacological interventions, innovative rapid diagnostic technologies have the potential to not only impact antimicrobial stewardship and outcomes of infectious diseases, but they can also address the imperfect information economic phenomenon associated with the use to antibiotics. These technologies are becoming more common in institutions and may eventually lead to real-time results that clinicians can use to optimize clinical decision making. By incorporating rapid diagnostics into antimicrobial stewardship programs, institutions have been able to decrease the amount of antibiotics used, including broad-spectrum agents, and therefore slow the emergence of resistance [60]. When employed, these technologies have successfully been able to shorten the time that a patient receives empiric antimicrobial therapy [61]. Eventually, the goal is to shorten empiric antibiotic therapy to be as short as possible or to eliminate empiric therapy altogether and replace with narrow spectrum agents if diagnostic data is received in a timely manner. The problem with such innovative technologies is their immense expense. Larger academic medical centers may be able to overcome this challenge, but it is a major deterrent for use in smaller community hospitals throughout the world. In order for these life-saving technologies to be employed to the broadest patient population possible, they must be economically attractive [17].

Non-antibiotic interventions have the potential to address externalities as well as the imperfect information associated with developing new antimicrobial agents. The effects of externalities would be diminished with the use of probiotics, vaccines, bacteriophages, or lysins because they have the potential to either decrease incidence or transmissibility of multidrug resistant infections which would benefit the broader population. The rapid diagnostic instruments would decrease the amount of imperfect information available to the clinician at the time the antimicrobial is being ordered or prescribed. Together these new agents and technologies have the potential to benefit the broader population while prolonging the time that the currently available standard antimicrobial treatments remain active.

PROGRESS MADE ON THE DRYING PIPELINE

Due to the many challenges that have disincentivized the pharmaceutical industry's interest in antibiotic development, several initiatives have been implemented that focus on mending the issues that have led to the dry antibiotic pipeline. Attention has concentrated on legislative acts that allow for incentives for pharmaceutical companies to recoup a return on investment as well as streamlining the regulatory hurdles that allow for a new antibiotic to be brought to market more efficiently. In addition, several public-private partnerships have developed innovative funding mechanisms and have acted as catalysts aimed at fixing the global market failure that incentivizes research in discovery and clinical development of new antibiotics. The different types of incentives that have been implemented and/or proposed are in Table **1**.

Table 1. Potential and Implemented Incentive Strategies Categorized into Push and Pull Incentives [36, 39, 50, 52, 62 - 66].

Push Incentives
Public-Private Partnerships • Combating Antibiotic-Resistant Bacteria Biopharmaceutical - Xccelerating global antibacterial innovation (CARB-X) • Antibacterial Resistance Leadership Group (ARLG) • New Drugs for Bad Bugs (ND4BB) • European and Developing Countries Clinical Trials Partnership (EDCTP)
Expedited Regulatory Pathways • Limited Population Antibacterial Development pathway (LPAD)
Clinical Trial Networks
Tax Credits • Reinvigorating Antibiotic and Diagnostic Innovation Act (READI)
Pull Incentives
Market Exclusivity • Generating Antibiotic Incentives Now Act (GAIN)
Reimbursement Changes • New Technology Add-on Payment (NTAP)
De-Link Return-on-Investment from Sales

Legislative Advances Affecting Antimicrobial Drug Development

There have been several legislative initiatives that have been implemented to reinvigorate the antibiotic development pipeline. The Generating Antibiotic Incentives Now (GAIN) Act was signed into law in 2012 which helped address one of the commercial concerns to antibiotic development [64]. The GAIN Act allows designation of qualified infectious disease products (QIDPs), which offers an additional 5-year extension on patent life which allows for a longer time period for companies to recoup their investment from costs incurred during their development program. Anti-infective agents with QIDP status receive fast track and priority review status from the FDA and undergo an expedited regulatory review process [67]. This advancement has provided a longer opportunity for developers to regain much of the cost associated with bringing a new antimicrobial to market and has already resulted in a meanginful amount of new antimicrobials that have qualified for this designation (Table **2**).

The 21st Century Cures Act (Cures Act) was signed into law in 2016 and is designed to help accelerate medical product development and bring new innovations and advancements to patients who need them faster and more efficiently [68]. The Antibiotic Development to Advance Patient Treatment (ADAPT) Act was modeled after the Cures Act but is aimed specifically at infectious diseases products. It accelerates the FDA approval process for antibacterial and antifungal therapies for the treatment of patients with serious or life threatening infections who have limited treatment options [69]. It achieves this by establishing an accelerated approval process, the Limited Population Antibacterial Drug approval pathway, which streamlines the regulatory path for antibacterial or antifungal agents that is intended to treat a serious or life-threatening infection in a limited population of patients with an unmet medical need [70, 71]. The end result of this accelerated regulatory pathway is new antibiotic and antifungal agents being available to providers and patients on a quicker timeline. Given the urgency of antimicrobial resistance, this advancement invaluable.

The Centers for Medicare & Medicaid Services (CMS) New Technology Add-on Payment (NTAP) program was designed to support timely access of innovative therapies used to treat Medicare beneficiaries in the inpatient setting. The NTAP program is only available to new technologies demonstrating a substantial clinical improvement from standard-of-care and would provide additional reimbursement to hospitals of up to 50% of the cost of the new technology when the diagnosis related group (DRG) is not sufficient. However, the NTAP reimbursement system has been criticized for its utility in supplementing payments for antibiotics [47, 65]. In response, the Developing an Innovative Strategy for Antimicrobial

Resistant Microorganisms (DISARM) Act was introduced in the House of Representatives in 2015 and was subsequently passed as a provision of the 21st Century Cures Act [72]. The DISARM act amends title XVIII (Medicare) of the Social Security Act to direct the Secretary of Health and Human Services to: recognize the costs of DISARM antimicrobial drugs under the Medicare payment system for the inpatient services, provide for additional payment with respect to discharges involving such drugs, publish in the Federal Register a list of the DISARM antimicrobial drugs, and make a proportional adjustment in standardized payment amounts to assure that the requirements of this act do not result in aggregate payments greater or less than those that would otherwise be made for a fiscal year. A DISARM antimicrobial drug is defined as a QIDP drug FDA approved on or after January 1, 2015, intended to treat an infection for which there is an unmet medical need, caused by a qualifying pathogen, and associated with high rates of morbidity and mortality. To date, DISARM has passed in the House of Representatives but has yet to be introduced in the US Senate [72]. The DISARM act is absolutely critical in addressing perhaps the most important disincentive to antimicrobial development- lack of meaningful reimbursement for valuable life-saving agents. Passing this legislation would be a major step in the fight towards a more robust antimicrobial pipeline and it is essential to continue to support its passage. In the meantime the NTAP program is one way to increase reimbursement. However, the infectious diseases community has signaled inefficiencies in applying for reimbursement as well as receiving payment and it is therefore not enough of a change to drive further antimicrobial development.

The Reinvigorating Antibiotic and Diagnostic Innovation (READI) Act was introduced to the House of Representatives in 2017 [63]. The READI Act amends the Internal Revenue Code to allow tax credits for 50% of the clinical testing expenses for infectious diseases products that are intended to treat a serious or life-threatening infection, including those caused by an antibacterial or antifungal resistant pathogens or a qualifying pathogen listed by the Department of Health and Human Services as having the potential to pose a serious threat to public health. It also includes *in vitro* diagnostic devices that can identify in less than four hours the presence, concentration, or characteristics of a serious or life-threatening infection. Decreasing the cost of antimibrobial development would provide a strong incentive to reinvest in this therapeutic area. The READI act would be a powerful addition to the many advancements that have either been enacted or considered and continued support is warranted.

Regulatory Advances Affecting Antimicrobial Drug Development

Prior to FDA approval, each drug marketed in the US must go through a detailed

FDA review process. Historically, the FDA has encouraged at least two rigorous clinical trials for antibiotics (preferably randomized, double-blind, placebo-controlled studies) that independently show a statistically and clinically meaningful benefit to obtain approval [11]. However, for drugs of clinical importance, the FDA maintains four expedited pathways intended to help shorten the drug development and approval timeline and make new antibiotics available quicker. The available expedited regulatory designations are listed in Table 2, and include fast track, breakthrough therapy, priority review and accelerated approval. Each of the designations is designed to facilitate drug development and/or expedite antibacterial or antifungal agents to market for serious infections considered for patients with unmet medical needs [73]. Under GAIN, a QIDP product is eligible for both priority review and a FDA fast track designation [67].

In 2015, the Limited Population Antibacterial Development pathway (LPAD) was established which expedited antibiotic development by allowing pharmaceutical companies to follow a streamlined development program [70]. A streamlined development program may involve smaller, shorter, or fewer clinical trials that meet the same safety and efficacy standards as any other drug. The determination of safety and efficacy would reflect the benefit/risk profile of the drug in the intended population that takes into account the severity, rarity, or prevalence of the infection the product is intended to treat. It would also take into account whether there are alternatives or treatment options available for the target population. Acceptable data for FDA approval could include a combination of non-clinical, *in vitro* susceptibility, PK/PD, phase II clinical trials, and any other data deemed applicable to obtain approval of the new anti-infective agent. To ensure that LPAD-approved agents are used only for the intended population, the product label must include the statement: "This drug is indicated for use in a limited and specific population of patients" and all related promotional materials related to the product must be reviewed by the FDA 30 days prior to dissemination [70].

The 505(b) [2] New Drug Application (NDA) is an existing pathway established in 1984 to help avoid unnecessary duplication of studies that have already been performed on previously approved drugs. The 505 (b) [2] pathway allows a manufacturer to submit their product for FDA review by including data and/or study results originally collected by another manufacturer or researcher. The applicant can rely on existing safety and efficacy data to reduce the amount of new, preapproval data required and thus streamline the regulatory approval process. To date, ceftazidime/avibactam and meropenem/vaborbactam are the only FDA approved antibiotics which have utilized this pathway to apply for approval. Ceftazidime/avibactam is a combination of the cephalosporin, ceftazidime, approved by the FDA in 1985, and a novel β-lactamase inhibitor, avibactam. The FDA review relied on the historical data of safety and efficacy for ceftazidime (including the finding for the cUTI and cIAI indications) alone as well as clinical data, animal models of infection, and *in vitro* data that support the role of avibactam in combination [74]. On initial approval, prescribing information stated that ceftazidime/avibactam should be limited to patients with limited to no alternative treatment options. However, after phase III studies in cUTI and cIAI were completed, the limited use language was removed from the prescribing information [75].

Table 2. FDA Regulatory Pathways Expediting Antimicrobial Development [11, 70, 71, 73, 76, 77] *Designates a Qualified Infectious Disease Product (QIDP).

Regulatory Pathway	Description	Antimicrobial (year of approval)
Accelerated Approval Pathway	▪ Designed to facilitate development and expedite FDA review based on a surrogate endpoint that must show advantage over existing therapies ▪ Phase 4 confirmatory trials must be conducted to verify clinical benefit o Approval can be withdrawn or the labeled indication can be changed	▪ Quinupristin/dalfopristin [1999] ▪ Bedaquiline [2012] ▪ Amikacin liposome inhalation [2018]
Priority Review	▪ Designed to expedite FDA review by shortening a review of an NDA from 10 months to 6 months ▪ Must show evidence of increased effectiveness in treatment or prevention of a condition or safety & effectiveness in a new subpopulation ▪ Designation does not affect the length of the clinical development period or alter the quality of evidence necessary for approval.	▪ Fidaxomicin [2011] ▪ Bedaquiline [2012] ▪ Dalbavancin [2014]* ▪ Oritavancin [2014]* ▪ Tedizolid [2014]* ▪ Ceftolozane/tazobactam [2014]* ▪ Ceftazidime/avibactam [2015]* ▪ Delafloxacin [2017]* ▪ Meropenem/vaborbactam [2017]* ▪ Omadacycline [2018]* ▪ Eravacycline [2018]* ▪ Amikacin liposome inhalation [2018]*

(Table 2) cont.....

Regulatory Pathway	Description	Antimicrobial (year of approval)
Fast Track Designation	• Designed to facilitate development and expedite FDA review of drugs to fill an unmet medical need in a serious condition that requires a review and decision within 60 days • Requires more frequent meetings and written communication with the FDA • Phase 3 clinical trials still required • Rolling NDA review	• Ceftaroline [2010] • Fidaxomicin [2011] • Bedaquiline [2012] • Dalbavancin [2014]* • Oritavancin [2014]* • Tedizolid [2014]* • Ceftolozane/tazobactam [2014]* • Ceftazidime/avibactam [2015]* • Delafloxacin [2017]* • Meropenem/vaborbactam [2017]* • Omadacycline [2018]* • Eravacycline [2018]* • Amikacin liposome inhalation [2018]*
Breakthrough Therapy Designation	• Designed to facilitate development and expedite FDA review of drugs intended to treat a serious condition and preliminary evidence demonstrate substantial improvement over available therapy on a clinically significant endpoint. • Designation receives a fast track designation and involves intensive FDA involvement during development (as early as Phase 1]	• Amikacin liposome inhalation [2018] *
Limited Population Antibacterial Drug	• Designed to facilitate development and approval of anti-infective agents to treat serious or life-threatening infections in a limited population of patients with unmet needs • May follow a streamlined development program • Requires prescribing information to include a statement indicating the limited population for which they are appropriate.	• Amikacin liposome inhalation [2018]* • Plazomicin [2018]*
505(b) [2]	• Expedites drug approvals involving changes to previously approved drugs (*e.g.* formulation, route, dosage, or strength) • Sponsors can rely on existing safety and efficacy data to reduce the amount of new, preapproval data required	• Ceftazidime/avibactam [2015]* • Meropenem/vaborbactam [2017]*

Public-Private-partnerships Incentivizing Antimicrobial Development

Public-private partnerships are initiatives that provide innovative funding mechanisms and shifts return-on-investment in ways that incentivizes companies to continue or re-start research in discovery and clinical development of new antibiotics. Two main government programs have emerged to aid in late-stage development of novel antibiotics: the US government's Broad Spectrum

Antimicrobial Program within BARDA, and the European Union's, New Drugs for Bad Bugs program under the Innovative Medicines Initiative. Together, both programs represent over $900 million in planned public funding [62].

BARDA was originally established to support late stage development of countermeasures against pandemic threats and bioterrorism [11]. Since 2010, BARDA's Broad Spectrum Antimicrobial Program has been forming public-private partnerships with the pharmaceutical industry to develop new antibiotics and diagnostics that can treat clinically relevant infections as well as products for biodefense indications consistent with the US Department of Homeland Security material threat list [78]. Funding from BARDA can be used by companies toward various aspects of drug development including clinical trials, manufacturing, or regulatory costs [62]. In 2016, BARDA established the world's largest global antibacterial private-public partnership, "Combating Antibiotic-Resistant Bacteria Biopharmaceutical Accelerator-Xcclerating global antibacterial innovation" (CARB-X) program. CARB-X is a collaboration between BARDA, the National Institute of Allergy and Infectious Diseases (NIAID), Boston University, Wellcome Trust, the UK Government's Global Antimicrobial Resistance Innovation Fund (GAMRIF), and the Bill & Melinda Gates Foundation as well as other academic, industry, and private organizations. The goal of the CARB-X program is to support projects in the early phases of development through Phase 1 so that they will attract additional funding to further clinical development and eventual approval. The scope of CARB-X funding is restricted to projects that target drug-resistant bacteria highlighted on the CDC's Antibiotic Resistant Threats list, or the Priority Bacterial Pathogens list published by the World Health Organization [7, 27]. To date, the CARB-X portfolio has 33 projects in seven countries and is actively managing $91.1 million in awards to research and development projects that accelerate the development of antibiotics and other products [79].

To address the necessity of new antibiotics and the regulatory hurdles for approval, the NIAID has been collaborating with the FDA and pharmaceutical companies to facilitate research on many aspects of drug development including: funding research projects, assisting with investigational new drug submissions, and exploring innovative and more feasible clinical trial infrastructures for new antibiotic development [80]. Established in 2013, the Antibacterial Resistance Leadership Group (ARLG) was formed by the NIAID to facilitate, implement, and manage a clinical research agenda that will increase knowledge of and mitigate the important factors that drive antimicrobial resistance. The ARLG has prioritized areas of research on infections caused by Gram-negative and Gram-positive bacteria, infection control/antimicrobial stewardship, and rapid diagnostics to either detect bacterial pathogens or antimicrobial susceptibility

[81]. In 2016, the NIAID released a funding opportunity for milestone-driven research aimed at advancing antibiotic development for select Gram-negative pathogens: Carbapenem-resistant Enterobacteriaceae (CRE), multidrug-resistant (MDR) *Acinetobacter*, and MDR *Pseudomonas aeruginosa*. The plan is to commit $9 million to fund 10 to 15 awards in 2018 that support projects that focus on developing novel predictive models and/or research tools and assays aimed at gaining a better understanding of the properties governing bacterial penetration and efflux of drug-like small molecules [82].

The Innovative Medicines Initiative is a public-private partnership between the European Union and the European Federation of Pharmaceutical Industries and Associations [83]. The Innovative Medicines Initiative's New Drugs for Bad Bugs (ND4BB) initiative was established in 2012 and is a platform of eight partially cross-linked research projects that address some of the biggest challenges in antibiotic development [84]. The overall vision of the ND4BB initiative is to create an innovative collaboration that will encompass all aspects from the discovery of new antibiotics to Phase II and III clinical trials to reimbursement and appropriate use with the aim of reinvigorating antibiotic research and development. The TRANSLOCATION and ENABLE projects specifically focus on the discovery and development of Gram-negative agents whereas COMBACTE focuses on clinical development of Gram-positive agents. The COMBACTE-CARE project focuses on clinical development of antibiotics for MDR Gram-negative pathogens and COMBACTE-MAGNET focuses on the clinical development of systemic molecules against healthcare associated infections due to clinically challenging Gram-negative pathogens. Lastly, DRIVE-AB will define a standard for the responsible use of antibiotics to minimize collateral damage and risk of emergence of antimicrobial resistance. DRIVE-AB will also develop, test and recommend innovative economic strategies and reward models to incentivize investment and development of new antimicrobial agents [85]. The total allocated budget in ND4BB is €660 million (~ $776 million) of which the pharmaceutical industry is contributing €347 million (~$397 million) [84].

The European and Developing Countries Clinical Trials Partnership (EDCTP) was formed in 2003, followed by EDCTP2 in 2014. The EDCTP is an evolving public–public partnership between 14 European countries, 14 African countries and the EU, in collaboration with the pharmaceutical industry [86]. The EDCTP provides a push incentive in the form of direct funding for research and development resources and infrastructure required to move a drug candidate through the clinical development phases that aims to support interventions in the prevention and treatment of of HIV/AIDs, tuberculosis, malaria and neglected infectious diseases, including certain bacterial infections, in sub-Saharan Africa [66].

The legislative and regulatory attention given to infectious diseases therapeutics is highly encouraging and represents a positive step in tackling the problems associated with increased microbial resistance. They have resulted in numerous accelerated drug approval pathways as well as public-private partnerships which were either formed or fortified. These advancements provide resources to developers, saves some of the costs of development, and lengthens the time that a company can recoup their investment. While these are very important measures, continued support is necessary for those advancements that have not yet been made, particularly as it pertains to the several legislative ideas that have been formulated but not yet been passed. Without additional legislative action the market failure described above will not be fully corrected. Addressing this issue broadly is what is ultimately going to drive companies towards investment into infectious diseases and development of new therapeutics.

CONCLUSION

Antimicrobials are an indispensable class of therapeutics in healthcare and are a miracle in modern medicine [87]. The unique qualities that they possess have changed the way that diseases are treated and have allowed many different parts of contemporary medicine to flourish [17]. However these positive outcomes have come at a cost, as higher use of antibiotics has resulted in bacterial evolution and antimicrobial resistance. There has been a simultaneous drastic reduction in the research and development of antimicrobials and therefore fewer new treatment options have become available to counter this problem. This phenomenon has progressed to the point where there are many infections today that are caused by bacteria for which there are no safe or effective treatment options. A public health crisis throughout the world has emerged as resistance is growing faster than the new antibiotic armamentarium [87].

Thankfully, there has been enough global awareness that governments and think tanks have sponsored research into the causes as well as potential solutions to alleviate the problem [11]. According to Pew Charitable Trusts, as of September 2018 there are 42 new antibiotics in development which have the potential to treat serious bacterial infections [88]. It is difficult to estimate the impact of new legislation or regulatory initiatives on development of these agents as many were in clinical development prior to implementation of the initiative, although this figure is encouraging nonetheless. Despite the advancements that have been made to alleviate the challenges of developing new agents, we are still in the beginning phases and there is much work to be done.

The future of healthcare is very much dependent on overcoming this public health crisis [87]. If enough of the disincentives to antibiotic development are removed, it is possible to gain an advantage over the rapid evolution of bacteria and formation of antimicrobial resistance. While it will not be easy to do so, it is entirely possible and may result in many novel safe and effective options that target multidrug resistant bacterial infections.

CONSENT FOR PUBLICATION

Not applicable.

CONFLICT OF INTEREST

The author(s) confirm that this chapter content has no conflict of interest.

ACKNOWLEDGEMENTS

Declared none.

REFERENCES

[1]   Prevention CfDCa. Antibiotic Resistance Threats in the United States, 2019. Atlanta, GA: U.S. Department of Health and Human Services, CDC 2019.

[2]   Infectious Diseases Society of America. The 10 x '20 Initiative: pursuing a global commitment to develop 10 new antibacterial drugs by 2020. Clin Infect Dis 2010; 50(8): 1081-3.
[http://dx.doi.org/10.1086/652237] [PMID: 20214473]

[3]   Norrby SR, Nord CE, Finch R. European Society of Clinical Microbiology and Infectious Diseases. Lack of development of new antimicrobial drugs: a potential serious threat to public health. Lancet Infect Dis 2005; 5(2): 115-9.
[http://dx.doi.org/10.1016/S1473-3099(05)70086-4] [PMID: 15680781]

[4]   Spellberg B, Powers JH, Brass EP, Miller LG, Edwards JE Jr. Trends in antimicrobial drug development: implications for the future. Clin Infect Dis 2004; 38(9): 1279-86.
[http://dx.doi.org/10.1086/420937] [PMID: 15127341]

[5]   Talbot GH, Bradley J, Edwards JE Jr, Gilbert D, Scheld M, Bartlett JG. Antimicrobial Availability Task Force of the Infectious Diseases Society of America. Bad bugs need drugs: an update on the development pipeline from the Antimicrobial Availability Task Force of the Infectious Diseases Society of America. Clin Infect Dis 2006; 42(5): 657-68.
[http://dx.doi.org/10.1086/499819] [PMID: 16447111]

[6]   A. Antibiotic Resistance: Implications for Global Health and Novel Intervention Strategies: Workshop Summary The National Academies Collection: Reports funded by National Institutes of Health Washington (DC)2010. 2010.

[7]   Prevention CfDCa. Antibiotic resistance threats in the United States 2013; 2013

[8]   Bugs IMINDfB https://www.imi.europa.eu/projects-results/project-factsheets/nd4bb [Available from]

[9]   Organization WH. Global Action Plan on Antimicrobial Resistance. Geneva, Switzerland 2015.

[10]   National Action Plan for Combating Antibiotic-Resistant Bacteria Washington DC 2015.

[11]   Luepke KH, Mohr JF III. The antibiotic pipeline: reviving research and development and speeding

drugs to market. Expert Rev Anti Infect Ther 2017; 15(5): 425-33.
[http://dx.doi.org/10.1080/14787210.2017.1308251] [PMID: 28306360]

[12]   Piddock LJ. The crisis of no new antibiotics--what is the way forward? Lancet Infect Dis 2012; 12(3): 249-53.
[http://dx.doi.org/10.1016/S1473-3099(11)70316-4] [PMID: 22101066]

[13]   Sengupta S, Chattopadhyay MK, Grossart HP. The multifaceted roles of antibiotics and antibiotic resistance in nature. Front Microbiol 2013; 4: 47.
[http://dx.doi.org/10.3389/fmicb.2013.00047] [PMID: 23487476]

[14]   UNITED States vital statistics, 1951-1952. Public Health Rep 1953; 68(1): 68-70.
[PMID: 13004224]

[15]   Levine DP. Vancomycin: a history. Clin Infect Dis 2006; 42 (Suppl. 1): S5-S12.
[http://dx.doi.org/10.1086/491709] [PMID: 16323120]

[16]   https://www.cdc.gov/drugresistance/about.html

[17]   O'Neill J. Tackling drug-resistant infections globally: final report and recommendations. Review on Antimicrobial Resistance 2016.

[18]   Ayukekbong JA, Ntemgwa M, Atabe AN. The threat of antimicrobial resistance in developing countries: causes and control strategies. Antimicrob Resist Infect Control 2017; 6: 47.
[http://dx.doi.org/10.1186/s13756-017-0208-x] [PMID: 28515903]

[19]   Okeke IN, Klugman KP, Bhutta ZA, *et al.* Antimicrobial resistance in developing countries. Part II: strategies for containment. Lancet Infect Dis 2005; 5(9): 568-80.
[http://dx.doi.org/10.1016/S1473-3099(05)70217-6] [PMID: 16122680]

[20]   Saleh N, Awada S, Awwad R, *et al.* Evaluation of antibiotic prescription in the Lebanese community: a pilot study. Infect Ecol Epidemiol 2015; 5: 27094.
[http://dx.doi.org/10.3402/iee.v5.27094] [PMID: 26112266]

[21]   de Kraker ME, Davey PG, Grundmann H. BURDEN study group. Mortality and hospital stay associated with resistant Staphylococcus aureus and *Escherichia coli* bacteremia: estimating the burden of antibiotic resistance in Europe. PLoS Med 2011; 8(10): e1001104.
[http://dx.doi.org/10.1371/journal.pmed.1001104] [PMID: 22022233]

[22]   de Kraker ME, Wolkewitz M, Davey PG, *et al.* Burden of antimicrobial resistance in European hospitals: excess mortality and length of hospital stay associated with bloodstream infections due to Escherichia coli resistant to third-generation cephalosporins. J Antimicrob Chemother 2011; 66(2): 398-407.
[http://dx.doi.org/10.1093/jac/dkq412] [PMID: 21106563]

[23]   Review on antimicrobial resistance. Securing New Drugs for Future Generations: The Pipeline of Antibiotics 2015. http://amr-review.org/sites/default/files/SECURING%20NEW%20DRUGS%20FOR%20FUTURE%20GENERATIONS%20FINAL%20WEB_0.pdf Available from

[24]   Organization   WH.   Antimicrobial   resistance: global   report   on   surveillance.   2014.
https://www.who.int/drugresistance/documents/surveillancereport/en/

[25]   Michael CA, Dominey-Howes D, Labbate M. The antimicrobial resistance crisis: causes, consequences, and management. Front Public Health 2014; 2: 145.
[http://dx.doi.org/10.3389/fpubh.2014.00145] [PMID: 25279369]

[26]   Organization WH. Global antimicrobial resistance surveillance system (GLASS) report: early implementation 2016-2017. Geneva 2017.

[27]   WHO. publishes list of bacteria for which new antibiotics are urgently needed [press release].

[28]   Hay M, Thomas DW, Craighead JL, Economides C, Rosenthal J. Clinical development success rates for investigational drugs. Nat Biotechnol 2014; 32(1): 40-51.
[http://dx.doi.org/10.1038/nbt.2786] [PMID: 24406927]

[29]   Kesselheim AS, Outterson K. Improving antibiotic markets for long-term sustainability. Yale J Health Policy Law Ethics 2011; 11(1): 101-67.
[PMID: 21381513]

[30]   Payne DJ, Miller LF, Findlay D, Anderson J, Marks L. Time for a change: addressing R&D and commercialization challenges for antibacterials Philos Trans R Soc Lond B Biol Sci 2015; 370(1670).
[http://dx.doi.org/10.1098/rstb.2014.0086] [PMID: 20140086]

[31]   Morel CM, Mossialos E. Stoking the antibiotic pipeline. BMJ 2010; 340: c2115.
[http://dx.doi.org/10.1136/bmj.c2115] [PMID: 20483950]

[32]   Spellberg B, Bartlett J, Wunderink R, Gilbert DN. Novel approaches are needed to develop tomorrow's antibacterial therapies. Am J Respir Crit Care Med 2015; 191(2): 135-40.
[http://dx.doi.org/10.1164/rccm.201410-1894OE] [PMID: 25590154]

[33]   Harbarth S, Theuretzbacher U, Hackett J. DRIVE-AB consortium. Antibiotic research and development: business as usual? J Antimicrob Chemother 2015; 70(6): 1604-7.
[http://dx.doi.org/10.1093/jac/dkv020] [PMID: 25673635]

[34]   Spellberg B. The future of antibiotics. Crit Care 2014; 18(3): 228.
[http://dx.doi.org/10.1186/cc13948] [PMID: 25043962]

[35]   Declaration by the pharmaceutical, biotechnology and diagnostics industries on combating antimicrobial resistance. 2016. https://amr-review.org/sites/default/files/Industry_Declaration_on_Combating_Antimicrobial_Resistance_UPDATED%20SIGNATORIES_MAY_2016.pdf

[36]   Luepke KH, Suda KJ, Boucher H, *et al.* Past, present, and future of antibacterial economics: increasing bacterial resistance, limited antibiotic pipeline, and societal implications. Pharmacotherapy 2017; 37(1): 71-84.
[http://dx.doi.org/10.1002/phar.1868] [PMID: 27859453]

[37]   Harbarth S, Samore MH. Antimicrobial resistance determinants and future control. Emerg Infect Dis 2005; 11(6): 794-801.
[http://dx.doi.org/10.3201/eid1106.050167] [PMID: 15963271]

[38]   Hollis A, Maybarduk P. Antibiotic resistance is a tragedy of the commons that necessitates global cooperation. J Law Med Ethics 2015; 43 (Suppl. 3): 33-7.
[http://dx.doi.org/10.1111/jlme.12272] [PMID: 26243241]

[39]   McDonnell A, Rex JH, Goossens H, Bonten M, Fowler VG Jr, Dane A. Efficient delivery of investigational antibacterial agents *via* sustainable clinical trial networks. Clin Infect Dis 2016; 63 (Suppl. 2): S57-9.
[http://dx.doi.org/10.1093/cid/ciw244] [PMID: 27481955]

[40]   Powers JH. Increasing the efficiency of clinical trials of antimicrobials: the scientific basis of substantial evidence of effectiveness of drugs. Clin Infect Dis 2007; 45 (Suppl. 2): S153-62.
[http://dx.doi.org/10.1086/519253] [PMID: 17683020]

[41]   Davido B, Bouchand F, Calin R, *et al.* High rates of off-label use in antibiotic prescriptions in a context of dramatic resistance increase: a prospective study in a tertiary hospital. Int J Antimicrob Agents 2016; 47(6): 490-4.
[http://dx.doi.org/10.1016/j.ijantimicag.2016.04.010] [PMID: 27208900]

[42]   DiMasi JA, Grabowski HG, Hansen RW. Innovation in the pharmaceutical industry: New estimates of R&D costs. J Health Econ 2016; 47: 20-33.
[http://dx.doi.org/10.1016/j.jhealeco.2016.01.012] [PMID: 26928437]

[43]   Sertkaya AEJ, Birkenbach A. Analytical Framework for Examining the Value of Antibacterial Products 2014. https://aspe.hhs.gov/report/analytical-framework-examining-value-antibacterial-products

[44]   America IDSo Infectious Diseases Society of America's (IDSA) Statement Promoting Anti-Infective

Development and Antimicrobial Stewardship though the US Food and Drug Administration Prescription Drug User Fee Act (PDUFA) Reauthorization Before the House Committee on Energy and Commerce Subcommittee on Health: Infectious Diseases Society of America 2012. http://emerald.tufts.edu/med/apua/index_363_626155726.pdf updated March 8, 2012. Available from

[45]   Gauthier TP, Suda KJ, Mathur SK, *et al.* Free antibiotic and vaccination programmes in community pharmacies of miami-dade county, FL, USA. J Antimicrob Chemother 2015; 70(2): 594-7.
[http://dx.doi.org/10.1093/jac/dku417] [PMID: 25331056]

[46]   Barlam TF, Cosgrove SE, Abbo LM, *et al.* Implementing an antibiotic stewardship program: guidelines by the infectious diseases society of America and the society for healthcare epidemiology of America. Clin Infect Dis 2016; 62(10): e51-77.
[http://dx.doi.org/10.1093/cid/ciw118] [PMID: 27080992]

[47]   Outterson K, Powers JH, Daniel GW, McClellan MB. Repairing the broken market for antibiotic innovation. Health Aff (Millwood) 2015; 34(2): 277-85.
[http://dx.doi.org/10.1377/hlthaff.2014.1003] [PMID: 25646108]

[48]   Outterson K, Powers JH, Seoane-Vazquez E, Rodriguez-Monguio R, Kesselheim AS. Approval and withdrawal of new antibiotics and other antiinfectives in the U.S., 1980-2009. J Law Med Ethics 2013; 41(3): 688-96.
[http://dx.doi.org/10.1111/jlme.12079] [PMID: 24088160]

[49]   Clinical Trial Network for Antibacterial Drugs. 2016. https://www.fbo.gov/index?s=opportunity &mode=form&id=c49bb f90a77767a69c9cdf148879f711&tab=core&_cview=0

[50]   Rex JH, Eisenstein BI, Alder J, *et al.* A comprehensive regulatory framework to address the unmet need for new antibacterial treatments. Lancet Infect Dis 2013; 13(3): 269-75.
[http://dx.doi.org/10.1016/S1473-3099(12)70293-1] [PMID: 23332713]

[51]   Boucher HW, Ambrose PG, Chambers HF, *et al.* Infectious Diseases Society of America. White Paper: Developing Antimicrobial Drugs for Resistant Pathogens, Narrow-Spectrum Indications, and Unmet Needs. J Infect Dis 2017; 216(2): 228-36.
[http://dx.doi.org/10.1093/infdis/jix211] [PMID: 28475768]

[52]   Rex JH, Outterson K. Antibiotic reimbursement in a model delinked from sales: a benchmark-based worldwide approach. Lancet Infect Dis 2016; 16(4): 500-5.
[http://dx.doi.org/10.1016/S1473-3099(15)00500-9] [PMID: 27036356]

[53]   Statement from fda commissioner scott gottlieb. 2018. https://www.fda.gov/NewsEvents/Newsroom/ PressAnnouncements/ucm610503.htm

[54]   https://assets.publishing.service.gov.uk/government/uploads/system/uploads/attachment_data/file/7730 65/uk-20-year-vision-for-antimicrobial-resistance.pdf

[55]   Tackling antimicrobial resistance 2019-2024 The UK's five-year national action plan 2019.
https://assets.publishing.service.gov.uk/government/uploads/system/uploads/attachment_data/file/7731 30/uk-amr-5-year-national-action-plan.pdf [Available from]:

[56]   https://aspe.hhs.gov/system/files/pdf/76891/rpt_antibacterials.pdf

[57]   Sharma P, Towse A. New drugs to tackle antimicrobial resistance: analysis of EU policy options 2011. https://www.ohe.org/publications/new-drugs-tackle-antimicrobial-resistance-analysis-eu-policy-options

[58]   Årdal C, Outterson K, Hoffman SJ, *et al.* International cooperation to improve access to and sustain effectiveness of antimicrobials. Lancet 2016; 387(10015): 296-307.
[http://dx.doi.org/10.1016/S0140-6736(15)00470-5] [PMID: 26603920]

[59]   Hoffman SJ, Outterson K. What will it take to address the global threat of antibiotic resistance? J Law Med Ethics 2015; 43(2): 363-8.
[http://dx.doi.org/10.1111/jlme.12253] [PMID: 26242959]

[60] Caliendo AM, Gilbert DN, Ginocchio CC, *et al.* Infectious Diseases Society of America (IDSA). Better tests, better care: improved diagnostics for infectious diseases. Clin Infect Dis 2013; 57 (Suppl. 3): S139-70.
[http://dx.doi.org/10.1093/cid/cit578] [PMID: 24200831]

[61] Perez KK, Olsen RJ, Musick WL, *et al.* Integrating rapid diagnostics and antimicrobial stewardship improves outcomes in patients with antibiotic-resistant Gram-negative bacteremia. J Infect 2014; 69(3): 216-25.
[http://dx.doi.org/10.1016/j.jinf.2014.05.005] [PMID: 24841135]

[62] Eichberg MJ. Public funding of clinical-stage antibiotic development in the United States and European Union. Health Secur 2015; 13(3): 156-65.
[http://dx.doi.org/10.1089/hs.2014.0081] [PMID: 26042859]

[63] Reinvigorating antibiotic and diagnostic innovation (READI) Act of 2017. 115th Congress, United States of America. 2017. ed. HR 18402017

[64] Generating Antibiotic Incentives Now (GAIN) Act. 112th Congress, United States of America ed S 3187, Title VIII2012.

[65] Renwick MJ, Brogan DM, Mossialos E. A systematic review and critical assessment of incentive strategies for discovery and development of novel antibiotics. J Antibiot (Tokyo) 2016; 69(2): 73-88.
[http://dx.doi.org/10.1038/ja.2015.98] [PMID: 26464014]

[66] European and Developing Countries Clinical Trials Partnership 2014.http://www.edctp.org/annualreport2014/EDCTP_Annual_Report_2014_-_EN.pdf

[67] (CDER) USDoHaHSFaDACfDEaR. Qualified Infectious Disease Product Designation Guidance for IndustryQuestions and Answers 20182018.

[68] 21st Century Cures Act (Cures Act) 114th Congress, United States of America, ed HR 34 2014.

[69] Antibiotic Development to Advance Patient Treatment Act (ADAPT) Act. 114th Congress, United States of America, ed. HR26292015.

[70] Administration UFaD 2018. https://www.fda. gov/downloads/Drugs/GuidanceComplianceRegulatory Information/Guidances/UCM610498.pdf

[71] Administration UFD. Antibacterial Therapies for Patients With an Unmet Medical Need for the Treatment of Serious Bacterial Diseases. 2017.

[72] Developing an Innovative Strategy for Antimicrobial Resistant Microorganisms (DISARM) 114th Congress, United States of America, ed HR 5122015

[73] Administration UFD. https://www.fda.gov/ForPatients/Approvals/Fast/default.htm

[74] Hwang TJ, Kesselheim AS. Leveraging novel and existing pathways to approve new therapeutics to treat serious drug-resistant infections. Am J Law Med 2016; 42(2-3): 429-50.
[http://dx.doi.org/10.1177/0098858816658275] [PMID: 29086648]

[75] Inc A AVYCAZ (ceftazidime and avibactam) for injection package insert 2014.

[76] FDA approves a new antibacterial drug to treat a serious lung disease using a novel pathway to spur innovation 2018. https://www.fda.gov/newsevents/newsroom/pressannouncements/ ucm622048.htm

[77] Administration UFaD. FDA approves new antibacterial drug 2017 [updated 03/27/2018]. 2018. https://www.fda.gov/newsevents/newsroom/pressannouncements/ ucm573955.htm

[78] Services USDoHaH. 2014 Public Health Emergency Medical Countermeasures Enterprise (PHEMCE). Strategy and Implementation Plan 2014.

[79] Combating Antibiotic Resistant Bacteria CARB-X. 2017.

[80] Services; DoHaH NIAID's antibacterial resistance program: current status and future directions Washington DC2014 2014.

[81]   (ARLG) ARLG. http://arlg.org/about-the-arlg/arlg-scientific-agenda

[82]   Services; UDoHaH. Partnerships for the Development of Tools to Advance Therapeutic Discovery for Select Antimicrobial-ResistantGram-Negative Bacteria (R01). 2016.

[83]   Kostyanev T, Bonten MJ, O'Brien S, Goossens H. Innovative Medicines Initiative and antibiotic resistance. Lancet Infect Dis 2015; 15(12): 1373-5.
[http://dx.doi.org/10.1016/S1473-3099(15)00407-7] [PMID: 26607115]

[84]   Initiave   IM.   Innovative   medicines   initiave: new   drugs   for   bad   bugs.
https://www.imi.europa.eu/projects-results/project-factsheets/nd4bb

[85]   Kostyanev T, Bonten MJ, O'Brien S, *et al.* The Innovative Medicines Initiative's New Drugs for Bad Bugs programme: European public-private partnerships for the development of new strategies to tackle antibiotic resistance. J Antimicrob Chemother 2016; 71(2): 290-5.
[http://dx.doi.org/10.1093/jac/dkv339] [PMID: 26568581]

[86]   Simpkin VL, Renwick MJ, Kelly R, Mossialos E. Incentivising innovation in antibiotic drug discovery and development: progress, challenges and next steps. J Antibiot (Tokyo) 2017; 70(12): 1087-96.
[http://dx.doi.org/10.1038/ja.2017.124] [PMID: 29089600]

[87]   Bartlett JG, Gilbert DN, Spellberg B. Seven ways to preserve the miracle of antibiotics. Clin Infect Dis 2013; 56(10): 1445-50.
[http://dx.doi.org/10.1093/cid/cit070] [PMID: 23403172]

[88]   Antibiotics   currently   in   global   clinical   development: pew   charitable   trusts.   2018.
https://www.pewtrusts.org/-/media/assets/2018/09/antibiotics_currently_in_global_clinical_development_sept2018.pdf?la=en&hash=BDE8590154A21A3167CB62A80D663534906C4308

SUBJECT INDEX

A

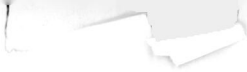

www.ingramcontent.com/pod-product-compliance
Lightning Source LLC
Chambersburg PA
CBHW050758220326
41598CB00006B/49